Drug Design

Volume II

MEDICINAL CHEMISTRY
A Series of Monographs

EDITED BY

GEORGE deSTEVENS

CIBA Pharmaceutical Company
A Division of CIBA Corporation
Summit, New Jersey

Volume 1. GEORGE deSTEVENS. Diuretics: Chemistry and Pharmacology. 1963

Volume 2. RUDOLFO PAOLETTI (ED.). Lipid Pharmacology. 1964

Volume 3. E. J. ARIËNS (ED.). Molecular Pharmacology: The Mode of Action of Biologically Active Compounds. (In two volumes.) 1964

Volume 4. MAXWELL GORDON (ED.). Psychopharmacological Agents. Volume I. 1964. Volume II. 1967

Volume 5. GEORGE deSTEVENS (ED.). Analgetics. 1965

Volume 6. ROLAND H. THORP AND LEONARD B. COBBIN. Cardiac Stimulant Substances. 1967

Volume 7. EMIL SCHLITTLER (ED.). Antihypertensive Agents. 1967

Volume 8. U. S. VON EULER AND RUNE ELIASSON. Prostaglandins. 1967

Volume 9. G. D. CAMPBELL (ED.). Oral Hypoglycaemic Agents: Pharmacology and Therapeutics. 1969

Volume 10. LEMONT B. KIER. Molecular Orbital Theory in Drug Research. 1971

Volume 11. E. J. ARIËNS (ED.). Drug Design. Volumes I and II. 1971. Volumes III and IV, *in preparation*

In Preparation
PAUL E. THOMPSON AND LESLIE M. WERBEL. Antimalarial Agents: Chemistry and Pharmacology

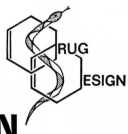

DRUG DESIGN

Edited by E. J. Ariëns

DEPARTMENT OF PHARMACOLOGY
UNIVERSITY OF NIJMEGEN
NIJMEGEN, THE NETHERLANDS

VOLUME II

ACADEMIC PRESS   New York and London   1971

ACADEMIC PRESS, INC.
111 Fifth Avenue, New York, New York 10003

United Kingdom Edition published by
ACADEMIC PRESS, INC. (LONDON) LTD.
24/28 Oval Road, London NW1 7DD

LIBRARY OF CONGRESS CATALOG CARD NUMBER: 72-127678

PRINTED IN THE UNITED STATES OF AMERICA

Contents

Chapter 1. Modulation of Pharmacokinetics by Molecular Manipulation

E. J. Ariëns

Chapter 2. Factors in the Design of Reversible and Irreversible Enzyme Inhibitors

Howard J. Schaeffer

Chapter 3.   The Design of Organophosphate and Carbamate Inhibitors of Cholinesterases

R. D. O'Brien

Chapter 4.   The Design of Reactivators for Irreversibly Blocked Acetylcholinesterase

I. B. Wilson and Harry C. Froede

Chapter 5.   Inhibition of Protein Biosynthesis: Its Significance in Drug Design

Arthur P. Grollman

Chapter 6. Enzymes and Their Synthesis as a Target for Antibiotic Action

M. H. Richmond

Chapter 7. The Rational Design of Antiviral Agents

Arthur P. Grollman and Susan B. Horwitz

Chapter 8. Design of Penicillins

A. E. Bird and J. H. C. Nayler

Chapter 9. The Design of Peptide Hormone Analogs

J. Rudinger

List of Contributors

Numbers in parentheses indicate the pages on which the authors' contributions begin.

E. J. ARIËNS (1), Department of Pharmacology, University of Nijmegen, Nijmegen, The Netherlands

A. E. BIRD (277), Beecham Research Laboratories, Brockham Park, Betchworth, Surrey, England

GEORGE DESTEVENS (421), CIBA Pharmaceutical Company, Summit, New Jersey

J. DE VISSER (437), N. V. Organon, Oss, The Netherlands

HARRY C. FROEDE (213), School of Pharmacy, University of Colorado, Boulder, Colorado

ARTHUR P. GROLLMAN (231, 261), Albert Einstein College of Medicine, Bronx, New York

SUSAN B. HORWITZ (261), Albert Einstein College of Medicine, Bronx, New York

M. MARTIN-SMITH* (453), Department of Pharmaceutical Chemistry, University of Strathclyde, Glasgow, Scotland

J. H. C. NAYLER (277), Beecham Research Laboratories, Brockham Park, Betchworth, Surrey, England

R. D. O'BRIEN (161), Section of Neurobiology and Behavior, Cornell University, Ithaca, New York

* Present address: School of Natural Resources, The University of the South Pacific, Suva, Fiji.

G. A. OVERBEEK (437), N. V. Organon, Oss, The Netherlands

M. H. RICHMOND (251), Department of Bacteriology, Bristol University Medical School, Bristol, England

J. RUDINGER (319), Pharmazeutisches Institut, Eidg. Technische Hochschule Zurich, Switzerland

HOWARD J. SCHAEFFER (129), Department of Organic Chemistry, The Wellcome Research Laboratories, Research Triangle Park, North Carolina

J. A. STOCK (531), Chester Beatty Research Institute, Institute of Cancer Research, Royal Cancer Hospital, London, England

J. VAN DER VIES (437), N. V. Organon, Oss, The Netherlands

I. B. WILSON (213), Department of Chemistry, University of Colorado, Boulder, Colorado

Preface

In Volume II of this treatise, special attention is given to the design of bioactive compounds interacting with enzymes and playing a role in enzyme synthesis as well as to topics such as modulation of pharmacokinetics by molecular manipulation and the design of bioactive polypeptides. As with Volume I, I hope the approach used will stimulate further research.

I am pleased that Dr. George H. Hitchings, a pioneer in the design of selectively acting enzyme inhibitors and responsible for many of the principles applied in this field, agreed to write an Introduction to this volume.

E. J. ARIËNS

Introduction

The designer of new drugs, as Professor Ariëns said in his Preface to Volume I of this treatise, seeks optimal rationalization of the process. Optimization implies not only "maximal reduction of trial and error" but also elimination of purposeless data gathering and of speculative considerations that cannot be tested. The practitioner will utilize whatever knowledge or technique advances his insight most economically. This will not only involve measurements and calculations of many parameters that might seem irrelevant to the pure empiricist, but will also involve trial and error (or trial and partial success) to ferret out answers to questions too abstruse or too complex for analysis. And ultimately it will involve tests at the preclinical and clinical levels to prove or disprove the soundness of an approach.

The ultimate question is: Does it work? Drug design has pragmatic goals and demands pragmatic answers. It is futile to reason, for example, that competitive enzyme inhibitors cannot produce useful growth inhibition in the face of examples of competitive inhibitors that do just that. The accumulation of precursor that is postulated to occur when an enzyme is blocked is thus revealed to have definable limits, and more information on the extent of accumulation and the processes that limit it (such as feedback control, diffusion and elimination, and chemical breakdown) could be useful to the design of future inhibitors. The potentiation of one inhibitor by another that acts at a different step in the same biochemical sequence implies that some accumulation does occur and that under some circumstances the accumulation can usefully be reduced by an inhibition of the biosynthesis of the precursor. The potential and limitations of this principle want further definition.

The concept of an active center or reactive site of an enzyme is old, but the recognition is relatively recent that it consists of amino acid residues that may be interspersed at intervals over a lengthy polypeptide chain and are brought into juxtaposition by convolutions and folding of the chain. It is becoming clear that function is an inadequate guide to structure, that the structures supporting the reactive site may vary widely with relatively little distortion of the functional parts of the molecule. This is illustrated by the various sequences of the hemoglobins, by the selective binding of small molecule inhibitors of dihydrofolate reductases, and by an increasing number of examples that encourage one to expect this to be a general phenomenon.

The key to the selectivity of the reductase inhibitors appears to be that their binding *loci* lie partly within and partly outside of the active center, and that it is the variations among these neighboring, supportive structures that give rise to selection among the reductases of different species. The exploration of these regions of enzymes is, therefore, a most promising avenue to specific inhibitors. It remains to be demonstrated that inhibitors capable of forming covalent bonds within such regions are necessarily the preferred tools for exploration, but such studies are important, in any case, for the insight they provide. As sequencing and conformational studies become easier and tools for the purification of enzymes improved, more detailed information of comparative enzyme structures is accumulating at an accelerated pace. Each increment of information increases the potential for design of active inhibitors.

Not all of useful therapeutic intervention can be achieved by inhibitors, yet the nature of agonistic action is very imperfectly perceived. Some progress is being made toward the description of the structures of specific cell receptors. Some features of the reactive centers of cellular transport structures are beginning to emerge from studies similar to those dealing with substrate and inhibitor specificities of enzymes. It seems probable that the concept and elucidation of facilitated transport mechanisms will have implications far beyond those currently apparent.

Professor Ariëns deserves a general vote of thanks and confidence for bringing together the outstanding contributions to this treatise. An overview of the struggle to bring into being rational approaches to the design is gaining momentum. In contrast to the sterility and stasis of pure empiricism, each increment of insight and competence begets the next.

GEORGE H. HITCHINGS

The Wellcome Research Laboratories
Burroughs Wellcome Co.
Research Triangle Park, North Carolina

Contents of Other Volumes

Drug Design

Volume II

Chapter 1 Modulation of Pharmacokinetics by Molecular Manipulation

E. J. Ariëns

I. Introduction

Drug design, as a rule, starts with a known bioactive compound, the mother compound, as a lead.

The main objectives of molecular manipulation in drug design are:

1. Modulation of the action in the strict sense of the mother compound. This implies elimination of particular components from the spectrum of action, conversion to antagonistic compounds, and possibly increase in potency.

2. Modulation of the pattern of action by modulation of the pharmacokinetics. This may concern realization of a particular time–response relationship, selectivity in action and possibly increase in potency (17). Often the aim is the development of compounds adapted to the specific requirements for optimal dosage regimens for therapeutics, application regimens for pesticides, etc.

In this chapter the modulation of pharmacokinetics by molecular manipulation will be discussed. In contrast to pharmaceutical formulation, in which the composition of the mixture used as the application form is adapted, here the term chemical formulation may be used indicating that the bioactive compound itself is adapted chemically. The design of drug mixtures (299) is a field of action for pharmacologists and pharmacists, not for the medicinal chemists who perform molecular manipulation (17).

For biological activity two types of chemical requirements can be differentiated (11, 12, 13):

1. The requirements for biological activity in the strict sense. These are the chemical properties necessary for the induction of the effect on the level of the specific receptors or sites of action (17).

2. The requirements for pharmacokinetics of the bioactive compounds. These are the chemical properties necessary for the uptake, transport, chemical conversion, and elimination of the drug. In general, the properties of the drug which determine the distribution over the multicompartment systems involved in individual and environmental pharmacokinetics (17).

In the efforts to modulate pharmacokinetics including environmental pharmacokinetics (17) there are two main approaches:

1. Modification of the characteristics of the biological or environmental multicompartment system. This may happen by modification of the capacity of the compartments for the drug, its transport mechanisms governing the uptake in, the exchange between and the elimination from the various compartments, and by modification of the turnover capacity of the processes governing its biochemical transformation involved in bioinactivation or bioactivation. This approach will not be discussed here. The reader is referred to the literature (7, 13, 21, 22, 55, 74, 78, 80, 92, 179, 291, 321, 341, 346).

2. Modification of the properties of the bioactive agent by modifying its partition coefficients or its affinity constants with respect to the various compartments, of the properties determinant for transportation, thus modifying its uptake in, exchange between, and elimination from the various compartments, and of the properties determining its sensitivity to biochemical conversion, i.e., bioinactivation or bioactivation. This in fact implies a modulation of the biological or physiological availability of the bioactive compounds by molecular manipulation (*15*, *16*).

The design of new compounds with chemical properties adapted to particular requirements with regard to pharmacokinetics opens wide perspectives.

On certain part-processes involved in pharmacokinetics, such as protein binding and enzymic biodegradation, information can be obtained from *in vitro* studies. Species differences for biological activity including toxicity of pharmaca appear more often to be due to differences in the pharmacokinetics, especially differences in the biodegradation, than to differences in biological activity in the strict sense (*46*, *47*). The design of bioactive compounds for application as therapeutic, food additive, pesticide, or whatever, will usually imply a compromise. The chemical properties required in one respect may be incompatible with those required in other respects. In the compromise the desiderata for pharmacokinetics as well as for the action and activity in the strict sense may be involved. As a rule the degree of freedom in molecular manipulation will be largest for pharmacokinetics. The drug distribution is mainly dependent on overall properties of the compound, such as partition over lipid/water phases, polarity, etc. The induction of the response, the drug–receptor interaction, often requires particular sterical properties and a particular charge distribution in the bioactive compound (*10*).

II. The Significance of the Chemical Structure of Bioactive Compounds with Regard to the Various Processes Involved in Pharmacokinetics

Efforts to modify the chemical structure of a bioactive compound in such a way that only or mainly its pharmacokinetics and not its pharmacological action in the strict sense are changed, imply a restriction of the chemical modification to particular groups or moieties of the molecule. The aim is modification of the chemical characteristics essential for one particular aspect of the biological action. This requires some insight into the relationship between structure and action, especially with regard to the various processes involved in pharmacokinetics (*13*, *17*, *343*).

With respect to the pharmacodynamic action of bioactive compounds rules for structure–action relationship are restricted to particular types of drugs. Chemical requirements can be formulated for the group of the cholinergic agents, histaminergic agents, indirectly acting anticoagulants, β-adrenergic agents, for the group of the tolbutamide-related oral antidiabetics, etc. The requirements are specific for each group or type of drugs and hold true only within that group.

The rules for the relationship between structure and pharmacokinetic properties may be expected to be characteristic for the particular steps or part-processes in pharmacokinetics and not necessarily dependent on the particular type of pharmacological action of the drug. For each of the part-processes, such as passive distribution, metabolic conversion, and active excretion, particular rules will hold true. For one compound different rules obtain, depending on the part-process concerned. These rules, however, have a more or less general character since they do not differ for the different types of drugs. Such rules are of special importance in efforts to modulate pharmacokinetics of bioactive compounds by molecular manipulation.

What can be said about the chemical structure of bioactive compounds in relation to the various part-processes in pharmacokinetics?

1. For the absorption in the biological object and the distribution over its various compartments if based on free diffusion of the drug molecules through hydrophilic and lipophilic media and through pores, the overall physico-chemical character of the drug is determinant. This character is the resultant of such properties as hydrophility, lipophility, polarity, size and shape, degree of ionization, etc. These properties in turn are the resultant of the contributions by the various parts or groups in the drug molecule. The balance between hydrophility and lipophility strongly depends, for instance, on the character of the various groups in the drug molecule. Also the localization of the groups, as in the case of substituents in aromatic nuclei, is of influence. Particular groups or moieties, such as highly ionized groups may play a predominant role. Consequently, for absorption, distribution, and excretion, insofar as these are processes based on free diffusion, certain general rules will hold true independently of the specific type of action of the drug. Strong bases or strong acids which are ionized for 100% will not, or only with difficulty, pass the various lipid membranes. They will restrict themselves in their distribution mainly to the extracellular compartment and will not or hardly penetrate the blood–brain barrier. For weak bases and acids distribution will be dependent on the degree of dissociation and therefore on the pH (Fig. 1). Strongly lipophilic compounds will accumulate in tissues rich in lipids (*10, 35, 48, 49, 234, 236, 293, 306, 326*).

2. The binding of the drug to more or less indifferent sites of binding on plasma proteins, mucopolysaccharides, and other body constituents also plays a role in its distribution. Although this binding to sites of loss, also called silent receptors (*336*), is related to the chemical properties of the drug

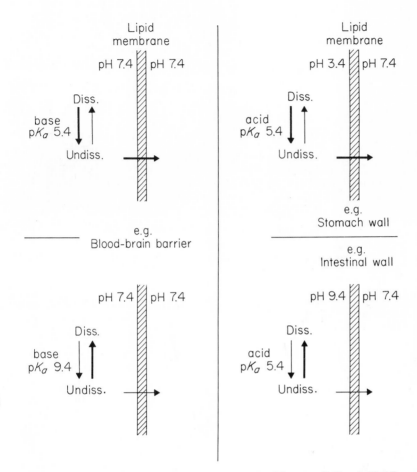

Fig. 1. Schematic representation of the influence of pK_a differences (left) and pH differences (right) on the penetration of lipid membranes by weak bases and acids.

molecule, as a rule the structural requirements for this type of binding are not very high (*201, 202, 252, 292*). This means that a great variety of compounds, as long as they have certain trivial chemical features such as, for instance, an anionic or a cationic group, and a hydrocarbon body, will be bound to, and possibly will compete for, common sites of binding, on, e.g., plasma proteins, irrespective of their specific pharmacological action (*17, 24a, 63, 127, 135, 157, 188, 223, 247, 252, 318*). Consequently also in this case certain general rules can be expected. Examples are the binding of drugs to plasma proteins which results in a mutual interference of drugs by displacement from common binding sites (*15–17*) and the binding of onium compounds such as curare to the acidic mucopolysaccharides. The consequence is that, for instance, curariform drugs may be potentiated by noncurariform bases as a result of the displacement of the curariform drug by these bases from such nonspecific binding sites (63).

3. If specific transport processes are involved which require binding of the drug to specific sites, for instance, on carrier molecules, the structure of the drug or the presence of particular groups in the drug molecule are important. Each specific transport system will have its own specific requirements with respect to the structure of the drug molecules transported. This implies a restriction in the applicability of the rules for structure and action that can be derived in this respect. In some cases the transport mechanisms are not highly selective, as, for instance, the system taking care of active excretion of a variety of organic acids and the system taking care of the active excretion of a variety of organic bases in the urine by the kidney and in the bile by the liver. Here certain general relations hold true, irrespective of the pharmacological character of the compounds involved. The acid-excreting system of the kidney, for instance, acts on certain types of organic acids such as antibiotic penicillin, radiopaque iodopyracet, diagnostic phenol red, and uricosuric probenecid (33, 34, 35, 112, 165, 258, 267, 292).

4. For metabolic changes in drugs, too, rules with a general applicability hold true. This means that they are not dependent on the specific type of action of the drug. Determinant is the occurrence of particular chemical groups in the drug molecule. If a drug contains an ester group, it may be hydrolyzed by plasma esterases or other esterases in the body independent of the pharmacological group to which the compound belongs. Local anesthetics, parasympatholytics, curariform drugs, and general anesthetics may, if containing a suitable ester group, be hydrolyzed by these esterases (10). Whether hydrolysis takes place is dependent on the characteristics of the ester moiety and not on the type of action of the drug (10, 53, 152, 192, 218, 224, 304, 322). The same holds for a number of other metabolic conversions such as oxidation of amines (298), reduction of azo compounds, and conjugation reactions (10, 132). The consequence is that also here general rules may be derived.

It can be concluded that for a number of fundamental steps in pharmacokinetics such as distribution and metabolic changes, rules may be derived for structure–action relationships applicable to drugs in general, irrespective of the specific type of effect induced by these drugs. For the final step, the induction of the specific effect, the rules for structure–action relationship will be restricted in their applicability to drugs with a particular type of action. Further elucidation and analysis of the more general rules mentioned will be fruitful for drug design, especially with regard to the efforts to modulate pharmacokinetics by molecular manipulation.

In this respect the analysis of the relationship between biological properties of drugs and their physicochemical properties on the basis of substituent constants as worked out in much detail by Hansch may be rewarding (*17, 145–148*). A regression analysis with respect to the various aspects of bioactivity, such as the activity in the strict sense to be tested on simple isolated test systems, the capacity to penetrate tissues, measured, e.g., by absorption experiments, the metabolic conversion tested in *in vitro* studies, etc., might indicate which type of molecular manipulation (substituents) may be expected to be most promising. The aim is the synthesis of new compounds with pharmacokinetics modulated as required but under maintenance of the pharmacological action.

III. Dissection of the Drug Molecule in Biofunctional Moieties

In the dissection of drug molecules into chemical groups or moieties, two approaches are possible. One can dissect the drug molecule into chemical groups on the basis of their contribution to the forces at action between drug and environment and more particularly between drug and receptor, such as the ionic groups, dipoles, inducible dipoles, groups able to contribute to hydrogen bonds, groups which contribute through van der Waals forces, and groups that contribute by means of hydrophobic aggregation forces (*131, 163, 270*). These may be called *chemofunctional moieties*. On the other hand, one can dissect the drug molecule on a more biological basis, namely by the distinction between various moieties on the basis of their significance for or predominance in particular aspects of the biological activity. These may be called *biofunctional moieties* (*11, 13, 14, 17, 122, 231*) (Table I).

The differentiation of the various biofunctional moieties has as a background the aim to modify certain biological properties or certain steps in the action

TABLE I
BIOFUNCTIONAL MOIETIES

Conducting moieties	Temporizing moieties
Moieties influencing the distribution of the drug in its active form over the various compartments	Moieties influencing the time–concentration relationship of the drug in its active form
Fixed moieties	*Disposable moieties*
Moieties which are part of the drug in its active form	Moieties which have to be disjuncted to get the drug free in its active form

of a bioactive compound by changing the moiety particularly involved, without essential interference with its other biological characteristics. It takes account of the multiconditionality of biological activity under the assumption that the requirements for the various steps or part-processes in the action may be fulfilled to a certain degree independently by different moieties in the drug molecule.*

The various biofunctional moieties in a biologically active compound cannot be considered to be fully independent. Therefore drug design is not simply the conjunction of various moieties potentially contributing to the wanted activity. The emphasis laid on particular aspects of drug action in relation to particular structural aspects can contribute, nevertheless, to a rational approach in the development of drugs. In the following sections various types of biofunctional moieties which play a role in pharmacokinetics, will be discussed.

Efforts to modulate pharmacokinetics and therewith the physiological availability of bioactive compounds can have as a purpose: (1) modulation of the distribution of the compound over the various compartments, e.g., to obtain a decrease in toxicity and a higher selectivity in action; and (2) modulation of the time–concentration relationship in the various compartments to obtain particular time–response relationships.

A. Biofunctional Moieties Involved in the Partition of Drugs over the Various Compartments

Certain moieties in a drug molecule have a predominant influence on the distribution over the various compartments. They are called *conducting moieties* (*11, 13, 14, 17*). In the case of transport by free diffusion the moieties governing the lipo-/hydrophility play a predominant role in distribution, since the compartments as a rule are separated by relatively lipid-rich barriers (the membranes) and also the compartments as such differ in lipo-/hydrophility. Highly hydrophilic, especially ionized groups in a drug will limit its rate of penetration through the biological membranes and thus restrict its distribution. They are called *restricting moieties*. Extreme lipophility of the drug too will limit its transport through the hydrophilic compartments and therefore restrict distribution. Moieties which confer to the drug a balanced lipo-/hydrophility will facilitate its penetration and its distribution. They are called *facilitating moieties*. If active transport processes are involved, selective

---

* The term drug molecule is used in this chapter in a broad sense, such that not only drugs, i.e., therapeutics, but also bioactive compounds in general are indicated, including toxons and biocides (*17*).

accumulation may take place. Particular chemical moieties in the drug molecule are required by the active transport system. These are called *selecting moieties.*

The various moieties mentioned may be part of the drug in its active form and are called *fixed moieties* or they may be only temporarily a part of the drug molecule being disjuncted under formation of the active compound (*98*), and are called *disposable moieties* then. As a rule in the disposable moieties there will be a larger degree of freedom with regard to molecular manipulation

TABLE IIA

Conducting Moieties

(Moieties influencing the distribution of the drug in its active form over the various compartments)

Restricting moieties	*Facilitating moieties*	*Selecting moieties*
Fixed or disposable, conferring to the drug extreme hydrophility or extreme lipophility, restricting its transport and distribution	Fixed or disposable, conferring to the drug a balanced lipo-/hydrophility, making it suitable for easy penetration into hydrophilic and lipophilic compartments, thus facilitating distribution	Fixed or disposable, adapting the chemical properties of the drug to the active transport mechanisms such that based on active transport selective accumulation in certain compartments takes place

Selective bioactivation	*Selective bioinactivation*
Introduction of vulnerable moieties may result in a selective bioactivation in the target tissue or target compartment and thus increase the therapeutic index and a selectivity in the action	Introduction of vulnerable moieties may result in a selective bioinactivation outside the target tissue or target compartment, and thus increase the therapeutic index and selectivity in the action

than in the fixed moieties which are part of the drug in its active form and therefore must fit to the sites of action or at least may not disturb drug–receptor interaction.

Introduction into a drug molecule of groups subject to enzymic attack, called *vulnerable moieties,* may result in a *selective bioinactivation* or in a *selective bioactivation* in those compartments which are rich in the enzyme concerned. Molecular manipulation by introduction of the biofunctional moieties indicated opens a possibility for modulation of drug distribution over the various compartments. Table IIA summarizes the various types of conducting moieties indicated (*11, 13, 14, 17*).

B. Biofunctional Moieties Involved in the Time–Concentration Relationship of Drugs in the Various Compartments

Certain moieties in the drug molecule have a predominant influence on its
rate of absorption, of inactivation or of excretion and thus on the time–
concentration relationship and the half-life time of the drug, e.g., in plasma.
Such moieties are called *temporizing moieties* (*17*).

The rate of absorption and thus the time–concentration relationship can be
modified by introduction into the drug molecule of fixed or disposable
desolubilizing moieties which strongly decrease water solubility and delay
uptake from the site of application, *facilitating moieties*, moderately lipophilic
moieties which enhance uptake in the tissues, or *solubilizing moieties*, which
increase water solubility such that by intravenous route rapidly high plasma
and possibly tissue concentrations can be obtained.

The half-life time can be modulated by introduction into the drug molecule
of *vulnerable moieties*—moieties which are easily subject to enzymic or, in
general, chemical attack—or by elimination or stabilization of such moieties.
Introduction of lipophilic moieties facilitating reabsorption from the tubulary
urine delays excretion. Introduction of highly ionized moieties, which act as
restricting moieties with regard to tubular reabsorption, enhance renal
excretion. In this way too the half-life time of a drug in the body can be
prolonged or shortened.

The time–concentration relationship of the drug in its active form can also
be controlled by introduction of disposable, and thus temporarily inactivating
or *masking moieties*. Table IIB summarizes these various biofunctional
moieties involved in the control of time–concentration relationship (*11, 13,
14, 17*).

As long as a drug molecule bears groups suitable for conjunction such as
OH— groups, NH_2— groups, SH— groups, or COOH— groups, the principle
of the disposable conducting moiety can be applied. There are various types
of links possible: e.g., such that can be broken by hydrolysis like in esters,
acetals, and amides, and such that can be broken by reduction like the diazo
link or the —S—S— link. Hydrolysis may occur in plasma or in cells like the
liver cells, rich in hydrolytic enzymes, such as esterases. Reduction is mainly
restricted to the intracellular compartment. Since the disposable moiety is
split off before the final induction of the effect, which implies that bioactivation
of the drug takes place, the conjugate of the active drug and the disposable
moiety can be looked at as a "transport form" (*45, 356*). Most of the time the
transport form of the drug is inactive, partly because groups in the drug
molecule essential for its action are masked by the disposable moiety and
partly because distribution is restricted. The transport form can be considered

as a precursor of the active drug. The bioactivation of the transport form may require some time, which implies a delay in action. The term "drug latentiation" (*151, 152*) is used in this respect.

Besides this form of bioactivation many other types of bioactivation of drugs are reported. These as a rule are incidental, however, and not the aim of drug design. In a number of cases after detection of such a bioactivation the active

TABLE IIB

TEMPORIZING MOIETIES

(Moieties temporizing the availability of the drug in its active form)

Desolubilizing moieties Usually disposable, conferring to the drug a very low water solubility, making it suitable as a depot preparation		*Solubilizing moieties* Usually disposable, conferring to the drug water solubility, such that, e.g., iv application is possible and high plasma concentrations are rapidly reached
Introduction or destabilization of vulnerable moieties Resulting in a shortening of the half-life time and thus in a shortening of the action	*Protection of vulnerable moieties* By disposable protecting moieties, resulting in a prolongation of the action	*Elimination or stabilization of vulnerable moieties* Resulting in a prolongation of the half-life time and thus a prolongation of the action
Facilitating moieties Conferring to the drug a balanced lipo-/hydrophility, thus enhancing absorption and renal reabsorption, the latter prolonging the action		*Masking moieties* Usually disposable, inactivating the drug temporarily, thus avoiding initial peaks in the plasma concentration and initial side effects

product itself or its derivatives are applied directly as drugs (*17, 47, 132, 324*).

In the following sections examples will be given and discussed for the application of the various types of moieties indicated, in the efforts to modulate pharmacokinetics of bioactive compounds. As a matter of fact changes in the distribution over the various compartments and changes in the time–concentration relationship are interrelated. In the various examples to be given the role of each of them is, however, clear enough to deal with both possibilities separately.

IV. Modulation of the Distribution of Pharmaca over the Various Compartments in Individual and Environmental Pharmacokinetics by Molecular Manipulation

Most compartments in the body consist of a solution in water of inorganic ions, proteins, and small organic compounds such as sugars, acids, and bases. The compartments are separated by lipid membranes with pores. Transport by free diffusion takes place for small water-soluble compounds through the pores. Further specific mechanisms take care of transport of particular groups of compounds between particular compartments. The passage by free diffusion via the lipid phase of the lipid membranes is restricted to sufficiently lipid-soluble compounds. Highly polar compounds such as sugars and ionized organic compounds do not pass. They can be objects of the active transport systems (*64, 291, 292, 347*).

Besides the compartments mainly consisting of water, compartments rich in lipids such as neural tissues and fat tissues exist. The compartments can differ with regard to their enzyme pattern and content. The intravascular compartment is of special importance since its content continuously circulates through the body. The vascular walls, especially the capillary walls, are freely penetrated by all the organic and inorganic components in the blood with the exception of larger polymers such as protein molecules and large polysaccharides. The fluid content of the gut, and that of the renal system have as characteristic the wide variation in pH allowed. Their fluid content belongs neither to extracellular nor to intracellular fluid.

In the modulation of the distribution of bioactive compounds over a multicompartment system by molecular manipulation there can be distinguished between four main possibilities: (1) adaptation of the size of the molecules of the drugs; (2) adaptation of the balance between hydrophility and lipophility in the drugs; (3) adaptation in the structure of the drugs with regard to the specific transport mechanisms at action between particular compartments; and (4) adaptation of the structure of the drugs with regard to bioactivation or bioinactivation in particular compartments.

A. Molecular Size as a Factor in the Restriction of Distribution of Drugs

Small water-soluble organic molecules and ions may pass through the pores filled with water if they are small enough and if they have suitable charges. The pores in the various lipid membranes have a diameter which varies from 4 to 40 Å. For water-soluble molecules of a molecular weight not higher than ±60 (such as urea and glycerol) passage through pores is possible (258). The capillary walls of the vascular system have a much higher tolerance. Here only large polymers with a molecular weight ±30,000 or higher are kept back. The membranes of the vascular loops involved in the ultrafiltration process in the renal glomeruli have about the same permeability as the capillary walls. In this respect one has to take into account that the binding of many smaller compounds to plasma proteins has a consequence that passage of such compounds through pores is not possible as long as they are present in the protein-bound form. The same holds for passage through lipid membranes. Only the free concentration has to be considered as far as the rate of penetration through the membranes is concerned.

The influence of molecular size on distribution is especially clear for the plasma volume extenders. These usually are polymers such as dextran, a glucose polymer, and polyvinylpyrrolidone, a purely synthetic polymer, or polypeptides of varying size such as gelatin. The effect of the plasma extenders, the colloid osmotic effect, is only dependent on the presence and retention in the vascular system of a certain number of molecular units. The further qualities of the compounds do not matter very much as long as toxicity is avoided. Therefore, such different substances as plasma proteins, e.g., albumin, simple proteins such as gelatin, polysaccharides such as dextran, and synthetic polymers such as polyvinylpyrrolidone can serve the purpose. The use of proteins like gelatin composed of the simple amino acid glycine has the advantage that because of lack of characteristic polar amino acid side chains the risk of antibody formation is low (253a). The essential variable with respect to retention is the size and therefore the molecular weight. In the design of plasma extenders control of molecular size is a main objective (5, 154, 170, 195, 294).

In some cases a retention of a drug in the plasma compartment is obtained by using compounds which are tightly bound to the plasma proteins, especially albumins. Examples are the azodyes Evans blue and congo red and the dye indocyanine green (cardiac green), compounds used to measure the plasma volume and to study cardiac output and circulation time. After intravenous injection these dyes are almost completely and tightly bound to protein (255).

Binding of drugs to plasma proteins also plays a role in the development of long-acting compounds. This principle will be discussed in the section on the modulation of the time–concentration relationship of drugs.

B. Hydrophility and Lipophility as Factors in the Restriction of Distribution

Molecules too large to pass the pores will have to pass the lipid phase of the membranes unless they are actively transported. In order to penetrate this phase they have to dissolve in it, which implies that only lipid-soluble compounds can pass (*35, 48, 258, 271a, 292, 293, 306*). The concentration gradient of the drug in the diffusable form and the diffusion constant are determinant for the rate of penetration.

What will be the consequences of a high degree of ionization of a drug? With respect to distribution on the basis of free diffusion, such a drug cannot, or only with difficulty, pass the various lipid barriers such as the outer cell membranes and the blood–brain barrier (*149, 190, 276, 292, 313*). The presence of ionized groups implies a restriction in the distribution. Such drugs as a rule are devoid of actions on the central nervous system also if applied in doses which are active on the peripheral tissues. Since the highly polar ions will not penetrate the cellular membranes or only penetrate relatively slowly, their actions will be mainly restricted to the cell surfaces.

Consequently, toxic effects dependent on intracellular actions may be reduced by introduction of ionized groups. Renal excretion of such drugs will be enhanced since there will be little or no passive diffusion from the renal tubules back into the plasma. The walls of the renal tubules have much in common with a lipid membrane and are comparable to the blood–brain barrier in this respect. They essentially differ from the membranes of the glomerular vessels through which ultrafiltration takes place (*190*). As a rule ionized and highly water-soluble drugs are excreted for a large fraction in a nonmetabolized form, partly because of their quick renal excretion and partly because of the impeded cellular penetration (*10, 258, 292, 293*).

If a variation in the pK_a value of ionizable groups or introduction of such groups into a drug is possible without interference with the pharmacological activity in the strict sense, chemical modification resulting in the modulation of the distribution is possible. In the case that weak bases or weak acids are involved changes in the pH of certain body compartments may help to obtain certain distribution characteristics (*35, 48*). Moderately lipophilizing groups may facilitate penetration of lipid membranes.

In the following sections a number of examples will be given of modification of the lipid/water solubility of drugs, aimed at a modulation of the distribution.

1. *Fixed or Disposable Restricting Moieties*

Organic compounds with basic or acidic groups, with a high or low pK_a value, respectively, which implies a 100% ionization at the pH of the body fluids, will be strongly restricted in transport by free diffusion since they cannot penetrate the lipid membranes separating the various compartments. They will mainly be restricted in their distribution to the extracellular fluid compartment. There can be differentiated between anionic groups and cationic groups as restricting moieties, whereas they can be fixed or disposable. Fixed restricting moieties of the highly water-soluble type such as ionized groups will, since they hinder the entry of the drug molecule into the cells and into the CNS, not be acceptable for drugs with intracellular sites of action, such as cytostatics or drugs acting on the CNS, unless they are actively transported. Disposable moieties—assumed as a matter of fact they are disjuncted before

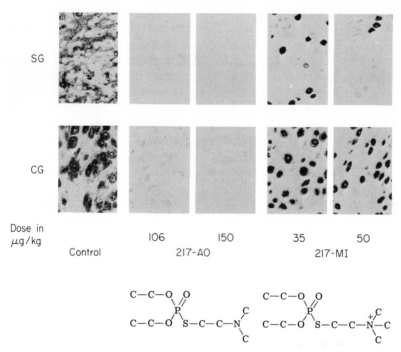

Fig. 2. The penetration of the acetylcholinesterase inhibitors 217-AO (tertiary base) and 217-MI (quaternary onium compound) in interstitial space and cells in the stellate ganglia (SG) and ciliary ganglia (CG) of cats. The preparations are stained on acetylcholinesterase activity. *Note*: The tertiary compound blocks the enzyme in the extracellular and intracellular space; the quaternary onium compound is restricted in its action to the extracellular space. After McIsaac and Koelle (*236*). Copyright (1959), The Williams & Wilkins Co., Baltimore, Maryland.

entry into the target cells or before entry into the CNS—give a larger degree of freedom for molecular manipulation in this respect. In those cases that cationic groups are introduced as fixed restricting moieties, this will often imply an introduction of a new component in the action, for instance, an anticholinergic, antihistaminic, or ganglion blocking action.

a. Cationic Groups as Fixed Restricting Moieties. Amines will, if the pK_a value is not too high, which implies that they are weak bases, be available at the pH of the body fluids partly in the un-ionized lipid-soluble form and therefore extend their actions also to the central nervous system. Quaternarization will eliminate these central actions. For certain drugs, e.g., anticholinergics or antihistamines, both tertiary amines and quaternary ammonium compounds are pharmacologically active. The consequence is that for these types of drug the action on the central nervous system can be far-reaching eliminated by developing quaternarized compounds. The differences in the distribution of quaternary ammonium compounds and their tertiary amino analogs, as expected, become manifest in the biological action of such compounds. Atropine, for instance, has clear-cut actions on the central nervous system and therewith on the behavior of animals, while methyl-atropine is devoid of such actions (137, 149, 190, 196, 197, 236, 340). Hansson et al. (149) studied the distribution of some tertiary and quaternary anti-histamines using radioactive labeled compounds and autoradiographic techniques. A clear difference is observed in distribution, especially as far as the central nervous system is concerned. A demonstration of this principle was also given by McIsaac and by Koelle in experiments with inhibitors of acetylcholine esterase. The quaternary compounds are restricted in their action to the extracellular phase of the neural tissues, the tertiary compounds extend their actions to extracellular and intracellular space (Fig. 2) (196, 197, 236, 340). This principle not only holds true for amines and ammonium compounds, but also for, e.g., sulfonium compounds (340). Drugs developed on this basis are antihistamines, such as the onium compounds thiazinamium and Aprobit (149) and quaternary anticholinergics such as propantheline and oxyphenonium which are devoid of CNS actions. Other examples are the reactivators of irreversibly blocked acetylcholinesterase such as the tertiary amines diacetyl monoxime (DAM) and monoisonitrosoacetone (MINA) which, contrary to the quaternary compounds such as pralidoxim, can reach the CNS. They therefore can also reactivate the acetylcholinesterase in the CNS after intoxication of the usually fat-soluble and therefore also centrally acting organic phosphates (137, 261, 308) (Table III).

An interesting example of the modulation of distribution by a shift in the balance between hydrophility and lipophility is the development of "systemic" insecticides, such as organic phosphates, taken up by the plants. To be taken up by the plant roots and transported by the sap stream throughout the plants, a relatively high hydrophility is required. The result is a certain degree of selectivity in the insecticidal action since only phytophagous insects, feeding on the plants concerned, will be affected. Highly lipid-soluble insecticides such as parathion are not transported in the plants. The introduction of amino groups into the organic phosphates resulted in the type of compound needed. Most systemic organic phosphorus insecticides, such as schradan and dimefox, are relatively weak bases, present partly in the hydrophilic,

TABLE III

COMPOUNDS WITH CATIONIC FIXED RESTRICTING MOIETIES DEVOID OF CNS ACTIONS

Anticholinergics

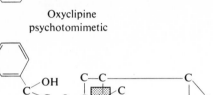

Oxyclipine
psychotomimetic

Oxyphenonium

Butylscopolamine

Hydroxythiospasmin

Antihistamines

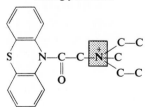

Promethazine
strongly sedative

Thiazinamium

Mephazin

Aprobit

TABLE III—*continued*

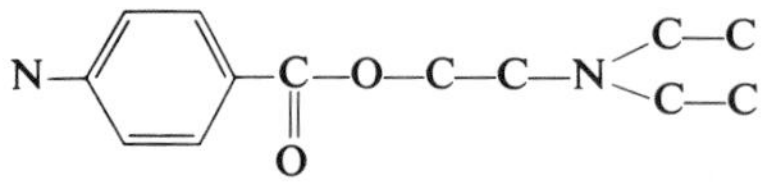

Procaine
local anesthetic action

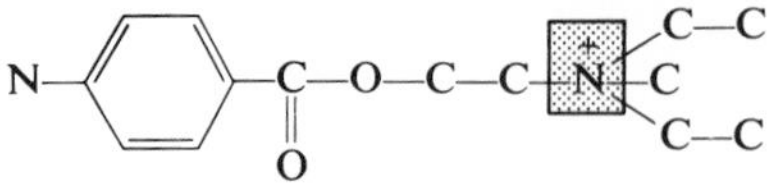

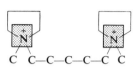

N-Methyl procaine
no local anesthetic action

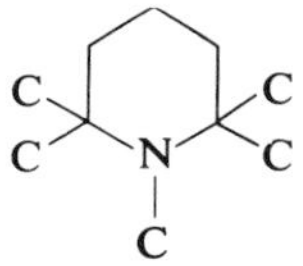

Pempidine
ganglionic blocker
side effects on CNS

Pentolonium
ganglionic blocker
no side effects on CNS

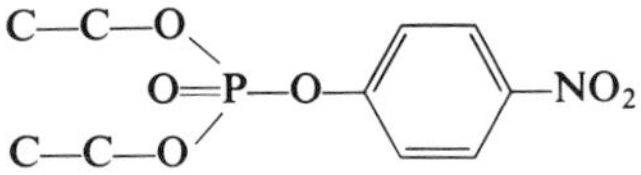

Paraoxon
irreversible
acetylcholinesterase inhibitor
active on CNS

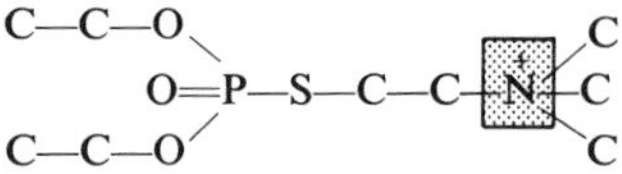

Ecothiopate
irreversible
acetylcholinesterase inhibitor
not active on CNS

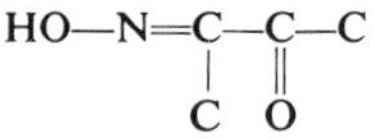

Diacetylmonoxime (DAM)
reactivator of acetylcholinesterase
also active on CNS

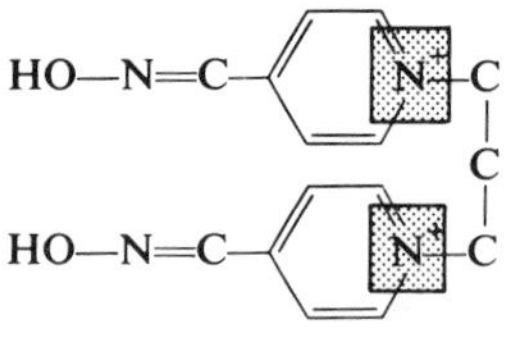

Trimedoxime
reactivator of acetylcholinesterase
not active on CNS

ionized, and partly in the lipophilic, nonionized form. This implies that they can penetrate into the leaves, are transported in the plants and are also taken up by the roots (*230, 256*). Amiton, which has a high pK_a value (8.4), is strongly ionized and therefore taken up readily by the roots but it only slightly penetrates into the leaves (*256*). The systemic compounds easily taken up by the roots can be used for the treatment of seeds to protect the seedlings against insects. They have the advantage that insects feeding on the crop plants concerned are eliminated already in an early stage (*24, 241, 256, 277, 279*).

   b. Anionic Groups as Fixed Restricting Moieties. An interesting group of compounds in this respect are the various food additives. To this group belong compounds used to ameliorate the color (eye appeal), taste and consistency of foods, conservatives, and other means used as expedients in processing and distribution of foods. For most food additives it holds that they should be pharmacologically inactive as far as the consumer is concerned. This implies that high polarity, by, e.g., introduction of onium groups or strong

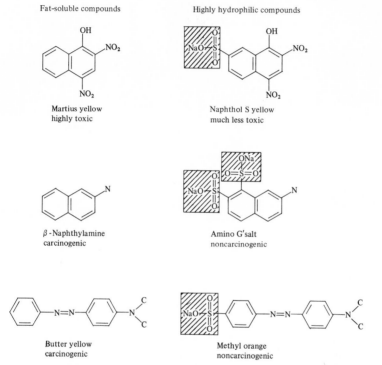

Fig. 3. Detoxification based on the introduction of highly ionized water-soluble restricting moieties. After Reith (276).

acidic groups, if compatible with the use of the compound as food additive, will be advantageous. The ionized compounds will be slowly absorbed from the gut, quickly excreted with the urine and will not or hardly penetrate into the cells (292). This may strongly reduce the toxic risks, including the risk of carcinogenesis (Fig. 3) (276). Introduction of ionic groups as a rule is compatible with the use as a food colorant. The use of quaternary ammonium compounds is not attractive since many of them find receptors for pharmacological action on cell surfaces or at least at sites easily reachable by highly polar compounds. Examples are the receptors for the muscle relaxant curare, the ganglionic blocker hexamethonium, and the anticholinergic propantheline.

The use of sulfonated compounds or other strong organic acids opens better perspectives.

Many of the dyes used as food additives are azo compounds. In the body, especially also under influence of the intestinal flora, splitting of the dyestuff molecule into two parts by reductive biochemical attack on the vulnerable azo group may easily take place, with the formation of toxic amines as a risk. The presence of sulfonic acid groups in the colorant gives no guarantee for nontoxicity, since after disjunction of the groups coupled via the diazo links

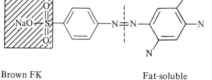

Trypan blue

3,3′-Dimethylbenzidine
fat-soluble
carcinogenic

Brown FK
suspicious fish colorant

Fat-soluble
potentially toxic amine

Fig. 4. Introduction of sulfonate groups in an azo dye in order to reduce toxicity requires the presence of such strongly polar groups in all moieties. Since the azo links can be broken by reduction, for instance by the intestinal flora, restriction of the sulfonation to only part of the moieties does not guarantee effective detoxification.

a nonsulfonated, fat-soluble toxic amine may be liberated (Fig. 4) (*85, 290*). It will be evident that for reasons of safety all sections of the dye molecule should bear sulfonate groups. This is in fact the case with practically all the azo dyes tolerated as food colorants (Table IV) (*64a, 117*). To obtain deep colors an extensive system of conjugated double bonds is needed, such that conjunction of more than two moieties via azo links is necessary. An example is brilliant black. Each of the three moieties in this food additive bears one or more sulfonate groups, which serve as fixed restricting moieties. The disjunction of the groups constituting the dye by reduction of the azo link has as an advantage a loss of color because of the decrease in the size of the system of conjugated double bonds. A transfer of the eye appeal of the foods concerned to the urine of the consumer is avoided in this way.

In chemical industries workers are often exposed to high risks as far as the toxicity of the chemicals used are concerned. A special discipline, industrial toxicology, is devoted to this subject (*111*, *144*, *263*). One of the examples is the carcinogenic action of β-naphthylamine, a compound used in the fabrication of synthetic dyestuffs and bringing about a high risk especially of bladder cancer. Also here the principles applied in drug design are applicable. Introduction of strong polar groups in β-naphthylamine eliminates its toxicity. Rearrangement of the steps in the synthetic procedure by an early introduction of the highly polar sulfonic acid groups eliminates the toxic risk (*290*) (Fig. 5). "Drug design" is extended here to the development of safe chemical procedures.

An example of efforts to modulate the distribution of a therapeutic by variation of the fat/water solubility ratio is the study of a variety of boron compounds to be used for the treatment of tumors. The isotope boron-10, not radioactive, has a high capacity for the absorption of thermal neutrons with as a result a nuclear reaction leading to a local destruction of the tissue.

$$^{10}_{5}B + ^{1}_{0}n \to (^{11}_{5}B) \to ^{7}_{3}Li + ^{4}_{2}He + 2.4 \text{ MeV}$$

Organic boron compounds were developed with a high ratio for the distribution in tumor tissue and adjacent brain tissue. Compounds restrained by the blood–brain barrier from entering the brain can relatively easily penetrate certain types of highly vascularized brain tumors, such as meningioma. High ratios for the concentration of the boron derivatives in such tumors and the surrounding brain tissue may be obtained on basis of a suitable choice in the balance between hydrophility and lipophility. Table V gives the relation for the partition coefficient and the tumor tissue/brain ratios for a series of benzeneboronic acid derivatives. Compounds with a high lipid solubility unvariably penetrate the brain tissue readily giving low tumor/brain tissue ratios and causing toxic symptoms from the central nervous system. For the compounds with a low lipid solubility high tumor/brain tissue ratios are obtained, while toxicity for the CNS is lower (*313*, *314*). In the case of the organic boronic acid derivatives discussed no damage to the hydrophilic peripheral tissues has to be feared since the radiation with thermal neutrons, resulting in the radioactive decay is restricted to the tumor-bearing area in the brain.

In the case of regional perfusion with cytostatics via the arteria carotis interna, the action of the cytostatics used is mainly restricted to the contents of the skull. In this case, too, a preferential action of the alkylating agent on relatively hydrophilic tumor tissue can be obtained by using compounds with a relatively high hydrophility, such as the phenylalanine mustard compound sarcolysine. Fat-soluble cytostatics such as thioTEPA (triethylenethio-

TABLE IV

FOOD COLORS WITH LOW TOXICITY REALIZED BY INTRODUCTION OF HIGHLY POLAR SULFONIC
ACID GROUPS AS FIXED RESTRICTING MOIETIES IN THE VARIOUS SECTIONS OF THE COMPOUNDS
(117)

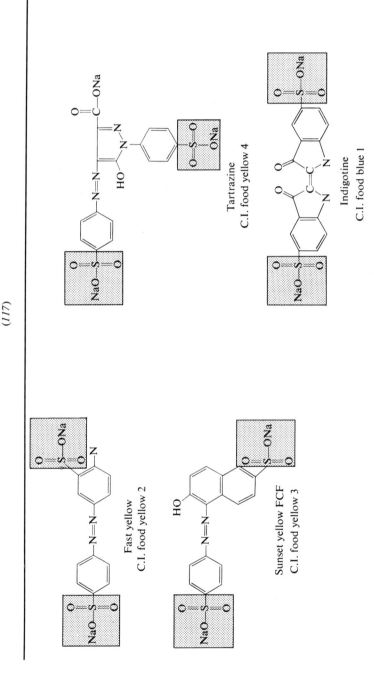

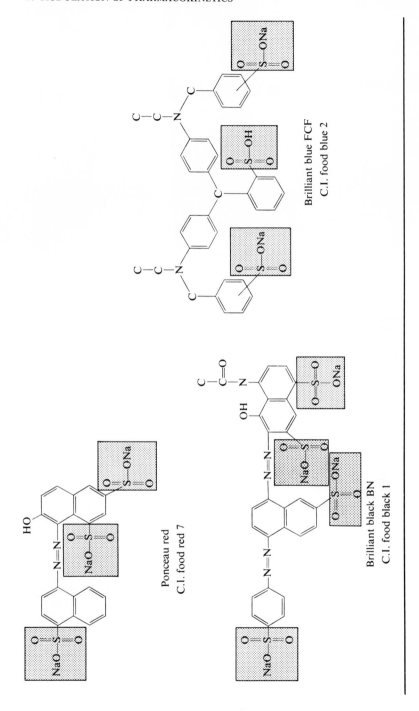

Brilliant blue FCF
C.I. food blue 2

Ponceau red
C.I. food red 7

Brilliant black BN
C.I. food black 1

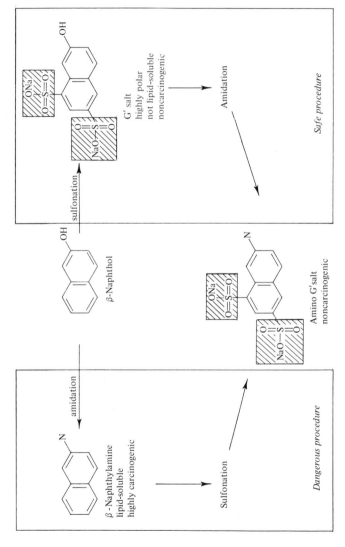

Fig. 5. Safe-guarding of industrial chemical procedure by adaptation of the route of synthesis, namely early introduction of toxicity-reducing fixed restricting moieties. After Scott (290).

phosphoramide) give no differences in the distribution between tumor and brain tissue (*312*). As a further example of fixed restricting moieties of the anionic type the sulfonic acid groups in certain isoquinolines such as chiniofon can be mentioned. This antiamoebal agent is for only a small fraction absorbed from the gut (*3a*). In this respect also can be mentioned the fixed restricting moieties introduced in hydroxyisoquinolines used as chelating agents (see Section IV,C,3 and Fig. 9).

TABLE V

MODULATION OF TUMOR/BRAIN DISTRIBUTION BY INTRODUCTION OF HYDROPHILIC FIXED RESTRICTING MOIETIES[a]

R	Partition coefficient water/benzene	Boron ratio tumor/brain
—S—C	0.7	0.2[b]
—Br	0.8	0.2[b]
—O—C	3	0.7
—H	6	0.7
—C=O	29	0.6
—COOH	67	4.8
—C—C—COOH $\quad\;\;$ | $\quad\;\;$ N	>200	8.5

[a] With an increase in the partition coefficient the tumor/brain ratio increases. After Soloway (*313*).
[b] Highly toxic.

c. Hydrocarbon Groups as Fixed Restricting Moieties. An interesting aspect of the shift in the balance between hydrophility and lipophility by means of introduction of hydrocarbon moieties into a drug is the shift from excretion of the drug in the urine to excretion in the bile. This principle can be used, for instance, in modulating the type of excretion of radiopaques (*9, 60*). Because of the relatively high lipophility of the α-alkyl or α-phenyl substituted acids renal excretion is strongly restricted and excretion via the bile facilitated (Table VI). An increase in the lipophility of the compounds used for pyelography by means of the introduction of hydrocarbon moieties makes them suitable for cholecystography (see Table VII) (*9, 60, 193, 194, 352*). The excretion by the liver via the bile may be enhanced by oral application, while intravenous application is an advantage for preferential renal excretion. Another example for changes in the distribution over the various compartments as a function of lipophility is the design of barbiturates accumulating rapidly in the lipid-rich tissues especially fat tissue. The thiobarbiturates such as thiopental and N-substituted barbiturates such as hexobarbital are

TABLE VI

THE EXCRETION IN URINE OR BILE OF X-RAY CONTRAST MEDIA[a]

R	Urine[b]	Bile[b]	Bile[c]
—H	+ + +	−	−
—C	+ + +	−	±
—C—C	+ +	+	+
—C—C—C	+	+ +	+ +
—C—C—C—C	−	+ + +	+ + +
—C—C—C—C—C	−	+ + +	

[a] With an increase of the size of the alkyl substituent R the excretion shifts from the urine to the bile. The alkyl moiety acts as a fixed restricting moiety with respect to urinary excretion and as a fixed facilitating moiety with respect to biliary excretion.

[b] After Archer et al. (9).

[c] After Cassebaum et al. (60).

examples. A main factor for the ultra-short action of these highly fat-soluble barbiturates is the redistribution after intravenous application, which results in a rapid disappearance of the barbiturate from the plasma and in an accumulation in the fat tissue (46, 48).

Since emphasis is put on the short action of these barbiturates they will be discussed more extensively in the sections on change in time–concentration relationship by molecular manipulation (Section V,C,1).

d. Anionic Groups as Disposable Restricting Moieties. The disposable moieties are disjuncted after serving their purpose of regulating uptake and/or

TABLE VII

RADIOPAQUES FOR PYELOGRAPHY AND CHOLECYSTOGRAPHY[a]

Used for pyelography

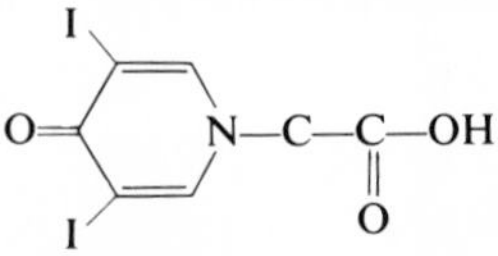

Diodone

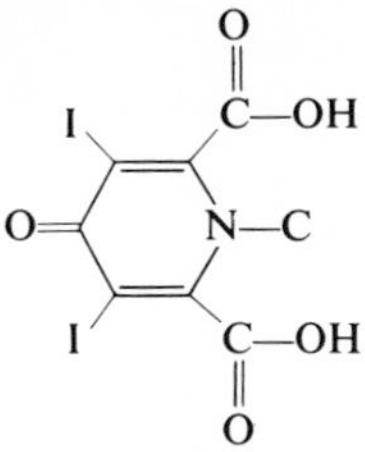

Iodoxyl

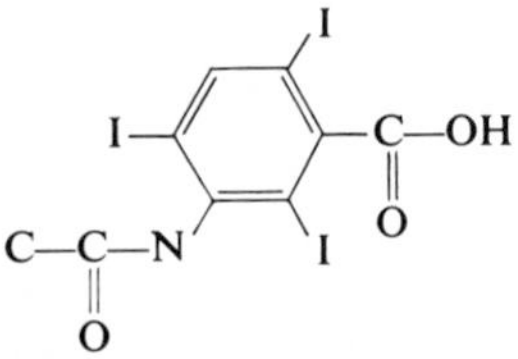

Acetrizoate

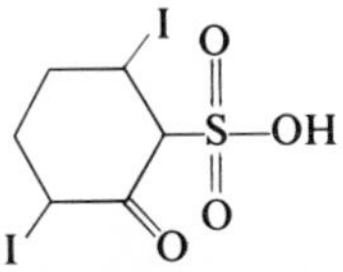

Renumbral

Used for cholecystography

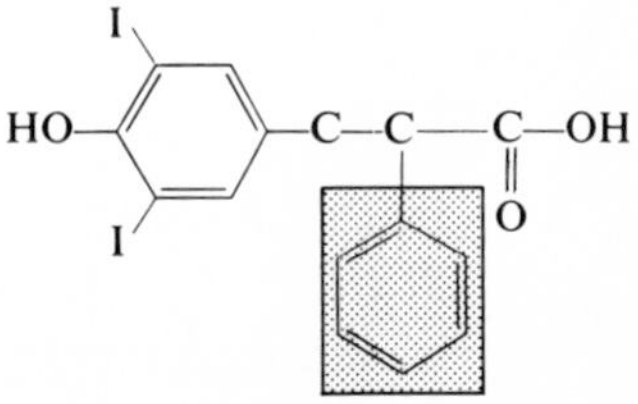

Pheniodol

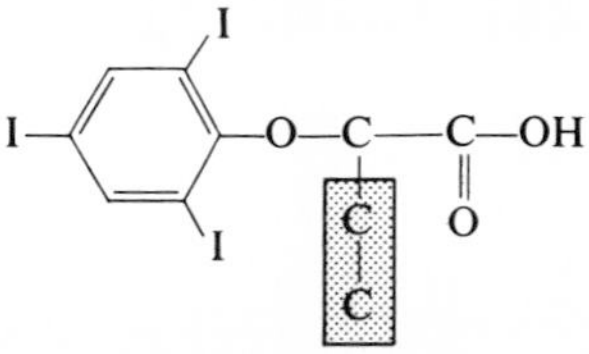

Phenobutiodil

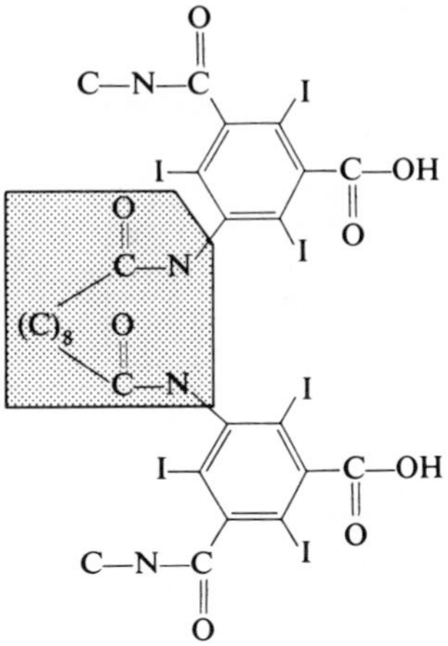

Iosefamic acid

[a] Note the presence of lipophilizing groups in the compounds used for cholecystography. These groups can be regarded as fixed facilitating moieties with respect to biliary excretion and as fixed restricting moieties with respect to urinary excretion.

distribution of the drug. The consequence is that the differentiation between the conducting moiety and the active moiety in the drug becomes especially clear. After disjunction the active moiety constitutes the drug in its active form; a bioactivation has taken place.

In the disposable moieties a relatively wide chemical variation is tolerated

TABLE VIII

RESTRICTION IN THE DISTRIBUTION OF SULFONAMIDES TO THE INTESTINAL TRACT BY INTRODUC-
TION OF STRONGLY HYDROPHILIC DISPOSABLE RESTRICTING MOIETIES[a]

	Succinylsulfathiazole
	Phthalylsulfathiazole
	Phthalylsulfacetamide
	Salazosulfapyridine

[a] ▢ Disposable restricting moiety.

since the groups involved are eliminated by disjunction before the final step of the action takes place. In this respect no incompatibility has to be feared therefore. The disposable carrier moiety must be adapted to the biochemical mechanism involved in its disjunction.

Examples of compounds with anionic restricting moieties disposed by hydrolytic processes are the sulfonamides used in the treatment of certain bacterial infections of the bowel. It mainly concerns combinations of sulfon-amides linked to dicarbonic acids via the NH_2— group in position 4 in such a way that only one of the carbonic acid groups is bound. The free carbonic acid group in the conducting moiety will be ionized in the gut, thus restricting the absorption of the drug (*348*), which thus remains available for a longer period in the intestinal tract. Table VIII represents examples of the application of this principle. In order to unfold its antibacterial activity, the amide link in these conjugation products has to be broken by hydrolysis so that the sulfonamides are set free.

e. Cationic Groups as Disposable Restricting Moieties. Although we have searched the literature in this respect we did not find any examples of disposable moieties on the basis of cationic groups. As was mentioned in the discussion on the anionic fixed restricting moieties, anionic moieties are preferable over cationic moieties such as onium groups, since the latter often tribute a pharmacological activity to the compounds. The consequence might be that the conjugate of the drug and the cationic group has curariform, anticholinergic, or antihistaminic activity or that after disjunction the isolated cationic moiety would be pharmacologically active. This makes it understandable that cationic groups are to be avoided in this respect.

f. Hydrocarbon Groups as Disposable Restricting Moieties. In the application of radiopaques for diagnostic purpose localization of the diagnostic agent in particular compartments is of special importance. Therefore a whole spectrum of such compounds with chemical properties adapted to particular distribution patterns has been developed. The strongly hydrophilic and the more lipophilic organic iodine-containing compounds used in pyelography and cholecystography, respectively, were discussed already. For part of these compounds also selective active excretion is involved in their localization (see Section IV,C,1). For particular purposes in which especially details of surfaces of cavities, as in bronchography, arthrography, and myelography, have to be studied, the radiopaques must be sufficiently lipid-soluble such that they do not mix too easily with the fluids in the cavities to be studied. They must have a certain viscosity such that they spread as a thick layer over and adhere to the surfaces to be made visible. The poor water solubility also means that strong hypertonicity, which is irritant especially in bronchography, can be avoided. A disadvantage of such poorly water-soluble compounds is their tendency to long-lasting local retention at the sites of application with as a consequence local reactions such as arachnoiditis after the use of iodinated vegetable oils in myelography. The problem is brought closer to a solution by introduction of readily disposable restricting hydrophobic moieties in radiopaques normally used in intravenous pyelography or cholecystography. This implies that after disjunction products are formed which are absorbed locally and quickly excreted then. Examples are the radiopaques developed for use in bronchography such as propyldiodone derived from diodone used in intravenous renography and the *n*-propylester of docetrizoic acid (Pulmidol)

TABLE IX
CONVERSION OF RADIOPAQUES FOR PYELOGRAPHY AND CHOLECYSTOGRAPHY TO RADIOPAQUES
FOR BRONCHOGRAPHY, MYELOGRAPHY, AND CYSTOGRAPHY BY INTRODUCTION OF LIPO-
PHILIZING DISPOSABLE RESTRICTING MOIETIES[a]

Diodone
used in renography

Propyliodone
used in bronchography

Acetrizoate
used in renography

Propyl docetrizoate
used in bronchography

Sodium iopodate
used in cholecystography

Ethyl iopodate
used in myelography and cystography

[a] The non-water-soluble derivatives do not mix with the fluids in the compartments, but
adhere to the walls of the compartments, the contours of which have to be visualized.

derived from docetrizoic acid used in intravenous cholecystography (*176*) (see
Table IX).

These radiopaques should, if used in bronchography, not be combined with
ether anesthesia or, in general, inhalation anesthesia with the ether-, halo-
thane-, or cyclopropane-type anesthetics. These organic solvents cause a
ready spreading of the fat-soluble bronchoradiopaques mentioned with as a
result that also the alveolar epithelium is covered by a layer of these substances
which may be fatal since gas exchange in the lungs is hampered seriously
then (*43*).

g. pH-Sensitive Moieties and Modulation of the Distribution of Drugs by Adaptation of the pH in the Various Compartments. For weak bases a decrease and for weak acids an increase in the pH in a compartment will result in an increase in the concentration of the drug in the ionized form there. Since the concentration of the un-ionized form which can pass the membranes is equal in the various compartments, the pH changes mentioned will lead to an increase in the total concentration of the drug in the compartment concerned. A change in the pH leading to a decrease in the degree of dissociation has the opposite effect. In this respect moieties in the drug molecule with a pK_a value in the range of biological pH values, the pH-sensitive moieties, play a predominant role (see Fig. 1). A shift in the pK_a value therefore may be the aim in drug design.

An example for the influence of pH differences in the various compartments on drug distribution is the accumulation of morphine in the acidic stomach fluid after parenteral application of the drug (*181*). Lavage of the stomach has been in the past a procedure to enhance elimination of morphine from the body. It will be clear that such a procedure only will be effective if a fluid with a relatively low pH is used for the lavage.

The influence of differences in and changes of the pH in the various compartments is not restricted to the intestinal fluid and urine, although there, because of the possibility of large variations in the pH as compared to the other compartments, the effects are most clear. There is, however, also a difference in the pH of the extracellular fluid: ± 7.2, and the intracellular fluid, which is about 0.4 pH unit more acidic. This implies that for drugs with a pK_a value of about 7.2 the intracellular concentration will be relatively high for bases and the extracellular concentration will be relatively high for acids, because of the larger ionized fraction of these drugs in the respective compartments. Induction of respiratory acidosis or alkalosis in the blood may level out or increase the pH differences between extra- and intracellular fluid and thus cause a shift in the distribution of drugs. The consequences thereof for the drug responses depend on the location of the sites of action. These may be located in the extracellular compartment, that is, the compartment outside the lipophilic membranes enclosing the intracellular compartment, which is the case, for instance, for quaternary ammonium compounds such as anticholinergics, ganglionic blocking agents, etc., or in the intracellular compartment like is the case for the barbiturates. For weak basic drugs like the ganglionic blocker mecamylamine, hypoventilation or inhalation of carbon dioxide, which lowers the plasma pH, results in an increase in the plasma/tissue level ratio of the drug with as a consequence an enhanced hypotensive action (*264*). For weak acids like the barbiturates the same procedure results in a decrease in the plasma/tissue level ratio, while hyperventilation or application of sodium bicarbonate raising the plasma pH, results in an increase of this ratio (*36b, 341*). The consequence is a decreased sedative action. Similar studies have been performed with salicylate (*159*).

Besides changes in the partition over the various compartments, pH differences and changes therein may also profoundly influence the rate of penetration through the lipid membranes and thus influence the rate of equilibration. Since the un-ionized fraction, the membrane-penetrating form of the drug, may greatly change with the pH, relatively small changes in the pH may bring about appreciable changes in the rate of exchange between the extracellular and the intracellular compartments.

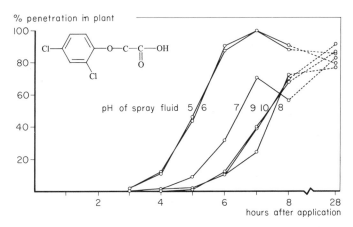

Fig. 6. Facilitation of the penetration in plant leaves of the weed killer 2,4-dichlorophenoxy-acetic acid. Note the enhanced penetration at lower pH values where a higher fraction of the weed killer is present in the undissociated lipid-soluble form. After Crafts (*74, 75*).

Application of the principle of the modulation of distribution of weak acids and weak bases by adaptation of the pH is not restricted to medicine. Many of the weed killers with an auxin-like activity are weak acids, such as the various ring-substituted phenoxyacetic acids. Spraying of the plants with these substances implies the necessity of the absorption of the weed killers by the leaves of the plants, especially the dicotyledons. As can be observed in the early morning from the dewdrops on the leaves, the cuticle thereof is more or less lipophilic. This implies that the various phenoxyacetic acids applied as weed killers will be absorbed the easier, the higher the fraction is of the undissociated, lipid-soluble form. A decrease in the pH of the spraying fluid may be expected to enhance the uptake of the weakly acidic weed killers by the plants. Figure 6 gives an example of the influence of the pH on the penetration of 2,4-dichlorophenoxyacetic acid into the plant tissues (*74, 75*). A decrease in the pH of the spray clearly enhances penetration. In the plant tissue the pH is higher, up to a value of around 7 in the phloem; here dissociation is practically complete again. The dissociation inside the plant steepens the gradient for the undissociated compound from outside to inside the plant, and thus further facilitates penetration. The significance of the pH for the distribution also manifests itself in the use of antimicrobial agents as preservatives for pharmaceutical preparations such as multidose containers. The cytoplasm of the microorganisms is surrounded by a lipid membrane which does not allow free passage to the various ionic organic compounds. The antiseptic action of ethylmercurithiosalicylic acid ($pK_a \pm 4$) is strongly pH-dependent. At pH 7 it is practically devoid of the bactericidal action present at pH 4. The phenols such as parachlorometacresol, and the esters of parahydroxybenzoic acid have pK_a values of about 8 which implies that they are suitable antiseptics for preparations with high pH values.

An example of the modulation of environmental pharmacokinetics by modification of the pH is the reduction of the fraction of ^{90}Sr (e.g., from radioactive fallout), present in a soluble form in acidic soils, by an increase in the pH, for instance by applying lime. This will result in a precipitation of a larger fraction of the ^{90}Sr in a poorly soluble form, which consequently may reduce the uptake in plants to about 50% of the original value (*214a, 221, 240*). Part of the ^{90}Sr is shifted to a compartment from which it is only slowly mobilized.

2. *Fixed or Disposable Facilitating Moieties*

As mentioned, balanced lipo-/hydrophilic properties are required for an easy distribution over the various body compartments, since transport is needed via hydrophilic phases such as the plasma compartments and the interstitial fluid, and via lipid phases such as the cell membranes and, in general, relatively lipophilic barriers such as the blood–brain barrier, the wall of the gut, etc. The consequence is that facilitating moieties have been introduced in a wide variety of drugs. For drugs such as antibiotics applied orally a rapid and complete absorption is the aim; for drugs which have to act intracellularly, such as cytostatics, penetration into the cell may be the limiting factor, etc.

A characteristic of the facilitating moieties is that they confer to the drug molecule a moderate or intermediate lipophility such that lipophilic barriers such as cell membranes as well as hydrophilic barriers such as the interstitial fluid can be passed. Consequently in a series of compounds ranging from hydrophilic to lipophilic an optimum may be expected with regard to the balance between hydro- and lipophility as required for facilitated transport. Here a regression analysis on basis of substituent constants for the contribution of the substituents to lipophility, the π constants as worked out by

TABLE XA
INTRODUCTION OF FIXED FACILITATING MOIETIES[a]

	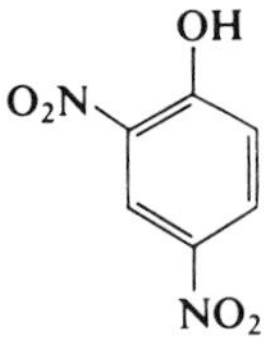 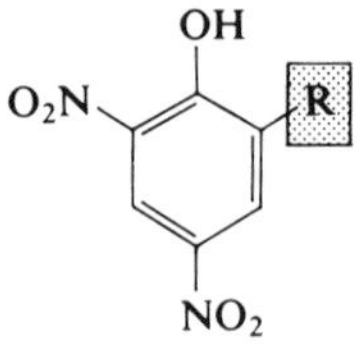 —C	DNC Dinitrocresol
	—C⟨C / C—C	Dinoseb
	⬡ (cyclohexyl)	Dinex

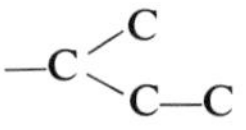

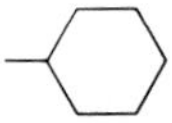

Dinitrophenol

Uncoupling agents used as pesticides (weed killers)

	R'	R″	
—C⟨phenyl	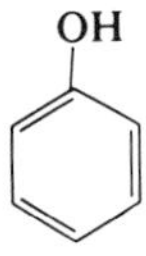 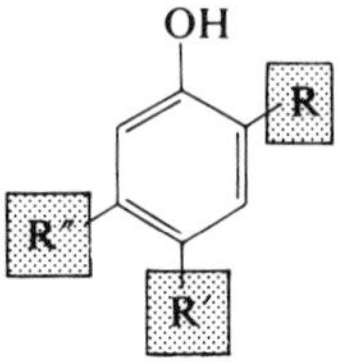 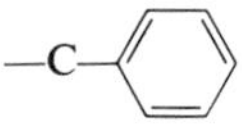 H	H	Delegol
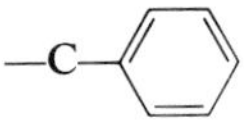 —C⟨phenyl	Cl	H	Septiphene
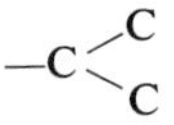 —C⟨C / C	Cl	C	Chlorothymol

Phenol

Phenols used as disinfectants

[a] The increase in lipophility results in an enhanced penetration of the compounds into the biological objects.

Hansch, may be helpful in selecting the substituents expected to be most promising for the synthesis of new compounds (*145, 146, 147, 148*).

  a. Fixed Facilitating Moieties. As a rule the use of disposable moieties has the advantage of a large degree of freedom in the chemical varieties allowed, since after disjunction the original active product is set free. For radiopaques, where besides a sufficient high density for x-rays, suitable pharmacokinetics and absence of specific pharmacodynamic activity are primary requirements, the objections against the use of fixed moieties for the modulation of pharmaco-

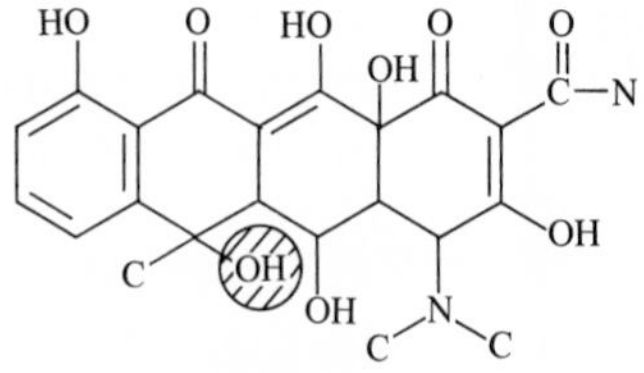

Oxytetracycline
poor intestinal absorption

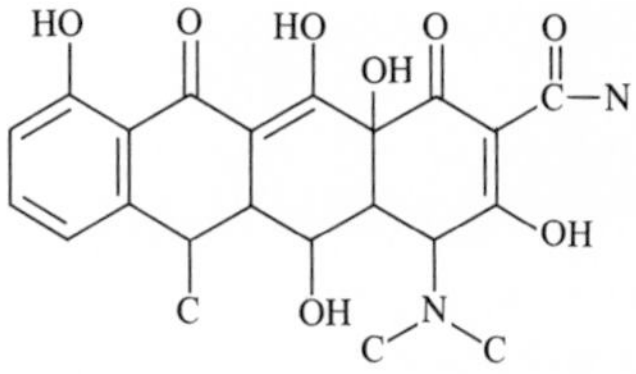

Doxycycline
good intestinal absorption

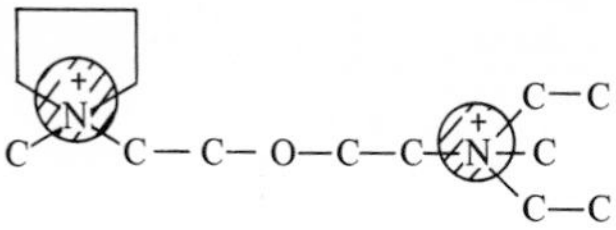

Plegarol
ganglionic blocker
poor intestinal absorption

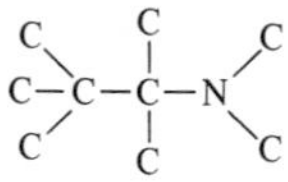

Penbutamin
ganglionic blocker
good intestinal absorption

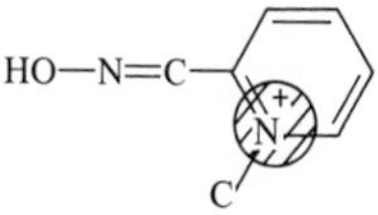

Pralidoxime
2-PAM
ACh-esterase reactivator
no penetration into CNS

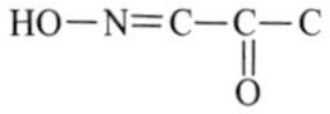

MINA
Monoisonitrosoacetone
ACh-esterase reactivator
penetration into CNS

Fig. 7. Elimination of hydrophilic, restricting moieties to facilitate uptake and distribution. ◉ Restricting moiety eliminated.

kinetics are less stringent. The shift in the excretion of the strongly hydrophilic renal radiopaques to an enhanced excretion by the liver into the bile by introduction of aryl or alkyl groups and therewith a shift toward lipophility is an example (see Tables VI and VII). The classification is a bit arbitrary here. The hydrocarbon groups in the various radiopaques used for cholecystography are restricting moieties with respect to the renal excretion and facilitating with respect to the excretion to the bile.

Also the alkyl groups and halogens in phenols used as disinfectants, which increase lipophility and thus facilitate penetration into biological targets, can be considered as fixed facilitating moieties (*176*). The same holds true for the alkyl groups in the nitrophenols used as weed killers such as dinoseb (*68*) (Table XA). An example of facilitation of transport, in this case absorption, by elimination of a polar moiety and thus lipophilization of the drug is the tetracycline derivative doxycycline (Fig. 7). This compound is more efficiently absorbed from the intestine partly because of a better lipid solubility and partly because of the decreased tendency to form poorly soluble complexes with Ca^{2+} and phosphate. The facilitated absorption decreases the risk of disturbance of the intestinal flora and of intestinal superinfections (*110*).

TABLE XB

INFLUENCE OF LIPID SOLUBILITY OF BARBITURATES ON THEIR
ABSORPTION IN RAT COLON[a]

Barbiturate	Absorption (%)	Partition coefficient chloroform/water
Barbital	12 ± 2	0.7
Aprobarbital	17 ± 2	4.9
Phenobarbital	20 ± 3	4.8
Butalbital	23 ± 3	10.5
Butethal	24 ± 3	11.7
Cyclobarbital	24 ± 2	13.9
Pentobarbital	30 ± 2	28.0
Secobarbital	40 ± 3	50.7
Hexethal	44 ± 3	>100

[a] After Schanker (*290a*).

Other cases in which a restricting moiety is eliminated to facilitate uptake and distribution are the ganglionic blocking agents of the onium type such as hexamethonium which are poorly and irregularly absorbed from the gut. By switching to tertiary amines such as mecamylamine and pempidine more steady and completely absorbed drugs were obtained. These tertiary amines, however, cause effects on the central nervous system contrary to the quaternary onium compounds which are devoid of such effects. In the case of the acetyl-cholinesterase reactivators penetration into the central nervous system is desired, since the irreversible acetylcholinesterase blockers, organic phosphates such as parathion, too penetrate the CNS. In the search for better antidotes one of the aims was the synthesis of reactivating oximes devoid of an onium group. The compounds diacetylmonoxime (DAM) and monoisonitroso-acetone (MINA) are examples (*308*) (see Fig. 7). The onium moieties which acted as restricting moieties with respect to the central nervous system were eliminated.

It will not always be easy to indicate in related drugs with clearly different lipid solubility the moieties responsible for these differences. A study of this relationship, however, is of utmost importance since the balance between lipo- and hydrophility has such a dominating influence on many aspects of drug action. Table XB gives an example for the relationship between intestinal absorption and the partition coefficients for a number of barbiturates (*290a*). The promises of an approach on basis of substituent contributions for sub-stituents in the various positions of the molecule to lipo-/hydrophility is self-evident.

b. Disposable Facilitating Moieties. The water-soluble vitamins which as essential nutrients should be readily absorbed have been the object of various efforts to facilitate absorption by introduction of disposable facilitating moieties.

The vitamin thiamine given orally is absorbed only slowly and partially; thiamine is a quaternary ammonium compound. Further the vitamin is attacked by the enzyme thiaminase produced by the bacterial flora of the gut. During preparation of food containing thiamine, part of the vitamin is lost because of extraction and instability at higher temperatures. Transport forms have been prepared with as an aim an increase in lipid solubility to facilitate intestinal absorption and to reduce extraction during food prepara-tion, an increase in heat stability, and resistance to thiaminase. For this purpose a rearrangement is brought about in the thiamine molecule by opening the thiazole ring so that an SH— group suitable for conjunction is obtained and the quaternary character of the nitrogen in the thiazole ring is lost. A variety of transport forms is obtained by conjunction of facilitating moieties with suitable groups on the SH— group and/or the OH— group in the molecule (Table XI). In the body regeneration of thiamine from the transport form takes place by reduction of the —S—S— links and by hydrolysis of the ester bonds in the transport form. The reduction can take place under influence of substances such as glutathion and is mainly located intracellularly, for instance in the erythrocytes and in the liver cells. The hydrolysis of the ester bonds partially takes place in the plasma, rich in various esterases, and partially intracellularly, especially in the liver (*36a, 102, 187, 233, 281*).

Extensive data on the various thiamine-transport forms can be found in a review written by Kawasaki (*187*). Data on the distribution in the body obtained with radioactively marked compounds are also available (*66*). For other water-soluble vitamins such as riboflavin and ascorbic acid fat-soluble derivatives have been prepared using disposable moieties, with as an aim enhanced absorption, reduced water extractability, heat stability, and pro-tracted action. Examples are riboflavin-2′,3′,4′,5′-tetrabutyrate (*99, 204*) pyridoxine-triaminobenzoate (*100*), 2-*O*-benzoyl-1-ascorbic acid (*99, 101, 173, 173a, 254a*), ascorbyl palmitate (*177*), etc. (*102*). In order to enhance

TABLE XI

THIAMINE TRANSPORT FORMS WITH AN ENHANCED INTESTINAL ABSORPTION,[a, b] OBTAINED BY
ELIMINATION OF THE STRONGLY HYDROPHILIC ONIUM GROUP, A RESTRICTING MOIETY,[c] AND
BY INTRODUCTION OF LIPOPHILIZING DISPOSABLE FACILITATING MOIETIES[d]

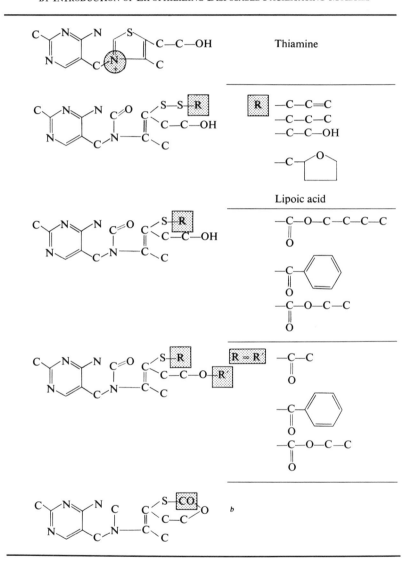

[a] After Kawasaki (*187*).

[b] Ref. (*102*).

[c] Restricting moiety eliminated.

[d] Facilitating moiety introduced.

penetration into the cells of 3′,5′-adenosine monophosphate (3′,5′-AMP), a metabolite holding a key position in the action of various hormones (*174*), esters such as dibutyryl-3′,5′-AMP and acetyl-3′,5′-AMP were prepared (*349*). To enhance absorption of 6-azauridine, an antimetabolite used in cancer chemotherapy and in treatment of psoriasis, its triacetyl derivative was successfully applied (*309*) (Table XIIA). Further disposable facilitating moieties are introduced into lincomycin and griseofulvin to enhance intestinal absorption. In the highly water-soluble antibiotic lincomycin lipophilizing moieties are used for this purpose (*116, 227*), while in the very poorly soluble compound griseofulvin hydrophilizing moieties were introduced to facilitate uptake (*115*). The use of amino acids such as tyrosine and dioxyphenylalanine and their derivatives to influence catecholamine synthesis in the central nervous system led to the synthesis of esters, such as the methyl ester of α-methyl-*p*-tyrosine (*4*), as transport forms for ready penetration of the blood–brain barrier. The esterification also protects the drug against ready decarboxylation by the liver decarboxylase. Hydrolysis is required as a matter of fact for action.

In a similar way, carbamates are formed of bioactive amines, such as amphetamine and ephedrine, to facilitate brain penetration and to protect the compounds against early enzymic inactivation in the liver. The compounds rapidly enter the central nervous system and are hydrolyzed therein. The stimulant action of these derivatives is preceded by a period of mild sedation (*336a*). This new component in the action may be ascribed to the carbamate moiety which is very common in sedatives.

For corticosteroid compounds to be applied on the skin lipophilizing disposable facilitating moieties are used to enhance skin penetration (*186*) (Table XIIB). Preparations of corticoid hormones to be used on the skin should be restricted in their actions to the skin, such that systemic actions are avoided. Therefore corticoid compounds should be used which are readily inactivated once they reach the general circulation. Consequently esters of, e.g., cortisol, a short-living compound, are to be preferred over esters of metabolically stable, longer living steroids. Further examples for the introduction of disposable facilitating moieties to enhance penetration of the skin are the various esters of salicylic acid, used as external antirheumatic rub and esters of nicotinic acid, used as rubefacients, which rubbed on the skin cause a local vasodilation (*176*) (see Table XIIB).

For chelating agents, used as therapeutics, antidotes, pesticides, or for other biological applications, besides the strength of the ligands between the chelating agent and the metals involved and thus selectivity with respect to the various metal ions, also the pharmacokinetics both of the chelating agent and of the chelate itself, are important (*2, 41, 61, 118, 120*). In the case of chelating agents, used as antibacterials or fungicides, a certain degree of fat solubility

TABLE XIIA

INTRODUCTION OF LIPOPHILIZING GROUPS AS DISPOSABLE[a] FACILITATING MOIETIES IN
EFFORTS TO FACILITATE DRUG ABSORPTION AND DISTRIBUTION

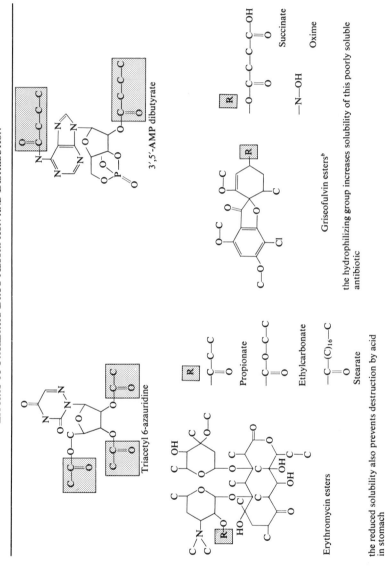

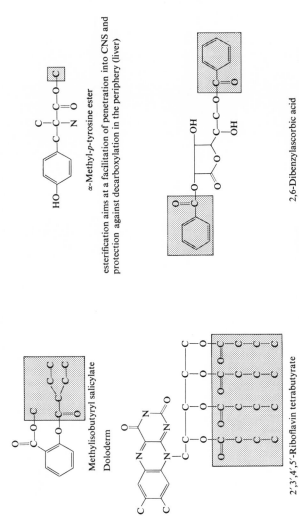

α-Methyl-p-tyrosine ester

esterification aims at a facilitation of penetration into CNS and
protection against decarboxylation in the periphery (liver)

2,6-Dibenzylascorbic acid

Methylisobutyryl salicylate

Doloderm

Carbimazole

2',3',4',5'-Riboflavin tetrabutyrate

if these esters are applied as food additives, the increased lipid solubility also decreases
the extraction of the vitamin during food preparation

MNFA

Pesticide

---

[a] Disjunction of the facilitating moieties before action is highly probable.

[b] In this case a hydrophilizing group is involved.

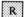

Hydrocortisone valerate
applied externally

Nicotinic acid esters
external rubefacientia

R

—C⟨TF⟩O
Nicotafuryl
Trafuril

—C⟨phenyl⟩
Benzylnicotinate
Rubriment

—C—C—C—C—C—C
Hexylnicotinate
Nicotherm

Salicylic acid esters
applied as external
antirheumatic

R

—C—C—OH
Rheumacyl

—C—C—O—C—C
  ‖
  O
Salenal

—C⟨TF⟩O
Tranvasin

Cinchophen derivatives
applied as external
antirheumatic

R

—C—C=C
Atoquinol

—N—C—O—C—C
   ‖
   O
Fantan

[a] Disjunction of the facilitating moieties before action is highly probable.

facilitating penetration into the target cells is required. If the aim is a depletion in the target organisms of certain essential metals the chelating agent as such should have a certain lipophility. If the aim is a poisoning of the target organisms by enhancement of the influx of certain toxic metals, the chelate (containing the metal) should have a certain lipid solubility. In the case distraction

TABLE XIII

INTRODUCTION OF DISPOSABLE FACILITATING MOIETIES IN CHELATING AGENTS[a]

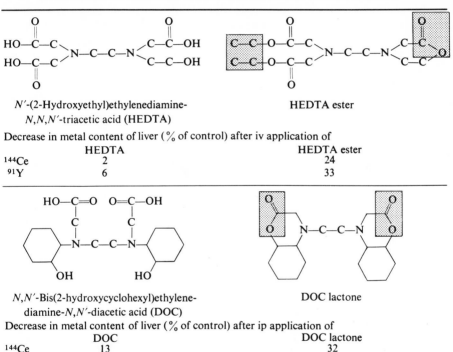

N′-(2-Hydroxyethyl)ethylenediamine-
N,N,N′-triacetic acid (HEDTA)

HEDTA ester

Decrease in metal content of liver (% of control) after iv application of

	HEDTA	HEDTA ester
^{144}Ce	2	24
^{91}Y	6	33

N,N′-Bis(2-hydroxycyclohexyl)ethylene-
diamine-N,N′-diacetic acid (DOC)

DOC lactone

Decrease in metal content of liver (% of control) after ip application of

	DOC	DOC lactone
^{144}Ce	13	32

[a] The decrease in the liver concentration of the metals to be eliminated is strongest after the use of the lipophilized transport forms of the chelating agents. After Catsch (61).

of toxic metals, e.g., lead, from the organism is the aim, the chelate should be hydrophilic so that it is excreted easily in the urine and does not penetrate into the cells or accumulate in lipid tissues. On the other hand, since the metal to be eliminated may be bound to a high degree intracellularly, it may be of advantage to use transport forms of chelating agents sufficiently lipid-soluble to penetrate into the tissue cells, being converted there to the chelating agent and sequentially to a chelate, hydrophilic enough to be readily excreted

by the kidney. For this purpose disposable facilitating moieties were introduced into chelating agents of the alkyldiamine-triacetic acid type, leading to
compounds such as the HEDTA ester and the DOC ester which are lipophilic
transport forms of chelating agents partly on the basis of intramolecular
lactone formation (*61*).

Table XIII represents some of the results obtained. The lipophilic transport
forms are more effective in distracting metal ions from weak tissue such as
the liver, enhancing renal excretion. The distraction from the slow compartment in bone is hardly influenced, which is expectable taking into account
the physicochemical properties of this compartment (*61*). The same principle
has been applied to the chelating agents of the oxyquinoline type used as antiinfectious agents. Esters of halogenated 8-oxyquinoline and 8-oxyquinolidine
because of their better balanced lipid and water solubility penetrate more
easily into the tissues and microorganisms, where after hydrolysis the active
chelating agent comes free (*41, 206*).

Other examples of hydrocarbon groups as disposable facilitating moieties
are found in the field of herbicides. For the uptake of the weed killer by the
leaves covered with a lipophilic cuticula a certain degree of lipid solubility is
required. In order to advance absorption by the leaves, esters of 2,4-dichloro-
phenolacetic acid and related acidic weed killers were produced. The esters
are better absorbed, while another advantage is that application can go on
even during rainfall. A disadvantage of the esters is that because of their
lipophility they are not readily transported in the plants to their site of action.
The esters of lower alcohols have as an extra disadvantage a high volatility.
Esters of higher alcohols, although not volatile, have the disadvantage of a
lack of distribution through the plant saps after uptake. For this reason
compounds were prepared using alcohols which are moderately lipophilic as
facilitating moieties. Examples are the butoxyethanol ester and the propylene-
glycol-butyl ester (*74–76*) (see Table XIV). In these compounds the balance
between lipophility and hydrophility is such that a ready uptake by the leaves
as well as transportation throughout the plant is guaranteed; further these
esters are not volatile. Before exerting their biological action the esters have
to be hydrolyzed such that the original phenoxyacetic acid derivative is set free.
The compound *N*-methyl-*N*(-1-naphthyl)monofluoro acetamide used as a
pesticide is a transport form of fluoroacetic acid, a highly toxic product. The
amide more efficiently penetrates into the biological targets since it is more
lipid-soluble. The naphthylamine group serves as a facilitating moiety. The
toxon fluoroacetic acid is released by hydrolysis in tissues such as the liver
(*104, 254*) (Table XII).

   c. Facilitating Moieties Disposed by Oxidative Degradation. An interesting
type of facilitating moieties are alkyl chains of varying length accessible to
biodegradation. The larger the chain the higher the lipid solubility of the

TABLE XIV

MODULATION OF THE DISTRIBUTION OF WEED KILLERS THROUGH ADAPTATION OF THE LIPO-/
HYDROPHILITY BY INTRODUCTION OF MODERATELY LIPOPHILIZING DISPOSABLE FACILITATING
MOIETIES[a]

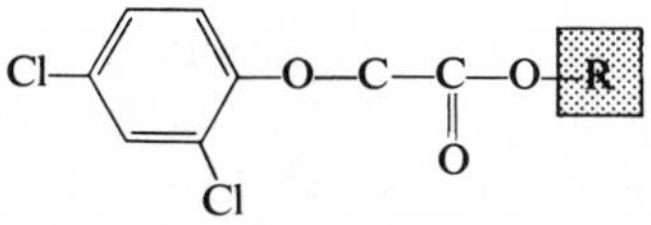

R	Absorption by the leaves	Transport in the plant	Low volatility
—C	+	±	−
—C⟨C C	+	±	−
—(C)$_3$—C	+	−	+
—(C)$_7$—C	+	−	+
—(C)$_2$—O—(C)$_3$—C	+	+	+
—C—C—C—O—(C)$_3$—C , OH	+	+	+

[a] After Crafts (75).

TABLE XV

ALTERNATION IN THE ACTIVITY OF AUXINS BASED ON THE NUMBER OF CARBON ATOMS IN THE
DISPOSABLE FACILITATING MOIETY: THE ALKYL CARBOXYL SIDE CHAIN, DISPOSED BY
β-OXIDATION[a]

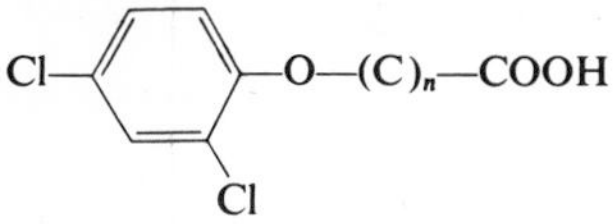

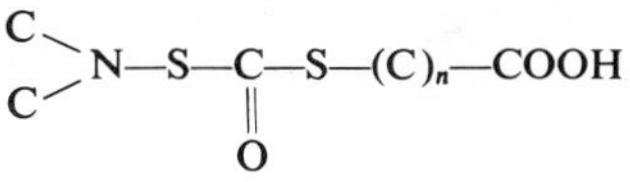

n	Auxin activity	n	Auxin activity
1	+ + +	1	+
2	−	2	−
3	+ + +	3	+
4	−	4	−
5	+ + +	5	+
6	−	6	−
7	+ + +		

[a] After Garraway and Wain (125) and Synerholm and Zimmerman (320).

compound is. In the body the chain is shortened stepwise by two carbon atoms, presumably β-oxidation. The end products of the degradation will depend on the number of carbon atoms in the chain and differ for chains with an odd and chains with an even number of carbon atoms. If these end products differ in their activity, the result will be an alternation in the activity of the series of homologous compounds. Examples are the alternating activity in various homologous series of compounds with an auxin-like activity (see Table XV) (125, 320). Another example are certain cytostatic nitrogen mustard derivatives bioactivated by alkyl chain oxidation (26, 107, 282, 283).

In the case of an alternation in the biological activity of series of homologous compounds with hydrocarbon chains one has not necessarily to assume an interference of β-oxidation in the chain. Physical properties such as melting points and water solubility alternate in a variety of series of homologous compounds such as dicarbonic acids and fatty acids. Since biological activity may be dependent on the partition of the compounds over lipophilic and hydrophilic phases in the biological object, the alternation in the activity with an odd or even number of carbon atoms in alkyl chains may be due to the alternation in such physicochemical constants as water and fat solubility (17, 58, 175, 185, 272).

C. SELECTING MOIETIES

A possibility to modulate the distribution of biologically active compounds is the use of selecting moieties. These are groups such as amino acids, sugars, etc. which are actively transported in the body by specific transport mechanisms. Also here there can be distinguished between fixed and disposable moieties. A condition is that the selecting moiety is still selectively processed by the specific transport mechanism involved notwithstanding its conjunction with the pharmacophoric moiety.

1. Fixed Selecting Moieties

The best-known examples of this principle are the various Röntgen-contrast means used for pyelography and cholecystography. For these purposes, as selecting moieties compounds are used which are excreted easily and at a high rate by the kidney into the urine or by the liver into the bile. p-Aminohippuric acid is an excretion product formed in the body after application of p-aminobenzoic acid. It is excreted in the urine by ultrafiltration and by active excretion by means of a transport system processing a variety of organic acids. Active excretion has as a result a practically 100% elimination of the compound from the blood passing the nephrons. There is little or no

TABLE XVI
COMPOUNDS EXCRETED IN URINE OR BILE OR ACCUMULATED IN PARTICULAR TISSUES USED AS
FIXED SELECTING MOIETIES IN DIAGNOSTICS[a]

Iodohippurate
used in renography

Iodophthalein
used in cholecystography

Bromophthalein
used in cholecystography

Phentetiothalein
used in cholecystography

Selenmethionine (^{75}Se)
used in pancreas scanning

Iodopyracet (^{131}I)
used in renal scanning

[a] Radiodense or radioactive principles conducted selectively to the target organ by the various compounds used as selecting moieties.

back-diffusion because of the high degree of dissociation of the acid. p-Amino-hippuric acid has been used as a selecting conducting moiety for iodine, an atom with a high density for the absorption of x-rays (Table XVI). With this compound as a lead a variety of organic acids with a high renal clearance has been developed as selecting conducting moieties for the iodine in radiopaques suitable for pyelography. The acid-excreting system of the kidney is especially suitable to transport highly water-soluble acids. In the liver there is an acid-excreting system suitable for the transport of more lipophilic acids. Therefore the hydrophilic or lipophilic character of the radiopaque molecule will be of influence on the active excretion of the compounds by the transport system in the kidney and that in the liver.

The role of lipophilizing α-alkyl substituents in radiopaques, enhancing excretion with the bile is demonstrated in Tables VI and VII.

The observation that phenolphthalein is excreted quickly via the bile, partly leading to a so-called enterohepatic circulation, resulted in the use of this compound as a selecting conductor for iodine in radiopaques for cholecystography. The radiopaque tetragnost thus obtained used as an orally applied radiopaque for cholecystography is an example (see Table XVI) (*194*).

Besides the acid-excreting systems in the kidney and in the liver there also are specific transport systems for the active excretion of organic bases (*112, 139, 258, 339*). This implies that strictly taken also such bases might be used as selecting conductors for iodine in radiopaques. As is well-known, however, many amines and quaternary ammonium compounds are pharmacologically active and for the radiopaques pharmacological activity has to be avoided. Avoidance of a pharmacological activity is evidently easier with organic acids than with bases. A particular aspect of chelate distribution is the potential use of stable metal chelates as x-ray contrast media. Here the chelating agent serves as a conducting moiety for the radiopaque metal. Increase in the hydrophility of the chelate will reduce soft tissue penetration and enhance renal excretion. A shift to a higher lipophility will enhance soft tissue penetration and biliary excretion. Here the same relations hold true as reported for the organic iodine compounds used as radiopaques (*9*). Chelates of iron with free carboxyl groups such as the iron chelate of diaminocyclohexane-N,N'-tetraacetic acid are mainly excreted by the renal way, while a shift in the properties of the compound towards lipophility results in a shift towards biliary and fecal excretion (*286*).

Another example of selecting conducting moieties are the localizing agents, which are in principle easily detectable agents, selectively bound to certain target tissues or sites of action. The use of tissue-specific antibodies as a carrier for radioactive isotopes or fluorescent labels is well-known in this respect (*105a*). Also drugs with a preferential uptake in particular tissues can be considered as conducting moieties. Examples are the use of radioactive melanine precursors and radioactive compounds showing a high binding to melanine for the localization of melanoma (*70*). Also the introduction of the conjugated system of double bonds as a chromophoric group into neuromuscular blocking agents to localize neuromuscular endplates can be mentioned here (*300, 301*).

The introduction of alkylating (covalently binding) moieties in suitable compounds such as enzyme substrates or drugs may result in active-site-directed irreversible blocking agents (*17, 19*). If radioactive, these may serve as a tool to localize the active sites or receptors for the particular compound used as conductor and possibly to identify the receptor molecules after extraction (*273*). This procedure is closely related to that followed in the design of active-site-directed irreversible enzyme blockers applied and discussed in a thoughtful way by Baker (*19*) and selective irreversible pharmacological antagonists in general (*17*). Not the modulation of pharmacokinetics but the design of new bioactive principles is the objective then.

Compounds with particular tissue binding are widely used as fixed selecting moieties for radioisotopes in efforts to design tumor-localizing agents and diagnostic agents for radio scanning of organs (*69, 71, 72, 73, 178, 342, 355*) (Table XVI). Also related to the procedure followed in the radiopaques is the incorporation of radioactive isotopes in compounds with a high affinity or specific binding-tendency to malignant tissues. Application of such radioactive compounds will have as a consequence a radiation especially of the tissues binding the drug. Efforts in this direction have been concentrated on dyes staining preferentially tumor tissues and on vitamin K derivatives especially 2-methyl-1,4-naphthalquinol (Sinkavit), a compound which when tested as a radiosensitizer was found to be concentrated in tumor tissue. Besides derivatives with radioactive halogen, phosphorus or carbon isotopes, especially the tritiated compound was extensively studied (*244*). An analogous approach is the use of cancer-specific antibodies as carriers for radioactive ^{131}I in order to restrict or localize preferentially the radiation to the target tissues (*130*). Both synthetic drug molecules and molecules of biological origin known to be actively transported, such as amino acids and sugars or particular groups present in such compounds, may be considered as selecting moieties. Ascites tumor cells, for instance, are reported to have a high capacity for the uptake of amino acids and sugars (*107*). There can be differentiated between the selecting moiety and the active moiety, which is the part of the drug essentially involved in the induction of the effect. The application of the principle of selecting conducting moieties is frequently mentioned in the literature on cytostatics of the biologically alkylating type (*107, 246, 283*). An example are the various nitrogen mustard derivatives where can be differentiated between the mustard moiety, the cytotoxic group or "warhead", and the "carrier" moiety for which amino acids, sugars, steroids, purine derivatives, etc. are used (*27, 28, 87, 172, 208, 211, 212, 246, 251, 266, 283, 307, 316, 335, 345a*) (Table XVII). Uracil mustard composed of the metabolite uracil and an alkylating nitrogen mustard moiety is an example (*134, 210, 226, 283*). Also essential amino acids such as phenylalanine are used as selecting moiety. In the rapidly proliferating tumor cells there is an enhanced uptake of these amino acids required for the protein synthesis. Phenylalanine mustard,

TABLE XVII

INTRODUCTION OF FIXED SELECTING MOIETIES IN EFFORTS TO OBTAIN COMPOUNDS SELEC-
TIVELY ACCUMULATED IN THE TARGET TISSUES

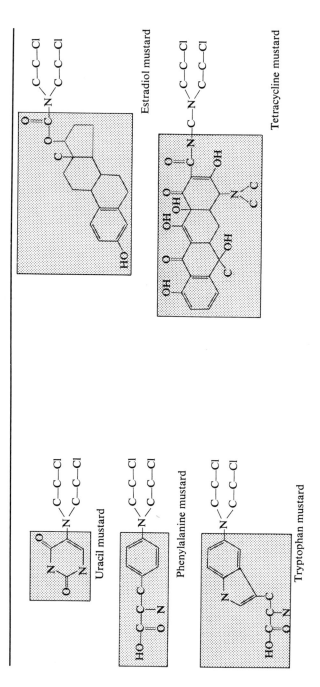

Uracil mustard

Phenylalanine mustard

Tryptophan mustard

Estradiol mustard

Tetracycline mustard

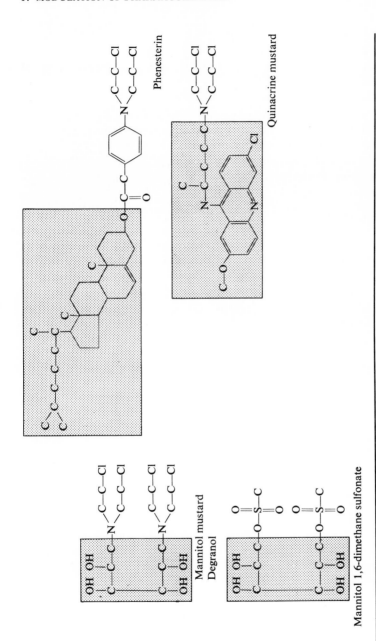

sarcolysine, was found to be effective in certain types of experimental tumors. An interesting aspect is the high activity of *l*-sarcolysine derived from the natural amino acid and the low activity of *d*-sarcolysine derived from the unnatural amino acid isomer (*198, 207, 316*). Besides phenylalanine also other natural amino acids are used as selecting conductors for alkylating moieties (*27, 164, 283, 316*). Not only derivatives of natural amino acids but also other compounds with an α-amino acid moiety such as the phenylbutyric acid analog of sarcolysine are found to be active as cytostatics (*225, 316*) (Table XVII). Also di-, tri-, and even polypeptides can be used as carriers for biologically alkylating moieties. Especially sarcolysine has been extended by conjunction with various amino acids (*27, 50, 209, 213, 246, 266, 283, 311, 316*). The compounds obtained appeared to be less toxic with respect to the hemopoietic system.

The cytostatic azaserine and diazooxonorleucine (DON) are amino acids carrying a diazo group as a potential alkylating group (Table XVII) (*275, 283*). The amino acids direct the diazo group to the enzyme transaminase which takes care of transamination reactions using glutamine as a substrate. The diazo group leads to an alkylating reaction on the enzyme with as a result an irreversible blockade thereof. From the carbohydrates used as conductors for alkylating groups mannitol has been most extensively studied (Table XVII). The sugar usually carries two alkylating groups, one at each end, and the compounds obtained are found to be active as cytostatics. Compounds derived from the stereoisomers of amino acids, peptides, and sugars are reported to differ in activity (*124, 246, 283, 333, 334*). Among the great variety of metabolites and metabolite-like compounds used as conductors for alkylating groups differences in the activities of stereoisomers are frequently reported (*107, 246, 283, 316, 333, 334*).

Not only metabolites such as amino acids and sugars have been studied as potential selecting moieties for alkylating groups but also hormones (*253, 344*) and a variety of drugs with an affinity to the cell nucleus, such as the antimalarials chloroquine and quinacrine, and tetracyclines (*77, 107, 180, 184, 246, 265, 283*) (Table XVII). In this respect the use as selecting moieties for alkylating groups of polynuclear aromatic hydrocarbons being carcinogenic themselves, may be mentioned (*265*). The examples given may be sufficient to demonstrate the principle of the introduction of fixed selecting moieties.

2. *Disposable Selecting Moieties*

Another example of efforts to apply this principle is the cytostatic mercasin. The essential amino acid moiety in this compound is assumed to enhance the uptake in protein-synthesizing cells to which the target tissues, the tumor cells, are counted. Disjunction is required for the activation of the mustard moiety.

TABLE XVIII

Introduction of Compounds Excreted in the Bile as Disposable[a] Selecting Moieties in an Effort to Concentrate Sulfanilamide in the Biliary System

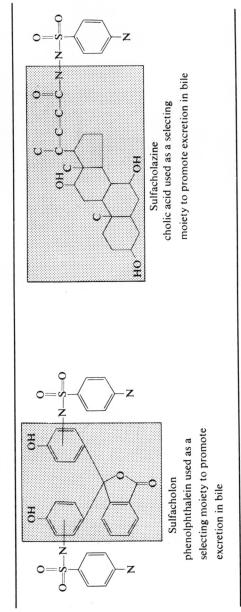

Sulfacholon
phenolphthalein used as a
selecting moiety to promote
excretion in bile

Sulfacholazine
cholic acid used as a selecting
moiety to promote excretion in bile

[a] Presumably the sulfanilamide is released for action.

Analogous to the use of phenolphthalein as a selecting conducting moiety for iodine in radiopaques, phenolphthalein and cholic acid are used as disposable selecting conducting moieties for sulfanilamide to obtain higher concentrations of that chemotherapeutic in the bile in case of infections in the biliary system (see Table XVIII) (*176*).

3. *Chelating Agents as Conducting Moieties for Metal Ions*

In a way also chelating agents can be considered as disposable or at least as nonfixed selecting moieties. They have to be selective with respect to the metal ions they bind, and the chelate formed must modulate the distribution of the metal in a particular way. Chelates are most easily formed if the metal together with the ligands forms a five- or six-membered ring (Fig. 7). Depending on the type of ligands and the valency of the metal, the chelate may be ionized and therefore relatively water-soluble, or un-ionized and fat-soluble. As a matter of fact also the structures R and R' bearing the ligand groups contribute to the lipid/water solubility of the chelate.

The action of the chelating agents may be based on:

(1) Binding such that the metal is un-ionized in a chelating agent in which R and R' guarantee water solubility with as a consequence the formation of a water-soluble chelate. This as a rule implies detoxification of the metal if toxic in the free ionized form, restriction of its distribution to the extracellular fluid and enhanced renal excretion and therefore elimination.

(2) Formation of un-ionized fat-soluble chelates (R and R' contribute to the lipid solubility). This may result in a facilitation of the penetration of lipid structures by the metal. The chelating agent then acts as an ionophore. The consequence may be an increased toxicity due to an intracellular accumulation of the chelate and possibly a release of the toxic metal there.

(3) The chelate as such may be toxic, for instance, because of its redox potential.

Usually accumulation in the urine and thus excretion of the chelate, which implies definite detoxification of the metals involved, is the aim (*2, 61, 62, 118*).

The best-known examples in this respect are the chelating agents used as antidotes of various toxic metal ions.

The primary requirement for detoxifying chelating agents is a high degree of selectivity and a high degree of binding with respect to particular metal ions such as Pb and Hg. This implies that the free concentration of these toxons in the extracellular fluid is kept extremely low by the chelating agent such that

Brain   Spleen   Kidney

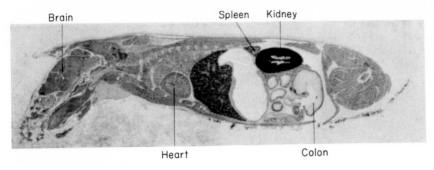

Heart   Colon

Brain   Spleen Pancreas Kidney

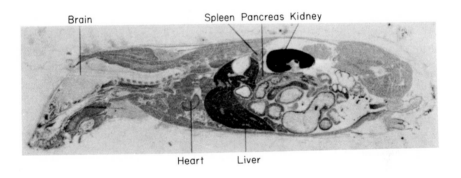

Heart   Liver

Fig. 8. Autoradiogram of whole-body sections of mice killed 24 hr after injection of methyl-^{203}Hg dicyandiamide alone (lower) and combined with dimercaprol (BAL) (upper). *Note*: In the presence of dimercaprol high ^{203}Hg levels are reached in brain tissue. The chelate is more lipid-soluble than Hg^{2+}. After Berlin *et al.* (*32*).

the concentration of the free metal ions in the "target" compartment—the tissue involved in the toxic effect—decreases below the toxic level. From the various tissue compartments in which the metal is present a flux following the concentration gradient of the free metal to the plasma should take place, leading to a mobilization of the stored toxon as a chelate, which can be considered as a masked, innocent transport form of the toxon. This implies that the chelating agent should be rather hydrophilic and contain for instance, free carboxylic groups like in fact is the case for most chelating agents used therapeutically as antidotes in the case of metal poisoning. If the chelate formed is more lipophilic in character, it may happen that the entry of the metal in its chelated form into the tissues is facilitated. This is in fact the case if dimercaprol (BAL = British antilewisite) is used as a chelating agent against, for instance, Hg^{2+} (see Fig. 8) (32). Dimercaprol appears to facilitate

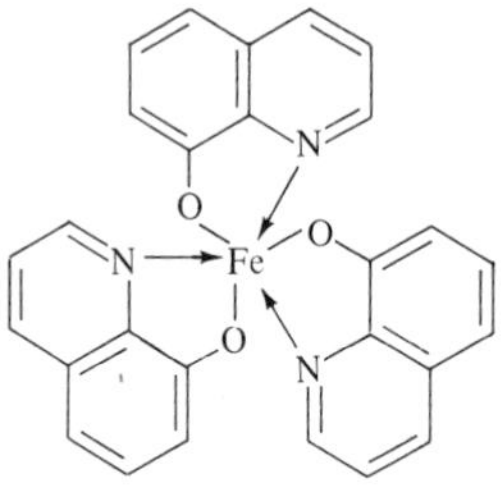

Tris-8-hydroxyquinoline-
Fe(III) complex

(a)

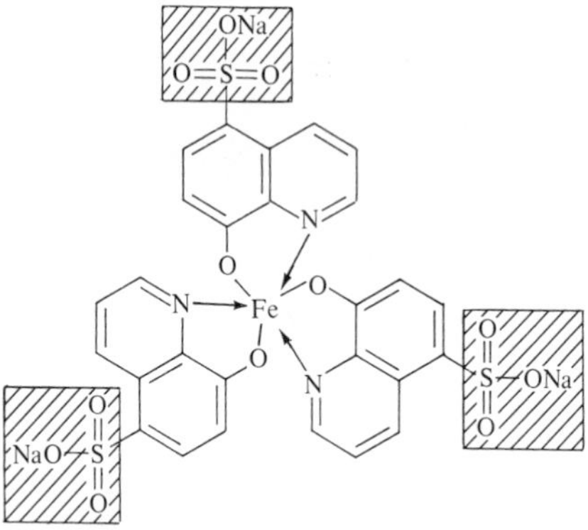

Tris-8-hydroxyquinoline-
5-sulfonic acid-Fe(III) complex

(b)

Fig. 9. The influence of the introduction of a fixed restricting moiety, an ionized sulfonic acid group, on the capacity of the chelating agent 8-hydroxyquinoline to prevent absorption of iron from the intestine. After Ewe (109). Percent of Fe^{3+} absorbed from intestine: (a) 70.2 ± 8.7; (b) 21.0 ± 18.3.

the penetration of the blood–brain barrier by Hg^{2+}. Conjugates of dimercaprol with a sugar molecule have been prepared to obtain more water-soluble products. These may, if the sugar moiety is nondisposable, show less tendency to facilitate the tissue penetration of the metals bound (84a, 317).

If the absorption of metals from the intestine has to be prevented, the use of highly ionized chelating agents forming highly ionized chelates, both poorly absorbed, will be of advantage over the use of more lipid-soluble chelating agents. Figure 9 gives an example of an effort to design chelating agents to be used for the prevention of the absorption of Fe^{3+} from the intestine. The sulfonate groups can be considered as fixed restricting moieties (109).

A secondary requirement for detoxication is that the chelate formed is water-soluble and is easily excreted in the urine by ultrafiltration and possibly by active excretion while no reabsorption in the kidney takes place. It will be clear that for the design of suitable chelating agents besides the selectivity and the strength of the ligands also the pharmacokinetics of the chelate formed are of great importance since these will determine the type of change obtained in the pharmacokinetics of the chelated toxon. Well-known examples of the application of chelating agents used clinically are dimercaprol binding Hg^{2+}, penicillamine binding Cu^{2+} and Ca-EDTA binding Pb^{2+} (*310a*). No definite evidence is available for an active excretion of the chelates by the renal tubules. Since penicillin is excreted actively this might as well be the case for penicillamine and its chelates. If this were so, drugs like probenecid might interfere with the effectivity of the chelates as far as excretion of the chelated metals in the urine is concerned.

Chelating agents not only are used to eliminate metals from biological systems. They may, if the chelate is sufficiently lipid-soluble, provide a transport mechanism to enhance the entrance of certain metals into the cells. This, for instance, appears to be the case with the various halogenated hydroxy-quinoline derivatives used against protozoal (amoebal) infections (*3*). These drugs form fat-soluble chelates with metal ions which then more easily penetrate the cell membranes of the protozoa, thus loading them up with the metal which is intracellularly taken over by other binding sites and thus leads to the amoebicidal action. The pharmacokinetics of the hydroxy-quinolines as chelating agents are not suitable to enhance the excretion of metals with the urine. Another example of the use of chelating agents as disposable facilitating moieties is the use of the chelate of copper and dimethyl-dithiocarbamate (DMDC) to fight fungal infections on plants. The selectivity in the uptake by the fungi of the thus chelated copper not taken up by the plants sprayed results in a selectivity of the action (*2*). The application of copper as a chelate is much more effective here than the use of the classical mixtures which contain copper sulfate. As discussed, chelating agents may have the character of restricting, facilitating or selecting conducting moieties for the metals they form chelates with. As mentioned, the chelating agent may act as an ionophore especially if the chelate formed is un-ionized and fat-soluble. Besides such chelating agents also other compounds acting as metal-including agents may act as ionophores. Examples are cyclic poly-peptides and the antibiotics of the inactine group. Such agents may show a remarkable degree of ion selectivity (*269a*). The design of programmed cyclic polypeptides with an ion-selective ionophoric capacity is an attractive goal (*302a*).

D. Vulnerable Moieties Involved in Selective Bioactivation or in Selective Bioinactivation

Bioactivation is not uncommon for drugs (*11, 17, 47, 132, 325*). In many cases the detection of such a process resulted in the introduction of the active metabolite or its derivatives as drugs. Bioinactivation is a very common process. With the exception of highly polar compounds such as various onium compounds, which are restricted in their distribution mainly to the extracellular fluid and are excreted very rapidly via the urine, and certain exceptionally stable fat-soluble drugs such as the insecticides of the halogenated alkane type, practically all drugs are inactivated and thus eliminated mainly by biochemical conversion. The processes involved are hydrolytic, oxidative and sometimes reductive, followed often by coupling of the products formed to body-own components such as glucuronic acid and glycocol (*10, 132, 353*). Drugs linked to disposable moieties have to be disjuncted. Usually enzymes are involved in this process. A conversion of the inactive compound, the "transport form" to an active one takes place. This too implies a bioactivation.

The chemical groups involved in biochemical conversion are called vulnerable moieties (*17*). The chemical character of the vulnerable moiety is determinant for the type of enzyme required in bioactivation or bioinactivation of the drug. The distribution of the enzymes in the various tissues will be determinant for the site of conversion and thus for distribution of the drug in its active form. Differences in the rate of bioactivation and bioinactivation in the various tissues play a role in drug distribution therefore.

1. *Vulnerable Moieties Involved in Selective Bioactivation*

One of the best-known efforts in this respect is the phosphorylation of diethylstilbestrol (Table XIX), suggested by Druckrey (*94*). Estrogens are used in the treatment of tumors of the prostate, an organ rich in the enzyme acidic phosphatase. Stilbestrol in the phosphorylated form is inactive since the phenolic OH— groups essential for the estrogenic activity of the drug are masked. The ester is a substrate for acidic phosphatase. Consequently one expected a more or less selective bioactivation in the target tissue, the prostate tissue. The formation of free diethylstilbestrol in the prostate tumor tissue of patients could be demonstrated; however, also other tissues such as bone and liver are rich in phosphatase able to split the ester, such that also in these tissues bioactivation takes place. This implies that bioactivation is not restricted to the target tissue. This was an effort in which disposable moieties are introduced with the aim a disjunction and thus bioactivation in the target tissue. A further example of this approach is the use of di- and tripeptides as disposable conducting moieties. The glycyl and phenylalanyl derivatives of β-(di-β-chloroethylamine)phenylamine are examples (*81, 83, 107*). Here, however, the selective activity aimed at is based on selective uptake and on the presence of particular peptidases in the target tissues releasing the active nitrogen mustard derivative from its transport form there. The distribution of the peptidases over the tissues plays a determinant role then for the distribution of the active compound. This principle of a selective bioactivation in particular tissues may play a role in the polypeptide mustards (*124, 164*) discussed in Section IV,C,1.

Another effort to obtain biological localization of the action of drugs by selective bioactivation in the target tissue is the formation of inactive transport forms from cytostatic biologically alkylating agents such as nitrogen mustard. The aim is an increase in the selectivity of these compounds with respect to the malignant tissue and therewith an increase in the therapeutic index. Compounds were prepared which are devoid of an alkylating activity but which become active in this sense when bioactivated by hydrolyzing or reducing enzymes. If the enzyme necessary for the bioactivation occurs especially in the tumor tissues a selective bioactivation would take place (*164, 283*). On basis of the lower oxidative capacity of certain cancer cells as compared to normal cells a number of transport forms of nitrogen mustard requiring reduction for the bioactivation were developed. Ross *et al.* worked out the principle of the "latent activity" or "transport form" of cytostatics in much detail. They synthesized a large series of derivatives of *N,N*-di-2-chloroethyl-aminoazobenzenes, and found a correlation between the rate of reduction and the biological activity (*164, 283, 284*). The occurrence of relatively high concentrations of the enzyme thioglucosidase in tumor tissues was the basis for the design of azathioprine. It was assumed that the enzyme in the target tissue might readily release the cytostatic mercaptopurine from its transport form (*105b*). Another example is the synthesis of glucuronides of anti-inflammatory steroids to be used in patients suffering from rheumatoid arthritis with as an aim selective bioactivation by the glucuronidases present in the synovial fluid (*163a*).

The occurrence of enzymes such as phosphamidase, carbamidase, and phosphatases in certain cancer tissues led to the synthesis of transport forms of nitrogen mustard to be bioactivated by these enzymes. Cyclophosphamide is an example of such cytostatics (*45, 141*). Although the selective bioactivation in the target tissue could not be verified, the formation of this type of transport forms of the biologically alkylating nitrogen mustard has certain advantages. The bioactivation, although not limited to the target tissue, is limited to certain tissues, sparing those tissues which are poor in the enzymes involved. Also the risk of an interaction of the alkylating agent with, e.g., plasma proteins is reduced as far as the enzymes involved in the bioactivation are restricted to the intracellular compartment.

An interesting approach to the idea of the selective bioactivation in the target tissue was developed by Danielli (*82, 84*). Certain carcinomas are sensitive to the cytostatic activity of urethanes. Often, however, a quick resistance to these cytostatics is developed, based on an increase in these tissues of the enzyme carbamidase, an enzyme which quickly inactivates the urethanes

TABLE XIX
INTRODUCTION OF PARTICULAR VULNERABLE MOIETIES IN EFFORTS TO DESIGN COMPOUNDS SELECTIVELY ACTIVATED IN THE TARGET TISSUE

Activating enzymes prevailing
in target tissue
in this case tumor tissue

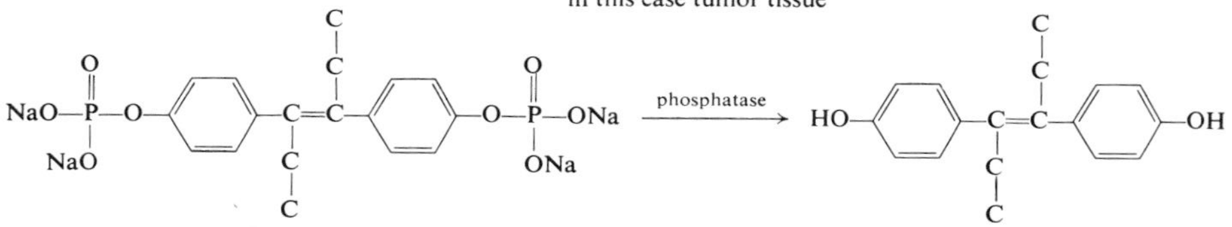

phosphatase

Honvan
inactive

Diethylstilbestrol
active

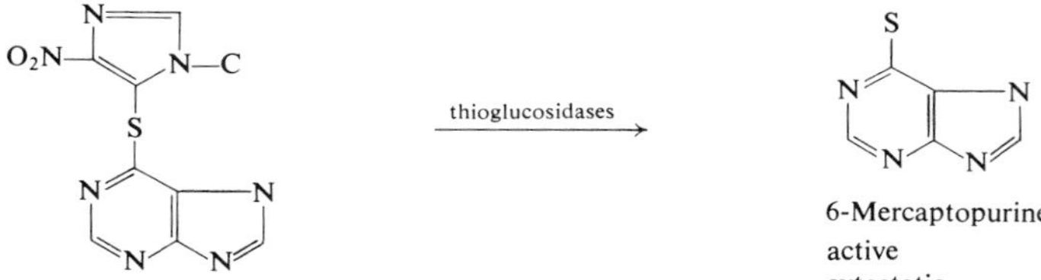

thioglucosidases

Azathioprine
inactive

6-Mercaptopurine
active
cytostatic
immunosuppressant

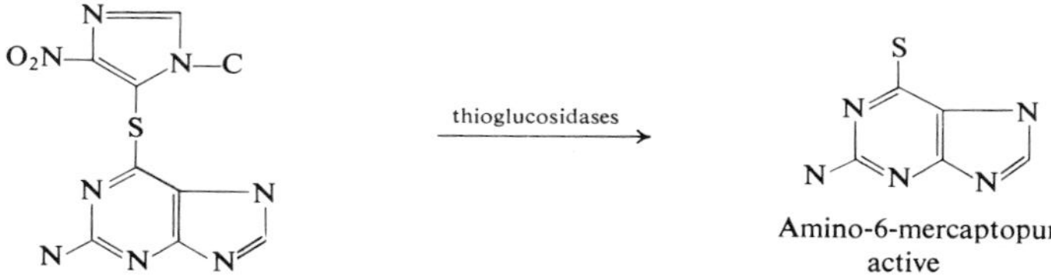

thioglucosidases

Thiamiprine
inactive

Amino-6-mercaptopurine
active
cytostatic

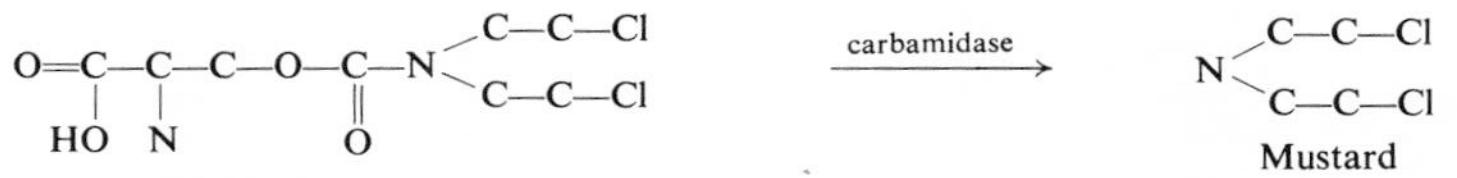

Mercasin
inactive

carbamidase →

Mustard
active
cytostatic

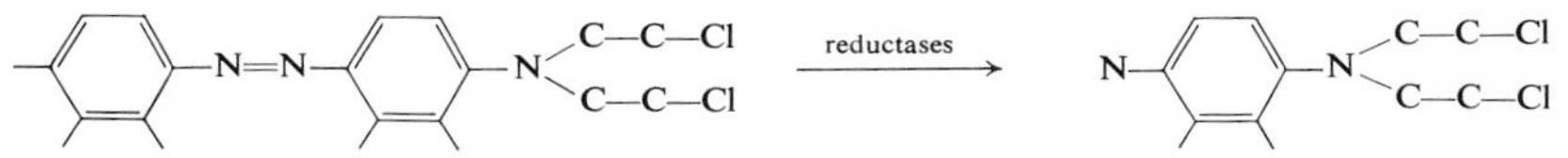

4-Di-β-chloroethylamino-
azobenzene derivative
inactive

reductases →

active
cytostatic

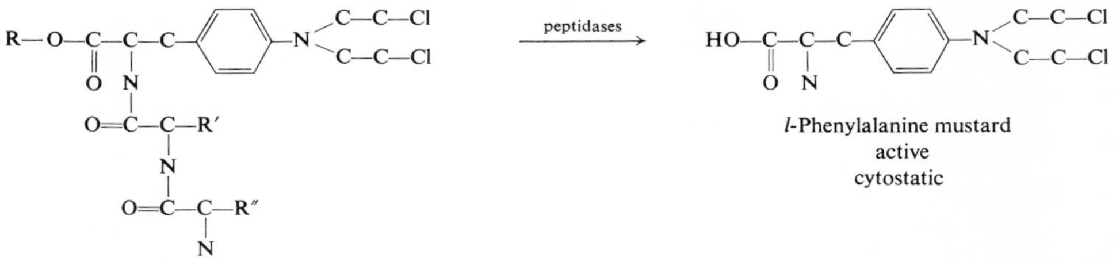

Tripeptide mustard
inactive

peptidases →

l-Phenylalanine mustard
active
cytostatic

The activating enzymes are, as a rule, not restricted to tumor tissue,
but often also present in liver and kidney

Systemic endometatoxic action of insecticide

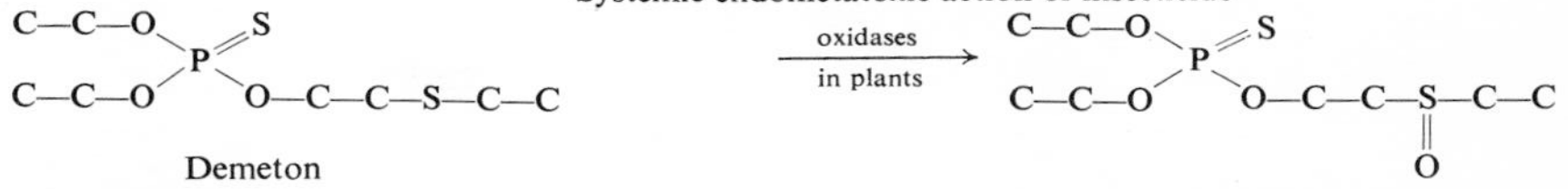

Demeton
slightly active

oxidases
in plants →

highly active
insecticide

by hydrolysis. Danielli's idea was to induce by means of urethanes a high concentration of the enzyme carbamidase in the tumor tissue followed by the application of a transport form of nitrogen mustard containing a carbamide group such that the transport form will be activated by the enzyme carbamidase. Applying the inductor, the urethane, and the transport form in sequence would lead to an induced selective bioactivation in the target tissue. As shown in Fig. 10 this principle could be experimentally verified. Again the fact has

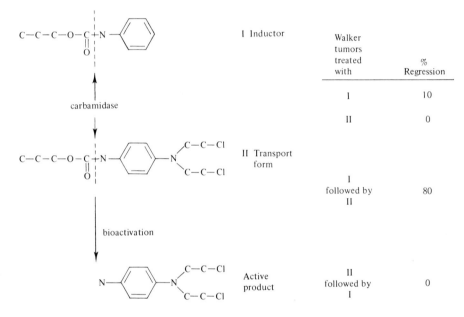

Walker tumors treated with	% Regression
I	10
II	0
I followed by II	80
II followed by I	0

Fig. 10. Selective bioactivation of a cytostatic agent based on introduction of a vulnerable moiety. The enzyme involved in the bioactivation of the transport form (II) by attack on the vulnerable moiety is induced by means of suitable inductor agents (I). After Danielli (*82, 84*).

to be accepted that not only the tumor tissues but also other tissues respond to urethane with an increase in the enzyme carbamidase. The principle of the induced bioactivation was demonstrated by Danielli for a variety of nitrogen mustard derivatives. The efforts to reach a selective activation in the target tissues are aimed at an increase in the therapeutic index. A differentiation in the action of the alkylating agents with respect to tumor and healthy tissue is essential in this respect.

Selectivity in the action is also required for such biologically active compounds as insecticides and weed killers. Low-hazard pesticides should be nontoxic for mammals and be specifically toxic to the insect or plant species

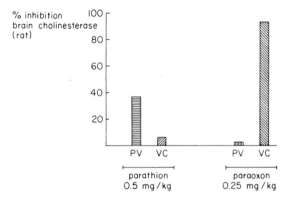

Fig. 11. Increase in the "selectivity" in the action by introduction of a vulnerable moiety. The use of the thiophosphonate, that means the introduction of the thio group, the vulnerable moiety involved in the bioactivation, implies a relatively high toxicity in the case of oral use (insects feeding on the plants sprayed) as compared to uptake via the skin (the farmer). *Note*: The precursor parathion is more active after infusion in the portal vein (bioactivation) and less active after infusion in the vena cava; the active product paraoxon is less active via the portal vein (bioinactivation) and more active via the vena cava. After Westermann (*350*).

that has to be eradicated. Strictly taken the selectivity can be based on differences in animal behavior or habit, differences in absorption or penetration of the toxon, differences in metabolism, bioactivation, or bioinactivation, differences in excretion, and differences in the sensitivity for the action of the pesticides in the strict sense. For compounds such as the insecticide parathion which is bioactivated in the liver under formation of the active compound paraoxon, toxicity after oral application is larger than the toxicity in the case of percutaneous absorption. Figure 11 shows the dependence of the activity of parathion and paraoxon on the way of application (*350*). The consequence is that as long as the pesticide is not put into the farmers' coffee there is a certain selective safety margin with respect to insects feeding on the plants sprayed. In the insects a to a certain degree selective bioactivation takes place.

The aim of the restriction of the action of bioactive compounds to particular compartments—the target compartments—is also common in environmental pharmacokinetics. The lack of selectivity is one of the main disadvantages of the chemical pesticides extensively used. One of the ways of reaching more selectivity in the action is the application of the principle of the selective bioactivation. An example is the use of nontoxic lipophilic compounds readily taken up by the plant leaves and converted in the plant to products with a high insecticidal activity. The aim is a restriction of the insecticidal activity to certain plant tissues and therewith a selectivity in the action for phytophagous insects feeding on the plants treated, and a more sustained action of the insecticide taken up by the plants. This principle is known as endometatoxic action of insecticides. An example is demeton (Cistox), a fat-soluble organic phosphate with a low insecticidal action. It is bioactivated in the plant tissues under formation of products which are 1000 times more active than the parent product (*156, 279*).

In the field of weed killers, too, the principle of selective bioactivation has been applied. Plants with an extensive foliage are exceptionally vulnerable to lipid-soluble weed killers because of the large surface available for the uptake. Highly water-soluble compounds, having a low lipid-solubility will be devoid of such an action since they cannot penetrate the lipophilic cuticula on the leaves. Hydrophilic compounds can be taken up easily by the plant roots, however. Highly water-soluble esters of compounds such as 2,4-dichloro-phenoxyethylalcohol, a precursor of the corresponding acid which acts as a weed killer, have been prepared (*75, 76*). These esters are not taken up by the plant leaves. After they reach the soil, where the esters are hydrolyzed, the alcohol is oxidized to the corresponding acid, which is a potent weed killer readily taken up by plant roots (Fig. 12). The consequence is a selectivity in the action. Plants with even an extensive foliage, if deeply rooted, will be protected and thus will be less sensitive than weeds with extensive superficial root systems. The latter will take up the weed killer more or less selectively and therefore be especially vulnerable to the treatment with this highly water-soluble type of esters.

An interesting example of selectivity in action based on selective bio-activation in particular species are the α-phenoxybutyric acids used as weed killers. These compounds have to be oxidized to the corresponding α-phenoxy-acetic acids for activity. They are highly active in many plant species and

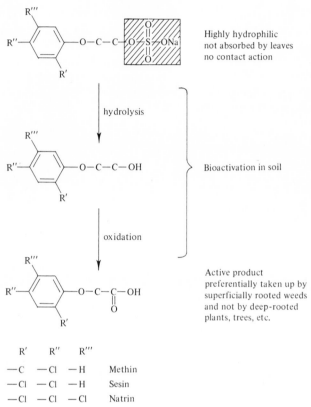

Fig. 12. Selectivity in action of weed killers obtained by introduction of a highly hydrophilic disposable restricting moiety in a precursor compound. After Crafts (75).

slightly active in Brassica species which apparently are less effective in this bioactivation (76, 76a) (Fig. 13).

2. Vulnerable Moieties Involved in Selective Bioinactivation

Local anesthetics should be restricted in their action to the site of application. Once absorbed into general circulation the compounds should be degraded and thus inactivated as soon as possible. For this purpose introduction of vulnerable moieties can be considered and has proved to be effective. The short-acting local anesthetic tolycaine obtained by introduction of a vulnerable moiety in the long-acting compound lidocaine (155) is an example (Fig. 14).

Besides the introduction of a vulnerable group in a drug in order to obtain short-acting compounds, also substitution of stable moieties by less stable moieties or labilization of suitable moieties already present can be considered. The introduction of suitable substituents in benzoic acid esters or anilides may result in labilization of the ester or amide bond. An example of this procedure is the development of butanilicaine, which is a more quickly hydrolyzed and therefore shorter acting analog of lidocaine (*322*) (Fig. 14). In this area application of Hammett constants may be helpful in selecting the right substituents (*13, 17, 292*).

2-Methyl-4-chlorophenoxyacetic acid
inactive in Galium aparine
due to rapid biodegradation

2-(2-Methyl-4-chlorophenoxy) propionic acid
active in Galium aparine
resistant to biodegradation

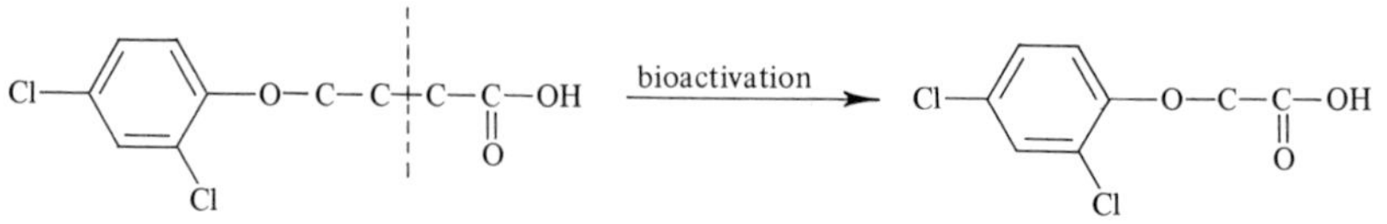

2, 4-Dichlorophenoxybutyric acid
inactive in Brassica species
probably due to lack in bioactivation
active in many other species

2, 4-Dichlorophenoxyacetic acid
active in Brassica and many other species

Fig. 13. Selectivity in action of weed killers related to the capacity for bioinactivation or bioactivation in the target tissues (*76*).

The introduction into cancer therapy of the technique of intra-arterial infusion and regional perfusion makes necessary the availability of cytostatics with a short action. In this way after passage of the region covered by the artery in which infusion takes place and after leakage into the general circulation in the case of regional perfusion, less harm is done to the healthy tissues by the cytostatic agent used. The fact that bifunctional alkylating agents as a rule are more active as cytostatics than monofunctional alkylating agents has been a basis for the development of short-acting cytostatics. Two alkylating groups, for instance, sulfur mustard groups, are conjugated by means of a vulnerable link such as a hydrolyzable amide or ester group. The disjunction caused by hydrolysis has as a result the formation of two monofunctional, only slightly active sulfur mustards, part of which with a free carboxyl group close to the sulfur atom. This implies a practically total loss of cytostatic

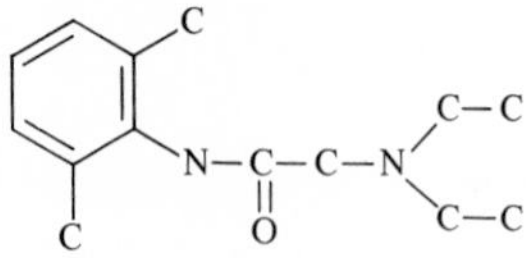

Lidocaine

stable local anesthetic

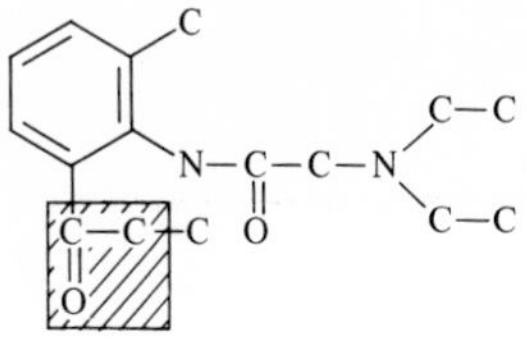

Tolycaine

introduction of the vulnerable
moiety implies rapid bioinactivation
once general circulation is reached

Butanilicaine

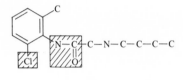

destabilization of the acylamide group
implies rapid bioinactivation once
general circulation is reached

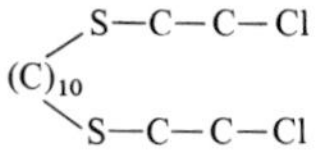

Cytostatic

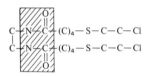

Cytostatic

designed for regional perfusion;
introduction of the vulnerable moieties
implies rapid hydrolysis by, e.g.,
liver amidase once general circulation
is reached

Fig. 14. Introduction of vulnerable moieties to avoid systemic actions in drugs locally
applied.

activity. For detailed information on this approach to the problem the reader
is referred to the papers of Witten (*358, 359*) and Williamson (*354*).

The incorporation into insecticidal organic phosphates of an ester group
which is easily hydrolyzed by carboxyesterases, resulting in compounds with
a free ionic carboxyl group close to the phosphate group, which implies an
inactivation, opens possibilities for a selective bioinactivation. The insecticides
concerned will be quickly inactivated by esterases occurring in plasma and
liver, especially of mammals. The insecticide malathion is an example. It
shows a remarkable safety margin.

Radioisotope studies with insects and mammals showed that two competing processes, the oxidative bioactivation to malaoxon and the hydrolytic bio-inactivation by splitting of the carboxy ester are involved (*121, 200, 256, 257*). The species with a slow conversion into the active oxoderivatives but a rapid

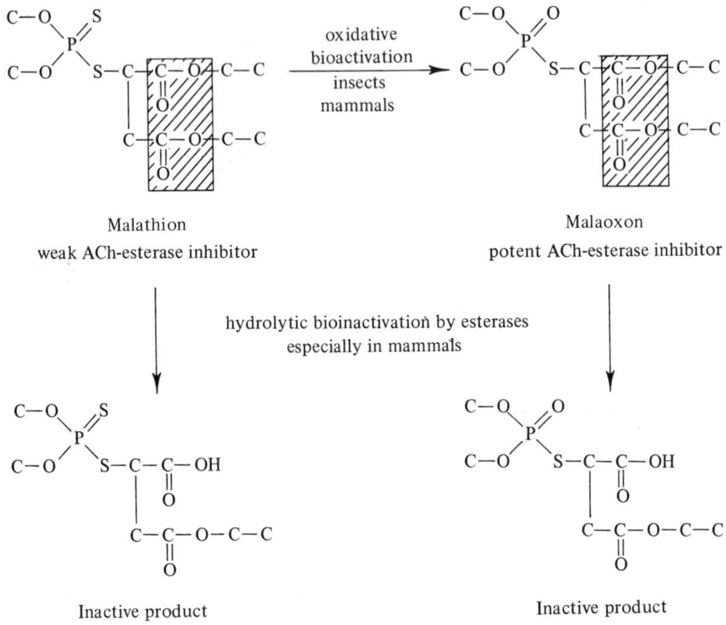

Fig. 15. Selectivity in action of insecticides obtained by introduction of vulnerable moieties. *Note*: The introduction of the vulnerable moiety results in a selective rapid bio-inactivation in mammals, which have as compared to insects, a high carboxyesterase activity in plasma and tissues (liver).

conversion by hydrolysis will be less susceptible than species where the relation between bioactivation and bioinactivation is the reverse. The differential toxicity of malathion with respect to insects and mammals seems to be due to a difference in the relation between bioactivation and bioinactivation. In this way in insects high levels of malaoxon are reached, in contrast to mammals, where because of the high rate of hydrolysis rapid inactivation takes place. The ester groups in malathion are the vulnerable moieties involved in selective bioinactivation (Fig. 15).

V. Modulation of the Time–Concentration Relationship in the Distribution of Drugs by Molecular Manipulation

The time–concentration relationship for the active form of a drug in the compartments, e.g., plasma, is dependent on the rate of uptake, the absorption, the rate of bioactivation of transport forms, and on the rate of elimination by excretion, redistribution, and by bioinactivation. The last three determine the half-life time of the active compound (*343*). Possibilities for modulation of the time–concentration relationship of a drug by its chemical modification are: (1) adaptation of the lipid- and water-solubility and therewith the rate of uptake, distribution, and excretion of the drug; (2) adaptation of the chemical, especially the metabolic stability of the drug; and (3) formation of a transport form by temporary inactivation.

The procedures indicated open a gamut of possibilities ranging from preparations with a protracted action such as depot preparations to ultra-short acting drugs.

A. PROTRACTION OF DRUG ACTION BY FORMATION OF POORLY SOLUBLE SALTS OR COMPLEXES

One of the best-known principles in this respect is the composition of pharmaceutical preparations for sustained release, usually called depot preparations. The aim is the maintenance of a certain effective concentration of the drug in the body for a longer period by means of a single dose.

We will not go into detail as far as the many pharmaceutical preparations designed to obtain sustained release of drugs in the intestinal tract are concerned. A variety of principles exists such as the use of granules of different size, granules with coatings of varying thickness or varying stability which have to be resolved in the intestinal tract, and, binding to resins (*114, 136, 166, 167, 219, 220, 250*). For parenteral application the use of suspensions of microcrystalline poorly soluble compounds or their solutions in oil can be mentioned. The rate of uptake varies with the size and type of crystal (*18, 182, 328*). This principle is applied extensively for various steroid hormone esters. The implantation of tablets can also be mentioned in this respect. The best-known examples of the formation of poorly soluble salts or complexes are the depot preparations of polypeptide hormones obtained by combining these hormones with suitable proteins resulting in complexes with a low solubility at the pH of the body fluids. The principle is applied in various depot preparations of insulin such as protamine-insulin. The relatively acidic polypeptide hormone—the isoelectric point of insulin is 5.5—is combined with the basic polypeptide protamine with an isoelectric point of 8.5. The complex formed has its isoelectric point at pH 7, the pH of the body fluids, which implies a low solubility of the complex at that pH (*10*). Addition of traces of certain metals such as zinc stabilizes the complex and enhances its crystallization. Other proteins such as globins (globin-insulin), gelatine (preparations of ACTH and parathyroid hormone) and small organic bases such as aminochinuridum (Surfen-insulin) too are used to obtain depot preparations of polypeptide hormones (*89, 205, 250, 274*). In the preparation of long-acting application forms under formation of poorly soluble salts, for basic drugs such as antimalarials and anthelmintics polycyclic dicarbonic acids such as pamoic acid are used (*106, 176, 324*), while for acidic drugs such as the penicillins dicyclic bases such as benethamine and benzathin are used (*176*).

Tannic acid has been used to obtain slowly absorbed preparations of vasopressin, vitamin B_{12} (*325*), amphetamine (*126*), and other biologically active amines. On the other hand, proteins such as albumins are used to obtain preparations which slowly release tannic acid. An example is tannalbin, which because of its astringent action is used for the treatment of diarrhea (*245*).

The procedure of the formation of poorly soluble salts and complexes cannot be regarded as molecular manipulation; it is pharmaceutical formulation.

B. Desolubilizing and Solubilizing Moieties

Since the many transport media in the body, especially the extracellular fluid, are strongly hydrophilic, a certain degree of water solubility is required for the uptake of the drug from the site of application especially in the case of intramuscular or subcutaneous injection. Consequently the conversion of drugs to highly lipophilic compounds results in a delay in the uptake after parenteral application. Drugs with alcoholic OH— groups can be converted, for instance, by esterification with monocarbonic acids to more lipophilic products. The increase in lipophility depends on the acid used. Often the esters as such are devoid of biological activity since OH— groups essential for the action are masked. Bioactivation by hydrolysis of the ester bond is required then to obtain the drug in its active form. The acid used in the ester formation can be considered as a disposable desolubilizing moiety.

If high plasma concentrations of a drug are required, the intravenous route is indicated. This implies that the drug must be available in a water-soluble form. A possibility is the "solubilization." Then poorly water-soluble drugs are brought into "solution" under formation of mixed micelles by means of Tween or other surface-active compounds used as additives. This procedure cannot be regarded as molecular manipulation. The formation of readily soluble compounds obtained by formation of hemiesters of dicarbonic acids and drugs, e.g., steroid hormones, can be regarded as molecular manipulation. The dicarbonic acid moiety is split off in the organism under release of the active compound. The acid moiety can be considered as a disposable solubilizing moiety. It is not always known whether the groups introduced as desolubilizing or solubilizing moieties are disjuncted. If not, they must be classified as fixed moieties. The introduction of desolubilizing and solubilizing moieties is one of the procedures most widely applied in efforts to modulate pharmacokinetics by molecular manipulation (*11, 13, 14, 250*).

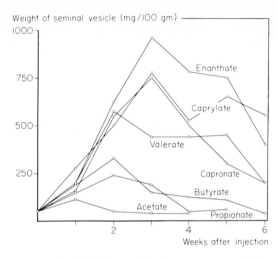

Fig. 16. Introduction of desolubilizing moieties in testosterone and the influence thereof upon the weight of the seminal vesicle of castrated rats after a single subcutaneous injection of 20 mg in 0.4 ml sesame oil. Note the increase in the effect obtained with the esters of larger fatty acids indicating that the protracted supply with the hormone is favorable and even required for the action. After Junkmann and Witzel (*182*).

1. *Disposable Desolubilizing Moieties*

The introduction of disposable desolubilizing moieties, that is lipophilizing moieties, is applied to a wide variety of steroid hormones which are converted into highly fat-soluble depot preparations on basis of this procedure (Fig. 16) (*18, 88, 91, 182, 289, 328, 330, 338*). The esters obtained can possibly be applied as a solution in oil or as a microcrystalline suspension in water. Because of the high fat-solubility there is only a slow release of the drug from the depot. In androgens and estrogens usually the alcoholic OH— group on C_{17} is involved in the esterification. The same holds for anabolic steroids. In progesterone no OH— group is available which implies that synthetic gestagens

TABLE XXA
INTRODUCTION OF DISPOSABLE[a] DESOLUBILIZING MOIETIES IN HORMONES AND HORMONOIDS
TO OBTAIN DEPOT PREPARATIONS

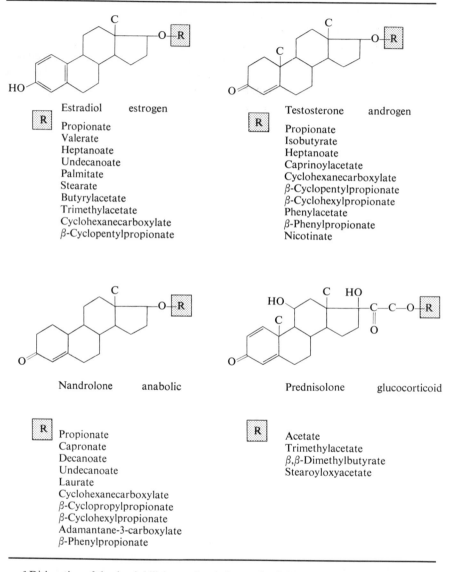

Estradiol   estrogen

R

Propionate
Valerate
Heptanoate
Undecanoate
Palmitate
Stearate
Butyrylacetate
Trimethylacetate
Cyclohexanecarboxylate
β-Cyclopentylpropionate

Testosterone   androgen

R

Propionate
Isobutyrate
Heptanoate
Caprinoylacetate
Cyclohexanecarboxylate
β-Cyclopentylpropionate
β-Cyclohexylpropionate
Phenylacetate
β-Phenylpropionate
Nicotinate

Nandrolone   anabolic

Prednisolone   glucocorticoid

R

Propionate
Capronate
Decanoate
Undecanoate
Laurate
Cyclohexanecarboxylate
β-Cyclopropylpropionate
β-Cyclohexylpropionate
Adamantane-3-carboxylate
β-Phenylpropionate

R

Acetate
Trimethylacetate
β,β-Dimethylbutyrate
Stearoyloxyacetate

[a] Disjunction of the desolubilizing moiety before action is highly probable.

with an alcoholic OH— group have to be used. In the synthetic gestagens usually the OH— group on C_{17} is used for esterification. Most corticosteroids have two alcoholic OH— groups suitable for esterification, one on C_{17} and one on C_{21}. The C_{21}-esters are preferred. Mineralocorticosteroid esters have been made of deoxycortone using the OH— group on C_{12} (Table XXA). As mentioned, hydrolysis of the esters will usually be necessary to obtain the hormone in its active form (90, 182, 338, 356). This implies that besides the increase in lipophility also the degree of stability of the esters with respect to hydrolysis may influence the depot effect. As is well known, steroid hormones such as androgens and gestagens induce a whole spectrum of effects. For certain components in the action short-lasting high concentrations of the hormone in its active form may be required. For other components in the action more sustained relatively low concentrations of the hormone may be required. The consequence is that the various transport forms may differ as far as the strength of the various components in the action is concerned. The rate of hydrolysis of the esters and therewith the rate of bioactivation depends, as mentioned, on the character of the desolubilizing moiety (259, 260, 338). Carboxy acids branched in the carbon atom next to the carboxyl group as a rule give esters which are more stable to hydrolysis than those of nonbranched acids.

Of great actuality are the extremely long-acting derivatives of progestatives used in oral contraceptives, such as the acetophenide of dihydroxyprogesterone (90, 153, 280, 363). The rate of uptake from the site of action as well as the rate of hydrolysis of long-acting steroid hormone preparations can be approached by model studies in vitro (338a). Other examples of the design of long-acting drugs by introduction of desolubilizing moieties are the esters of larger fatty acids and phenothiazines widely used as tranquillizers in psychiatry, e.g., fluphenazine enanthate (191, 243). Further, the possibility to use esters of certain antimalarial 4-aminoquinolines and 9-aminoacridines as repository drugs has been probed (106) (Table XXB). The sulfonamide–formaldehyde copolymers demonstrate another chemical principle applied to desolubilize drugs (90a).

The principle of prolongation of the action based on an esterification of alcoholic OH— groups is also applied in the field of vitamins. Esters of vitamin A such as the palmitate (176) and the α,α-dimethylvaleric acid and α-methyl-α-ethylbutyric acid esters can be mentioned in this respect (119) (see Section V,C,2 and Table XXVIII). In this case the prolongation of the action is partly based on a protection of the vitamin against bioinactivation. Also in the field of the herbicides the principle of the formation of esters to obtain derivatives with a prolonged action based on a sustained release is applied. An example is the compound tris(2,4-dichlorophenoxyethyl)phosphite, a highly lipophilic viscous fluid which after hydrolysis releases 2,4-dichlorophenoxyethanol

TABLE XXB

INTRODUCTION OF DISPOSABLE[a] DESOLUBILIZING MOIETIES IN DRUGS TO OBTAIN DEPOT PREPARATIONS

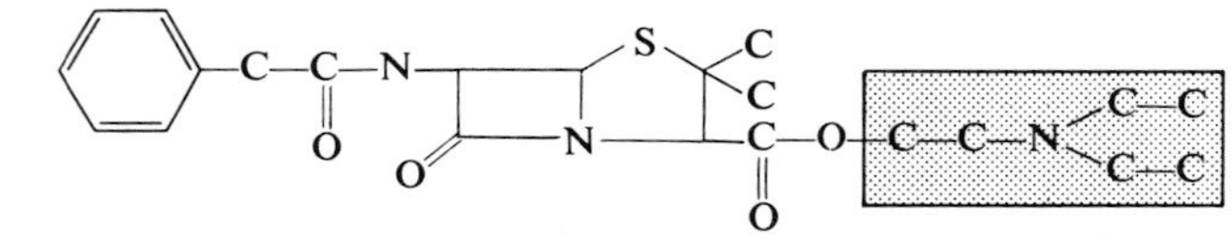

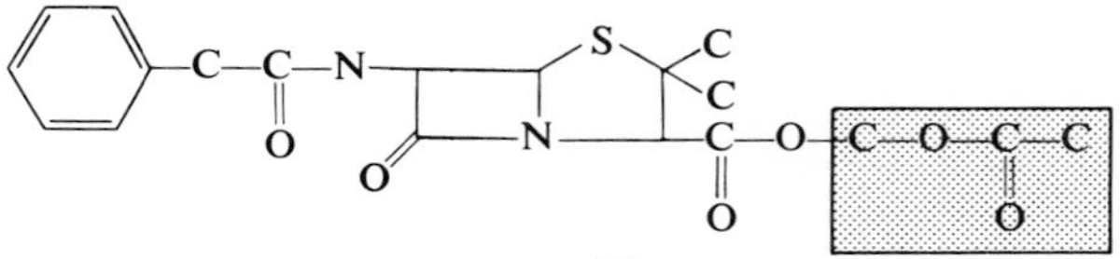

Penamecillin

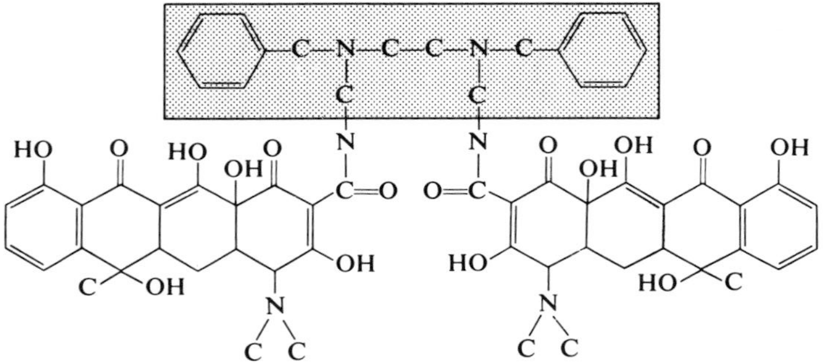

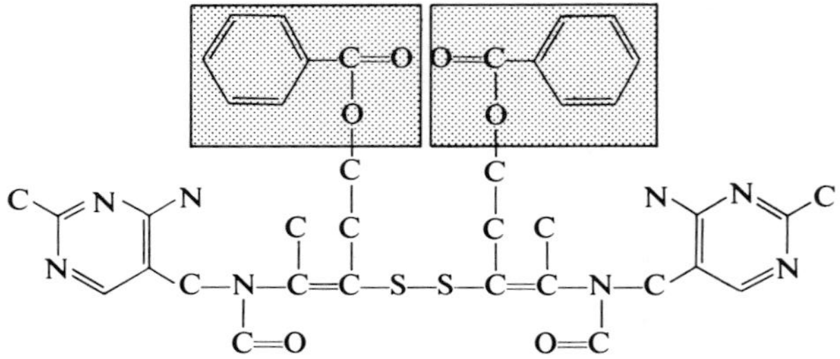

Beprocin
"oral" depot preparation of thiamine

Penethacillin

Ditetracycline

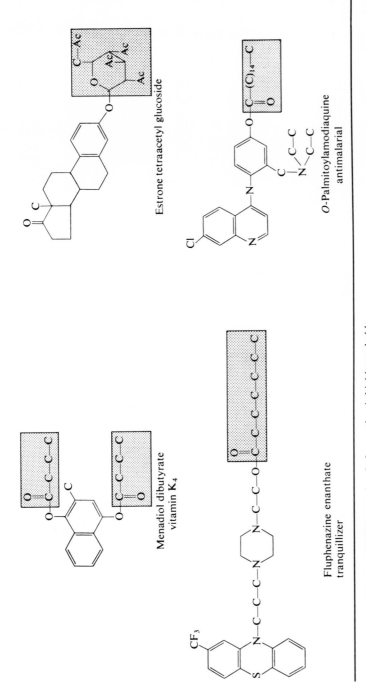

Estrone tetraacetyl glucoside

O-Palmitoylamodiaquine
antimalarial

Menadiol dibutyrate
vitamin K₄

Fluphenazine enanthate
tranquillizer

[a] Disjunction of the desolubilizing moiety before action is highly probable.

which has to be oxidized then to the corresponding acid to obtain the active weed killer 2,4-dichlorophenoxyacetic acid (Fig. 17). After application of this compound to the soil it remains active for 3–7 weeks (75).

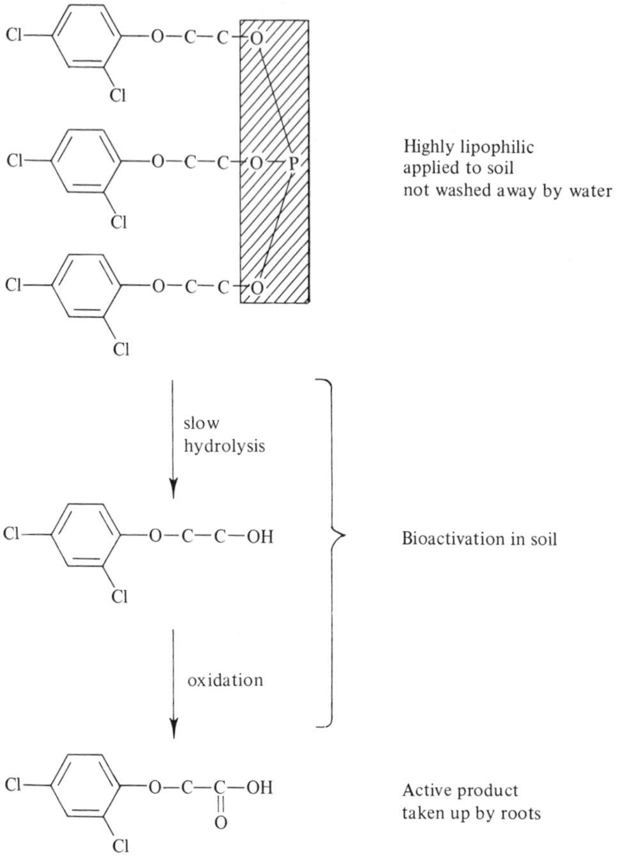

Fig. 17. Highly lipophilic depot preparation of a weed killer with a protracted action (3–7 weeks) after application to the soil.

2. Disposable Solubilizing Moieties

A classical example of a disposable solubilizing moiety is found in prontosil solubile, a chemical modification of prontosil rubrum. It was prepared with the aim to increase water solubility in order to obtain a drug suitable for intravenous application (343a). As is well known, prontosil rubrum (Fig. 18a) as well as prontosil solubile are bioactivated by reduction of the azo link with as a result a disjunction of the antibacterial sulfanilamide and the rest of the

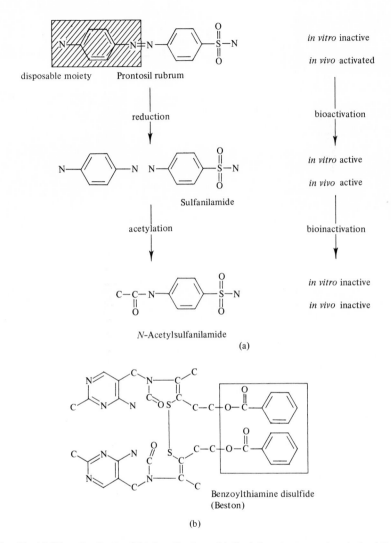

disposable moiety · Prontosil rubrum

in vitro inactive

in vivo activated

reduction · bioactivation

Sulfanilamide

in vitro active

in vivo active

acetylation · bioinactivation

N-Acetylsulfanilamide

(a)

in vitro inactive

in vivo inactive

Benzoylthiamine disulfide
(Beston)

(b)

Fig. 18. (a) Bioactivation and bioinactivation. (b) Oral depot preparation derived from thiamine.

molecule. Introduction of the sulfonate groups used for the solubilization in the sulfanilamide moiety would as well have resulted in a water-soluble product. Nevertheless, it would have been the wrong procedure since disjunction would not have resulted in the formation of an active sulfanilamide. In prontosil solubile a correct procedure was followed. The solubilization was performed by introduction of sulfonate groups in the disposable moiety.

TABLE XXIA

INTRODUCTION OF DISPOSABLE[a] SOLUBILIZING MOIETIES IN ANTIINFECTIOUS CHEMOTHERA-
PEUTICS TO OBTAIN WATER-SOLUBLE COMPOUNDS

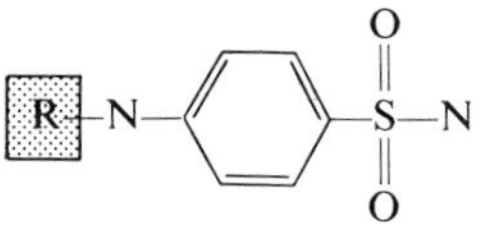

Sulfanilamide

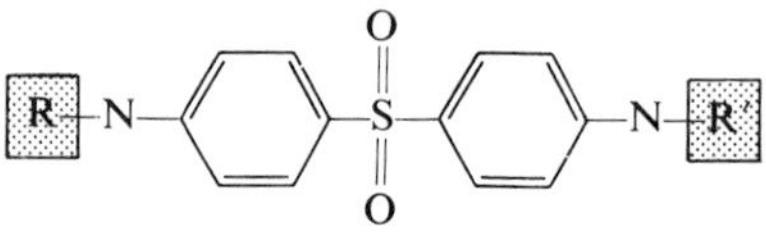

Diaphenylsulfone

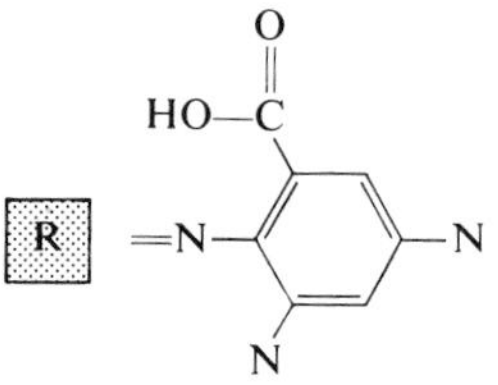

Rubiazole II

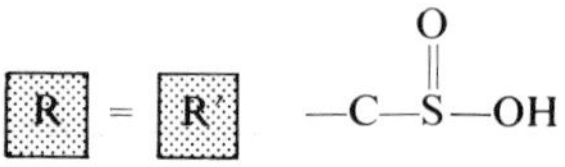

Aldesulfone

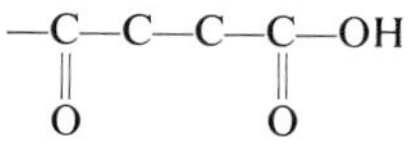

Ambesid soluble

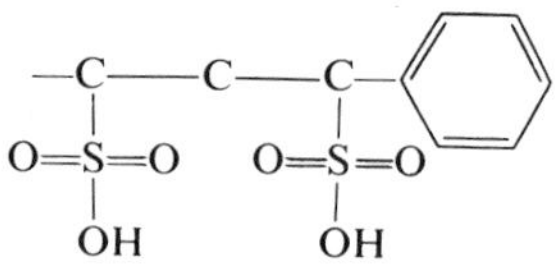

Solasulfone

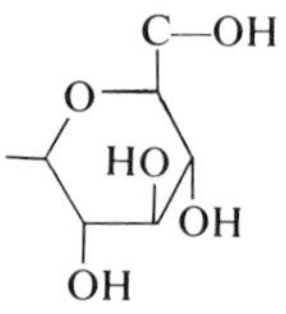

Glucosyl sulfanilamide

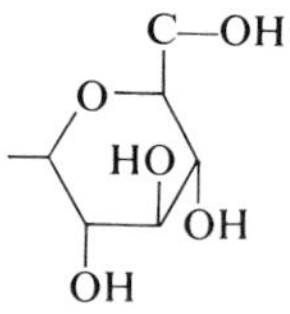

Tibatin

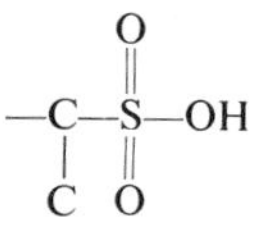

Septosil

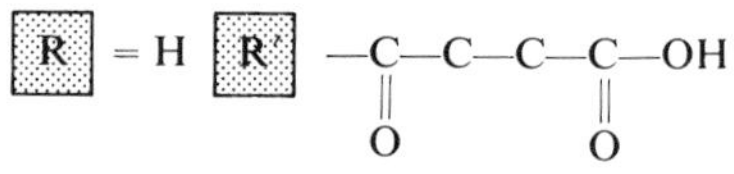

Succisulfone

[a] Disjunction of the solubilizing moiety before action is highly probable.

The reader may object that at the time prontosil solubile was developed it was not yet known that a disjunction and consequential bioactivation takes place. All right, this demonstrates that it is worthwhile to analyze closely those instances where the trial-and-error procedure has been successful. The success may be based upon the fact that incidentally a valuable principle, worth to

INTRODUCTION OF DISPOSABLE[a] SOLUBILIZING MOIETIES IN HORMONES AND HORMONOIDS TO
OBTAIN WATER-SOLUBLE COMPOUNDS

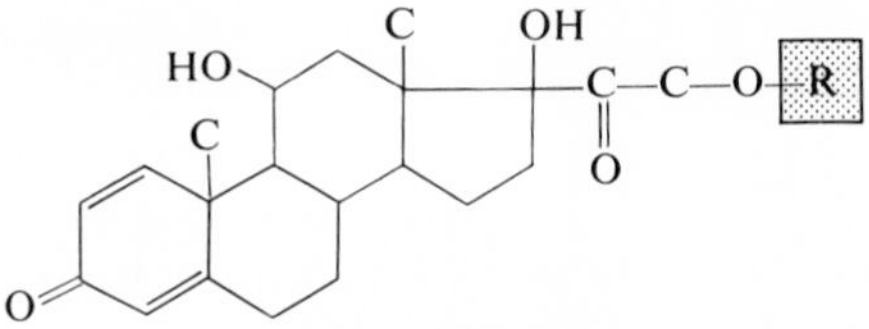

Prednisolone

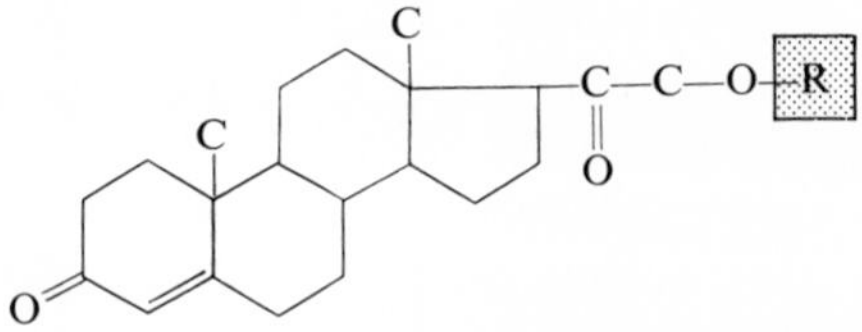

Deoxycortone

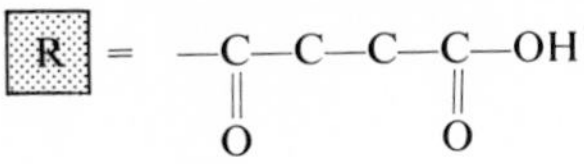

R =

Soludacortin

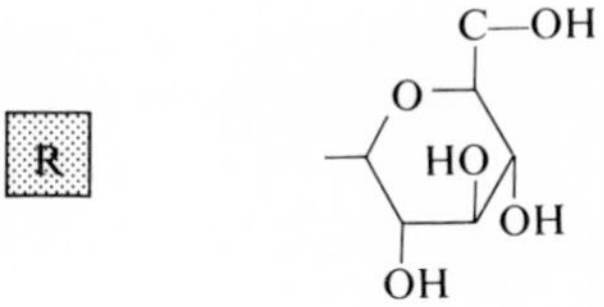

Docaquosum

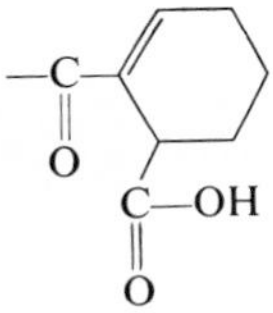

Ultracorten soluble

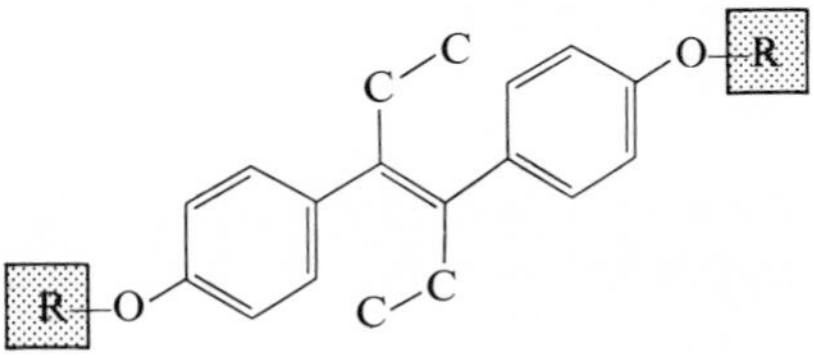

Diethylstilbestrol

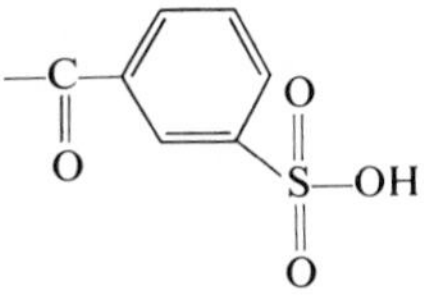

Corticosol

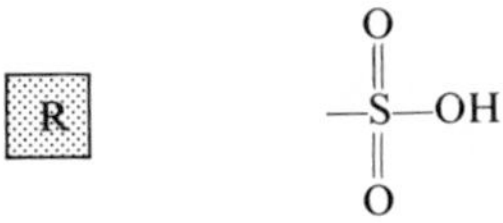

Idroestril

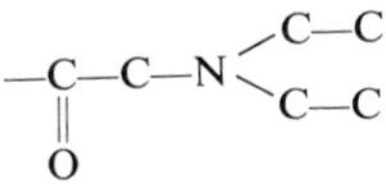

Magnadelt

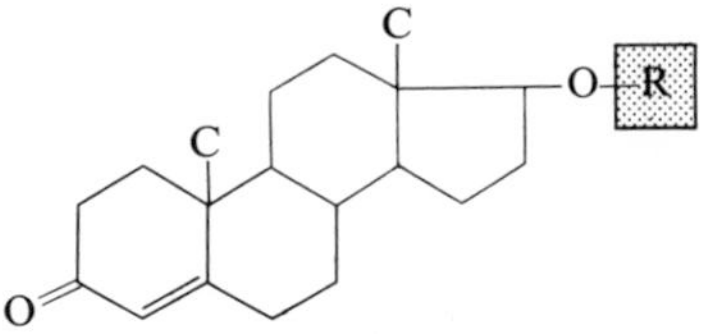

Testosterone

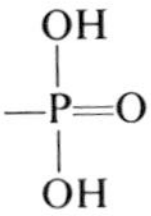

Solucort

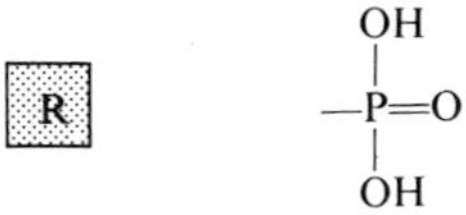

Testosterone phosphate
Telipex aquosum

[a] Disjunction of the solubilizing moiety before action is highly probable.

be recognized, was applied. Recognition of such principles may in the long run contribute essentially to the advancement of drug design more so than the development of the drug in which the principle was incidentally, unwittingly applied.

The sulfonamide sulfacarboxychrysoidine (Table XXIA), also a good water-soluble product, was designed on basis of the insight gained with prontosil and prontosil rubrum (95, 217). Here too disjunction is based on a reduction of the azo link which results in the liberation of the active drug sulfanilamide. Various water-soluble acidic derivatives of sulfanilamides are still in use (52a, 176, 235a). Also for the related sulfones used against leprosy, water-soluble derivatives have been developed by introduction of disposable solubilizing moieties (93) (Table XXIA). Another example are the tuberculostatics thiosemicarbazone and isonicotinic acid hydrazide (52a, 176, 235a). Besides dicarbonic acids also other hydrophilic moieties such as sugars are used as disposable solubilizing moieties (Table XXIA).

In order to obtain water-soluble preparations of, e.g., steroid hormones, hemiesters of dicarbonic acids can be used. If the aim is to reach without much delay high concentrations of the hormone the esters used should easily be hydrolyzed to release the steroid hormone in its active form (90, 356). The dicarbonic acid groups serve as disposable solubilizing moieties then (Table XXIB). Steroid hormones such as androgens and gestagens induce a whole spectrum of effects. For certain components in the action short-lasting high concentrations of the hormone in its active form may be required. For other components in the action longer lasting, relatively low concentrations of the hormone may be required. Consequently, the various transport forms may differ as far as the proportion of the various components in the action is concerned (259, 260, 338). The principle of the introduction of disposable solubilizing moieties is widely applied. Examples chosen from a great variety of poorly water-soluble drugs are the hemisuccinates of estriol, a hemostatic, of hydroxydione, an intravenous anesthetic (176), of oxazepam, a tranquillizer (345), of griseofulvin (115), erythromycin, and chloramphenicol (176, 249), antibiotics, of tocopherol, a vitamin (176), of glycyrrhizinic acid, a plant product with glucocorticoid action (176), etc. (Table XXIC).

3. Fixed Desolubilizing Moieties

Although for a number of the steroid esters used as depot preparation, disjunction of the lipophilizing moiety has been made probable, it is definitely not excluded that in a number of cases, the ester or the acetals are active as such and not split in the body. In that case the groups attached to the steroid serve as fixed desolubilizing moieties. Strictly taken, only in a few cases definite proof is given for the disjunction of the desolubilizing and solubilizing moieties discussed in the foregoing sections. In many cases the information available on structure–action relationship of the mother compound gives an indication. So for instance the fact that N_4-substituted sulfanilamides are found to be antibacterially inactive *in vitro* allows the classification "disposable" for the various moieties linked to the amino group concerned. Definite information in this respect on existing drugs is extremely scarce. It may be expected that the more detailed analysis of pharmacokinetics applied to new drugs will ameliorate this situation in the future. Systematic studies in this field are badly needed, since they may well contribute to the rational approach in drug design. A stimulating effort in this respect is presented by Eckert *et al.* (98). A special type of protracted action, obtained by introduction of lipophilizing moieties is reported for ethers of steroid hormones such as the 3-cyclopentyl ether of methyltestosterone (239) and of ethynylestradiol (238). The ethers taken orally are much longer acting than the mother compounds, not only because of the higher metabolic stability, but also since the ethers are, after absorption, stored in the body fat and gradually released then.

With the ultra-short acting barbiturates too storage in the body fat of these highly lipophilic compounds takes place. Here, the rapid fall in the originally high plasma concentrations obtained by intravenous application implies that introduction of lipophilizing moieties—the thio group in thiobarbiturates and the *N*-alkyl substituents in short-acting barbiturates such as hexobarbital—leads to a shortening of the action (46, 48, 261). The storage in the body fat may especially after repeated application result in a long lasting sedation as aftereffect (160, 261, 327).

The alkyl substituents in the steroid ethers probably must be regarded as fixed desolubilizing moieties; a disjunction is not very feasible. The same holds true for the "thio groups" of thiobarbiturates used in intravenous anesthesia. The alkyl substituents in the *N*-alkyl-substituted barbiturates appear to be rapidly eliminated.

4. *Fixed Solubilizing Moieties*

Since a high hydrophility is incompatible with an easy penetration into the cells, fixed solubilizing moieties are rare. If they are applied, they as a rule only cause a modest shift in the balance from lipid solubility in the direction of water solubility. The best-known examples are the water-soluble derivatives of the tetracyclines. Here secondary or tertiary amino groups are used as solubilizing moieties. This implies that as salts these compounds are well water-soluble; at the pH of the body fluids a sufficiently high fraction is available in the undissociated form to guarantee tissue penetration (176) (see Table XXIIA).

TABLE XXIC

INTRODUCTION OF DISPOSABLE[a] SOLUBILIZING MOIETIES TO OBTAIN WATER-SOLUBLE COMPOUNDS

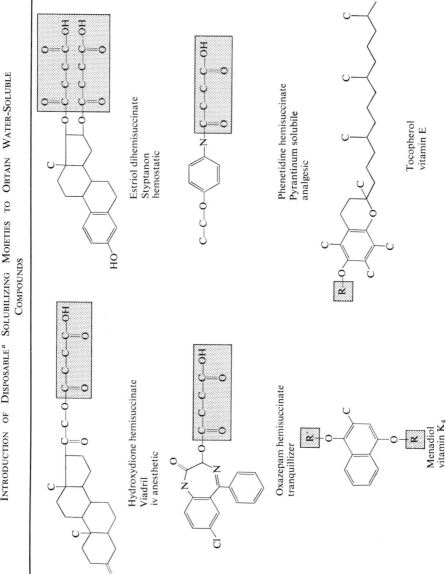

Estriol dihemisuccinate
Styptanon
hemostatic

Hydroxydione hemisuccinate
Viadril
iv anesthetic

Phenetidine hemisuccinate
Pyrantinum soluble
analgesic

Oxazepam hemisuccinate
tranquillizer

Tocopherol
vitamin E

Menadiol
vitamin K₄

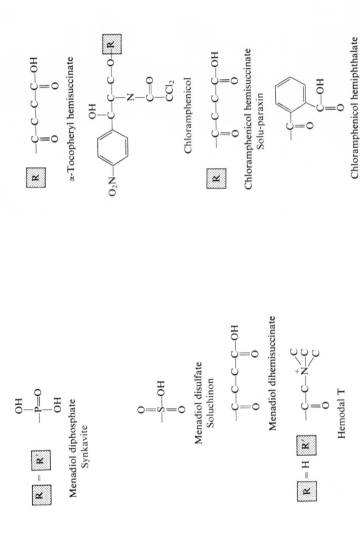

^a Disjunction of the solubilizing moiety before action is highly probable.

TABLE XXIIA

INTRODUCTION OF FIXED SOLUBILIZING MOIETIES IN DRUGS TO ENHANCE WATER SOLUBILITY

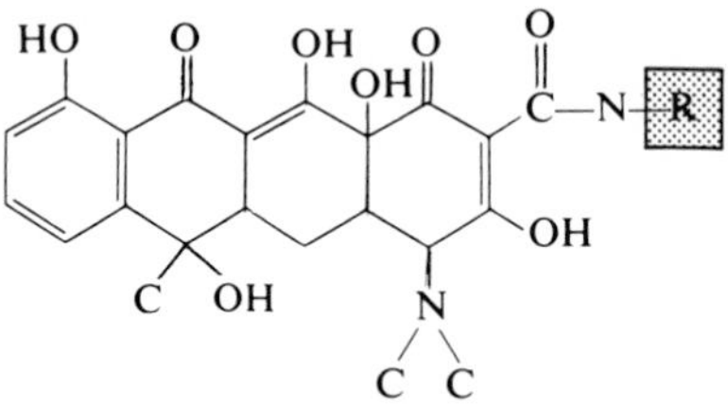

Tetracycline

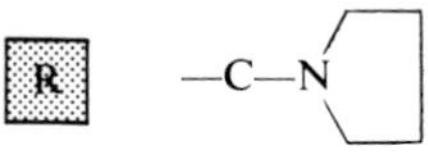

R: $-C-N\langle$ (pyrrolidine)

Rolitetracycline
Reverin

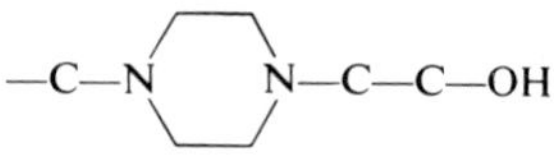

$-C-N\langle$ (piperazine) $N-C-C-OH$

Pipacycline
Tetrasolvina

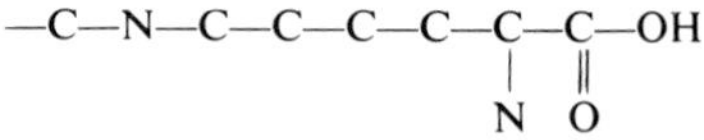

$-C-N-C-C-C-C-C-C-OH$ with N and O substituents

Lymecycline
Tetralysine

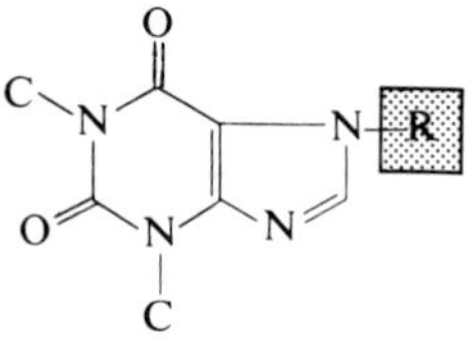

Theophylline

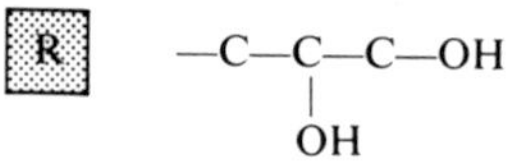

R: $-C-C-C-OH$ with OH

Diprophylline
Solufylin

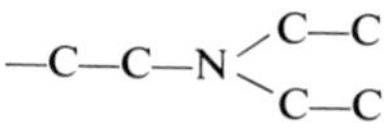

$-C-C-N\langle \begin{array}{c} C-C \\ C-C \end{array}$

Etamiphyllin
Soluphyllin

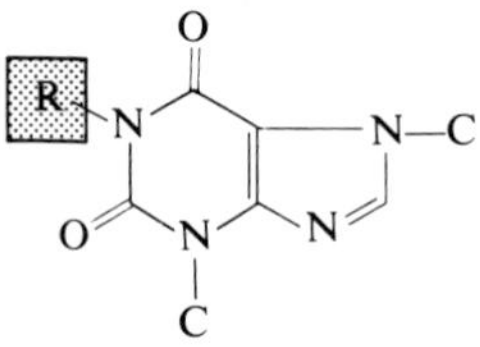

Theobromine

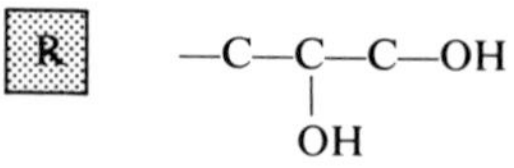

R: $-C-C-C-OH$ with OH

Isobromin

The poorly water-soluble compounds theophylline and theobromine have been subject to a wide variety of efforts to increase the water solubility by introduction of fixed solubilizing moieties (*176*) (see Table XXIIA).

5. *Protraction of Drug Action by Introduction of Facilitating Moieties*

There is one particular aspect in the increase in the lipophility of drugs to be discussed more in detail, namely the increased tendency to retention in the organism and thus to prolonged action. The retention may be due to storage in fat as in the case of the highly fat-soluble chlorinated alkanes such as DDT, used as pesticides. Also the enhanced renal reabsorption which takes place for fat-soluble compounds in the unionized form and the biliary excretion of such compounds possibly combined with enteral reabsorption will contribute to the retention and therefore a prolongation of the action. Plasma protein binding, which implies protection of the drug from renal excretion by ultrafiltration, is another factor in this respect. The plasma protein binding in a series of compounds as a rule increases with their hydrophobic character. The protein can be considered as a temporary protecting adsorbent. A high degree of protein binding has as a consequence that the concentration of the free diffusable drug is kept low. This free concentration must be regarded as the active concentration. This holds for the pharmacological action including the action on microorganisms.

The implications of drug binding to plasma proteins and other more or less indifferent sites of binding are the object of intensive study (*6, 31, 42, 127, 135, 157, 201, 252, 295, 296, 315*). It has many aspects also beyond the delay of elimination and the depot function of the drug in its bound form. In case of combinations of drugs, for instance, mutual displacement from the sites of binding may take place resulting in changes in the "active" concentration, and therewith an enhancement of degradation and excretion and possibly also changes in the absorption of the drug (*7, 8, 202, 351*). Not only other drugs but also compounds inactive if applied singly may be of interest as inhibitors of protein binding of drugs (*202, 203*). Further not only displacement of drugs from carrier proteins but also displacement of endogenous compounds such as hormones and other biocatalysts from their carrier proteins may be involved (*247, 337*). We will not go into further detail in this respect. It will be clear that the study of the various implications of drug–protein binding, etc., not only will contribute to drug design but may also help us in understanding many complications observed in the action of combinations of drugs (*11, 15, 16*).

For the long-acting sulfonamides such as sulfaphenazole and sulfadimethoxine, the high degree of binding to plasma protein, up to 99%, was assumed to play a role in the protracted action of these compounds. As is shown, however, in Table XXIIB the short- and long-acting compounds are much more clearly differentiated by differences in their lipid solubility than by differences in protein binding (*317a*). The long-acting compounds have high lipid solubility. This indicates that renal reabsorption may well be a determinant factor. The fact that there are exceptions such as sulfadimidine (compound 9) which also has a high lipid solubility may be attributed to metabolic inactivation, which, as a matter of fact, complicates the picture. The same holds true for the pH of the urine which determines the degree of ioniza-

TABLE XXIIB

PHYSICOCHEMICAL CHARACTERISTICS OF SULFANILAMIDES IN RELATION TO THE HALF-LIFE TIME[a]

Compound	pK_a	Protein binding (%)	Lipid solubility % drug in ethylene chloride at pH 7.4	Half-life time man (hr)
		Short-acting		
4	7.1	77	15.3	4
14	4.9	86	4.8	6
13	7.4	86	19.0	7
8	5.6	99	6.2	7
9	7.4	80	82.6	7
		Long-acting		
20	6.7	85	69.6	35
17	7.2	90	70.4	37
24	7.0	87	64.0	37
19	6.1	99	78.7	40

[a] After Struller (*317a*).

tion and thus influences reabsorption, as will be discussed in the next section. No doubt, the adaptation in the lipid solubility of drugs by suitable substitutions, possibly on guidance of the substituent contributions to this parameter as outlined by Hansch and others (*17, 145, 146, 147, 148*), constitutes a promising approach in drug design. A systematic analysis for the detection in the drug molecule of sites with a certain bulk tolerance and thus a reasonable degree of freedom for molecular manipulation, followed by an introduction of substituents, selected on basis of their substituent constants (*17*) may be expected to become one of the main lines of approach in drug design.

Besides promotion of renal reabsorption to obtain drugs with a protracted action, enhancement of an intermediate storage of the drug, namely in fat tissue constituting a suitable store for highly lipid-soluble drugs, may be considered. Again introduction of suitable lipophilizing groups and possibly elimination or masking of polar groups conferring a too high water-solubility to the drug will be the task of the medicinal chemist. The principle apparently is applied already.

For certain orally long-acting steroid ethers, such as the methyltestosterone-3-cyclopentylenol ether, after absorption storage in the body fat is supposed to be involved from which a slow release takes place, and which implies a protection against quick bioinactivation (239). The compounds can be considered as "oral" depot preparations. An intermediate storage in fat tissue takes possibly place too in the case of the "oral" depot preparation derived from thiamine (Beston) (see Fig. 18b). These are examples of retention based on lipophilizing moieties which facilitate storage in lipid compartments. In case of the short-acting barbiturates which rapidly escape from the plasma into the fat tissues, such a storage phenomenon leads to unwanted aftereffects.

Intermediate storage in particular compartments for orally taken long-acting drugs is also reported for various antimalarials such as mepacrine and chloraquine where tissue concentrations being 500-fold the plasma concentrations are found. Here not storage in lipophilic compartments but binding to other tissue components, presumably nucleic acids, is involved. A somewhat different approach to temporary compartmentalization is found in the use of poorly water-soluble esters of erythromycin, which, since they pass the stomach unsolved, are protected there against the inactivation by acid hydrolysis. The esters are solved in the gut and absorbed partly after hydrolysis there (250). A pharmaceutical approach to the problem of protection against the acid medium in the stomach is the use of enteric-coated preparations.

6. pH-Sensitive Moieties and the Modulation of the Rate of Absorption and Excretion of Drugs by Adaptation of the pH in the Various Compartments

Besides elimination of the active drug as a result of metabolic degradation also renal excretion may be a factor of importance in the determination of time–concentration relationships. As was indicated already, reabsorption of drugs from the renal tubules back to the plasma depends on the lipophility of the drug and the degree of ionization. The higher the percentage of the drug present in the un-ionized form and the higher the lipophility of the un-ionized compound the higher the degree of reabsorption and the longer effective plasma concentrations may be maintained. Adaptation of the pK value of the ionizable groups in a drug by suitable chemical modification may result in an enhanced reabsorption and thus lead to a more protracted action.

As was shown in Fig. 1 the rate of penetration of weak acids and weak bases through lipid membranes is determined by the fraction of the compounds present in the undissociated form and therefore dependent on the pH in the

TABLE XXIIIA

COMPARISON OF GASTRIC ABSORPTION AT pH 1 AND 8 IN THE RAT[a]

	pK_a	% absorption at	
		pH 1	pH 8
Acids			
5-Sulfosalicylic	Strong	0	0
5-Nitrosalicylic	2.3	52	16
Salicylic	3.0	61	13
Thiopentone	7.6	46	34
Bases			
Aniline	4.6	6	56
p-Toluidine	5.3	0	47
Quinine	8.4	0	18
Dextrorphan	9.2	0	16

[a] After Brodie and Hogben (*48*).

TABLE XXIIIB

COMPARISON OF INTESTINAL ABSORPTION IN THE RAT AT SEVERAL pH
VALUES[a]

	pK_a	% absorption at			
		pH 4	pH 5	pH 7	pH 8
Acids					
5-Nitrosalicylic	2.3	40	27	0	0
Salicylic	3.0	64	35	30	10
Acetylsalicylic	3.5	41	27	—	—
Benzoic	4.2	62	36	35	5
Bases					
Aniline	4.6	40	48	58	61
Amidopyrine	5.0	21	35	48	52
p-Toluidine	5.3	30	42	65	64
Quinine	8.4	9	11	41	54

[a] After Brodie and Hogben (*48*).

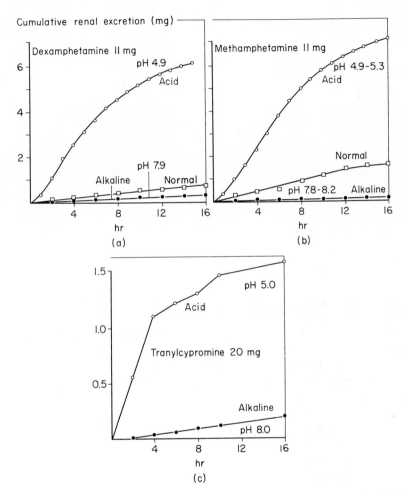

Fig. 19. Cumulative urinary excretion under normal (□), alkaline (●), and acidic (○) urine conditions after oral administration of (+) amphetamine (a), methamphetamine (b), and tranylcypromine (c). Note the enhanced excretion in the acidic urine as a result of an increase in the degree of dissociation of the drugs at lower pH. (a, b) After Beckett *et al.* (*23*); (c) after Turner *et al.* (*329*).

medium. Classical examples for the demonstration of this principle are represented in Tables XXIIIA and XXIIIB representing the absorption of weak acids and weak bases from the stomach and from the intestinal tract respectively at different pH values (*1, 3, 35, 48, 292, 306*).

The principle of enhancing the excretion of drugs by adaptation of the pH of the urine is clinically applied. In the case of barbiturate poisoning, for instance, alkalinization of the urine of the patients enhances the excretion of the weakly acidic barbiturates (214, 250a). The delay in the excretion of amphetamine and tranylcypromine by alkalinization of the urine can be considered as a relative decrease in the capacity of that compartment for the drug (21, 22, 23, 310, 329).

In their desire for a better performance, sportsmen or their coaches often resort to combinations of drugs. One of the most clear-cut examples is the combination of an alkalosis-inducing diet or alkaline salts such as sodium bicarbonate with psychostimulants, such as amphetamine. The induction of alkalosis is practiced to avoid or reduce the lactacidemic acidosis, which normally develops during strong physical exertion (10a). During this alkalosis alkaline urine (pH ±8) is formed with as a consequence that practically no excretion of amphetamine takes place anymore (Fig. 19). A given dose of amphetamine therefore will cause a prolonged effect. Consequently, accumulation of amphetamine in the body takes place then if sequential doses of amphetamine are used, even with dose intervals of hours. This implies that doses of amphetamine normally nontoxic may now result in toxic levels of the drug in the body and therefore in intoxication.

Another aspect of the combination of amphetamine with alkalinizing means is that the strong reduction in the excretion of amphetamine in the urine makes its detection in the urine of offenders of the rules against the use of doping more difficult. Since amphetamine remains in the circulation it will, although slowly, be mainly degraded biochemically now in the liver, with as an end product hippuric acid (353). This product, however, is also formed from benzoic acid, which in a concentration of 0.1 % enjoys a wide use as preservative in foods and especially drinks. Changes in the pH of body fluids, especially of the urine may disturb the therapeutic application of weakly basic drugs such as quinidine (129).

An insight in the role of pH-sensitive moieties in pharmacokinetics is important in drug design. From the ultrafiltrate formed in the glomerulus reabsorption of water up to 98 % takes place. This results in a very high concentration gradient of the drug between plasma and urine in the collecting tubules. The low diffusable concentration in plasma as a result of possible protein binding may further contribute to this gradient. A high degree of renal reabsorption will take place if the drug has the properties required for the passage of the wall of the tubules which implies fat-solubility and a low degree of dissociation, and a high degree of plasma binding which also correlates with the hydrophobic character of the drug (36, 199, 242).

C. INTRODUCTION, STABILIZATION OR PROTECTION, AND ELIMINATION OF VULNERABLE MOIETIES

Since biochemical degradation plays a predominant role in the elimination and therewith the inactivation of drugs, adaptation in its metabolic stability is a means of modulating the pharmacokinetics especially with respect to the relationship between the time and the concentration in the various compartments and therewith to the modulation of the time–response relationship. The moieties in the drug molecule attacked by the degradative enzymes, the vulnerable moieties, require special attention here. New vulnerable moieties may be introduced, existing moieties may be stabilized or protected, or they may be eliminated. In order to obtain ultra-short-acting compounds it may be of advantage to rely on the plasma enzymes as a degradative system for drugs. Usually the microsomal enzyme systems in the liver perform the bioinactivation of foreign body compounds (*52b, 353*). With respect to the influence of various substituents on the stability of vulnerable moieties, e.g., ester groups, linked to phenyl rings, information can be gained and to a certain degree predictions can be made on basis of the Hammett-Taft substituent constants. First, it is decided whether a particular moiety should be stabilized or labilized. Then a regression analysis must be made on the relation between the sensitivity to enzymes or metabolic stability of a number of substituted compounds and the Hammett substituent constants as worked out in much detail by Hansch (*17, 145–148*). This may indicate which of the substituents will be most promising in the synthesis of new compounds. This holds true in general for molecular manipulation on biofunctional moieties.

As far as stabilization or protection of vulnerable moieties is concerned, it may be mentioned that stabilization as a rule implies introduction of fixed protecting groups, often small alkyl groups on the carbon atoms next to the vulnerable moiety. This procedure is indicated as packing of the vulnerable moiety (*10*). In the case of a protection the vulnerable moiety may be masked by a disposable protecting moiety. This approach may be followed if the vulnerable moiety as such is required for action.

1. *Introduction of Vulnerable Moieties*

A possibility in this respect is the introduction as vulnerable moieties of ester groups, sensitive to carboxyesterases present in abundance in plasma and liver of mammals. Also a labilization of existing ester groups may be considered. Introduction of a vulnerable moiety, for instance an ester group, may have as a consequence that the molecule concerned breaks apart under

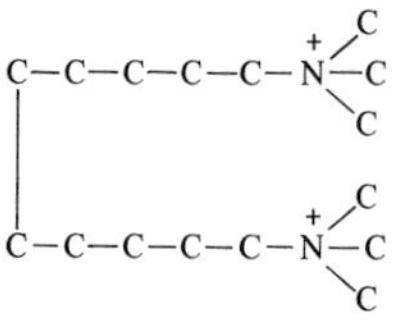

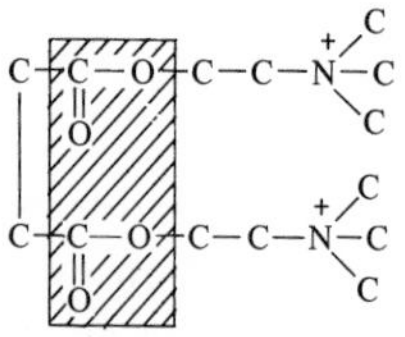

Suxamethonium

ultra-short acting muscle relaxant;
rapid hydrolysis by plasma esterases
results in inactivation due to breaking
apart of the drug molecule

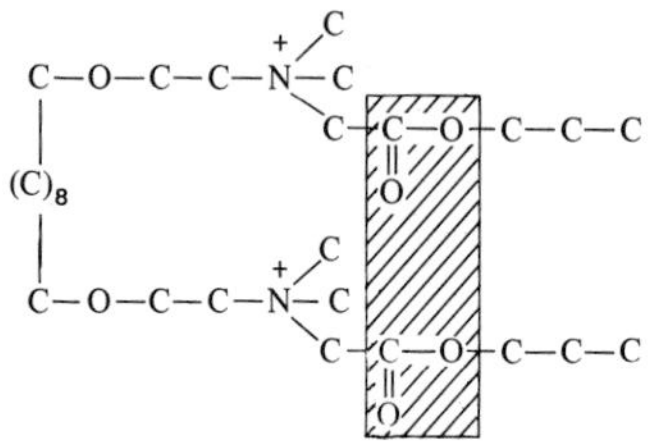

Decamethonium

muscle relaxant

Prodeconium

ultra-short acting muscle relaxant
rapid hydrolysis by plasma esterases
results in inactivation due to unmasking
of carboxyl groups in the drug molecule

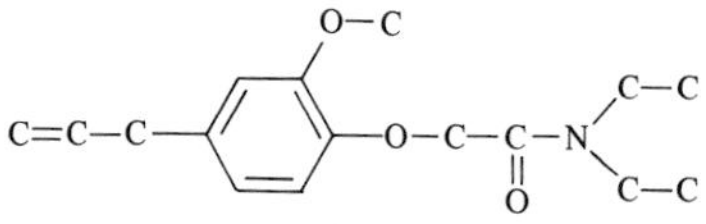

G 29505

iv anesthetic

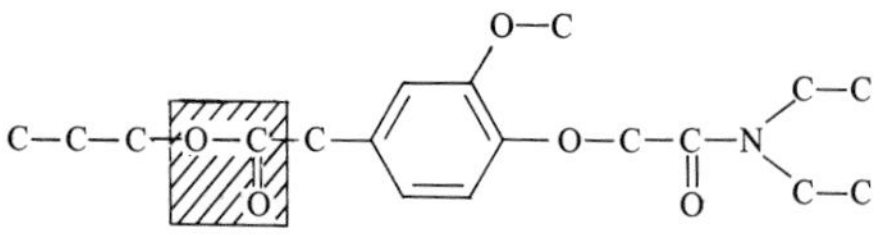

Propanidid

ultra-short acting iv anesthetic;
rapid hydrolysis by esterases
results in inactivation due to
unmasking of a carboxyl group
in the drug molecule

Fig. 20. Introduction of vulnerable moieties to obtain short-acting compounds.

influence of the esterases and thus is inactivated, or that the hydrolysis results
in the unmasking of strongly hydrophilic carboxy groups in the drug molecule
which are incompatible with its action. As a rule the aim of such preparations
is a short or ultrashort and controllable action. One of the best-known examples
of the introduction of vulnerable groups resulting in a shortening of the action
is the synthesis of the muscle relaxant succinylcholine which as compared to
the related compound decamethionium can be considered as a short-acting

compound (Fig. 20). Hydrolysis of the ester groups by plasma esterases and esterases in the liver cells results in a rapid inactivation of the drug which is broken apart. A comparable procedure is followed in the curariform drug prodeconium where the vulnerable group is introduced into one of the substituents on the onium group (*140, 285*). Hydrolysis results in an unmasking of the carboxy groups in the remaining bisonium compound, which is the cause of the loss of action (Fig. 20). The ultra-short-acting intravenous general anesthetic propanidid can be considered to be a derivative of the short-acting intravenous anesthetic G 29505 (*327*). The introduction of a vulnerable group, the ester group, which is readily hydrolyzed, results in a compound with an ultrashort action (Fig. 20). The short action of the intravenous anesthetic G 29505 is found to be due to its rapid oxidation in the allyl side-chain, converting the compound to an inactive product (*44, 169, 271, 327, 357*).

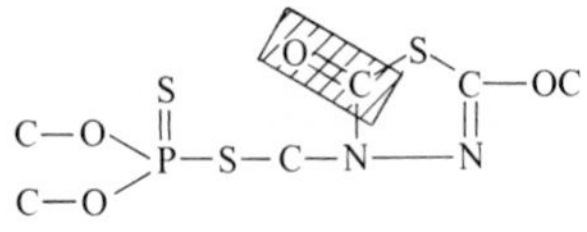

GS 13005 (Supracid)

Fig. 21. Pesticide with a reduced residue-risk obtained by introduction of a vulnerable moiety leading to a quick bioinactivation in plant and mammalian tissue. After Esser and Müller (*108*).

Although thousands of barbiturates differing in the C_5 substituents have been made, no clear-cut rules for a preferential structure of the side-chain leading to short-acting compounds have emerged (*319*). This may be due to the fact that not only the rate of oxidative degradation, but also the fat solubility is changed by variation in the C_5 substituents. Various thiobarbiturates being highly fat-soluble have an ultrashort general anesthetic action based on a quick redistribution in the body, resulting in accumulation of the drug in fat tissue and a steep fall of the concentration in plasma (*46, 48*). The advantage of the barbiturates with an ultrashort action based on metabolic degradation is that no cumulation of the active drug in fat tissue occurs, thus avoiding a protracted sedation after intravenous anesthesia (*160, 327*). In many of the ultra-short-acting thiobarbiturates allyl substituents or related unsaturated groups are present. This means that often probably both principles, that of the redistribution and that of the rapid metabolic degradation may contribute then to the short action. The metabolic component then reduces the risk of a protracted sedation (*57, 232, 235, 305*).

A special aspect of rapid inactivation of bioactive compounds is the need for avoidance of pesticide residues in food products and avoidance of accumulation of pesticides in the body. The avoidance of pesticide residues implies that the compound must be eliminated or degraded to nontoxic products by the time that the agricultural products are used for consumption. A possibility is the introduction in the pesticide of a vulnerable moiety such that already in the plant tissues or on the plants inactivation takes place at such a rate that by the time of consumption the residues can be neglected. An example is GS 13005 (Supracid), an organic phosphate with a labile heterocyclic ring, a substituted thiadiazole ring, easily cleaved under formation of carbon dioxide and a metabolite that is inactive (Fig. 21) (*108*). This degradation is performed

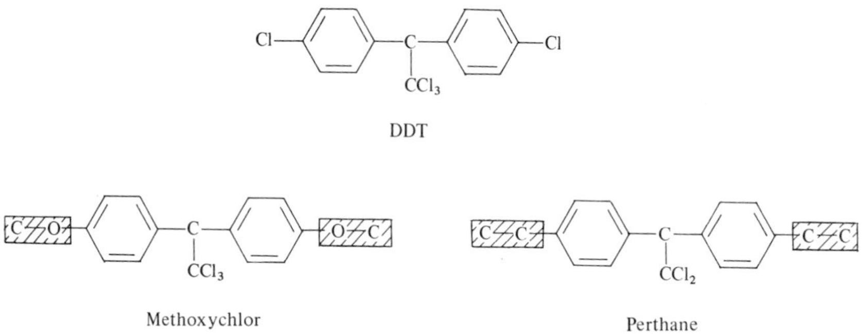

DDT

Methoxychlor   Perthane

Fig. 22. Introduction of vulnerable moieties in highly lipophilic chlorinated hydrocarbon insecticides. *Note*: DDT is highly resistant against oxidative degradation and due to its lipophility has a strong tendency to persistent accumulation. The presence of vulnerable moieties in methoxychlor and perthane which can be converted by oxidation followed eventually by conjugation into water-soluble groups implies a decrease in the tendency to accumulation for these insecticides.

very readily in mammals, but also in the plant tissues. Within a period of 14 days up to 95 % of the pesticide originally taken up by the plant is inactivated.

A particular problem is the tendency of the highly lipophilic chlorinated hydrocarbons such as DDT, which are resistant to metabolic degradation, to accumulate in body fat (*353*). The accumulation is progressive since these lipophilic products are concentrated also in the lipid phases of various food products. Animal products, such as fish, are enriched in DDT (*59*). The tendency to accumulation becomes especially clear in animals at the end of the food chains such as preying birds (*17, 359a*). Introduction into the chlorinated hydrocarbons of vulnerable groups suitable for biodegradation leading to an increase in the hydrophility will result in a conversion of these products in the body, with as a consequence an increased tendency for excretion, for instance, in the urine, and a decreased tendency for accumulation. In this respect the introduction in DDT of alkyl or alkoxy groups in the rings in the *meta* or *para* position can be considered. Such substituted compounds maintain their insecticidal activity while on the other hand the oxidation of the alkyl or alkoxy groups will lead to metabolites with more hydrophilic carboxyl groups or phenolic OH— groups. These groups will make the compounds more hydrophilic and thus enhance excretion and reduce the tendency to accumulation in the body fat (Fig. 22). The objection that the metabolic products obtained are inactive as an insecticide and that also the insects will bio-inactivate the insecticide only holds if the insects do this quick enough. This seems not to be the case since the substituted derivatives still have a reasonable insecticidal activity (*79, 278*). Examples are the compounds Perthane and

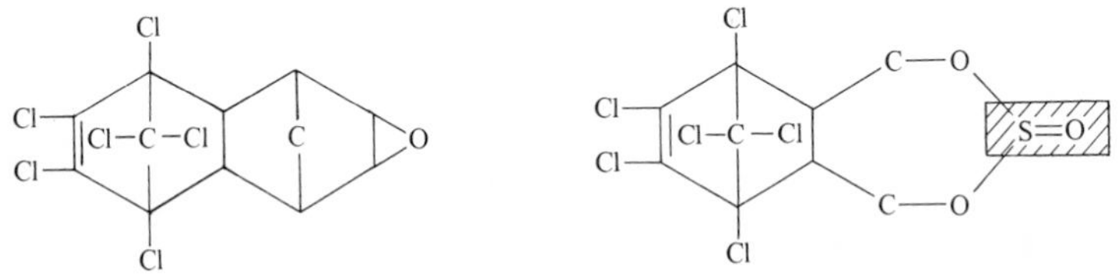

Dieldrin

(a)

Endosulfan

(b)

Fig. 23. Introduction of a vulnerable moiety in the highly lipophilic chlorinated hydro-carbon dieldrin with as a consequence an enhanced biochemical conversion to water-soluble products and a decrease in the tendency to accumulation. Accumulation in body-fat (sheep) after 20 days application of 15 mg/day: (a) 13.7 ppm; (b) 0.1 ppm. After Maier-Bode (*228*).

methoxychlor (*114a*). In an analogous way derivatives of dieldrin, also a metabolically stable highly fat-soluble insecticide, have been prepared. The derivative endosulfan bearing a vulnerable moiety has much less tendency to accumulate than dieldrin (*228*). It appears to be rather toxic, however, to fish (Fig. 23). Sensitization of a compound to metabolic degradation may be realized also by substitution of branched alkyl chains in a compound which are relatively resistant to biological degradation with straight alkyl chains which, as a rule, are more easily oxidized by, e.g., β-oxidation. The influence of branching of alkyl chains on the biological oxidation is demonstrated in Table XXIV. It can be seen that the branched alcohols which are more resistant to oxidative degradation appear to a higher degree as glucuronic acid conjugation products in the urine. Another example of destabilization especially for aromatic compounds is the introduction of, e.g., a methyl group in the ring which then, unless other substituents interfere, as a rule is easily converted to the corresponding carboxyl group, which may result in a loss or at least an essential change in the activity. Table XXV gives some examples.

The presence of easily oxidizable alkyl groups—methyl groups or straight alkyl chains—in the aromatic rings makes them more suitable for oxidative degradation under formation of carboxylic acids. Consequently only a smaller fraction is converted to phenols. Introduction of the vulnerable groups (methyl groups, etc.) therefore results in a decrease in the excretion of

TABLE XXIV

Glucuronide Conjugation of Primary, Secondary, and Tertiary Alcohols in Rabbits[a,b]

Primary alcohol	Secondary alcohol	Tertiary alcohol
$\overset{\alpha}{C-C}-OH$ 0.5	$C-\overset{\underset{\mid}{C}}{\overset{\mid}{C}}-OH$ α 10	$C-\overset{\underset{\mid}{C}}{\overset{\overset{\mid}{C}}{C}}-OH$ α 24
C—C—C—OH 0.9	$C-C-\overset{\underset{\mid}{C}}{\overset{\mid}{C}}-OH$ 14	$C-C-\overset{\underset{\mid}{C}}{\overset{\overset{\mid}{C}}{C}}-OH$ 58
C—C—C—C—OH 1.8	$C-C-C-\overset{\underset{\mid}{C}}{\overset{\mid}{C}}-OH$ 45	$C-C-C-\overset{\underset{\mid}{C}}{\overset{\overset{\mid}{C}}{C}}-OH$ 57
C—C—C—C—C—OH 6.7	$C-C-C-C-\overset{\underset{\mid}{C}}{\overset{\mid}{C}}-OH$ 54	

[a] Stabilization of the vulnerable alcoholic OH-group by α-alkyl substitution results in a slowing-down of the oxidative degradation with as a consequence an increase in the fraction excreted as glucuronide conjugate. After Williams (353).

[b] The numbers indicate the glucuronidation in percentage.

organic sulfate. An interesting aspect of the influence of the character of alkyl groups on biological degradation is found in the field of detergents. These surface-active compounds, mostly sulfonated alkyl or aralkyl derivatives, cause much trouble via pollution of water, partly because many of the detergents used are resistant against biological attack by the microorganisms normally taking care of the clearance of polluted water. Examples of resistant detergents, also called "hard" detergents, are given in Fig. 24. They contain a sulfonated benzene ring and a branched hydrocarbon chain. The substitution of the branched chain by a straight hydrocarbon chain makes the detergents more vulnerable to biological attack with as a consequence that for this type of detergents indicated as "soft" detergents, biological self-clearance of polluted water is possible (*54, 161, 162, 171, 331*). The fact that straight-chain detergents are biodegraded rather rapidly does not mean that such products are nontoxic. The highly surface-active straight-chain ($C_{11}-C_{15}$) alkylbenzylsulfonates are even more toxic to fish than the corresponding branched-chain products with

TABLE XXV

THE INFLUENCE OF VARIOUS SUBSTITUENTS IN PHENYL RINGS ON THE EXCRETION OF SULFATE CONJUGATED PHENOLIC METABOLITES (ORGANIC SULFATES)[a,b]

94   28   94

19   52   1

[a] Low percentages of organic (phenolic) sulfate are found for those compounds with vulnerable alkyl groups which are easily converted by oxidation of the alkyl groups to polar hydrophilic carboxyl derivatives. For those compounds which are not easily converted to carboxy acids formation of phenolic metabolites is more predominant with as a result an increase in the excretion of organic sulfate. After Gerarde (*128*).

[b] The figures indicate the mean values for the urinary organic sulfate excretion expressed as a percentage of the total sulfate excretion, measured 24, 48, and 72 hours after dosing the rats subcutaneously with the substances (5 ml/kg).

a somewhat lower surface activity (*161, 162*) (Table XXVI). The preferred biodegradative attack on straight alkyl chains in detergents is reminiscent of the fact that for the production of amino acids and proteins by microbiological conversion of oil products the straight-chain hydrocarbons, especially the $C_{10}-C_{25}$ chains, are most suitable as starting product. The branched compounds, the isoparaffins, are not or only very slowly converted (*158, 158a, 179a, 222*). An important aspect is that the isoparaffins do not interfere with the conversion of the straight-chain paraffins.

A situation reminiscent of that described for hard detergents and hard insecticides such as DDT is reported in the field of plasticizers used in plastics. These lipid-soluble additives can migrate into foods that are packaged in

Hard detergents			Soft detergents		
structure	residue left %	after days	structure	residue left %	after days
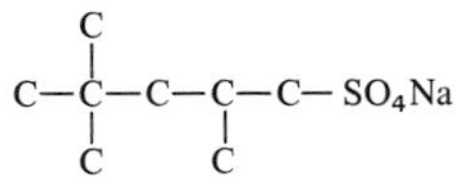 $C-C-C-C-SO_4Na$ (branched)	100	18	$C-(-C-)_n-SO_4Na$	0	1-3
$C-C-C-C-C-SO_4Na$ (branched)	100	18	$C-(-C-)_n-SO_3Na$	0	3
benzene ring with SO_3Na (branched chain)	97	28	benzene ring with SO_3Na, $C-(-C-)_n$	0	4
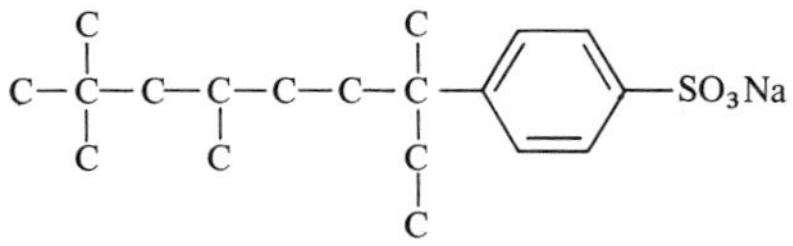			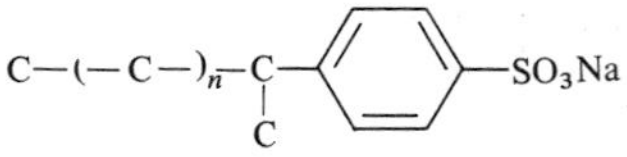 benzene ring with SO_3Na, $C-(-C-)_n-C$	0	5-11

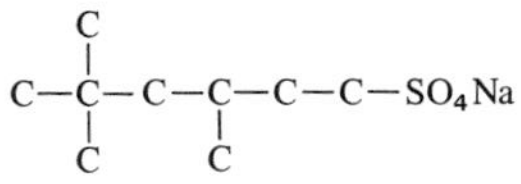

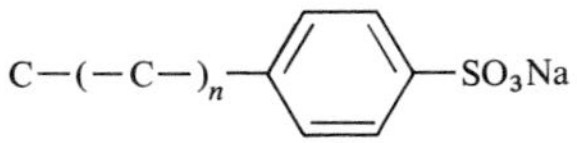

$n = 10\text{-}14$

storage test in river water 20°C, dark, open bottles

Fig. 24. The introduction of vulnerable moieties as an effort to obtain soft detergents. *Note*: The detergents with branched alkyl chains (hard detergents) are resistant to biodegradation and therefore cause persistent water pollution. The detergents with straight alkyl chains (soft detergents) are biologically degraded such that persistent pollution is avoided. After Huyser (*171*).

plastics, or into blood during transfusions that utilize plastic devices. Metabolic stability and fat solubility, again, are the factors which determine accumulation of these substances in the tissues. A comparison of two plasticizers in a metabolic study with rat liver revealed that the compound DEHP is metabolically stable and accumulates in the tissue, whereas the compound BGBP is readily converted to water-soluble products (Fig. 24a) (*178a*). The compound DEHP occurred in concentrations up to 0.27 mg/g of dry weight in abdominal fat of patients who received blood transfusions.

TABLE XXVI
ACUTE TOXICITY OF "SOFT" AND "HARD" DETERGENTS FOR FISH[a]

Straight-chain alkylbenzene sulfonates "soft" detergents		Branched-chain alkylbenzene sulfonate "hard" detergent
n	LD_{50} for golden orfe (mg/liter)	LD_{50} for golden orfe (mg/liter)
6	125	
7	90	
8	17	14
9	7	
10	3	
11	0.6	

[a] "Soft" detergents may still have a relatively high acute toxicity. "Hard" detergents may have a relatively low toxicity. Their drawback is the resistance against biodegradation with as a consequence a progressive persistent pollution. After Hirsch (*161, 162*).

In view of the above considerations, it is evident that those plasticizers containing vulnerable moieties, which are metabolically converted to water-soluble substances (hence rendering them suitable for rapid excretion), are preferred for use in plastics which find utility in the packaging of lipophilic foods (meat products, butter, oils, etc.), as blood storage containers, or as components of transfusion devices.

2. Stabilization or Protection of Vulnerable Moieties

The time–concentration relationship for a drug in its active form depends on the rate of bioinactivation. A variety of biochemical processes may be involved. The most common ones are hydrolysis of ester and amide bonds and oxidation of alkyl groups possibly bearing particular groups such as OH— or NH$_2$— groups. A bioinactivation will be the consequence if a group essential for the action is eliminated, for instance, if an amino group is eliminated by oxidative deamination, or if polar groups are introduced such as carboxyl groups, which may be incompatible with the activity of the drug.

Drugs containing an ester group may be sensitive to degradation by enzymic hydrolysis. The rapid inactivation of acetylcholine and procaine by esterases

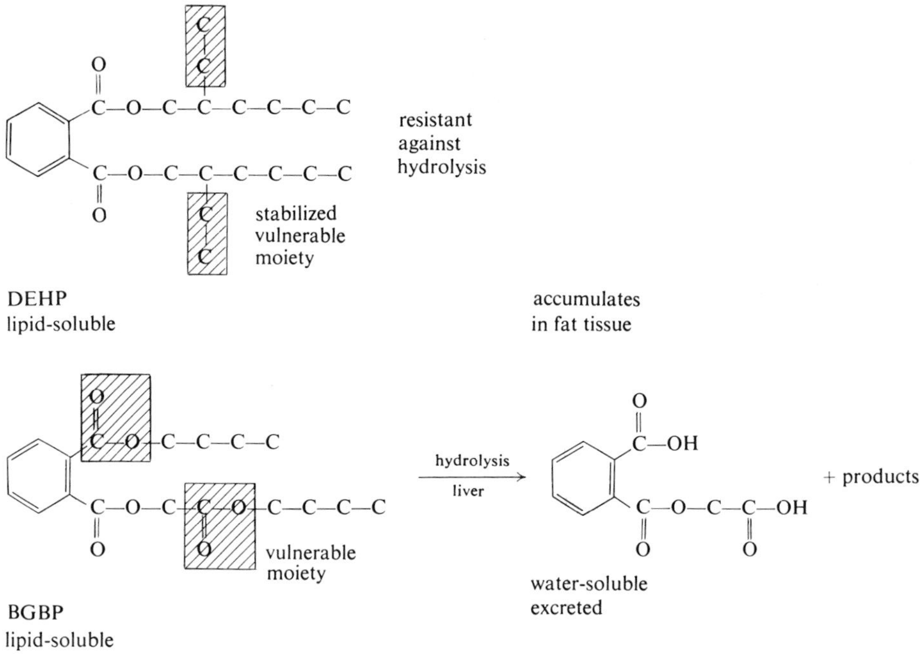

Fig. 24a. Influence on the stability of the vulnerable moieties in plasticizers on the pharmacokinetics.

of plasma and cells, especially liver cells, is an example. Introduction of suitable substituents, especially small alkyl groups close to the vulnerable group, in this case the ester group, often results in an increased resistance to metabolic attack. This procedure is indicated as packing of the vulnerable moiety (10). Sometimes the stabilized compounds act as competitive inhibitors of the enzymes involved (20, 218). As a cause for this type of stabilization of vulnerable groups a sterical hindrance by the alkyl groups on the active site of the enzymes involved is feasible. In many cases, however, the protection against enzyme action also implies a protection against alkaline hydrolysis which means that also a stabilization of the ester bond as such may be involved. The introduction of a methyl group next to the ester group of acetylcholine gives acetyl-β-methylcholine, which is much more stable than acetylcholine against acetylcholinesterase. A clear-cut difference is found for the rate of hydrolysis of both isomers of acetyl-β-methylcholine. One of the isomers even acts as a competitive inhibitor of acetylcholinesterase (Fig. 25) (20). A variety

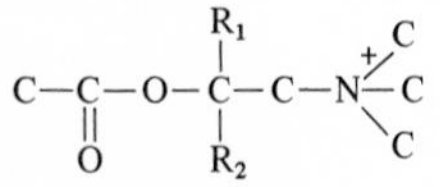

$$C-C-O-\overset{R_1}{\underset{R_2}{C}}-C-\overset{+}{N}\overset{C}{\underset{C}{\diagdown}}C$$

	Introduction of stabilizing moieties		Relative rate of hydrolysis (acetylcholinesterase)
	R_1	R_2	
Acetylcholine	—H	—H	100
L (+)-acetyl-β-methylcholine	—C	—H	54.5
D (-)-acetyl-β-methylcholine	—H	—C	Inhibitor

(a)

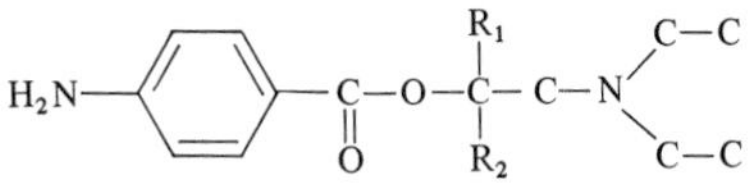

$$H_2N-\langle\!\!\!\rangle-C-O-\overset{R_1}{\underset{R_2}{C}}-C-N\overset{C-C}{\underset{C-C}{\diagdown}}$$

Introduction of stabilizing moieties		Relative rate of hydrolysis (human serum)
R_1	R_2	
—H	—H	500
—H	—C	15
—C	—C	0

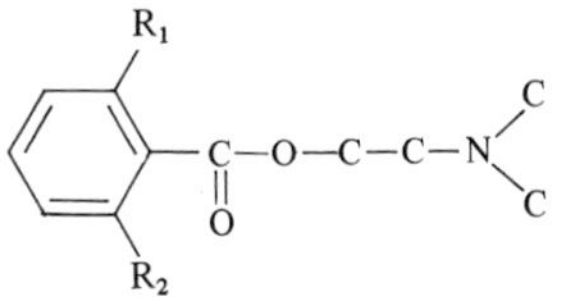

(b)

Introduction of stabilizing moieties		Relative rate of hydrolysis (horse serum)
R_1	R_2	
—H	—H	100
—H	—C	65
—C	—C	0

(c)

Fig. 25. Stabilization of vulnerable moieties by alkyl substitution adjacent to the vulnerable moiety, also called packing of the vulnerable moiety. (a) After Beckett (20); (b) after Levine and Clark (218); (c) after Thomas and Stoker (323).

of examples for the principle of stabilization of ester groups by alkyl substitution close to these groups, a "packing" of the vulnerable groups, are reported by Levine and others (10, 123, 133, 192, 218, 304) (see Fig. 25). If esters or amides of benzoic acid are involved, the vulnerable group is linked directly to the system of conjugated double bonds in the ring. By introduction of suitable substituents shifts in charge distribution may be induced resulting in

TABLE XXVII

INTRODUCTION OF PROTECTING GROUPS RESULTING IN COMPOUNDS ACTING AS ENZYME INHIBITORS[a]

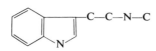

Phenylethylamine
substrate MAO

Phenylisopropylamine
MAO inhibitor

N-Methyltryptamine
substrate MAO

N-Methyl α-methyltryptamine
MAO inhibitor

Dopamine
substrate dopamine β-hydroxylase

α-Methyl dopamine
inhibitor dopamine β-hydroxylase

Dopa
substrate dopa decarboxylase

α-Methyl dopa
inhibitor dopa decarboxylase

Glutamic acid
substrate glutamic acid decarboxylase

α-Methyl glutamic acid
inhibitor glutamic acid decarboxylase

Histidine
substrate histidine decarboxylase

α-Methyl histidine
inhibitor histidine decarboxylase

TABLE XXVII—*continued*

N | HO—C—C—C—C—OH ‖ ‖ O O	N | HO—C—C—C—C—OH ‖ C ‖ O O
Aspartic acid converted in urea synthesis	α-Methyl aspartic acid inhibitor argininosuccinate synthetase in urea synthesis

C
             |+
C—C—O—C—C—N—C
   ‖ |
   O   C
	C
	             |+
	C—C—O—C—C—N—C
	   ‖ C C
	   O

Acetylcholine substrate acetylcholinesterase	D(−)-Acetyl-β-methylcholine inhibitor acetylcholinesterase

[a] Some of the inhibitors are converted at a slow rate themselves.

stabilization or destabilization of the ester bond (*323*). The approach based on the Hammett substituent constants may be helpful in selecting the substituents most promising for the characteristics aimed at. The type of substituent and the site of substitution in the ring will be determinant (*138, 142, 224*). Alkyl substitution in the *ortho* position usually has a stabilizing effect (*53, 304*). Introduction of a halogen in the *ortho* position, however, has a destabilizing influence and makes the ester bond more sensitive to hydrolysis (*322*).

The stabilized compounds not only are resistant against the enzymic attack but often also act as inhibitors of the enzymes concerned. The affinity to the enzyme is maintained then but the turnover is reduced to practically zero ($V_{max} \to 0$). Even if the turnover is not reduced to zero, the protected compounds may on basis of substrate competition act as enzyme inhibitors. The consequence is that for a large variety of substrates for enzymes the procedure of the α-alkyl (usually methyl) substitution is applied in efforts to obtain enzyme inhibitors (see Table XXVII) (*20, 218, 280a, 293a, 320a, 323*).

Reminiscent of the "packing procedure" in efforts to stabilize or protect vulnerable moieties is the situation for the penicillinase-resistant penicillins. Although the lactam ring is opened by the enzyme, it appears that *ortho* substitution on the acid moiety in the adjacent carbamide group plays a predominant role here (*168a*) (Table XXVIIA). Some of the resistant penicillins act as inhibitors of the penicillinase.

In the foregoing the stabilization and protection of vulnerable ester bonds against hydrolysis was discussed. Another type of vulnerable moieties are alkyl groups possibly bearing terminal amino or hydroxyl groups which may be involved in oxidative degradation. An example is phenylethylamine, a

TABLE XXVIIA

STRUCTURE ACTION IN PENICILLINASE-SUSCEPTIBLE AND -RESISTANT PENICILLINS

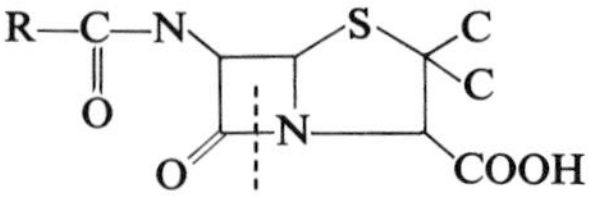

Penicillinase

susceptible	resistant	Penicillins

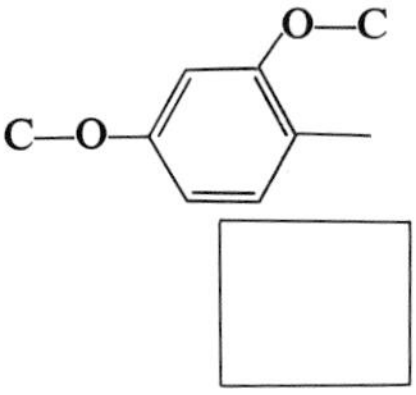

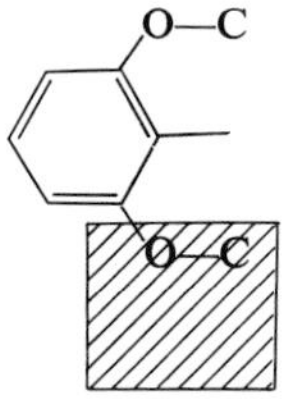

Methicillin

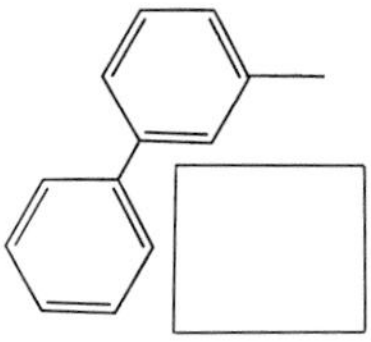

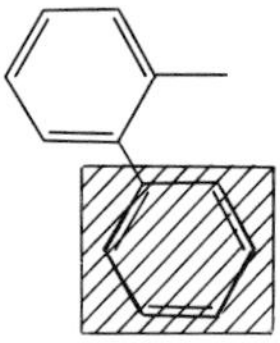

Diphenicillin

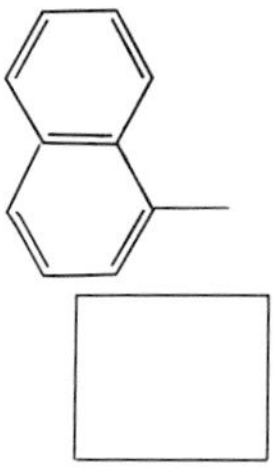

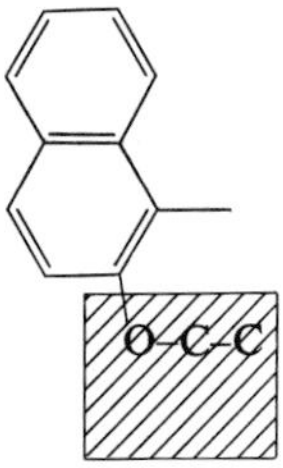

Nafcillin

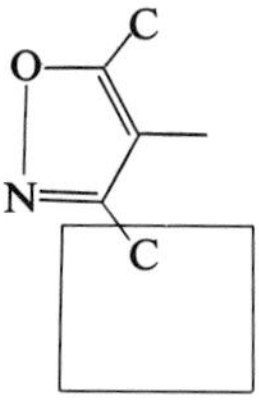

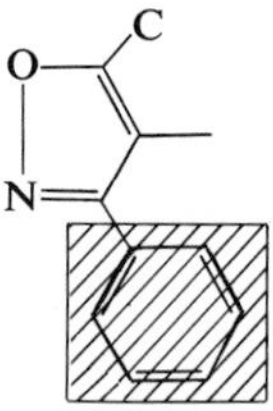

Oxacillin

TABLE XXVIIA—*continued*

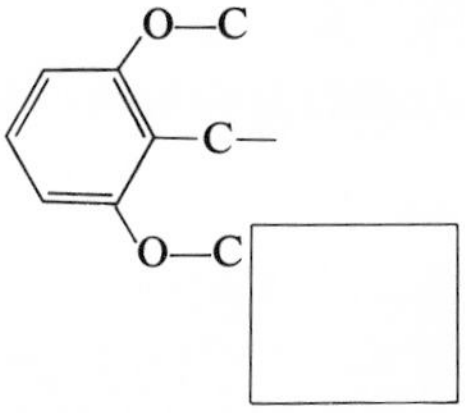

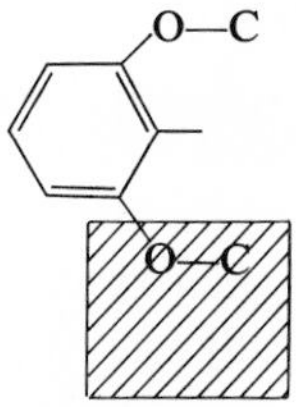

Methicillin

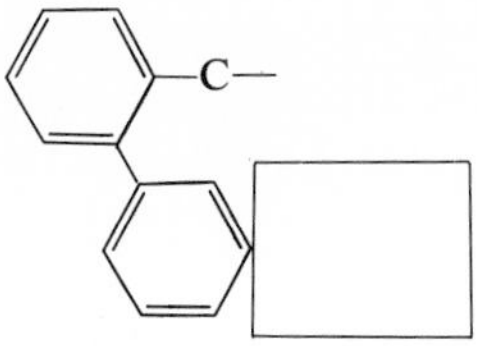

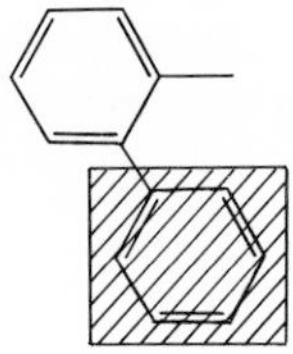

Diphenicillin

compound with a weak sympathomimetic activity and nearly devoid of central nervous system stimulant activity. Introduction of methyl groups next to the amino group results in a stabilization of the vulnerable moiety. Highly effective central nervous system stimulants such as amphetamine and mephentermine are obtained, compounds which also have prolonged vascular effects. Application of phenylethylamine to animals in which the amine oxidase is inhibited by suitable monoamine oxidase inhibitors shows that under these circumstances phenylethylamine is about as active as amphetamine as far as central nervous system stimulant action is concerned and that the vascular effects are prolonged (*297*). The rapid oxidative deamination of phenylethylamine and the stability in this respect of amphetamine and mephentermine in which the vulnerable amino group is protected appear to be the basis for the differences in the action of these compounds (*297, 298*).

Examples of α-substitution leading to protection of a vulnerable group are found in the field of herbicides. The herbicide 4-chloro-2-methylphenoxy-acetic acid is inactive with respect to certain dicotyledonous weeds. This appears to be due to a rapid oxidation of the acetic acid group. Introduction of an α-methyl group in the acetic acid moiety of the compound blocks this degradation. The compound then is active in controlling the weeds mentioned (*216*). For the eradication of woody plants with weed killers α-methyl sub-stituted phenoxyacetic acids are more suitable than the phenoxyacetic acid derivatives. This seems to be due to the greater stability of the α-methyl substituted compounds against oxidative degradation leading to inactive phenols (*75*) (Fig. 26).

The principle of α-alkyl substitution in the case of terminal amino groups, carboxyl groups, etc. is comparable to the principle of terminal branching in vulnerable alkyl groups. An increasing stability against oxidative dealkylation is observed for alkoxy and alkylamine groups of drugs in the series *O*-methyl, *O*-ethyl, *O*-isopropyl, *O*-*t*-butyl and *N*-methyl, *N*-ethyl, *N*-isopropyl, and *N*-*t*-butyl (*56, 67*). Further examples of an increased resistance of alkyl groups against oxidative degradation obtained by suitable branching in the alkyl groups are reported in the literature (*10, 97, 128, 183, 353*).

Approaches similar to those outlined before are followed in the efforts to protect biologically active polypeptides against bioinactivation. Small polypeptides such as angiotensin II and oxytocin are rapidly inactivated by specific polypeptidases in plasma such as angiotensinase and oxytocinase. The inactivating enzymes are polypeptidases attacking particular peptide links. As long as the amino acids constituting the vulnerable peptide link in

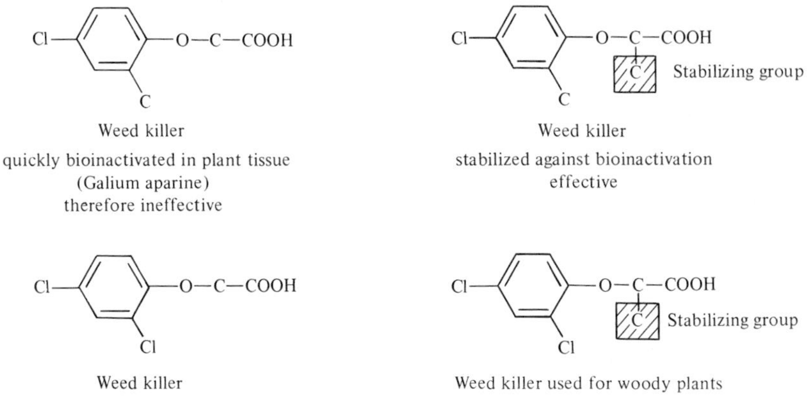

Fig. 26. Protection of weed killers against biodegradation by stabilization of the vulnerable moiety by α-alkyl substitution. After Leafe (*216*) and Crafts (*75*).

the polypeptide allow changes in structure, such as substitution by other amino acids, without a loss of the activity, the possibility for a stabilization is given (*51, 215, 302*). An example is the substitution of the terminal L-amino acid in angiotensin by the unnatural D-amino acid resulting in a protection of the still active polypeptide obtained against angiotensinase (*51, 215*).

Besides the specific degrading enzymes in plasma also enzymes in liver and kidney play a role in the inactivation of the polypeptide hormones. Poly-peptidases breaking peptide links and hydrogenases breaking the —S—S— bonds which occur in the cyclic polypeptides such as oxytocin and vasopressin can be mentioned in this respect. Various types of derivatives of polypeptide hormones have been prepared to obtain stable compounds (*287, 288*).

The procedures followed are: modification of the peptide bond attacked by the enzyme, as indicated before; modification of the terminal hemicystine residue by methylation, by acylation of the free amino group or by replacing the terminal L-hemicystine group by its D isomer; coupling of additional amino acids to the free amino group of the terminal hemicystine group.

Especially the derivatives of the last type show a prolonged action. The amino acids attached to the hormone have to be split off by polypeptidases in order to obtain the hormone in its active form. This enzymatic removal of the groups attached implies a gradual bioactivation of the compound and therefore a protracted action. The rate of activation depends on the amino acids attached. The hormone analogues stabilized by protecting moieties will usually be only slightly active or inactive *in vitro*, but active *in vivo* (*25, 215*) (Table XXVIIB). The procedures just outlined were also applied to anti-diuretic hormone leading to derivatives with a protracted action (*362*).

As expected the biologically active structural analogs of the polypeptide hormones obtained by exchange of amino acids often will not be suitable as substrates for the specific degrading enzymes. Consequently, these too will have a prolonged action (*361*). In this case, however, the compounds will be active *in vitro* and *in vivo*. Examples are the various vasopressin analogs with a protracted action (*362*).

A decrease in the activity of a bioactive compound as a result of a change in its chemical structure often will imply a prolongation of the effect if equiactive doses are compared, since the larger quantity of the less active derivative usually will require more time for degradation or elimination, especially when the enzyme system involved is saturated.

The protection of the vulnerable groups in polypeptide hormones such as oxytocin and vasopressin by introduction of protecting substituents which have to be removed in order to set the active drug free, resulting in a sustained release of the drug in its active form, can be regarded as a temporary protection of the drug against degradation, by masking of the vulnerable group. The application of the principle of the disposable conducting moieties discussed before will often also imply a temporary protection of the drug against degradation. Certain drugs are unstable because of the presence of particular vulnerable groups, for instance easily oxidizable groups. If such groups are essential for the action, a temporary masking by a disposable moiety may result in a protected transport form from which the active compound is gradually released. Examples of this procedure are the esterification of the terminal OH— group in vitamin A to acetyl or palmityl esters and of the OH— group of tocopherol to the acetyl ester (Table XXVIIIA). Also the various conjugation products formed by the introduction of disposable moieties of other vitamins such as thiamine (*187*), riboflavin (*360*), and *l*-ascorbic acid (*99, 173*) partially serve the purpose of increasing stability. Attention is paid also to the stability of the ester link between the protecting moiety and vitamins. α,α-Dialkyl substitution in the acids used as usual

TABLE XXVIIB

STRUCTURE AND ACTIVITY OF OXYTOCIN ANALOGS[a]

R-CyS-Tyr-iLeu-Glu(NH$_2$)-Asp(NH$_2$)-CyS-Pro-Leu-Gly-NH$_2$

Peptide R	Activity on rat uterus (IU/μmole)		Activity ratio in vivo/in vitro
	in vitro	*in vivo*	
H-	450	450	1
Leu-Leu-	9	80–100	10
Gly-Gly-	0.6	5–11	10–20
Phe	2	46–57	25
Leu-Gly-Gly-	0.2	18–24	100

[a] From (25).

stabilize the ester group (see Table XXVIIIA) (119). The protecting action may partly be based on the high lipophility and thus complete lack of water solubility of the vitamin A esters. This situation is reminiscent of the protection of erythromycin against destruction by the acid in the stomach through formation of poorly water-soluble esters such as the propionate or stearate, which are hydrolyzed in the gut under release of the antibiotic (176).

The principle of the protection of vulnerable moieties is also applied to bioactive amines. Examples are the esters of α-methyl-p-tyrosine which is protected thusly against rapid decarboxylation in the liver (4), and, the carbamates of amphetamine and ephedrine which protect against rapid bioinactivation of the free amines in the liver (336a). In both cases the derivatives, because of the increased lipid solubility, also readily penetrate the central nervous system such that the ester and carbamate formation not only implies introduction of a protecting moiety but at the same time implies the introduction of disposable facilitating moieties in the bioactive amines concerned. The p-aminosalicylic acid derivative ethopabate, a potent coccidiostat with improved feed stability, is another example (281a). Both stabilization and facilitated transport are realized by introduction of suitable disposable moieties (Fig. 26a).

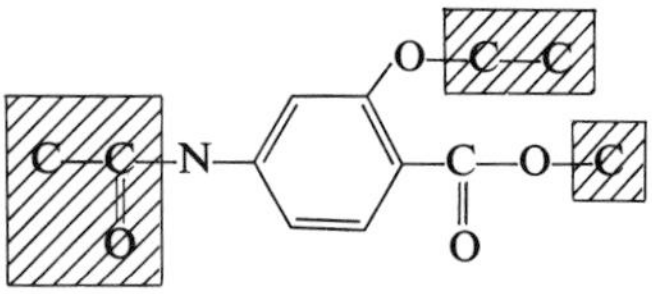

Ethopabate

Fig. 26a. Stabilized p-aminosalicylic acid derivative with facilitated penetration used as coccidiostat.

3. *Elimination of Vulnerable Moieties*

Another possibility for the protection of a drug against metabolic degradation is the elimination of the vulnerable group from the drug molecule possibly through substitution by a more stable group. In fact some of the procedures discussed for the stabilization of polypeptide hormones can be considered as such a substitution.

Substitution of an amide link for an ester link often implies a stabilization of the drug with respect to hydrolysis. This change in the structure leads, however, to the introduction of a new opportunity for hydrogen bond formation, namely by the hydrogen on the amide nitrogen. Often this appears not to be compatible with the action of the drug in the strict sense. The amide analog of, for instance, acetylcholine, is practically devoid of cholinergic action. In the case of procaine the switch to procainamide has been successful, at least as far as antiarrhythmic action is concerned. On the whole in local anesthetics substitution of an amide link for an ester link is well tolerated (*52, 150, 229, 332*). An analogous procedure is followed in the development of meprobamate. 2,2-Diethyl-1,3-pronanediol and related diols have an anticonvulsant and muscle relaxing action which is of only short duration due to the quick metabolic degradation. Conversion to esters results in a prolongation of the action. The carbamates have a still more prolonged action. Of the compounds thus obtained meprobamate was chosen for therapeutic use (*29, 30, 303*). With the carbamate formation besides the muscle relaxant action also a sedative action, common to many carbamates and carbamides, was introduced. A similar approach was followed in the development of carbamates of muscle relaxants such as mephenesin (*39, 176*) (Table XXVIIIB).

The conversion of the relatively short-acting oral antidiabetic tolbutamide to the longer acting chlorpropamide is an example of the avoidance of oxidative degradation by elimination of the vulnerable moiety. Such an elimination nearly always implies substitution of the vulnerable moiety by another one. Substitution of the methyl group of tolbutamide and its analogs by less easily oxidized groups such as Cl leads to a prolongation of the action (*237*) (see Table XXIX). Orciprenaline is a stabilized isoprenaline analog (*168*).

A special aspect of the procedure under discussion is the substitution by fluorine of those H atoms in a drug molecule that are involved—that have to be mobilized—in the case of oxidative degradation. Among the halogens fluorine is most closely related to hydrogen. It has about the same atom radius and the same internuclear distance to the carbon atom as hydrogen in hydrogen–carbon bonds. The binding energy in the fluorine–carbon bonds, however, is higher than that for the hydrogen–carbon bond, or other halogen–carbon bonds. The consequence is that as far as the size and shape are concerned the fluorine-substituted derivatives are isosteric with the hydrogen

TABLE XXVIIIA

DISPOSABLE MOIETIES INTRODUCED TO PROTECT VULNERABLE MOIETIES IN VITAMINS

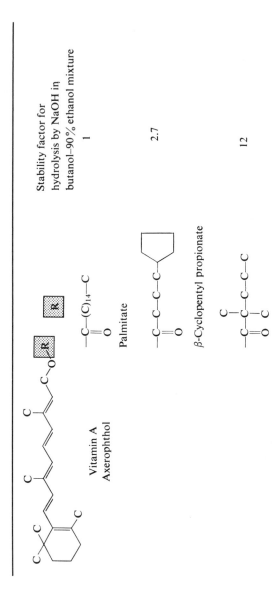

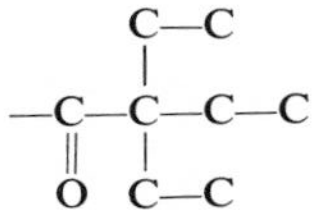

20

26.3

Triethylacetate

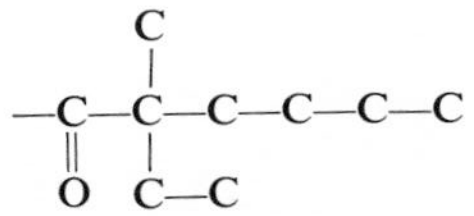

α-Methyl-α-ethylcaproate

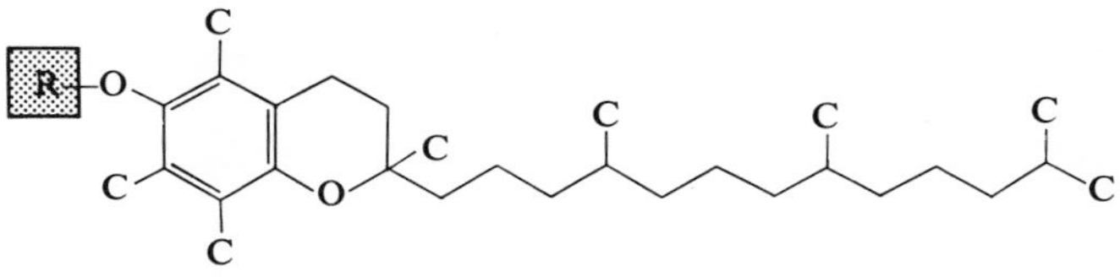

D-L-α-Tocopherol

R

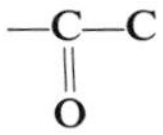

Acetate

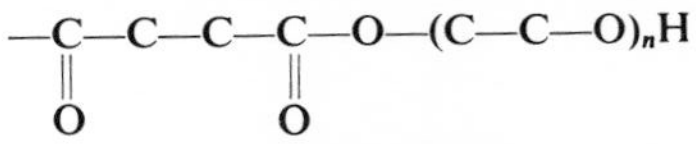

Polyoxyethylene succinate

$n \sim 22$

TABLE XXVIIIB
PROTECTION AND SUBSTITUTION OF VULNERABLE MOIETIES TO OBTAIN PROLONGED
ACTION

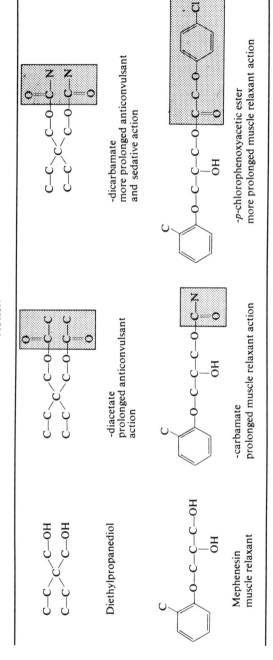

TABLE XXIX

Conversion of Short-Acting Oral Antidiabetics to Longer Acting Compounds by Substitution of the Vulnerable Moieties by Stable Groups [a]

	Half-life time (hr)		Half-life time (hr)
Short-acting		Long-acting	
Tolbutamide	5.7	Chlorpropamide	33
Cycloheptolamide	4.7	Carbutamide	36
U-17,835	7.2	U-12,504	16–18
Acetohexamide	1.3	Metahexamide	22
vulnerable moiety		stable moiety	

derivatives; they are more resistant, however, to oxidative degradation (262). If the fluorine is situated close to double bonds a shift in charge distribution interfering with the activity may take place (131). A substitution of fluorine for hydrogen under the circumstances outlined may result in a stabilization of the drug. There are, however, some pitfalls in this procedure. If the biological activity of the compound involved is based on an assimilation in the chemical constituents of the biological object, a "lethal" synthesis (268, 269), known, for instance, for fluoroacetic acid and p-fluorophenylalanine, may take place. In other cases the compounds obtained may act as competitive antagonists, or antimetabolites. An example is 5-fluorouracil (38, 65, 96, 107).

Avoidance of vulnerable moieties in drug development may play a major role in future drug design. It would greatly reduce the embarrassing species differences and patient-to-patient variations in responses mainly due to genetic and drug-induced differences in drug metabolism. For the adaptation of time–concentration relationships partition coefficients and pK_a values are more reliable parameters.

D. Masking Moieties

The various efforts to modulate distribution of bioactive compounds, described before, had as a main goal to obtain a time–concentration pattern optimal for the action, in plasma or particular target compartments. The avoidance of side effects, however, by avoiding high concentrations of the active compound in certain compartments or by avoiding initial peak concentrations may also be the aim. The efforts to keep the free concentration of iron and calcium ions in preparations of these metals low to avoid irritation at the sites of application in casu the sites of injection are examples. For this purpose poorly ionized compounds such as calcium gluconate or levulinate for intravenous injection and iron-sorbitol citrate for intramuscular injection are used (30). Quinidine polygalacturonate is used to avoid gastric irritation by quinidine (40, 143, 189). The use of disposable masking moieties which temporarily eliminate the properties of the drug responsible for the unwanted side effects, which, however, often also implies a temporary inactivation in the therapeutic sense, is another possibility. In this respect there can be mentioned the application of salicylic acid as acetosalicylic acid in which the phenolic OH— group is masked. This has as a result a decrease in the gastrointestinal irritation. Salicylic acid is set free partly in the gut and further after absorption in plasma by plasma esterases. Another example are the acetates of trioxyanthracene, used against psoriasis, which have a local irritating action and a strong staining tendency if applied on the skin. The compound triacetoxyanthracene is found to be less irritating and less staining. By hydrolysis the diacetoxy compound is formed, which is assumed to be the active product (103). The masked acetylated polyphenols used as laxatives,

TABLE XXX

Introduction of Readily Disposed Masking Moieties to Obtain Compounds with a "Latency" in Their Action and to Avoid Local "Actions" at the Site of Application

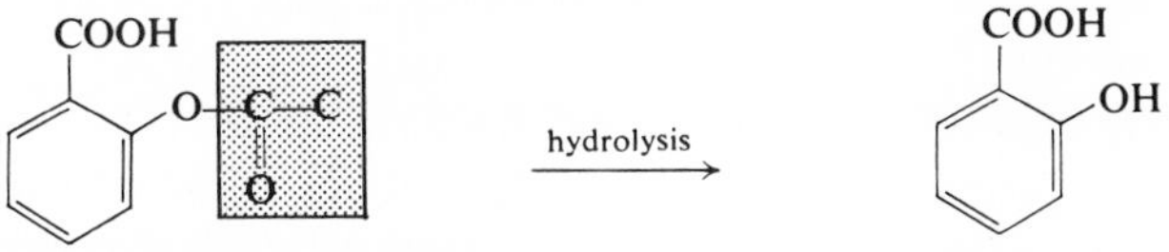

Acetylsalicylic acid
phenolic OH-group masked to
reduce stomach irritation

$\xrightarrow{\text{hydrolysis}}$

Salicylic acid
analgesic

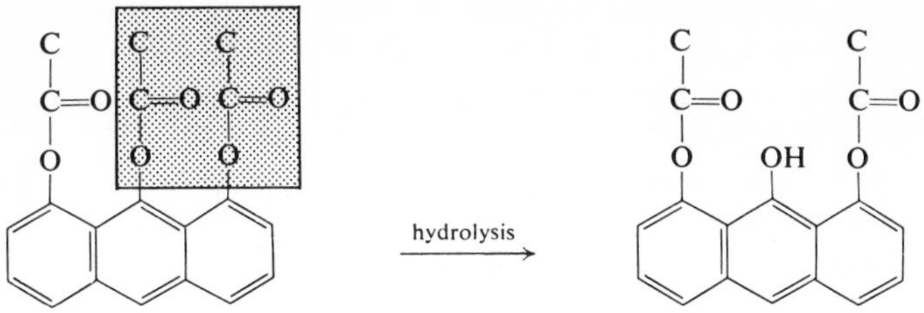

Triacetoxyanthracene
phenolic OH-groups masked
to avoid skin irritation and
tissue staining

$\xrightarrow{\text{hydrolysis}}$

Diacetate (and monoacetate)
active antipsoriatic

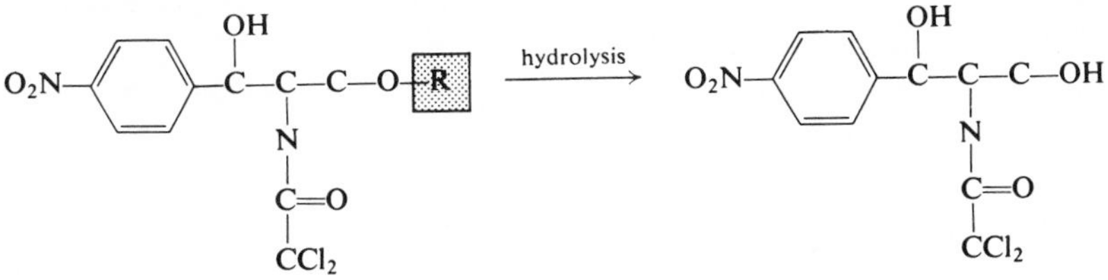

$\xrightarrow{\text{hydrolysis}}$

Chloramphenicol

R | Palmitate
Cinnamate
Glycinate
N-Alkyl carbamate

Chloramphenicol esters
devoid of bitter taste

$\xrightarrow{\text{hydrolysis}}$

2 S—C—C

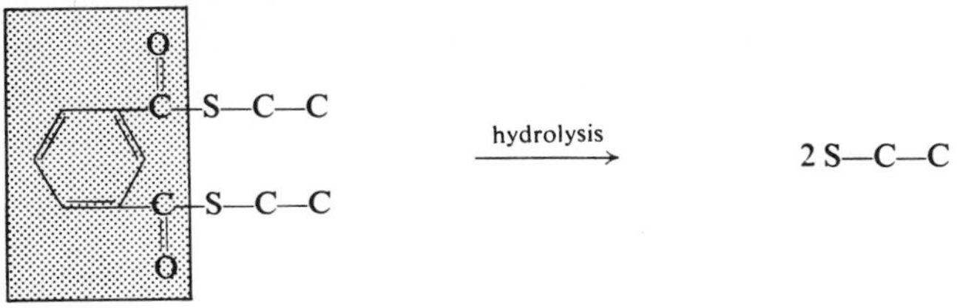

Ditophal
devoid of bad mercaptan smell

Ethyl mercaptan
tuberculostatic

such as acetphenolisatin and biscacodyl, which are converted in the intestinal tract to the more irritating polyphenols which are in fact the effective laxatives are another example for the use of disposable masking moieties (*37, 113, 265a*).

Examples for the avoidance of untolerable taste or smell by formation of esters are also known; for instance, by formation of the palmitate or *N*-alkylcarbamates of chloramphenicol the bitter taste of this antibiotic is avoided. In the gut and after absorption the antibiotic is liberated by hydrolysis of the ester. The same holds true for the ester of lincomycin; its enzymically labile esters taste less bitter than the antibiotic itself (*105, 116, 248*). Ethyl-mercaptan, a very evil smelling compound, used as tuberculostatic and for the treatment of leprosy, is applied as an ester of phthalic acid to obtain a non-volatile odorless product releasing the active mercaptan gradually in the body (Table XXX) (*86*).

In the field of pharmaceutical formulation a variety of examples of transport forms suitable to correct for bad taste, evil smell, local irritation, etc. can be found. Besides molecular changes in the drug—chemical formulation—also pharmaceutical formulation by the use of adjuvants such as corrigents for taste and smell and by enteric-coating can be applied for this purpose. With respect to the time–concentration relationship, avoidance of initial high peak concentrations in plasma and other body fluids at the moment of intravenous or intramuscular application is a problem especially for relatively short-acting compounds where relatively high doses are required to cover a certain period of action. For drugs applied orally, pharmaceutical sustained-release formulations have been developed, containing the drug in different granulation forms giving a sequential release. The use of transport forms of the drug which gradually release or generate the active product is another possibility. An example of such a compound with a "latentiation" (*151, 152*) in its action is the immunosuppressive agent azothioprine. Its action is based on a gradual release of mercaptopurine, the active cytostatic moiety in the drug. Initial peak concentrations of mercaptopurine and therewith the risk for strong cytostatic effects can be reduced in this way. The group attached to the mer-captopurine molecule too can be regarded as a masking moiety. The compound was originally designed on basis of the principle of the selective bioactivation in the target tissue. Tumors are rich in thioglucosidases which might release the cytostatic mercaptopurine by splitting the *S*-linkage in azathioprine (*105a*). The lesser degree of toxicity observed with the cytostatic cyclophosphamide—a transport form which is activated in the body cells—may be ascribed to a latency in the action. The compound is inert during its transportation via plasma and extracellular fluid, thus reducing damage in these compartments. Originally the aim of this cytostatic was a selective bioactivation in the target tissues (the cancer tissues) but the activation takes place also in healthy tissues such as liver tissue (*45, 141*).

VI. Summary

In this chapter the classical approach to the modulation of pharmacokinetics on basis of molecular manipulation is presented. The differentiation of various types of biofunctional moieties in the drug molecule, such as restricting moieties, facilitating moieties, selecting moieties, desolubilizing and solubilizing moieties, and masking moieties, all fixed or disposable, and the differentiation between introduction, stabilization, protection, and elimination of vulnerable moieties in the drug molecule allow a rational schematization of various possibilities and limitations in this section of drug design. Examples from such diverse fields as therapeutics, toxons, food additives, pesticides, and environmental pollutants are presented to elucidate the various principles applied. Successful application but also less successful but instructive efforts are discussed, to provoke thoughts and discussion and thus to stimulate progress in drug design, which implies a reduction to the possible minimum of the trial-and-error factor in the development of new useful bioactive compounds.

REFERENCES

1. A. Albert, *Pharmacol. Rev.* **4**, 136 (1952).
2. A. Albert, *Federation Proc.* **20**, 137 (1961).
3. A. Albert, "Selective Toxicity." Methuen, London, 1968.
3a. E. C. Albright, D. L. Tabern, and E. S. Gordon, *Amer. J. Trop. Med. Hyg.* **27**, 553 (1947).
4. N. E. Andén, H. Corrodi, A. Dahlström, K. Fuxe, and T. Hökfelt, *Life Sci.* **5**, 561 (1966).
5. R. A. Anderson and E. Hardenbergh, *J. Surgical Res.* **5**, 256 (1965).
6. A. H. Anton, *J. Pharmacol. Exp. Ther.* **129**, 282 (1960).
7. A. H. Anton, *J. Pharmacol. Exp. Ther.* **134**, 291 (1961).
8. A. H. Anton, *Federation Proc.* **20**, 171 (1961).
9. S. Archer, J. O. Hoppe, T. R. Lewiis, and M. N. Haskell, *J. Pharm. Sci.* **40**, 143 (1951).
10. E. J. Ariëns, "Molecular Pharmacology," Vol. I. Academic Press, New York, 1964.
10a. E. J. Ariëns, *in* "Doping" (A. De Schaepdryver and M. Hebbelinck, eds.), p. 27. Pergamon Press, Oxford, 1965.
11. E. J. Ariëns, *Progr. Drug. Res.* **10**, 431 (1966).
12. E. J. Ariëns, *Ann. Ist. Super. Sanità* **3**, 412 (1967).
13. E. J. Ariëns, *Farmaco (Pavia) Ed. Sci.* **24**, 6 (1969).
14. E. J. Ariëns, *Pure Appl. Chem.* **19**, 187 (1969).
15. E. J. Ariëns, *J. Mond. Pharm.* **3**, 263 (1969).
16. E. J. Ariëns, *Progr. Drug Res.* **14**, 11 (1970).
17. E. J. Ariëns, *in* "Drug Design" (E. J. Ariëns, ed.), Vol. I. Academic Press, New York, 1971.
18. E. B. Astwood, *in* "The Pharmacological Basis of Therapeutics" (L. S. Goodman and A. Gilman, eds.), 3rd ed., p. 1540. Macmillan, New York, 1965.

19. B. R. Baker, "Design of Active-Site Directed Irreversible Enzyme Inhibitors." Wiley, New York, 1967.
20. A. H. Beckett, *in* "Enzymes and Drug Action" (J. L. Mongar and A. V. S. de Reuck, eds.), pp. 15 and 238. Churchill, London, 1962.
21. A. H. Beckett, *Dansk Tidsskr. Farm.* **40**, 197 (1966).
22. A. H. Beckett and M. Rowland, *J. Pharm. Pharmacol.* **17**, 628 (1965).
23. A. H. Beckett, J. A. Salmon, and M. Mitchard, *J. Pharm. Pharmacol.* **21**, 251 (1969).
24. S. H. Bennett, *Ann. Rev. Entomol.* **2**, 279 (1957).
24a. H. Bennhold, *West-European Symp. Clin. Chem.* **5**, 1 (1966).
25. Z. Beránková-Ksandrova, I. Rychlik, and F. Sorm, *Proc. 2nd Int. Pharmacol. Meet. 1963* Vol. 10, p. 181 (1964).
26. F. Bergel, *J. Pharm. Pharmacol.* **7**, 297 (1955).
27. F. Bergel, "Chemotherapy of Cancer," *Proc. Int. Symp. Lugano*, p. 21 (1964).
28. F. Bergel, J. M. Johnson, and R. Wade, *J. Chem. Soc.* p. 3802 (1962).
29. F. M. Berger, *Proc. Soc. Exp. Biol. Med.* **71**, 270 (1949).
30. F. M. Berger, *J. Pharmacol. Exp. Ther.* **104**, 229 (1952).
31. H. Berlin and E. Krüger-Thiemer, *Nord. Med.* **72**, 1358 (1964).
32. M. Berlin, L. A. Jerksell, and G. Nordberg, *Acta Pharmacol. Toxicol.* **23**, 312 (1965).
33. K. H. Beyer, H. F. Russo, S. R. Gass, K. M. Wilhoyte, and A. A. Pitt, *Amer. J. Physiol.* **160**, 311 (1950).
34. K. H. Beyer, V. D. Wiebelhaus, E. K. Tillson, H. F. Russo, and K. M. Wilhoyte, *Proc. Soc. Exp. Biol. Med.* **74**, 772 (1950).
35. T. B. Binns, "Absorption and Distribution of Drugs." Livingstone, Edinburgh, 1964.
36. A. E. Bird and A. C. Marshall, *Biochem. Pharmacol.* **16**, 2275 (1967).
36a. K. U. Blum and L. Thomas, *Pharmacol. Clin.* **2**, 177 (1970).
36b. D. Boerner and U. J. Jovanovic, *Naunyn-Schmiedebergs Arch. Pharmakol.* **266**, 299 (1970).
37. D. D. Bonnycastle, *in* "Drill's Pharmacology in Medicine" (J. R. DiPalma, ed.), p. 747. McGraw-Hill, New York, 1965.
38. L. Bosch, E. Harbers, and C. Heidelberger, *Cancer Res.* **18**, 335 (1958).
39. F. Bottari, M. F. Saettone, and M. F. Serafini, *J. Med. Chem.* **11**, 904 (1968).
40. D. Boyle, A. W. Dellipiani, J. A. Owen, D. A. Seaton, and R. W. Tonkin, *Brit. Med. J.* **1**, 285 (1964).
41. N. Brack, *Arzneimittel-Forsch.* **12**, 133 (1962).
42. E. Brandl, R. Brunner, and F. Knauseder, *Arzneimittel-Forsch.* **14**, 883 (1964).
43. G. Ch. F. Brinkbok, H. G. A. Charbon-Boon, H. van Genderen, W. Lammers, A. T. H. van der Meulen, N. J. Poulie, J. G. Voerman, and E. van der Voort Maarschalk, *Ned. Tijdschr. Geneesk.* **102**, 479 (1958).
44. J. C. Brinling, T. D. Shopiro, and E. B. Sigg, *Arch. Int. Pharmacodyn.* **136**, 113 (1962).
45. N. Brock, *Proc. 2nd Int. Symp. Chemotherapy 1961* Part III, p. 1 (1963).
46. B. B. Brodie, *Federation Proc.* **11**, 632 (1952).
47. B. B. Brodie, *Pharmacologist* **6**, 12 (1964).
48. B. B. Brodie and C. A. M. Hogben, *J. Pharm. Pharmacol.* **9**, 345 (1957).
49. B. B. Brodie, H. Kurz, and L. S. Schanker, *J. Pharmacol. Exp. Ther.* **130**, 20 (1960).
50. S. S. Brown, *Advan. Pharmacol.* **2**, 243 (1963).
51. H. Brunner and D. Regoli, *Experientia* **18**, 504 (1962).
52. J. Büchi, P. Labhart, and L. Ragaz, *Helv. Chim. Acta* **30**, 507 (1947).
52a. J. Büchi, "Grundlagen der Arzneimittelforschung und der synthetischen Arzneimittel." Birkhäuser, Basel, 1963.
52b. J. Büchi, *Pharm. Acta Helv.* **41**, 1 and 65 (1966).

53. K. Bullock and J. Grundy, *J. Pharm. Pharmacol.* **7**, 755 (1955).
54. J. Burgers, *Chem. Weekblad* **66**, 55 (1970).
55. J. J. Burns and A. H. Conney, *Proc. Roy. Soc. Med.* **58** (11), Part 2 (1965).
56. J. J. Burns and R. A. Salvador, Conference on New Adrenergic Blocking Drugs, February 24–26, 1966. N.Y. Acad. Sci., New York, 1966.
57. M. T. Busch, *in* "Physiological Pharmacology" (W. S. Root and F. G. Hofmann, eds.), Vol. 1, p. 185. Academic Press, New York, 1963.
58. A. G. Caldwell and O. D. Standen, *Brit. J. Pharmacol.* **11**, 372 (1956).
59. R. Carson, "Silent Spring." Houghton-Mittlin, Boston, 1962.
60. H. Cassebaum, K. Dierbach, and H. Bekker, *Pharmazie* **22**, 470 (1967).
61. A. Catsch, *Federation Proc.* **20**, Suppl. 10, Part II, 206 (1961).
62. M. B. Chenoweth, *Clin. Pharmacol. Ther.* **9**, 365 (1968).
63. J. Cheymol and F. Bourillet, *Actualités Pharmacol.* **13**, 63 (1960).
64. H. N. Christensen, "Biological Transport." Benjamin, New York, 1962.
64a. D. B. Clayson, "Chemical Carcinogenesis," p. 263. Churchill, London, 1962.
65. S. S. Cohen, J. G. Flaks, H. D. Barner, M. R. Loeb, and J. Lichtenstein, *Proc. Nat. Acad. Sci. U.S.* **44**, 1004 (1958).
66. Y. Cohen, A. Uzan, and G. Valette, *Biochem. Pharmacol.* **11**, 721 (1962).
67. A. H. Conney, M. Sansur, F. Soroko, R. Koster, and J. J. Burns, *J. Pharmacol. Exp. Ther.* **151**, 133 (1966).
68. G. von Corduan, *Arch. Pharm.* **303**, 30 (1970).
69. R. E. Counsell, R. E. Willette, and W. DiGuilio, *J. Med. Chem.*, **10**, 975 (1967).
70. R. E. Counsell, P. Pocha, J. O. Morales, and W. H. Beierwaltes, *J. Pharm. Sci.* **56**, 1042 (1967).
71. R. E. Counsell, T. D. Smith, W. DiGuilio, and W. H. Beierwaltes, *J. Pharm. Sci.* **57**, 1958 (1968).
72. R. E. Counsell, V. V. Ranade, L. K. Lala, and B. H. Hong, *J. Med. Chem.* **11**, 380 (1968).
73. R. E. Counsell, B. H. Hong, R. E. Willette, and V. V. Ranade, *Steroids* **11**, 817 (1968).
74. A. S. Crafts, *Science* **108**, 85 (1948).
75. A. S. Crafts, *Advan. Pest Control Res.* **1**, 39 (1957).
76. A. S. Crafts, "The Chemistry and Mode of Action of Herbicides." Wiley (Interscience), New York, 1961.
76a. A. S. Crafts and W. W. Robbins, "Weed Control," p. 293. McGraw-Hill, New York, 1962.
77. H. J. Creech, *Ann. N.Y. Acad. Sci.* **68**, 868 (1958).
78. S. A. Cucinell, A. H. Conney, M. Sansur, and J. J. Burns, *Clin. Pharmacol. Ther.* **6**, 420 (1966).
79. P. A. Dahm, *Advan. Pest Control Res.* **1**, 86 (1957).
80. F. E. van Dam and M. J. H. Gribnau-Overkamp, *Folia Med. Neerl.* **10**, 141 (1967).
81. J. F. Danielli, *Ann. Rept. Brit. Empire Cancer Campaign* **34**, 398 (1956).
82. J. F. Danielli, *Ann. Rept. Brit. Empire Cancer Campaign* **37**, 575 (1959).
83. J. F. Danielli, *Ann. Rept. Brit. Empire Cancer Campaign* **38**, 693 (1960).
84. J. F. Danielli, *Biol. Approaches Cancer Chemotherapy, Symp. Louvain, 1960* p. 2 (1961).
84a. J. F. Danielli, M. Danielli, J. B. Fraser, P. D. Mitchell, L. N. Owen, and G. Shaw, *Biochem. J.* **41**, 325 (1947).
85. H. Dannenberg, *Physiol. Chem.* **2**, 342 (1959).
86. T. F. Davey, *Proc. Int. Congr. Leprosy, Tokyo, 1958*
87. W. Davis, *12ᵉ Jaarboek Kanderonderzoek en Kankerbestrijding in Nederland*, p. 113 (1962).

88. E. Dicfalusy, O. Fernö, H. Fex, and B. Högberg, *Acta Chem. Scand.* **17**, 2536 (1963).
89. J. R. DiPalma, "Drill's Pharmacology in Medicine," 3rd ed. McGraw-Hill, New York, 1965.
90. W. Dirscherl and H. L. Krüskemper, *Biochem. Z.* **323**, 520 (1953).
90a. L. G. Donaruma and J. Razzano, *J. Med. Chem.* **14**, 244 (1971).
91. G. Dörner and E. Kleinert, *Acta Biol. Med. Ger.* **11**, 77 (1963).
92. F. H. Dost, *Deut. Med. Wochschr.* **92**, 264 (1967).
93. L. Doub, *Med. Chem.* **5**, 360 (1961).
94. H. Druckrey, *Klin. Wochschr.* **30**, 882 (1952).
95. P. Durel, "La Thérapeutique Sulfamidée." Baillière, Paris, 1940.
96. R. Duschinsky, E. Pleven, and C. Heidelberger, *J. Amer. Chem. Soc.* **79**, 4559 (1957).
97. D. D. Dziewiatkowski and H. B. Lewis, *J. Biol. Chem.* **158**, 77 (1945).
98. Th. von Eckert, I. Reimann, and K. Krisch, *Arzneimittel-Forsch.* **20**, 487 (1970).
99. Editorial, *Japan. Med. Gazette* **2**, 15 (1965).
100. Editorial, *Japan. Med. Gazette* **2**, 12 (1965).
101. Editorial, *Japan. Med. Gazette* **3**, 12 (1966).
102. Editorial, *Japan. Med. Gazette* **4**, 13 (1967).
103. Editorial, *Brit. Med. J.* **1**, 682 (1967).
104. Editorial, *Japan. Med. Gazette* **5**, 8 (1968).
105. Editorial, *Japan. Med. Gazette* **5**, 13 (1968).
105a. Editorial, *Sci. J.* **4/8**, 9 (1968).
105b. G. B. Elion, S. Callahan, R. W. Rundles, and G. H. Hitchings, *Cancer Res.* **23**, 1207 (1963).
106. E. F. Elslager, *Progr. Drug Res.* **13**, 170 (1969).
107. P. Emmelot, *in* "Molecular Pharmacology" (E. J. Ariëns, ed.), Vol. II, pp. 53 and 143. Academic Press, New York, 1964.
108. H. D. Esser and P. W. Muller, *Experientia* **22**, 38 (1966).
109. K. Ewe, *Klin. Wochschr.* **46**, 296 (1968).
110. J. Fabre, J. S. Pitton, J. P. Kunz, S. Rozbroj, and R. M. Hungersbuehler, *Chemotherapia* **11**, 73 (1966).
111. R. Fabre, *Actualités Pharmacol.* **10**, 117 (1957).
112. A. Farah, M. Frazer, and E. Porter, *J. Pharmacol. Exp. Ther.* **126**, 202 (1959).
113. E. Fingl, *in* "The Pharmacological Basis of Therapeutics" (L. S. Goodman and A. Gilman, eds.), 3rd ed., p. 1008. Macmillan, New York, 1965.
114. P. Finholt, *Pharm. Ztg.* **109**, 616 (1964).
114a. J. K. Finnegan, G. R. Hennigar, R. Blackwell Smith, P. S. Larson, and H. B. Haag, *Arch. Int. Pharmacodyn.* **103**, 404 (1955).
115. L. J. Fischer and S. Riegelman, *J. Pharm. Sci.* **56**, 469 (1967).
116. H. P. Fletcher, H. M. Murray, and T. E. Weddon, *J. Pharm. Sci.* **57**, 2101 (1968).
117. *Food Agr. Organ. U.N.*, Specifications for Identity and Purity of Food Additives, Vol. II (Food Colors, F.A.O.). Rome, 1963.
118. H. Foreman, *Drugs Enzymes* **4**, 95 (1966).
119. A. J. Forlano, C. I. Jarowski, and H. F. Hammer, *J. Pharm. Sci.* **57**, 1184 (1968).
120. W. O. Foye, *Federation Proc.* **20**, Suppl. 10, Part II, 147 (1961).
121. J. P. Frawley, H. N. Fuyat, E. C. Hagan, J. R. Blake, and O. Garth Fitzhugh, *J. Pharmacol. Exp. Ther.* **121**, 96 (1957).
122. H. L. Friedman, Symposium on Chemical-Biological Correlation. Natl. Acad. Sci., Natl. Research Council publ. No. 206, p. 295. Washington D.C., 1951.
123. S. C. J. Fu, S. M. Birnbaum, and J. P. Greenstein, *J. Amer. Chem. Soc.* **76**, 6054 (1954).
124. S. C. J. Fu, H. Terzian, C. L. Maddock, and V. M. Binns, *J. Med. Chem.* **9**, 214 (1966).

125. J. L. Garraway and R. L. Wain, *Ann. Appl. Biol.* **50**, 11 (1962).
126. T. A. Garrett, *Clin. Med.* **3**, 1185 (1956).
127. E. Genazzani, L. J. Bononi, G. Pagnini, and R. Dicarlo, *Antimicrobial Agents Chemotherapy*, p. 192 (1965).
128. H. W. Gerarde, "Toxicology and Biochemistry of Aromatic Hydrocarbons." Elsevier, Amsterdam, 1960.
129. R. E. Gerhardt, R. F. Knouss, P. T. Thyrum, R. J. Luchi, and J. J. Morris, Jr., *Ann. Internal Med.* **71**, 927 (1969).
130. T. Ghose, M. Cerini, M. Carter, and R. C. Nairn, *Brit. Med. J.* **1**, 90 (1967).
131. E. W. Gill, *Progr. Med. Chem.* **4**, 39 (1965).
132. J. R. Gillette, *Progr. Drug Res.* **6**, 13 (1963).
133. D. J. Glick, *Biol. Chem.* **125**, 729 (1938); **130**, 527 (1939); **137**, 357 (1941).
134. A. Goldin and H. B. Wood, *Ann. N.Y. Acad. Sci.* **163**, 954 (1969).
135. A. Goldstein, *Pharmacol. Rev.* **1**, 102 (1949).
136. J. A. L. Gorringe and E. M. Sproston, *in* "Absorption and Distribution of Drugs" (T. B. Binns, ed.), p. 184. Livingstone, Edinburgh, 1964.
137. J. A. Gosling and T. C. Lu, *J. Pharmacol. Exp. Ther.* **167**, 56 (1969).
138. H. Grasshof, *Progr. Drug Res.* **4**, 354 (1962).
139. R. E. Green, W. E. Ricker, W. L. Attwood, Y. S. Koh, and L. Peters, *J. Pharmacol. Exp. Ther.* **126**, 195 (1959).
140. H. R. Griffith, W. C. Cullen, and P. Welt, *Can. Anaesthetists Soc. J.* **3**, 346 (1956).
141. H. Grunicke, M. Liersch, H. Holter, and H. Arnold, *Biochem. Pharmacol.* **14**, 1495 (1965).
142. V. Hach, *Cesk. Farm.* **2**, 159 (1953).
143. A. Halpern, N. Shaftel, and A. J. Monte Bovi, *Amer. J. Pharm.* **130**, 190 (1958).
144. A. Hamilton and H. L. Hardy, "Industrial Toxicology," 2nd ed. Hoeber, New York, 1949.
145. C. Hansch, *Ann. Rept. Med. Chem.*, p. 347 (1967).
146. C. Hansch, *Phys. Chem. Aspects Drug Action* **7**, 141 (1968).
147. C. Hansch, *in* "Drug Design" (E. J. Ariëns, ed.), Vol. I. Academic Press, New York, 1971.
148. C. Hansch and T. Fujita, *J. Amer. Chem. Soc.* **86**, 1616 (1964).
149. E. Hansson and C. G. Schmiterlöw, *Arch. Int. Pharmacodyn.* **131**, 309 (1967).
150. M. Häring and G. Stille, *Helv. Chim. Acta* **44**, 642 (1961).
151. N. J. Harper, *J. Med. Pharm. Chem.* **1**, 467 (1959).
152. N. J. Harper, *Drug Res.* **4**, 221 (1962).
153. A. A. Haspels, *Ned. Tijdschr. Geneesk.* **114**, 61 (1970).
154. L. Havers, I. von Borgstede, and H. Breuer, *Deut. Med. Wochschr.* **87**, 730 (1962).
155. D. Haunfelder and G. Kodel, *Deut. Zahnaerztebl. Z.* **15**, 339 (1961).
156. D. F. Heath, P. O. Park, L. A. Lickerish, and E. F. Edson, Pest Control, Ltd. (Mimeo Report), 1953.
157. E. Heinz, *Deut. Med. Wochschr.* **87**, 1829 (1962).
158. J. W. Heringa, R. Huybregtse, and A. C. van der Linden, *Antonie van Leeuwenhoek, J. Microbiol. Serol.* **27**, 51 (1961).
158a. J. K. C. Hessels, *Chem. Tech. Amsterdam* **20**, 861; 915; 952 (1965).
159. J. B. Hill, *Federation Proc.* **29**, 411 (1970).
160. R. Hiltmann, H. Wollweber, W. Wirth, and F. Hoffmeister, *in* "Berichte Arbeitstagung der Deutschen Gesellschaft für Anaesthesie" (K. Horatz, R. Frey, and M. Zindler, eds.), p. 1. Springer, Berlin, 1965.
161. E. Hirsch, *Vom Wasser* **30**, 249 (1963).
162. E. Hirsch, *15th Int. Hygiene-Kolloquium*, p. 52 (1965).

163. J. Hirschfelder, *in* "Molecular Biophysics" (B. Pullman and M. Weisbluth, eds.), p. 325. Academic Press, New York, 1965.

163a. R. Hirschmann, R. G. Strachan, P. Buchschacher, L. H. Sarett, S. L. Steelman, and R. Silber, *J. Amer. Chem. Soc.* **86**, 3903 (1964).

164. G. H. Hitchings and J. J. Burchall, *Advan. Enzymol.* **27**, 417 (1965).

165. R. Höber, "Physical Chemistry of Cells and Tissues." Blakiston, Philadelphia, 1945.

166. L. E. Hollister, *New Engl. J. Med.* **266**, 281 (1962).

167. L. E. Hollister, S. L. Kanter, and D. J. Clyde, *Clin. Pharmacol. Ther.* **4**, 612 (1963).

168. P. Holtz and D. Palm, *Rev. Physiol. Biochem. Exptl. Pharmacol.* **58**, 56 (1966).

168a. J. R. E. Hoover and R. J. Stedman, *in* "Medicinal Chemistry" (A. Burger, ed.), 3rd ed., p. 371. Wiley, New York, 1970.

169. K. Horatz, R. Frey, and M. Zindler, "Berichte Arbeitstagung der Deutschen Gesellschaft für Anaesthesie." Springer, Berlin, 1965.

170. W. C. Hueper, *J. Nat. Cancer Inst.* **26**, 229 (1961).

171. H. W. Huyser, Original Lectures 3rd Int. Congr. of Surface Activity, Cologne, 1960. Vol. III, Section C, p. 295.

172. L. A. Ignatova and M. I. Goriaev, *Vest. Akad. Nauk Kaz. SSR* **6**, 207 (1960).

173. Y. Imai, *Chem. Pharm. Bull.* **14**, 1045 (1966).

173a. Y. Imai, H. Matsumura, and Y. Aramaki, *Japan. J. Pharmacol.* **17**, 330 (1967).

174. H. Imura, S. Matsukura, H. Matsuyama, T. Sitsuda, and T. Miyaka, *Endocrinology* **76**, 933 (1965).

175. H. R. Ing, *Progr. Drug Res.* **7**, 305 (1964).

176. H. Ippen, "Index Pharmacorum." Thieme, Stuttgart, 1968.

177. O. Isler, *Experientia* **26**, 225 (1970).

178. G. L. Jackson, M. L. Corson, and J. Dick, *J. Nucl. Med.* **8**, 611 (1967).

178a. R. J. Jaeger and R. J. Rubin, *Science* **170**, 460 (1970).

179. L. Johnson, F. Sarmiento, W. A. Blanc, and R. Day, *A.M.A. J. Diseases Children* **97**, 591 (1959).

179a. M. J. Johnson, *Science* **155**, 1515 (1967).

180. R. Jones, U. Jonsson, M. Browning, H. Lessner, C. C. Price, and A. K. Sen, *Ann. N.Y. Acad. Sci.* **68**, 1133 (1958).

181. S. E. de Jongh, "Inleiding tot de Algemene Farmacologie." N.V. Noord-Hollandsche Uitgevers Mij., Amsterdam, 1959.

182. K. Junkmann and H. Witzel, *Z. Vitamin-, Hormon-, Fermentforsch.* **9**, 227 (1958).

183. I. A. Kamil, J. N. Smith, and R. T. Williams, *Biochem. J.* **53**, 137 (1953).

184. M. A. Kaplan, W. T. Bradner, F. H. Buckwalter, and M. H. Pindell, *Nature* **205**, 399 (1965).

185. P. Karrer, "Lehrbuch der organischen Chemie," p. 216. Thieme, Stuttgart, 1959.

186. M. Katz and Z. I. Shaikh, *J. Pharm. Sci.* **54**, 591 (1965).

187. C. Kawasaki, *Vitamins Hormones* **21**, 69 (1963).

188. P. M. Keen, *Brit. J. Pharmacol.* **26**, 704 (1966).

189. A. I. Kertesz, "The Pectic Substances," p. 393. Wiley (Interscience), New York, 1951.

190. K. A. Khavari and R. P. Maickel, *Int. J. Neuropharmacol.* **6**, 301 (1967).

191. E. Kingstone, *Int. J. Clin. Pharmacol.* **1**, 413 (1968).

192. M. C. Kloetzel, S. J. Davis, U. Pandit, C. R. Smith, and H. Nishihara, *J. Med. Pharm. Chem.* **1**, 197 (1959).

193. P. K. Knoefel, "Radiopaque Diagnostic Agents." Thomas, Springfield, Ill., 1961.

194. P. K. Knoefel, *in* "Drill's Pharmacology in Medicine" (J. R. DiPalma, ed.), 3rd ed., p. 1429. McGraw-Hill, New York, 1965.

195. P. K. Knoefel and G. Lehmann, *J. Pharmacol. Exp. Ther.* **83**, 185 (1945).

196. G. B. Koelle, *in* "Bioelectrogenesis" (C. Chagas and A. Paes de Carvalho, eds.), p. 314. Elsevier, Amsterdam, 1961.
197. G. B. Koelle, "Handbuch der experimentellen Pharmakologie," Vol. 15, p. 187. Springer, Berlin, 1963.
198. P. C. Koller and U. Veronesi, *Brit. J. Cancer* **10**, 703 (1956).
199. J. Krieglstein, *Klin. Wochschr.* **47**, 1125 (1969).
200. H. R. Krueger and R. D. O'Brien, *J. Econ. Entomol.* **52**, 1063 (1959).
201. E. Krüger-Thiemer, W. Diller, L. Dettli, P. Bünger, and J. Seydel, *Antibiot. Chemotherapia* **12**, 171 (1964).
202. C. M. Kunin, *J. Lab. Clin. Med.* **65**, 406, 416 (1965).
203. C. M. Kunin, *Clin. Pharmacol. Ther.* **7**, 166, 180 (1966).
204. K. Yagi, J. Okuda, A. A. Dmitrovskii, R. Honda, and T. Matsubara, *J. Vitaminol.* **7**, 4 (1961).
205. J. Kuntze and H. Otto, *Deut. Med. Wochschr.* **76**, 472 (1951).
206. W. Kunz, *Progr. Drug Res.* **10**, 360 (1966).
207. L. F. Larionov, *Brit. J. Cancer* **10**, 26 (1956).
208. L. F. Larionov, *Vest. Akad. Med. Nauk SSSR* **4**, 29 (1960).
209. L. F. Larionov, "Cancer Progress," p. 211. Butterworth, London, 1960.
210. L. F. Larionov, *Cancer Chemotherapy Rept.* **12**, 205 (1961).
211. L. F. Larionov, *Biol. Approaches Cancer Chemotherapy Symp. Louvain, 1960,* p.139 (1961).
212. L. F. Larionov and G. N. Platonova, *Vop. Onkol.* **1**, 36 (1955).
213. L. F. Larionov and Z. P. Sofina, *C.R. Acad. Sci. URSS* **114**, 1070 (1957).
214. N. A. Lassen, *Lancet* **2**, 338 (1960).
214a. G. H. Lathe, P. Lord, and C. Toothill, *West-European Symp. Clin. Chem.* **5**, 129 (1965).
215. H. D. Law, *Progr. Med. Chem.* **4**, 86 (1965).
216. L. E. Leafe, *Nature* **193**, 485 (1962).
217. C. Levaditi, *Pathol. Microbiol.* **1**, 365 (1938).
218. R. M. Levine and B. B. Clark, *J. Pharmacol. Exp. Ther.* **113**, 272 (1955).
219. G. Levy and T. Matsuzawa, *J. Pharm. Sci.* **54**, 1003 (1965).
220. G. Levy and L. E. Hollister, *J. Pharm. Sci.* **54**, 1121 (1965).
221. S. Lewis, *Brit. Vet. J.* **113**, 380 (1957).
222. A. C. van der Linden and G. J. E. Thijsse, *in* "Symposium on Marine Microbiology" (C. H. Oppenheimer, ed.), Chapter 44, p. 475. Thomas, Springfield, Ill., 1963.
223. F. Linneweh, "Erbliche Stoffwechsel Krankheiten," p. 35. Urban & Schwarzenberg, Munich, 1962.
224. N. Löfgren and B. Lundquist, *Svensk. Kem. Tidskr.* **58**, 206 (1946).
225. J. M. Luck, *Cancer Res.* **17**, 1071 (1957).
226. D. A. Lyttle and H. G. Petering, *J. Amer. Chem. Soc.* **80**, 6459 (1958).
227. B. J. Magerlein, R. D. Birkenmeyer, and F. Kagan, *J. Med. Chem.* **10**, 355 (1967).
228. H. Maier-Bode, *Naturwissenschaften* **55**, 470 (1968).
229. L. C. Mark, H. J. Kayden, J. M. Steele, J. R. Cooper, I. Berlin, E. A. Rovenstine, and B. B. Brodie, *J. Pharm. Exp. Ther.* **102**, 5 (1951).
230. H. Martin, *Symp. Soc. Exp. Biol.* No. 3 (1949).
231. C. Martius and D. Nitz-Litzow, *Biochem. Z.* **327**, 1 (1955).
232. H. S. Mathewson, *Structural Forms Anesthetic Comp.*, p. 86 (1961).
233. T. Matsukawa, S. Yurugi, and Y. Oka, *Ann. N.Y. Acad. Sci.* **98**, 31 (1962).
234. S. Mayer, R. P. Maickel, and B. B. Brodie, *J. Pharmacol. Exp. Ther.* **127**, 205 (1959).

235. E. W. Maynert, *in* "Drill's Pharmacology in Medicine" (J. R. DiPalma, ed.), 3rd ed., p. 188. McGraw-Hill, New York, 1965.
235a. E. Mayr, *Pharmazie*, Beil. **7**, 163 (1967).
236. R. J. McIsaac and G. B. Koelle, *J. Pharmacol. Exp. Ther.* **126**, 9 (1959).
237. F. G. McMahon, *Advan. Chem. Ser.* **45**, 102 (1964).
238. A. Meli, A. Wolff, and W. L. Honrath, *Steroids* **2**, 417 (1963).
239. A. Meli, W. L. Honrath, and A. Wolff, *Endocrinology* **74**, 79 (1964).
240. R. G. Menzel, *Federation Proc.* **22**, 1398 (1963).
241. R. L. Metcalf, Plant Protect. Conference 1956, *Proc. 2nd Int. Fernhurst Research Sta.*, p. 129 (1957).
242. M. C. Meyer and D. E. Guttman, *J. Pharm. Sci.* **57**, 895 (1968).
243. J. Mishkinsky, K. Khazen, and F. G. Sulman, *Neuroendocrinology* **4**, 321 (1969).
244. J. S. Mitchell, *Proc. Roy. Soc. Med.* **56**, 561 (1963).
245. K. O. Møller, "Pharmakologie als theoretische Grundlage einer rationellen Pharmakotherapie," p. 203. Benno Schwabe, Basel, 1958.
246. J. A. Montgomery, *Progr. Drug Res.* **8**, 438 (1965).
247. P. de Moor, R. Deckx, and O. Steeno, *J. Endocrinol.* **27**, 356 (1963).
248. W. Morozowich, D. J. Lamb, H. A. Karnes, F. A. Mackellar, C. Lewis, K. F. Stern, and E. L. Rowe, *J. Pharm. Sci.* **58**, 1485 (1969).
249. P. Münchow, *Pharmazie*, Beil. **11**, 299 (1967).
250. K. von Munzel, *Progr. Drug Res.* **10**, 206 (1966).
250a. A. Myschetzky and N. A. Lassen, *Danish Med. Bull.* **10**, 97 (1963).
251. L. Nemeth, B. Kellner, and K. Lapis, *Ann. N.Y. Acad. Sci.* **68**, 879 (1958).
252. B. B. Newbould and R. Kilpatrick, *Lancet* **1**, 887 (1960).
253. I. Niculescu-Duvăz, A. Cambanis, and E. Tărnăuceanu, *J. Med. Chem.* **10**, 172 (1967).
253a. Hs. Nitschmann and H. R. Stoll, *Pharm. Ztg.* **42**, 1594 (1968).
254. T. Noguchi, Y. Hashimoto, and H. Miyata, *Toxicol. Appl. Pharmacol.* **13**, 189 (1968).
254a. H. Nomura and K. Sugimoto, *Chem. Pharm. Bull.* **14**, 1039 (1966).
255. P. Novack, *in* "Drill's Pharmacology in Medicine" (J. R. DiPalma, ed.), p. 1437. McGraw-Hill, New York, 1965.
256. R. D. O'Brien, "Toxic Phosphorus Esters." Academic Press, New York, 1960.
257. R. D. O'Brien, *Ann. N.Y. Acad. Sci.* **123**, 156 (1965).
258. G. A. J. van Os, E. J. Ariëns, and A. M. Simonis, *in* "Molecular Pharmacology" (E. J. Ariëns, ed.), Vol. I, p. 7. Academic Press, New York, 1964.
259. G. A. Overbeek, *Symp. Anabolic Therapy*, Michigan and Wayne County Acad. Gen. Practice, March 21, 1962. Detroit, 1962.
260. G. A. Overbeek, J. van der Vies, and J. de Visser, *Proc. Intern. Symp. Protein Metabolism*, p. 185 (1962).
261. E. M. Papper, R. C. Peterson, J. J. Burns, E. Bernstein, P. Lief, and B. B. Brodie, *Anesthesiology* **16**, 544 (1955).
262. F. L. M. Pattison, "Toxic Aliphatic Fluorine Compounds." Elsevier, Amsterdam, 1959.
263. F. A. Patty, "Industrial Hygiene and Toxicology," Vol. 2, 2nd ed. Wiley (Interscience), New York, 1962.
264. J. P. Payne and G. G. Rowe, *Brit. J. Pharmacol.* **12**, 457 (1957).
265. R. M. Peck, A. P. O'Connell, and H. J. Creech, *J. Med. Chem.* **13**, 284 (1970).
265a. H. Pelzer, *Humangenetik* **9**, 278 (1970).
266. N. J. Perevodchikova and N. N. Blokhin, "Amino Acids and Peptides with Antimetabolic Activity," p. 110. Churchill, London, 1958.
267. L. Peters, *Pharmacol. Rev.* **12**, 1 (1960).

268. R. A. Peters, *Discussions Faraday Soc.* **20**, 189 (1955).
269. R. A. Peters, *Bull. Johns Hopkins Hosp.* **97**, 21 (1955).
269a. B. C. Pressman, *Proc. 4th Int. Congr. Pharmacol. 1969.* **4**, 383 (1970).
270. B. Pullman, "Electronic Aspects of Biochemistry," p. 559. Academic Press, New York, 1964.
271. J. Putter, *in* "Berichte Arbeitstagung der Deutschen Gesellschaft für Anaesthesie" (K. Horatz, R. Frey, and M. Zindler, eds.). Springer, Berlin, 1965.
271a. J. Raaflaub, *Experientia* **26**, 457 (1970).
272. C. G. Raison and O. D. Standen, *Brit. J. Pharmacol.* **10**, 191 (1955).
273. H. P. Rang, *Ann. N.Y. Acad. Sci.* **144**, 756 (1967).
274. J.-G. Rausch-Stroomann and R. Petry, *Deut. Med. Wochschr.* **93**, 1938 (1968).
275. H. Ch. Reilly, "Amino Acids and Peptides with Antimetabolic Activity," p. 62. Churchill, London, 1958.
276. J. F. Reith, "Kleur van Levensmiddelen," p. 15. D. B. Centen's Uitg. Mij., Hilversum, Netherlands, 1960.
277. H. T. Reynolds, *Advan. Pest Control Res.* **2**, 135 (1958).
278. R. Riemschneider, *Advan. Pest Control Res.* **2**, 315 (1958).
279. W. E. Ripper, *Advan. Pest Control Res.* **1**, 307 (1957).
280. T. H. Rizkallah and M. L. Taymor, Advances in Planned Parenthood. Int. Congr. Series no. 138, 111, 1967. Excerpta Med. Found., Amsterdam.
280a. O. Rochovansky and S. Ratner, *Arch. Biochem. Biophys.* **127**, 688 (1968).
281. E. F. Rogers, *Ann. N.Y. Acad. Sci.* **98**, 412 (1962).
281a. E. F. Rogers, R. L. Clark, H. J. Becker, A. A. Pessolano, W. J. Leanza, E. C. McManus, F. J. Andriuli, and A. C. Cuckler, *Proc. Soc. Exp. Biol. Med.* **117**, 488 (1964).
282. W. C. J. Ross, *Acta Unio Int. Contra Cancrum* **10** (2), 159 (1954).
283. W. C. J. Ross, "Biological Alkylating Agents." Butterworth, London, 1962.
284. W. C. J. Ross, *Biochem. Pharmacol.* **13**, 969 (1964).
285. J. M. van Rossum, E. J. Ariëns, and G. H. Linssen, *Biochem. Pharmacol.* **1**, 193 (1958).
286. M. Rubin and G. di Chiro, *Ann. N.Y. Acad. Sci.* **78**, 764 (1959).
287. J. Rüdinger and K. Jošt, *Proc. 2nd Int. Pharmacol. Meet., 1963.* **10**, 3 (1964).
288. I. Rychlik, *Proc. 2nd Int. Pharmacol. Meet., 1963.* **10**, 153 (1964).
289. F. J. Saunders, *Proc. Soc. Exp. Biol. Med.,* **123**, 303 (1966).
290. T. S. Scott, "Carcinogenic and Chronic Toxic Hazards of Aromatic Amines." Elsevier Monographs on Toxic Agents. Elsevier, Amsterdam, 1962.
290a. L. S. Schanker, *J. Pharmacol. Exp. Ther.* **126**, 283 (1959).
291. L. S. Schanker, *Pharmacol. Rev.* **14**, 501 (1962).
292. L. S. Schanker, *Advan. Drug Res.* **1**, 71 (1964).
293. L. S. Schanker, P. A. Shore, B. B. Brodie, and C. A. M. Hogben, *J. Pharmacol. Exp. Ther.* **120**, 528 (1957).
293a. R. W. Schayer, *Handbook Exp. Pharmacol.* **18**, 687 (1966).
294. I. Schechter and S. Hestrin, *J. Lab. Clin. Med.* **61**, 962 (1963).
295. W. Scholtan, *Arzneimittel-Forsch.* **11**, 707 (1961).
296. W. Scholtan, *Arzneimittel-Forsch.* **14**, 348, 469, 1139 (1964).
297. J. B. van der Schoot, "Central Stimulating Phenylethylamines," Ph.D. Thesis, University of Nijmegen. Nijmegen, 1961.
298. J. B. van der Schoot, E. J. Ariëns, J. M. van Rossum, and J. A. Th. M. Hurkmans, *Arzneimittel-Forsch.* **12**, 902 (1962).
299. F. W. Schueler, "Chemobiodynamics and Drug Design," p. 336. McGraw-Hill, New York, 1960.
300. F. W. Schueler, *Bull. Tulane Univ. Med. Fac.* **24**, 7 (1964).

301. F. W. Schueler, *Bull. Tulane Univ. Med. Fac.* **24**, 19 (1964).
302. R. Schwyzer, *Proc. Int. Congr. Pharm. Chem. 1962* (1963).
302a. R. Schwyzer, *Experientia* **26**, 577 (1970).
303. A. Sekera, *Actualités Pharmacol.* **14**, 197 (1961).
304. A. Sekera, J. Sova, and V. Vrba, *Experientia* **11**, 275 (1955).
305. S. K. Sharpless, *in* "The Pharmacological Basis of Therapeutics" (L. S. Goodman and A. Gilman, eds.), p. 105. Macmillan, New York, 1965.
306. P. A. Shore, B. B. Brodie, and C. A. M. Hogben, *J. Pharmacol. Exp. Ther.* **119**, 361 (1957).
307. E. N. Shkodinskaya, O. S. Vasina, A. Ya. Berlin, Z. P. Sofina, and L. F. Larionov, *Zh. Obshch. Khim.* **32**, 324 (1962).
308. M. van Sim, *in* "Drill's Pharmacology in Medicine" (J. R. DiPalma, ed.), p. 971. McGraw-Hill, New York, 1965.
309. M. Slavik, J. Elis, H. Raskova, M. Gutova, M. Duchkova, M. Kubikova, and V. Seycek, *Pharmacol. Clin.* **2**, 120 (1970).
310. J. V. Smart and P. Turner, *Brit. J. Pharmacol. Chemotherapy* **26**, 468 (1966).
310a. A. Soffer, "Chelation Therapy." Thomas, Springfield, Ill., 1964.
311. Z. P. Sofina, *Tr. 2nd Vses. Konf. Onkol.*, p. 773 (1959).
312. A. H. Soloway, *J. Med. Pharm. Chem.* **5**, 1371 (1962).
313. A. H. Soloway, *Progr. Boron Chem.* **1**, 203 (1964).
314. A. H. Soloway, B. Whitman, and J. R. Messer, *J. Pharmacol. Exp. Ther.* **129**, 310 (1960).
315. K. J. Sterling, *Clin. Invest.* **43**, 1721 (1964).
316. J. A. Stock, "Amino Acids and Peptides with Antimetabolic Activity," p. 89. Churchill, London, 1958.
317. L. A. Stocken and R. H. S. Thompson, *Physiol. Rev.* **29**, 168 (1949).
317a. T. Struller, *Progr. Drug Res.* **12**, 389 (1968).
318. M. I. Surks and J. H. Oppenheimer, *Endocrinology* **72**, 567 (1963).
319. E. E. Swanson, W. R. Gibson, and W. J. Doran, *J. Amer. Pharm. Assoc. Sci. Ed.* **44**, 152 (1955).
320. M. E. Synerholm and P. W. Zimmerman, *Contrib. Boyce Thompson Inst.* **14**, 369 (1947).
320a. D. H. Tedeschi, R. E. Tedeschi, P. J. Fowler, H. Green, and E. J. Fellows, *Biochem. Pharmacol.* **11**, 481 (1962).
321. T. R. Tephly, R. E. Parks, and G. J. Mannering, *J. Pharmacol. Exp. Ther.* **143**, 296 (1964).
322. L. Ther, *Med. Chem.* **6**, 399 (1958).
323. J. Thomas and J. R. Stoker, *J. Pharm. Pharmacol.* **13**, 129 (1961).
324. P. E Thompson, B. J. Olszewski, E. F. Elslager, and D. F. Worth, *Amer. J. Trop. Med. Hyg.* **12**, 481 (1963).
325. R. E. Thompson and R. A. Hecht, *Amer. J. Clin. Nutr.* **7**, 311 (1959).
326. J. M. Thorp, *in* "Absorption and Distribution of Drugs" (T. B. Binns, ed.), p. 64. Livingstone, Edinburgh, 1964.
327. M. J. Thuillier and R. Domenjoz, *Anaesthesist* **6**, 163 (1957).
328. R. H. Travis and G. Sayers, *in* "The Pharmacological Basis of Therapeutics" (L. S. Goodman and A. Gilman, eds.), 3rd ed., p. 1608. Macmillan, New York, 1965.
329. P. Turner, J. H. Young, and J. Paterson, *Nature* **215**, 881 (1967).
330. H. Ueberberg, U. Chuchra, and K. Liebrich, *Arzneimittel-Forsch.* **16**, 487 (1966).
331. N. Valery, *Discovery* **25**, 26 (1964).
332. H. Vanderhaeghe, P. Kolosy, and M. Claesen, *J. Pharm. Pharmacol.* **6**, 119 (1954); **7**, 477 (1955).

333. L. Vargha, *Ann. N.Y. Acad. Sci.* **68**, 875 (1958).
334. L. Vargha, L. Toldy, O. Feher, and S. Lendvai, *J. Chem. Soc.*, p. 805 (1957).
335. L. Vargha, L. Toldy, O. Feher, T. Horvath, E. Kaztreiner, J. Kuszmann, and S. Lendvai, *Acta Physiol. Acad. Sci. Hung.* **91**, 305 (1961).
336. H. Veldstra, *Pharmacol. Rev.* **8**, 339 (1965).
336a. A. J. Verbiscar and L. G. Abood, *J. Med. Chem.* **13**, 1176 (1970).
337. A. Vermeulen, Thesis, University of Ghent, Belgium, 1960.
338. J. van der Vies, *Acta Endocrinol.* **49**, 271 (1965).
338a. J. van der Vies, *Acta Endocrinol.* **64**, 656 (1970).
339. R. L. Volle, L. Peters, and R. E. Green, *J. Pharmacol. Exp. Ther.* **129**, 377 (1960).
340. Z. Votava, J. Metỹs, J. Metỹsová-Srámková, *Pharmacotherapeutica 1950–1959. Anniversary Res. Inst. Pharm. Biochem. 10th Prague 1960*, p. 307 (1961).
341. W. J. Waddell and T. C. Butler, *J. Clin. Invest.* **36**, 1217 (1957).
342. H. N. Wagner, Jr., *Clin. Pharmacol. Ther.* **4**, 351 (1963).
343. J. G. Wagner, *J. Pharm. Sci.* **50**, 359 (1961).
343a. Th. Wagner-Jauregg, "Therapeutische Chemie," p. 160. Hans Buber, Bern, 1949.
344. C. R. Walk, T. C. Chou, and H. H. Lin, *J. Med. Chem.* **10**, 255 (1967).
345. S. S. Walkenstein, R. Wiser, C. H. Gudmundsen, H. B. Kimmel, and R. A. Corradino, *J. Pharm. Sci.* **53**, 1181 (1964).
345a. M. E. Wall, G. S. Abernethy, F. I. Carroll, and D. J. Taylor, *J. Med. Chem.* **12**, 810 (1969).
346. I. M. Weiner, *Ann. Rev. Pharmacol.* **7**, 39 (1967).
347. I. M. Weiner, J. A. Washington, and G. H. Mudge, *Bull. Johns Hopkins Hosp.* **106**, 333 (1960).
348. L. Weinstein, *in* "The Pharmacological Basis of Therapeutics" (L. S. Goodman and A. Gilman, eds.), 3rd ed., p. 1144. Macmillan, New York, 1965.
349. A. D. Welch, *Cancer Res.* **21**, 1475 (1961).
350. E. O. Westermann, *Proc. 1st Int. Pharmacol. Meet. 1961.* **6**, p. 205 (1963).
351. U. Westphal, *in* "Mechanism of Action of Steroid Hormones" (C. A. Villee, ed.), p. 33. Pergamon Press, New York, 1961.
352. O. v. St. Whitelock, *Ann. N.Y. Acad. Sci.* **78**, 705 (1959).
353. R. T. Williams, "Detoxication Mechanisms." Wiley, New York, 1959.
354. C. E. Williamson, J. I. Miller, S. Sass, J. Casanova, S. P. Kramer, A. M. Seligman, and B. Witten, *J. Nat. Cancer Inst.* **31**, 273 (1963).
355. J. Winkelman, *Experientia* **23**, 949 (1967).
356. Ch. A. Winter and C. C. Porter, *J. Amer. Pharm. Assoc. Sci. Ed.* **46**, 515 (1957).
357. W. Wirth and F. Hoffmeister, *in* "Berichte Arbeitstagung der Deutschen Gesellschaft für Anaesthesie" (K. Horatz, R. Frey and M. Zindler, eds.), p. 17. Springer, Berlin, 1965.
358. B. Witten, C. E. Williamson, S. Sass, J. I. Miller, R. Rest, G. E. Wicks Jr., S. P. Kramer, T. Weinberg, R. D. Solomon, L. E. Goodman, and A. M. Seligman, *Cancer* **15**, 1041 (1962).
359. B. Witten, S. Sass, J. I. Miller, C. E. Williamson, H. Guerrero, S. P. Kramer, R. D. Solomon, L. E. Goodman, and A. M. Seligman, *Cancer* **15**, 1062 (1962).
359a. G. M. Woodwell, *Sci. Amer.* **216**, 24 (1967).
360. K. Yagi, J. Okuda, A. A. Dmitrovskii, R. Honda, and T. Matsubara, *J. Vitaminol. (Kyoto)* **7**, 4 (1961).
361. M. Zaoral, V. Pliška, K. Režábek, and F. Sorm, *Collection Czech. Chem. Commun.* **28**, 747 (1963).
362. M. Zaoral and F. Sorm, *Proc. 2nd Int. Pharmacol. Meet. 1963.* **10**, 167 (1964).
363. E. R. Zartman, Advances in Planned Parenthood. Int. Congr. Series no. 138, 116, 1967. Excerpta Med. Found., Amsterdam.

Chapter 2   Factors in the Design of Reversible and Irreversible Enzyme Inhibitors

Howard J. Schaeffer

I. Introduction

We have reached the stage where the theories concerning the action of enzyme or receptor systems have been removed from an aura of mysticism. It is now recognized, although not yet fully understood, that mechanisms of enzymic or receptor systems obey the laws of chemistry. The unique property of enzymes is their extraordinary ability to catalyze chemical reactions. A general mechanism by which enzymes function can be depicted in the following manner (1):

$$E + S \underset{k_{-1}}{\overset{k_1}{\rightleftharpoons}} E \cdots S \overset{k_2}{\longrightarrow} E + P$$

where E = free enzyme, S = substrate, E$\cdots$S = the initial enzyme–substrate complex, and P = product. In the simplest case, the process may be a two-step reaction. In the more complex case, the formation of the E$\cdots$S complex and its conversion to products may be a multistep procedure which is controlled by the rate-limiting step. In all cases, however, attractive forces exist between the enzyme and the substrate which control the formation of the initial reversible ES complex. The specificity of enzymic reactions is initially governed by the formation of the ES complex. The second phase of enzyme specificity is controlled when reactive functional groups on the enzyme and the substrate are properly juxtapositioned in the ES complex to allow reaction to occur. In the reaction step, covalent bonds may or may not be formed between the enzyme and substrate. However, in the formation of the initial ES complex, noncovalent interactions between the enzyme and the substrate are involved. The types of bonds that may be involved in the initial ES complex are charge–charge interactions, hydrogen bonding, protein–water interactions, and hydrophobic bonding (2). The types of interactions, the number of each type, the strength of each interaction, and the stereochemical relationship of the various types of interaction are sufficient to control whether or not an ES complex will form. Furthermore, if the ES complex does form, these non-covalent interaction parameters will determine whether or not the potentially reactive groups on the substrate and enzyme will be properly oriented to allow chemical reaction to occur. Certain enzymes can, in fact, utilize more than one small molecule as their substrate. However, in these cases there exists a striking similarity of structure in those compounds which serve as substrates so that the enzyme exhibits a specificity by virtue of the class of chemical compounds which will undergo enzymic reaction. Thus, the conclusion emerges that the binding of small molecules to enzymes need not be absolutely specific. When an enzyme and a molecule form a reversible complex which does not yield a product; i.e., $k_2 = 0$, inhibition of the enzymic reaction results.* This equilibrium can be depicted as:

$$E + I \underset{k_{-1}}{\overset{k_1}{\rightleftharpoons}} EI$$

In the simplest cases, reversible inhibitors can be classified into two main types: (1) competitive and (2) noncompetitive inhibitors.† Irreversible enzyme inhibitors will be discussed in a later section of this chapter. Competitive inhibitors react reversibly with the free enzyme to form an EI complex which

* For a description of the isolation and purification and for a discussion of mechanism of reaction and inhibition of enzymes, see, for example, Dixon and Webb (3), Webb (4), and Hochster and Quastel (5).

† There are, in fact, many types of reversible inhibitors such as uncompetitive and various mixed types of mechanisms. For a more complete discussion, see Dixon and Webb (3) and Webb (4).

prevents the enzyme from combining with the substrate. This is not to say that the competitive inhibitor and substrate complex to the same site on the enzyme; it does say that the binding of the substrate and competitive inhibitor is mutually exclusive (6). Too often the assumption has been made that competitive inhibitors complex at the active site of the enzyme. While it is true that a competitive inhibitor *might* complex at the active site, it is equally true that a competitive inhibitor might complex at a different site. Unless experimental evidence is presented to support one possibility or the other, it is clearly unwarranted to make the assumption that competitive inhibitors complex at the active site of the enzyme. Noncompetitive enzyme inhibitors react with the enzyme in such a way that the formation of the ES complex is not prevented; rather, noncompetitive inhibitors function by inhibiting the breakdown of the ES complex into products.

From considerations concerning enzyme specificity and substrate-binding requirements, the classical antimetabolite theory was developed.* This theory suggests that it is best to prepare inhibitors that exhibit only minor variations in structure compared to the natural substrate. This concept is based on classic work of Woods (8) and Fildes (9) on the relationship of sulfanilamide (I) and *p*-aminobenzoic acid (II) in bacterial systems. These investigators recognized that the structural similarity of the antimetabolite (I) compared

$$H_2N\!-\!\!\langle\quad\rangle\!-\!SO_2NH_2 \qquad\qquad H_2N\!-\!\!\langle\quad\rangle\!-\!COOH$$

I II

to the metabolite (II) was responsible for the antibacterial action. Since 1940 considerable effort has been expended making small structural changes in metabolites, but the number of clinically successful compounds which have evolved from the classical antimetabolite theory has been disappointingly small. Part of the problem has been the paucity of biochemical information concerning the mechanism of the various disease processes. Such information has become more readily available during the past decade, which should result in a greater frequency of success in the future.

An additional problem with classical antimetabolites revolves around the question of selective toxicity.† Suppose that a single substrate is used by several different enzymes. It is highly probable that the active site, or more specifically the site required for binding the substrate to the various enzymes, will be

---

* For an extensive review, see Wooley (7).

† For an extensive discussion of the many factors involved in selective toxicity, see Albert (10).

either identical or at least extremely similar. Therefore, the chances of designing a reversible inhibitor of only one of these enzymes are small. Recently, a new approach to this problem of selectivity of enzyme inhibition has been advanced by B. R. Baker (*11, 12*). It has been suggested that an extra dimension of biological specificity could be obtained by the preparation of inhibitors which, after the initial formation of a reversible enzyme–inhibitor complex, irreversibly inactivate the enzyme by means of a covalent bond between the enzyme and the inhibitor. Such a mechanism can be depicted in the following manner:

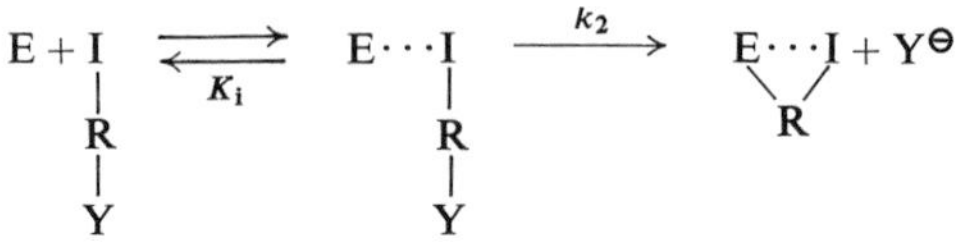

$$
\begin{array}{ccc}
\underset{\substack{|\\ R\\ |\\ Y}}{E+I} & \underset{K_i}{\rightleftharpoons} & \underset{\substack{|\\ R\\ |\\ Y}}{E\cdots I} \xrightarrow{k_2} \underset{\substack{\diagdown\diagup\\ R}}{E\cdots I}+Y^{\ominus}
\end{array}
$$

where

E = free enzyme

$\underset{\substack{Y}}{\overset{\substack{I\\ |}}{\underset{|}{R}}}$ = an inhibitor bearing a reactive grouping $\left(\begin{array}{c}R\\ |\\ Y\end{array}\right)$

$\underset{\substack{|\\ Y}}{\overset{\substack{I\\ |}}{E\cdots R}}$ = the initial reversible enzyme–inhibitor complex

$\underset{\substack{\diagdown\diagup\\ R}}{E\cdots I}$ = the inhibitor covalently bound to the enzyme

Reactions with macromolecules which occur by this mechanism have been termed active site-directed irreversible inhibition (*11, 12*), affinity labeling (*13*), and inhibition with bifunctional reagents (*14–17*).

The theoretical basis for active site-directed irreversible inhibitors has been summarized by Baker in the following three points (*11, 12*): "(a) enzymes are macromolecules that can form complexes with substrates and inhibitors; (b) enzymes have functional groups on their surfaces which can be attacked by chemical reagents with the formation of a covalent linkage; and (c) neighboring group reactions can be accelerated 1,000–10,000-fold compared to the same chemical reaction occurring by a bimolecular process."

A second concept which will probably have tremendous implications for selective toxicity is the bridge principle of specificity for active site-directed irreversible enzyme inhibitors. Baker has stated this concept as "Compared to a reversible inhibitor, the active site-directed type of irreversible inhibitor can have an extra dimension of specificity; this extra specificity is dependent upon the ability of the reversibly bound inhibitor to bridge to and form a covalent bond with a nucleophilic group on the enzyme surface and upon the nucleophilicity of the enzymic group being covalently linked" (6).*

II. Mechanism of Action of Selected Drugs

Most of the clinically useful drugs which are available today probably exert their biological response by reversible interactions with enzyme or receptor systems. While the molecular mechanism of action of many drugs is not yet completely understood, detailed descriptions of the mechanism of action of certain compounds have recently been presented. One of the compounds which has been extensively studied is the antileukemic agent, 6-mercaptopurine (III).† It has been established rather firmly that 6-mercapto-purine (III) must be activated *in vivo* before it exerts its biological effect. This activation is catalyzed by the enzyme, inosinic pyrophosphorylase, which normally causes the formation of inosinic acid (VII) from hypoxanthine (IV) and 5-phospho-D-ribofuranosyl-1-pyrophosphate (V). When III is utilized as a substrate for this enzyme, it is converted into thioinosinic acid (VI). Studies with thioinosinic acid (VI) revealed that a number of enzymes that normally utilized purine ribonucleotides as their substrates were significantly inhibited. However, none of these inhibitions appeared to be large enough

III	R = S	VI	R = S
IV	R = O	VII	R = O

* See Baker (12, p. 173).

† For a comprehensive review, see Bennett and Montgomery (18).

to define the primary site of action of **VI**. It is known that in mammalian cells the normal biosynthetic pathway to the purine ribonucleotides did not usually employ preformed purines; rather, the purine ring is constructed in a multistep biosynthesis from a 5-phosphoribofuranosyl nucleus and that the first purine ribonucleotide product which is formed is inosinic acid (**VII**). The first step in the *de novo* synthesis of purine ribonucleotides is the condensation of 5-phospho-D-ribofuranosyl-1-pyrophosphate (**V**) with glutamine (**VIII**) to give 5-phosphoribosylamine (**IX**). The enzyme, glutamine ribosyl-pyrophosphate-5-phosphate amidotransferase, which catalyzes this reaction is subject to feedback inhibition by purine ribonucleo-

tides. By studying incorporation patterns into the nucleic acids of a series of isotopically labeled precursors in the presence and absence of 6-mercapto-purine (**III**) in neoplasms grown in mice, it was found that the key blockade of the biosynthetic pathway was prior to the formation of formylglycine-amide ribotide. Precursors further along the biosynthetic pathway were incorporated into the nucleic acids even in the presence of effective doses of 6-mercaptopurine. Since the first enzyme in this biosynthetic pathway is subject to feedback inhibition by purine ribonucleotides, it appears that the primary locus of action of **VI** is as a feedback inhibitor of glutamine ribosyl-pyrophosphate-5-phosphate amidotransferase (*19*). In fact, studies on the isolated enzyme have shown that thioinosinic acid (**VI**) is a potent feedback inhibitor of this enzyme (*18*).

One of the pathways by which 6-mercaptopurine is metabolized is by the enzyme, xanthine oxidase (XO). This enzyme reacts with 6-mercaptopurine (**III**) to give initially 6-thioxanthine (**X**) which undergoes further oxidation to 6-thiouric acid (**XI**). It was reasoned that by coadministration of a xanthine oxidase inhibitor with 6-mercaptopurine (**III**) it should be possible to lower the dose of 6-mercaptopurine (**III**) due to the sparing action of the xanthine oxidase inhibitor (*20*). The xanthine oxidase inhibitor which was employed was 4-hydroxypyrazolo 3,4-*d* pyrimidine (**XII**) which is also called allopurinol. When allopurinol was coadministered with 6-mercaptopurine, it did, in fact, exhibit a considerable protective effect toward 6-mercaptopurine (*20*). How-

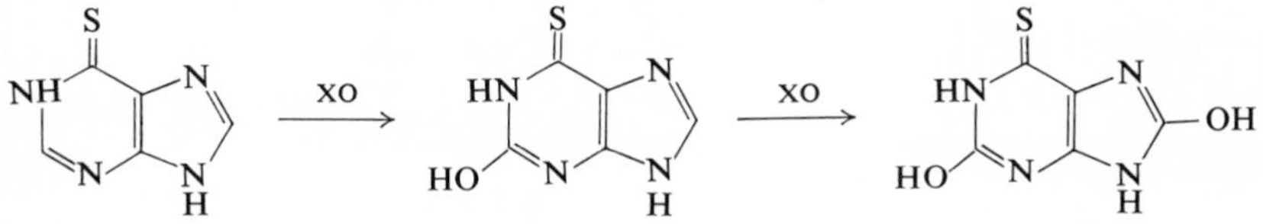

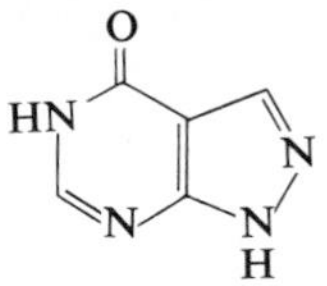

XII

ever, allopurinol (**XII**) exhibited a second effect which ultimately led to a new concept in the treatment of hyperuricemia as is found, for example, in gout (*21*). Individuals with primary gout tend to produce excessive quantities of the uric acid. The major catabolic pathway of the purine ribonucleotides is outlined in Scheme 1. Allopurinol (**XII**) functions in several different ways

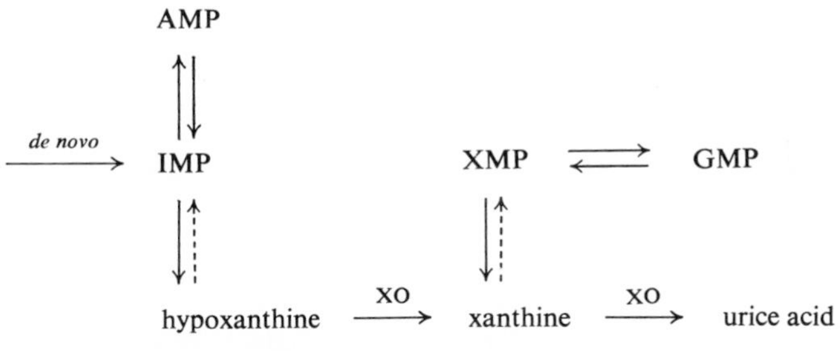

Scheme 1

which ultimately results in the control of uric acid production by utilizing the normal control mechanism present in the cell. As we have already in-dicated, allopurinol (**XII**) inhibits xanthine oxidase and therefore inhibits the formation of xanthine from hypoxanthine and the formation of uric acid from xanthine. Allopurinol (**XII**) is also a substrate of xanthine oxidase which leads to the formation of alloxanthine (**XIII**). Alloxanthine (**XIII**) is also an

inhibitor of xanthine oxidase but its ability to form complexes with the enzyme
is less than that of allopurinol (**XII**). Nevertheless, **XIII** exerts significant
activity because its renal elimination rate is lower than that of **XII**. Finally,

XIII

when xanthine oxidase is inhibited by **XII** and **XIII**, the increased levels of
hypoxanthine and xanthine are partly excreted and partly utilized in the
enzymic resynthesis of inosinic and xanthylic acids which, in turn, probably
results in the feedback inhibition of the first enzyme in the purine ribonucleotide biosynthesis; i.e., the enzyme that converts 5-phospho-D-ribofuranosyl-1-
pyrophosphate (**V**) to 5-phosphoribosylamine (**IX**). Thus, by utilizing the
control mechanism present in the cell, the production of uric acid can be
controlled without interfering with the other metabolic pathways required
by the cell (*21*).

There are a number of examples of compounds that exert their biological
effect by the mechanism of irreversible inhibition; probably the best known
of these is penicillin. Early studies on the anti-bacterial action of penicillin
suggested that the primary locus of action was at the level of the synthesis of
the cell wall. In general, penicillin kills gram-positive bacteria which are
rapidly growing and is relatively ineffective on cells in the resting state. Following exposure to penicillin, the morphology of the cell changes with the eventual
lysis of the cell. Elegant studies on the constitution of the cell wall have
established the structures of the major components of the cell wall as well as
elucidated the pathways of biosynthesis of these components (*22–24*).

In *Staphylococcus aureus*, the synthesis of the cell wall is initiated by the
formation of a linear polymer consisting of alternating units of *N*-acetyl-
glucosamine (**XIV**) and a pentapeptide derivative of *N*-acetylmuramic acid
(**XV**) containing L-alanine, D-isoglutamic acid, L-lysine, D-alanine, and D-

$$O{=}C \rightarrow \text{L-Ala} \rightarrow \text{D-isoGlu} \rightarrow \text{L-Lys} \rightarrow \text{D-Ala} \rightarrow \text{D-Ala}$$

XIV   **XV**

alanine. To the ϵ-amino group of lysine in the glycopeptide is added a penta-glycine chain. Finally, cross-linking occurs between adjacent linear glyco-peptides which produces the three-dimensional network of the cell wall. The cross-linking occurs by a transpeptidation between the terminal amino group of the pentaglycine chain on one polymer to the penultimate D-alanine residue of an adjacent glycopeptide resulting in the expulsion of the terminal D-alanine from that chain. Using partial structures, one can visualize the reaction in the manner shown in Scheme 2. By repetition of the transpeptidation

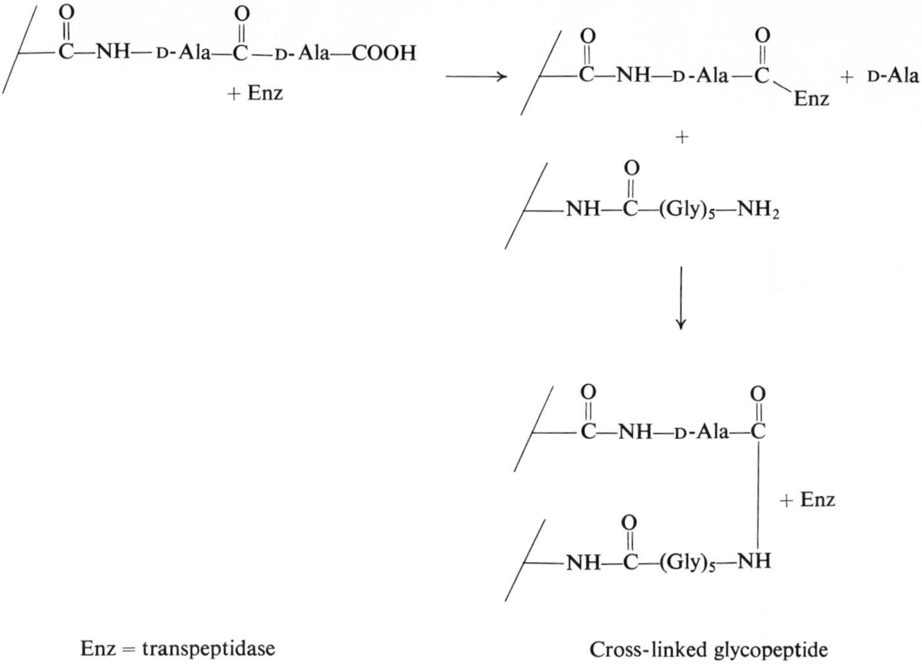

Enz = transpeptidase   Cross-linked glycopeptide

Scheme 2

reaction, one can easily visualize the biosynthesis of a highly cross-linked polymer which provides the appropriate physical properties of the cell wall. It has now been shown that penicillin is irreversibly bound to a component of the bacterial cell which results in an inhibition of the cross-linking reaction. It is postulated penicillin (**XVI**) acylates the transpeptidase enzyme with the formation of an acyl enzyme intermediate (23, 24). This covalently bound acyl enzyme intermediate is not susceptible to nucleophilic attack by the terminal amino group of the pentaglycine chain thereby causing irreversible inhibition of the cross-linking reaction as outlined in Scheme 3.

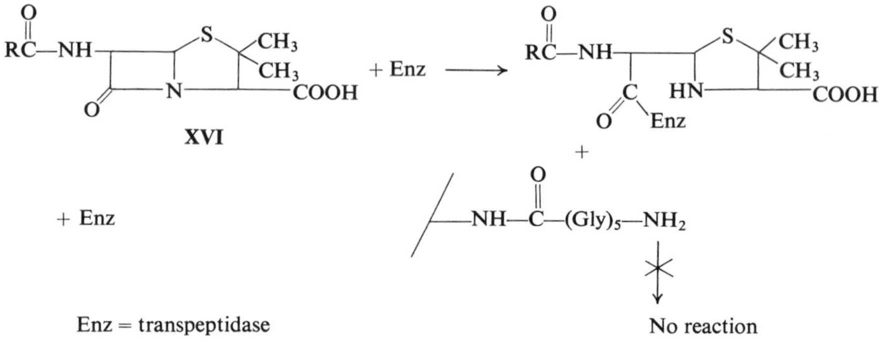

Enz = transpeptidase   No reaction

Scheme 3

III. Factors Involved in the Reversible Inhibition of Selected Enzymes

The biological specificity exhibited by enzymes must be a function of at least two processes. Initially, the specificity is controlled by the formation or lack of formation of the ES complex and secondly, if an ES complex is formed, reactive functional groups on the enzyme and the substrate must be properly positioned in the ES complex to allow reaction to occur. Since the formation of the initial reversible ES complex involves noncovalent interactions, one can prepare inhibitors by the synthesis of compounds that contain functional groups closely related to those found on the substrate. In this way, one would expect that the inhibitor could utilize the same binding regions on the enzyme as does the substrate. This type of inhibitor would have relatively small changes in structure compared to the natural substrate and, therefore would be best described as a classical antimetabolite. Generally, if an inhibitor and substrate have similar binding groups and form complexes with the same sites on the enzyme, one would not expect the inhibitor to form significantly better complexes than does the substrate. Consequently, the K_i of this type of inhibitor would usually be equal to or larger than the K_s of the substrate.* One way to overcome this difficulty is to probe the enzyme surface with inhibitors that contain functional groupings which are not present on the substrate in the hope of finding additional binding regions adjacent to the active site of the enzyme. By this procedure, it is theoretically possible to prepare inhibitors that are capable of forming a greater number of non-covalent bonds with the enzyme than does the substrate; therefore, the K_i of this type of inhibitor could be considerably smaller than the K_s of the substrate. Such inhibitors could be termed nonclassical antimetabolites (11).

We have not reached the stage where accurate predictions can be made

---

* K_s is the enzyme–substrate dissociation constant (k_{-1}/k_{+1}) and should not be confused with the Michaelis constant, $K_m[(k_{-1} + k_{+2})/k_{+1}]$.

concerning the number and types of accessory binding regions on various enzymes. X-ray crystallography has provided a tool which, in the future, may greatly improve such predictions of accessory binding regions (25). For the present, however, the most rapid procedure involves the synthesis of a series of potential inhibitors substituted by different types of functional groups.

During the past two decades, a number of interesting studies on the reversible inhibition of enzymes has been completed. No attempt will be made to survey all of this research; rather, one study will be described in detail that illustrates important points in the design and evaluation of enzyme inhibitors.

The importance of synthesizing inhibitors that can form complexes with accessory binding regions on the enzyme can be well illustrated by some studies on adenosine deaminase. Early studies have shown that neither adenine nor adenylic acid were inhibitors of this enzyme. However, a variety of 6-substituted purine nucleosides have been shown to be either substrates or inhibitors of adenosine deaminase (26–30). In a study of some nonnucleosidic 6-substituted purines, it was found that for a given 9-substituent, the adenine derivative was always the most potent inhibitor (31); therefore, our discussion will be limited to adenine derivatives and, in particular, to the effect that change in structure of the 9-substituent has on the inhibition of adenosine deaminase by some 9-substituted adenines. When a series of 9-(hydroxy-cycloalkyl)adenines was evaluated as inhibitors of adenosine deaminase, it was found that a hydroxyl group on the 2'-position of the cycloalkyl group makes a contribution to binding but hydroxyl groups located at other positions on the cycloalkyl group did not significantly influence inhibitory properties (31–34). Based on this data, it was concluded that there is a hydroxyl binding site on the enzyme and that the hydroxyl binding site is removed by two carbon atoms from the site to which the 9-position of adenine is complexed. In order to probe the enzyme for additional accessory bind areas, a series of 9-(ω-hydroxyalkyl)adenines (XVII–XXII) was prepared because the 9-substituent of these compounds would have more conformational freedom than would the cyclic analogs (35, 36). The interesting observation was made that for this series of compounds (XVII–XXII) as the ω-hydroxyalkyl chain was lengthened, the inhibitors initially became more potent, then less potent, and finally more potent again (Table I).* These effects were clearly distinct from those found

* The data in Tables I–V refer to adenosine deaminase which was obtained from calf intestinal mucosa. The assay was performed in 0.05 M phosphate buffer at pH 7.6. Unless otherwise noted, the substrate concentration was 0.066 mM. Those inhibitors which were only slightly soluble in phosphate buffer were dissolved in phosphate buffer containing 10% dimethyl sulfoxide.

The inhibition index $(I/S)_{0.5}$ = the ratio of the mM concentration of the inhibitor for 50% inhibition to the mM concentration of the substrate; i.e., the I_{50} divided by the substrate concentration. The I_{50} was determined from a plot of V_0/V vs. [I] where V_0 = initial velocity of the uninhibited reaction, V = initial velocity of the inhibited reaction at various inhibitor concentrations, and [I] = the various concentrations of inhibitor.

TABLE I[a]

Inhibition of Adenosine Deaminase by

Compound no.	R	$(I/S)_{0.5}$
XVII	HO—CH$_2$—CH$_2$—	1.1
XVIII	HO—CH$_2$—(CH$_2$)$_2$—	0.70
XIX	HO—CH$_2$—(CH$_2$)$_3$—	1.9
XX	HO—CH$_2$—(CH$_2$)$_4$—	3.0
XXI	HO—CH$_2$—(CH$_2$)$_5$—	1.7
XXII	HO—CH$_2$—(CH$_2$)$_7$—	0.64

[a] See footnote on page 139.

with the 9-(hydroxycycloalkyl)adenines; furthermore, in the 9-(ω-hydroxy-alkyl)adenines, it was found that the most potent inhibitor was obtained when the hydroxyl group was located on the 3-position of the alkyl chain. The variation in activity of the 9-(ω-hydroxyalkyl)adenines suggested that at least two factors were important in the complexation of the 9-substituent of the inhibitor with the enzyme. In addition to the hydroxyl binding site, adenosine deaminase possesses a hydrophobic region to which the 9-substituent of certain 9-(substituted) adenines can complex. To test this hypothesis, a series of 9-(n-alkyl)adenines (XXIII–XXX) were prepared (Table II), and it was found that the enzyme does, in fact, possess a rather large hydrophobic region (37).

Belleau and Lacasse have presented an excellent discussion on the importance of hydrophobic bonds in the formation of enzyme–inhibitor complexes. Based on their work (38) and the work of others (39), they conclude that the affinity of an inhibitor for the enzyme can be increased by hydrophobic transfer forces by a maximum of approximately −730 cal/methylene group. From quantitative solubility measurements on compounds that differ by a methyl or methylene group, it has been found that the transfer of a methyl or methylene group from an aqueous to a nonaqueous phase is accompanied by a maximum change in free energy of approximately −730 cal. The elegant studies of Hansch and his co-workers also support this figure; for example, $\pi = +0.52$ for a methyl group (40). Therefore, if a series of enzyme inhibitors differs by a methylene group, it would be expected that the maximum change in free energy due to the transfer of the inhibitor for the aqueous phase to the enzyme surface (nonaqueous phase) would be approximately −730 cal/ methylene group. Smaller changes in free energy/methylene group might be observed with enzyme inhibitors because the transfer of the inhibitor to the enzyme surface may not be ideal, as it could be in the transfer from, for example, water to octanol-1. Because of the change in free energy for each additional methylene group in **XXV–XXIX**, it is postulated that there is a nonpolar region on the enzyme to which the 9-alkyl substituent binds. This nonpolar

TABLE II[a]

Inhibition of Adenosine Deaminase by

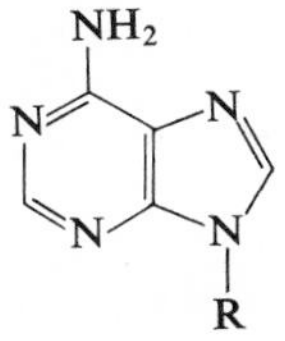

NH$_2$

R

Compound no.	R	$(I/S)_{0.5}$	ΔG (cal)/additional —CH$_2$—
XXIII	CH$_3$—	7.3	—
XXIV	CH$_3$—CH$_2$—	6.2	−98
XXV	CH$_3$—(CH$_2$)$_2$—	3.3	−362
XXVI	CH$_3$—(CH$_2$)$_3$—	2.3	−215
XXVII	CH$_3$—(CH$_2$)$_4$—	1.4	−292
XXVIII	CH$_3$—(CH$_2$)$_5$—	0.70	−408
XXIX	CH$_3$—(CH$_2$)$_6$—	0.32	−459
XXX	CH$_3$—(CH$_2$)$_7$—	0.24	−168

[a] See footnote on page 139.

region on the enzyme has a dimension which corresponds to a distance from the terminal carbon atom of the 9-*n*-propyl group (**XXV**) through the additional four carbon atoms of the 9-*n*-heptyl chain (**XXIX**). This conclusion is based on the observation that the change in free energy per methylene group is small when the 9-substituent is modified from methyl to ethyl (**XXIII → XXIV**) or from heptyl to octyl (**XXIX → XXX**) (*37*).

The second observation concerning the dimension of the hydrophobic region is based on the variation of the inhibition caused by the 9-(ω-hydroxy-alkyl)adenines. When the 9-position of the adenine group is substituted with a 2-hydroxyethyl (**XVII**) or a 3-hydroxypropyl group (**XVIII**), the compounds complex with the enzyme considerably better than the corresponding non-hydroxylated derivatives (**XXIV** and **XXV**) (*27*). It appears that a significant driving force for the formation of a complex between the enzyme and the 9-substituent of **XVII** or **XVIII** is the formation of a bond between the hydroxyl group of **XVII** and **XVIII** and the hydroxyl binding site on the enzyme. There is, however, a smaller contribution of a hydrophobic nature by the alkyl chain of **XVII** or **XVIII**. As the carbon chain of the 9-(ω-hydroxyalkyl)-adenines is lengthened, the hydroxyl group loses its ability to bind to the

TABLE III^a

INHIBITION OF ADENOSINE DEAMINASE BY

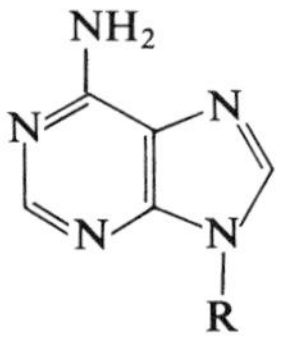

NH$_2$

R

Compound no.	R	$(I/S)_{0.5}$
XVII	HO(CH$_2$)$_2$—	1.1
XVIII	HO(CH$_2$)$_3$—	0.70
XXXI	DL—CH$_3$CH(OH)CH$_2$—	0.245
XXXII	D—CH$_3$CH(OH)CH$_2$—	1.48
XXXIII	L—CH$_3$CH(OH)CH$_2$—	0.148
XXXIV	C$_2$H$_5$CH(OH)CH$_2$—	1.2
XXXV	C$_5$H$_{11}$CH(OH)CH$_2$—	2.8
XXXVI	C$_6$H$_{13}$CH(OH)CH$_2$—	3.2
XXXVI	C$_6$H$_{13}$CH(OH)CH$_2$—	3.2

^{a} See footnote on page 139.

enzyme with the result that hydrophobic forces become the main driving force for the formation of a complex between the 9-substituent of the adenine derivatives and the enzyme. Note that in **XX** the hydroxyl group causes a decrease in binding relative to the nonhydroxylated derivative, a result which would be expected if the major driving force for the formation of a complex between the enzyme and the long carbon chain were hydrophobic in nature (*36*).

If there is a single hydroxyl binding site for the cycloaliphatic and acyclic derivatives, then the most effective position for a hydroxyl group in the acyclic derivatives should also be at the 2-position. Therefore, 9-(2-hydroxypropyl)-adenine (**XXXI**) was prepared (*41*), and it was found to be a better inhibitor of adenosine deaminase than **XVIII** (Table III). In the acyclic as well as the cyclic derivatives of adenine, it has been found that the strongest bonds can be formed between the hydroxy group and the enzyme when the hydroxyl group is located at the 2-position of the 9-substituent (*41*). In order to determine if the enzyme exhibits a stereoselectivity in complex formation with inhibitors, the D and L isomers (**XXXII** and **XXXIII**) of 9-(2-hydroxypropyl)adenine were prepared (*42*). It was found the L isomer (**XXXIII**) was a much better inhibitor than the D isomer (**XXXII**). Calculations of the change in free energy of binding of **XXXIII** compared to **XVII** show that the difference is −1.15 kcal, a value which cannot be accounted for only on the basis of hydrophobic transfer forces for a methyl group (*38*). Therefore, a positive involvement of van der Waals forces is invoked which occurs in a specific methyl binding site on the enzyme. That this region is specific for a methyl group and is different from the main hydrophobic area can be seen from the inhibition indices of **XXXIV**, **XXXV**, and **XXXVI** (Table III) (*43*). Compounds which possess a group larger than methyl on the carbon atom bearing the hydroxyl group are weaker inhibitors than **XXXI**. Consequently, there must be two nonpolar regions on the enzyme: a specific methyl binding region closely associated with the hydroxyl binding site and a second nonpolar region of considerably larger dimensions (*43*).

It is often an unstated assumption that two competitive inhibitors will form EI complexes at the same site on the enzyme. The fact that inhibitors act in a competitive manner does not prove this assumption, but it does establish that the binding of the two inhibitors is mutually exclusive.

One pathway to establish that two different reversible inhibitors bind to the same site is to combine in one molecule two or more of the different structural groups present in the separate inhibitors, each of which makes its own special contribution to the formation of an enzyme–inhibitor complex. Such a combined inhibitor will result in a compound with exceedingly strong inhibitory properties if the original two inhibitors were reversibly complexed in approximately the same manner at the same site. If, however, the original two inhibitors were complexed at different sites on the enzyme, one would not expect such an inhibitor to have greatly enhanced activity. For example, it is known that adenosine deaminase has a hydroxyl binding site and hydrophobic region. The presence of these sites has been demonstrated with compounds such as 9-(2-hydroxyethyl)adenine (**XXVII**) and the 9-*n*-alkyladenines (**XXV**–**XXX**). If the adenine moieties of **XVII** and **XXV**–**XXX** are complexed in a similar manner to the same site on adenosine deaminase, one would predict that the 9-(1-hydroxyl-2-alkyl)adenines should be potent enzymic inhibitors, since the 9-substituent of these compounds could bind to both the hydroxyl binding site as well as the hydrophobic region. The experimental verification of this prediction is shown in Table IV (*44*). In general, this series of inhibitors exhibits much greater inhibition than either of the two original inhibitors separately. For example, the $(I/S)_{0.5}$ of **XLIII** which may be viewed as an inhibitor combining structural features of **XVII** and **XXX** is 0.0047. This dramatic increase in potency of inhibition would be observed if the adenine moiety of both **XVII** and **XXX** complexed with the same site on the enzyme. An inspection of the change in free energy of binding per methylene unit reveals that the large hydrophobic area appears to terminate at approximately seven carbons in length since the ΔG/methylene group for **XLII** is

TABLE IV[a]

INHIBITION OF ADENOSINE DEAMINASE BY

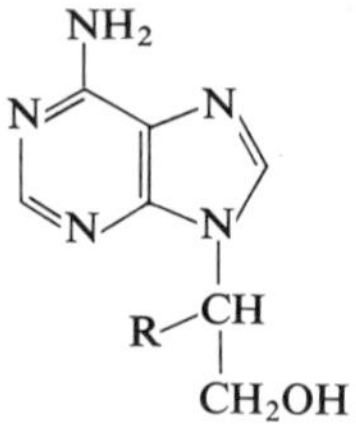

NH$_2$

R—CH
|
CH$_2$OH

Compound no.	R	$(I/S)_{0.5}$	ΔG(cal)/CH$_2$ unit
XVII	H—	1.1	—
XXXVII	CH$_3$—	1.2	—
XXXVIII	C$_2$H$_5$—	0.49	−521
XXXIX	C$_3$H$_7$—	0.071	−1140
XL	C$_4$H$_9$—	0.033	−451
XLI	C$_5$H$_{11}$—	0.015	−467
XLII	C$_6$H$_{13}$—	0.0062	−521
XLIII	C$_7$H$_{15}$—	0.0047	−163
XLIV	C$_8$H$_{17}$—	0.0039	−110
XLV	C$_9$H$_{19}$—	0.0030	−155

[a] See footnote on page 139.

−521 cal, whereas further increase in the carbon chain (**XLII–XLV**) gave near-minimum changes in free energy. Note the unusually large change in free energy for the addition of one methylene unit by comparing **XXXVIII** with **XXXIX**. The magnitude of this change in free energy is clearly beyond simple hydrophobic transfer forces (*38*) and may reflect a conformational change in the enzyme. It may well be that the large change in free energy in comparing **XXXVIII** to **XXXIX** will be the resultant of the entropy term since the inhibitors were designed to complex simultaneously with three regions on the enzyme (a purine binding region, a hydroxyl binding site, and a hydrophobic region). Experimental work on the thermodynamics of inhibition is needed before this question can be answered.

Once it had been shown that it was possible to obtain potent inhibitors by combining several binding moieties into a single molecule, it became apparent that the 9-(2-hydroxy-3-alkyl)adenines should be even more effective inhibitors. This type of compound would combine on the adenine nucleus the functions required to complex with the main hydrophobic region, the hydroxyl binding site and the specific methyl binding region. Studies with certain

TABLE V^a

INHIBITION OF ADENOSINE DEAMINASE BY

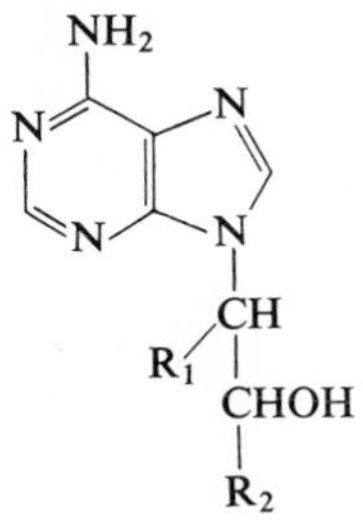

Compound no.		R_1	R_2	$(I/S)_{0.5}$
XVII		H—	H—	1.1
XXXI		H—	CH_3—	0.245
XLII		C_6H_{13}—	H—	0.0062
XLVI	(erythro)	C_6H_{13}—	CH_3—	0.00029
XLVII	(threo)	C_6H_{13}—	CH_3—	0.0045

^{a} See footnote on page 139.

optically active inhibitors suggested that of the 9-(2-hydroxy-3-alkyl)adenines the most potent inhibitors would have the *erythro* configuration (45). The data in Table V clearly demonstrate the effect of combining the various binding moieties into one molecule (45). The *erythro* derivative (XLVI) is an extremely potent inhibitor; the ratio of the $(I/S)_{0.5}$ of XVII and XLVI is almost 4000. The effect of steric configuration is also seen in a comparison of the *erythro* with the *threo* isomer (XLVI and XLIV).

By the stepwise alteration of the 9-substituent of adenine, information has been obtained concerning the size of the main hydrophobic area, the position of the hydroxyl binding site, and the presence of a specific methyl binding region. This data offers strong evidence that the adenine portion of these inhibitors all bind to the same site on adenosine deaminase and that the hydrophobic region, the hydroxyl binding site, and the specific methyl binding region are closely associated with the site to which adenine binds.

There are now a large number of studies on the reversible inhibition of various enzymes. Belleau has carried out extensive studies on the thermodynamics involved in the formation of EI complexes between acetylcholinesterase and n-alkyltrimethylammonium ions (46). A correlation was found between the entropies of binding of n-alkyltrimethylammonium ions on acetylcholinesterase and the corresponding pharmacological properties of the quaternary ions. Koshland has advanced the idea of an "induced fit" of the active site of an enzyme (47). Since the protein is a flexible molecule, the active site of the enzyme on complexation with substrates or inhibitors could assume different conformations. This conformational adaptability of the active site provides a number of interesting interpretations on the differences between substrates and inhibitors. An excellent discussion of reversible inhibition of dihydrofolic reductase, thymidine kinase and thymidine phosphorylase, chymotrypsin, trypsin, and guanine deaminase has recently been published (12).

IV. Irreversible Inhibition of Selected Enzymes

The formation of a covalent bond between a small molecule and an enzyme has previously been used primarily to perform end-group analyses or amino acid sequences on the protein. During the past ten years, however, there has been a rather rapid development of selective irreversible enzyme inhibitors that have been designed and synthesized to label the active site of the enzyme, to study the mechanism of the enzymic reaction, to serve as a reporter group (48), or to control the enzymic reaction with the hope of preparing chemotherapeutic agents. The remainder of this chapter will be devoted to a description of the studies carried out with several types of irreversible enzyme inhibitors.

An elegant example of the design and evaluation of an irreversible enzyme inhibitor comes from the work of Lawson and Schramm on the enzyme, chymotrypsin (14, 15). In order to take advantage of the enzymes' specificity, a bifunctional reagent was designed which would first form an acyl enzyme intermediate with the active site and after attachment to the enzyme, the second reactive function on the inhibitor could form a covalent bond with another amino acid which would be in close spatial proximity to the active site of the enzyme. The reagent which was prepared by Lawson and Schramm was p-nitrophenyl N-bromoacetyl-α-aminoisobutyrate (**XLVIII**). Incubation of chymotrypsin with **XLVIII** gave an initial rapid burst of p-nitrophenol corresponding to the formation of an acyl enzyme intermediate. The bromo-acetyl moiety of the covalently linked inhibitor was then selectively attacked by the sulfur atom of methionine-192. Finally, cleavage of the initial acyl enzyme bond occurred with the formation of an irreversible modified chymo-trypsin which retains approximately 20% of the original enzymic activity. Interestingly, this modified chymotrypsin with 20% activity is capable of reacting with diisopropylphosphorfluoridate (DFP) in a 1:1 ratio to give a totally inactive enzyme establishing that in the modified enzyme (20% activity) the hydroxyl group of serine-195 has been completely regenerated. The specificity of this inhibitor was shown by a variety of methods. Two of these methods were (1) if chymotrypsin was inactivated by DFP, the inactivated enzyme did not react with **XLVIII** and (2) the acid, N-bromoacetyl-α-amino-

XLVIII

isobutyric acid, which corresponds to the hydrolysis product of **XLVIII** was not capable of causing irreversible inhibition of chymotrypsin even though it was incubated at higher concentrations and longer times than was **XLVIII**. These and other data firmly establish that the mechanism of irreversible inactivation of chymotrypsin by **XLVIII** occurs through the formation of an acyl enzyme intermediate at serine-195 through which an intramolecular alkylation of methionine-192 occurs by the bromoacetyl moiety (*14, 15*).

A second approach to the design of a selective irreversible inhibitor of chymotrypsin is taken from the excellent work of Schoellmann and Shaw (*16, 17*). These authors utilized the concept of incorporating into the inhibitor two types as structural features; one type to provide affinity toward the enzyme and the second type to provide a functional group which is capable of forming a covalent bond with nucleophilic groups on the enzyme. Since it was known that the ethyl ester of N-tosyl-L-phenylalanine (**XLIX**) was a substrate for chymotrypsin, Schoellmann and Shaw selected the structurally related chloro-methyl ketone (**L**, TPCK) as a candidate irreversible inhibitor. Incubation of **L** with chymotrypsin did, in fact, cause irreversible enzyme inactivation. It was found that there was a 1:1 ratio of incorporation of **L** to enzyme, and it was shown by various hydrolytic procedures that histidine-57 had been alkylated by **L** and that the alkylation occurred at the 3-position of histidine-57. Furthermore, **L** did not react with DFP-inactivated chymotrypsin. In addition, if the inhibition of chymotrypsin by **L** was performed in the presence

XLIX   L (TPCK)

of the reversible inhibitor, β-phenylpropionic acid, the rate of irreversible inactivation was slowed. These and other data provide strong experimental evidence that the mechanism of irreversible inactivation of chymotrypsin by **L** proceeds via an initial reversible EI complex through which covalent bond formation with histidine-57 occurs.

Trypsin is a proteolytic enzyme that catalyzes the hydrolysis of peptides and esters from the carboxyl group of basic amino acids, arginine and lysine. Because the active centers of chymotrypsin and trypsin are quite similar, a candidate irreversible inhibitor was designed related to **L** but modified in such a way that it was a structural analog of lysine; the compound is 1-chloro-3-tosylamido-7-amino-2-heptanone (**LI**, TLCK) (*49*). Incubation of **LI** with trypsin resulted in an irreversible inactivation of the enzyme. By criteria similar to that used for TPCK (**L**) and chymotrypsin, it was shown that only one of the three histidines in trypsin was alkylated. Furthermore, it was

LI   (TLCK)

shown that TLCK (**LI**) did not react with chymotrypsin and that TPCK (**L**) did not react with trypsin. Such specificity of reaction is almost certainly due to the formation of an initial reversible EI complex; i.e., TLCK (**LI**) forms such a complex with trypsin but not chymotrypsin whereas the reverse is true for TPCK (**LI**).

V. Kinetics of Irreversible Enzyme Inactivation

When an enzyme is irreversibly inhibited by an alkylating or acylating agent, at least two different mechanisms can be visualized: a bimolecular attack of the inhibitor on the enzyme [Eq. (1)] or the initial formation of a reversible enzyme–inhibitor complex through which covalent bond formation occurs [Eq. (2)].* These two mechanisms are kinetically distinguishable since in the case of the bimolecular mechanism [Eq. (1)], increases in the

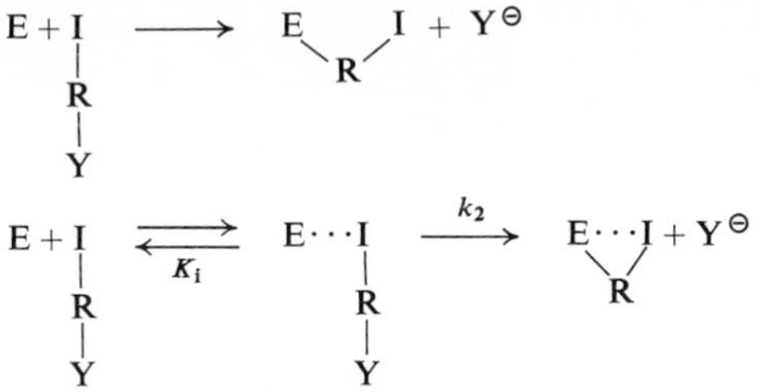

$$
\begin{array}{c}
E + I \longrightarrow E \diagdown_{R} I + Y^{\ominus} \\
\mid \\
R \\
\mid \\
Y
\end{array}
\tag{1}
$$

$$
\begin{array}{c}
E + I \underset{K_i}{\rightleftarrows} E\cdots I \xrightarrow{k_2} E\cdots I + Y^{\ominus} \\
\mid \qquad\quad \mid \qquad\quad \diagup_{R} \\
R \qquad\quad R \\
\mid \qquad\quad \mid \\
Y \qquad\quad Y
\end{array}
\tag{2}
$$

inhibitor concentration would result in corresponding increases in the rate of inactivation for all concentrations of inhibitor. However, when an initial reversible enzyme–inhibitor complex is formed, increases in the concentration of the inhibitor would result in an increase in the rate of irreversible inactivation only until the enzyme became saturated with inhibitor in the reversible $E\cdots I$ complex [Eq. (2)]. Further increases in the concentration of the inhibitor would not affect the rate of irreversible inactivation. This phenomenon has been termed the "rate-saturation effect" (50). In order to evaluate the "rate-saturation effect," Baker, Lee, and Tong have derived Eq. (5) in the following way (50)†:

$$
K_i = [E][I]/[EI]
\tag{3}
$$

$$
[E_t] = [E] + [EI]
\tag{4}
$$

Substituting Eq. (4) into Eq. (3) gives Eq. (5)

$$
[EI] = \frac{E_t}{(K_i/[I]) + 1}
\tag{5}
$$

where [E] is the concentration of free enzyme, [I] the concentration of inhibitor, [EI] the concentration of the reversible enzyme–inhibitor complex, K_i the dissociation constant of this complex, and [E_t] the total enzyme concentration.

---

* For a discussion of other mechanisms for irreversible inhibition, see Baker (12, p. 122).
† See Baker (12).

Because an irreversible enzyme inactivation proceeding by the mechanism shown in Eq. (2) depends on both K_i and k_2, an expression has been derived which separates these two kinetic parameters in order to gain a more complete understanding of the reaction mechanism (51). If an irreversible inactivation of an enzyme proceeds through an initial reversible enzyme–inhibitor complex and follows apparent first-order kinetics, the rate of irreversible inactivation (R) is described by Eq. (6).

$$R = k_2[EI] \tag{6}$$

Substituting Eq. (5) into Eq. (6) gives Eq. (7)

$$R = \frac{k_2[E_t]}{(K_i/[I]) + 1} \tag{7}$$

Since $\qquad\qquad\qquad R/[E_t] = k_{obs} \tag{8}$

where k_{obs} is the observed first-order rate constant for enzyme inactivation at the various concentrations of inhibitor, then

$$k_{obs} = \frac{k_2}{(K_i/[I]) + 1} = \frac{k_2[I]}{K_i + [I]} \tag{9}$$

Taking the reciprocal of (9) gives (10).

$$\frac{1}{k_{obs}} = K_i/k_2 \cdot 1/[I] + 1/k_2 \tag{10}$$

Therefore, if a series of irreversible enzyme inactivations are performed at various concentrations of inhibitor, a plot of $1/k_{obs}$ vs. $1/[I]$ should give a straight line whose intercept would be $1/k_2$ and whose slope would be K_i/k_2. The use of this procedure allows one to evaluate both the reversible dissociation constant (K_i) and the first-order rate constant for the alkylation of the enzyme by the inhibitor (k_2) (51).

The utility of this kinetic procedure is well illustrated by a study of the irreversible inhibition of adenosine deaminase. As was described previously, adenosine deaminase has a hydrophobic region on the enzyme to which the 9-substituent of some 9-substituted adenines complexes. Since it had been found that 9-benzyladenine was a good reversible competitive inhibitor of adenosine deaminase, 9-(o-,m-, and p-bromoacetamidobenzyl)adenines (LII, LIII, and LIV) were prepared as candidate irreversible inhibitors (52–54). By performing short-term enzyme experiments, it was found that all three compounds were initially competitive inhibitors of adenosine deaminase and that the effectiveness of the initial reversible inhibition decreases in the following order: para isomer (LIV) > meta isomer (LIII) > ortho isomer (LII). When these compounds were incubated with adenosine deaminase, it was found that the *ortho* and *para* isomers (**LII** and **LIV**) caused a rapid irreversible inactivation whereas the rate of enzymic inactivation with the *meta* isomer (**LIII**) was extremely low. These results suggest that the irreversible enzyme inactivation proceeds through an initial, reversible EI complex and that **LII** and **LIV** alkylate different amino acids on the enzyme; when **LIII** forms an initial, reversible EI complex with the enzyme, the bromoacetamido moiety is not easily able to bridge to either of the amino acids alkylated by **LII** or **LIV**. Therefore the rate of inactivation by **LIII** is extremely slow. In order to

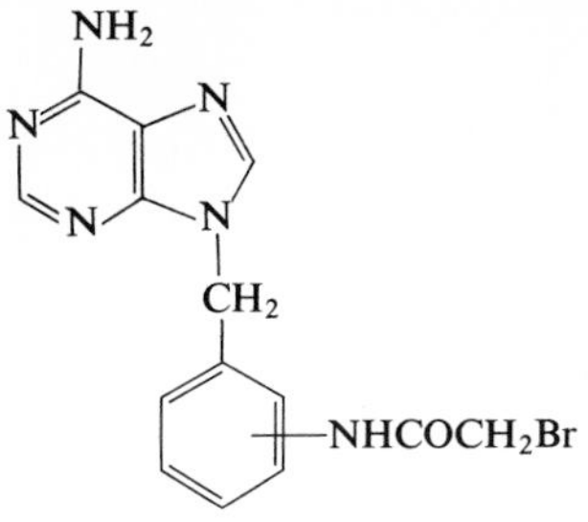

LII, *ortho* isomer
LIII, *meta* isomer
LIV, *para* isomer

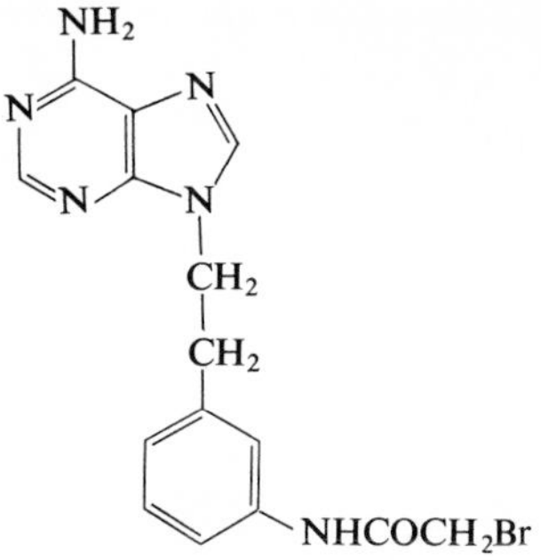

LV

test this hypothesis, 9-(*m*-bromoacetamidophenethyl)adenine (**LV**) was synthesized (*55*). Thus, compared to **LIII**, lengthening the chain by one carbon atom might allow the bromoacetamido group of **LV** to bridge and react more readily with a nucleophilic group on the enzyme. When **LV** was evaluated as an inhibitor of adenosine deaminase, it was found to be a weaker reversible inhibitor than **LIII**, but when it was incubated with the enzyme, a rapid irreversible inactivation occurred.

When **LII** and **LIV** were incubated with the enzyme, it was found that they caused greater than 95% enzyme inactivation; however, **LV** irreversibly inactivated the enzyme only to an extent of $80 \pm 5\%$. That the enzyme has been completely alkylated by **LV** was shown in the following way. The enzyme and **LV** were allowed to react until there was no further decrease in the rate of inactivation at which time an additional volume of freshly prepared inhibitor solution (**LV** or **LIV**) was added. Incubation of this solution *did not* result in a further decrease of enzymic activity (see Fig. 1). However, when the enzyme was irreversibly inactivated with **LV** until no further decrease in the rate was observed and then a freshly prepared solution of **LII** was added, an additional decrease in the rate of enzymic activity was noted (see Fig. 2).

Based on these results, it is postulated that **LIV** and **LV** alkylate the same amino acid, whereas **LII** alkylates a different amino acid on the enzyme. Furthermore, when **LV** has completely alkylated the enzyme, there remains a residual enzyme activity of 20%. These results have a bearing on the mechanism of inhibition. When the enzyme has been alkylated in the initial reversible enzyme–inhibitor complex by **LII** or **LIV**, it is postulated that

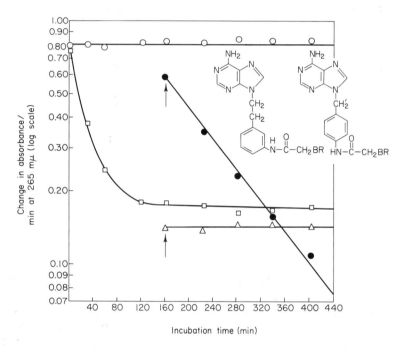

Fig. 1. Irreversible inhibition of adenosine deaminase by 9-(*m*-bromoacetamidophen-ethyl)adenine (**LV**): ○ = enzyme control; □ = **LV**. At 160 min, 9-(*p*-bromoacetamidoben-zyl)adenine (**LIV**) was added to aliquots of the control (●) and the inhibited enzyme solution (△).

the adenine moiety of the inhibitor is either juxtapositioned over the active site of the enzyme or the adenine moiety still forms a tight reversible complex with the active site. Thus, for steric reasons the substrate can no longer complex with the active site of the enzyme. When adenosine deaminase has been inactivated by **LV**, the additional methylene group in the 9-substituent of the inhibitor does not allow the adenine moiety to be ideally juxtapositioned over the active site. Consequently, there remains a residual enzymic activity of 20% (*55*).

In order to determine the kinetic constants for the irreversible inhibition for **LII**, **LIV**, and **LV**, the amount of irreversible inactivation was measured at various timed intervals for a variety of concentrations of each inhibitor. From these data, the k_{obs} for each inhibitor concentration was calculated. A plot of $1/k_{obs}$ vs. $1/[I]$ is shown in Fig. 3, and a comparison of the constants calculated from Fig. 3 is given in Table VI. The excellent agreement of the

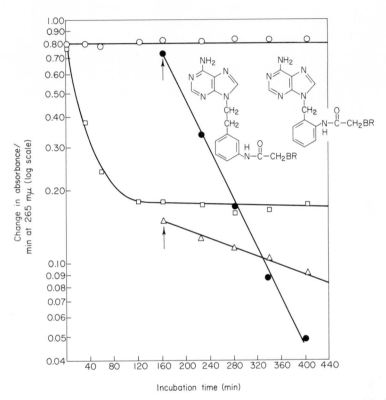

Fig. 2. Irreversible inhibition of adenosine deaminase by 9-(*m*-bromoacetamidophenethyl)adenine (**LV**): ○ = enzyme control; □ = **LV**. At 160 min, 9-(*o*-bromoacetamidobenzyl)adenine (**LII**) was added to aliquots of the control (●) and the inhibited enzyme solutions (△).

values obtained for the K_i from the irreversible inactivation experiments compared with those obtained by the Lineweaver-Burk method from the short-term experiments offers strong experimental support for the mechanism as outlined in Eq. (2), especially in view of the observation that iodoacetamide had little or no effect on the enzyme even at concentrations of 1.6 mM.

Finally, the results of irreversible inactivation of adenosine deaminase by **LII**, **LIV**, and **LV** demonstrate an important principle which must be considered when comparisons are made between irreversible inhibitors. If comparisons are made at only one inhibitor concentration, it is possible to draw erroneous conclusions concerning the relative effectiveness of the inhibitors. For example, if irreversible inactivations were performed with 0.1 mM concentration of the inhibitors, the following order of effectiveness would be found: $LV > LII > LIV$. If, however, similar inactivation were performed at 0.03 mM, the apparent order of effectiveness would be $LV > LIV > LII$ (see Fig. 3). This apparent change in the order of effectiveness occurs because the observed first-order loss of enzyme activity is a function of both K_i and

TABLE VI[a]

KINETIC CONSTANTS FOR THE REVERSIBLE AND IRREVERSIBLE INHIBITION OF
ADENOSINE DEAMINASE

Compound no.	$k_2 \times 10^2$ (min^{-1})	$K_i \times 10^5\ M$[b]	$K_i \times 10^5\ M$[c]
LII	7.7	43	44
LIV	1.1	1.4	1.3
LV	28	72	—

[a] Data taken from *51* and *55*.
[b] Calculated from irreversible inactivation experiments.
[c] Calculated from Lineweaver-Burk plots with short-term experiments.

k_2. It is clear that in comparing irreversible inhibitors, the observed first-order inactivation should not be used unless the K_i's of the compounds are equal. Rather, the comparison should be made by the procedure described in this chapter so that both K_i and k_2 are evaluated.

Several other studies of the kinetics of irreversible inhibition have been reported. Main and co-workers have measured the affinity and phosphorylation constants of some irreversible inhibitors of choline esterases (*56, 57*). Gold and Fahrney have studied the irreversible inhibition of chymotrypsin (*58*) and recently Brox and Hampton have studied the kinetics of irreversible inhibition of inosine 5'-phosphate dehydrogenase with the 6-chloro analog of inosine 5'-phosphate (*59*).

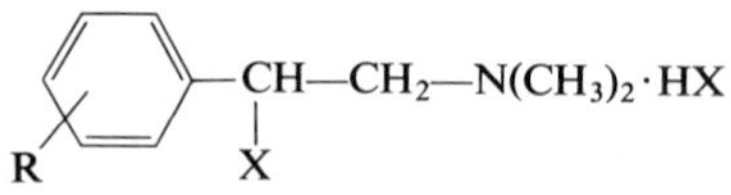

$$\text{R} \overset{}{\underset{}{\bigcirc}} - \text{CH} \underset{\overset{|}{\text{X}}}{} - \text{CH}_2 - \text{N(CH}_3)_2 \cdot \text{HX}$$

(R = H, *m*- or *p*- Br, OMe)

LVI

An examination of the kinetics of irreversible enzyme inhibition reveals that subtle changes in chemical structure can affect either K_i, k_2, or both parameters. For example, Belleau and Tani have prepared some substituted N,N-dimethyl-2-halo-2-phenethylamines (**LVI**) as irreversible inhibitors of acetylcholine (*60*). Incubation of these compounds with the enzyme revealed that only the unsubstituted phenyl derivative (**LVI, R = H**) was an irreversible inhibitor. The substituted phenyl derivatives did form complexes with the

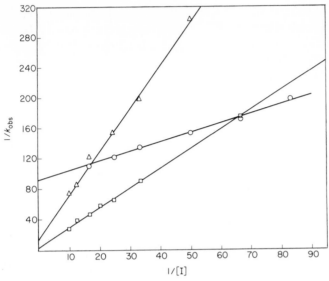

Fig. 3. Plot of $1/k_{obs}$ for irreversible inactivation of adenosine deaminase vs. $1/[I]$; $\triangle = 9$-(*o*-bromoacetamidobenzyl)adenine, $\square = 9$-(*m*-bromoacetamidophenethyl)adenine, $\bigcirc = 9$-(*p*-bromoacetamidobenzyl)adenine.

enzyme since they were shown to be competitive inhibitors of acetylcholinesterase. Based on these results, it was suggested that only the unsubstituted phenyl derivative (**LVI, R = H**) can induce in the anionic site of the enzyme the type of fit which is necessary to allow covalent bond formation. Such subtle effects make the task of preparing irreversible enzyme inhibitors a formidable challenge, but it also suggests that irreversible inhibitors can be designed that will be target enzyme-specific.

VI. Tissue-Specific Irreversible Enzyme Inhibitors

One of the most exciting concepts in the design of selective enzyme inhibitors has been advanced by the prolific research worker, B. R. Baker (*61*). This concept is based on the observation that the structure of enzymes that utilize identical substrates may vary from one animal to another or from one tissue to another in the same animal. For these substrate-identical enzymes, it is reasonable to assume that the binding requirements for the substrate at the active site will be either identical or nearly so. Thus, it is not likely that the active sites of the substrate-identical enzymes isolated from different sources will be largely different; rather, it is more probable that the differences which exist in substrate-identical enzymes will be found in the amino acid sequence outside of the active site. Consequently, if classical antimetabolites are employed, i.e., compounds which utilize the same binding sites as the substrate, one would not expect much selectivity in the inhibition of substrate-identical enzymes from different sources since the active sites of these enzymes will probably be identical. Based on the structural differences outside of the active site in substrate-identical enzymes, Baker proposed that it should be possible to select a target enzyme and by the use of the bridge principle of selectivity, irreversibly inhibit the target enzyme while leaving another substrate-identical enzyme functional. This unique proposal will undoubtedly have tremendous importance in chemotherapy.

In the short span of ten years, Baker and his co-workers have synthesized and studied reversible inhibitors, and in many cases, irreversible inhibitors of the following enzymes: lactic dehydrogenase (*12*), glutamic dehydrogenase (*12*), thymidine kinase (*12, 62*), thymidine phosphorylase (*12, 63*), thymidylate synthetase (*12, 64*), chymotrypsin (*65*), trypsin (*66*), succinoadenylate kinosynthetase (*12*), guanine deaminase (*12, 67*), xanthine oxidase (*12, 68*), cytosine nucleoside deaminase (*69*), 5,10-methylene-1-tetrahydrofolate dehydrogenase (*12*), and dihydrofolate reductase (*12, 69*). Clearly, the review of all of this work is beyond the scope of this chapter; rather, as has been done previously, selected examples will be discussed which demonstrate important concepts and principles.

In a brilliant series of experiments, Baker has designed compounds which cause selective irreversible inhibition of substrate-identical enzymes (*11, 12*). After a comprehensive study of the reversible and irreversible inhibition of lactic and glutamic dehydrogenase, Baker selected the rabbit skeletal muscle and beef heart isozymes of lactic dehydrogenase for further development of irreversible inhibitors of substrate-identical enzymes. 4-(Iodoacetamido)-salicylic acid (**LVII**) was found to be an irreversible inhibitor of skeletal muscle, but not heart lactic dehydrogenase. When the bridge carrying the alkylating function was lengthened as in **LVIII** both lactic dehydrogenases were irreversibly inhibited but at different absolute rates. Crossover of specificity was observed with the 5- and 4-(phenoxycarbonylamino)salicylic acids (**LIX** and **LX**). The 5 isomer (**LIX**) irreversibly inhibited the heart, but not the skeletal muscle lactic dehydrogenase, whereas the 4 isomer (**LX**) was

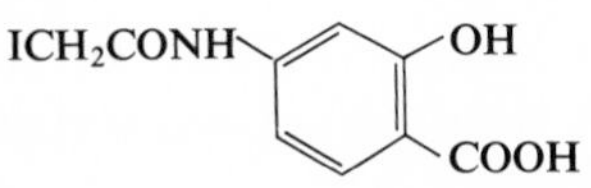

$$ICH_2CONH-\underset{COOH}{\overset{OH}{\bigcirc}}$$

LVII

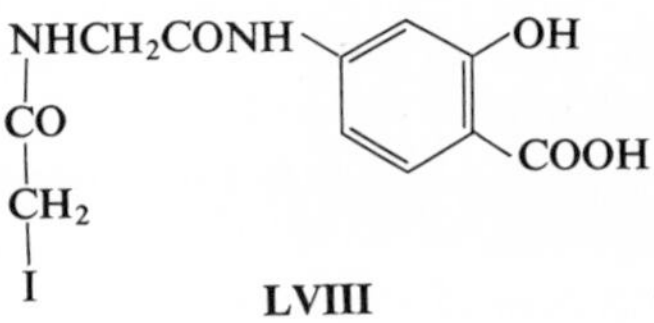

$$NHCH_2CONH-\underset{COOH}{\overset{OH}{\bigcirc}}$$
$$\underset{\underset{\underset{I}{\overset{|}{CH_2}}}{\overset{|}{CO}}}{}$$

LVIII

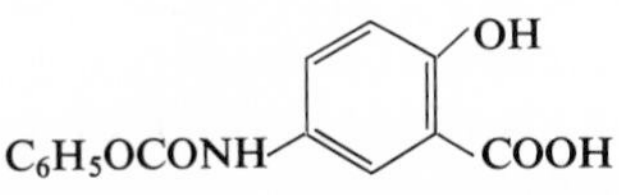

$$C_6H_5OCONH-\underset{COOH}{\overset{OH}{\bigcirc}}$$

LIX

$$C_6H_5OCONH-\underset{COOH}{\overset{OH}{\bigcirc}}$$

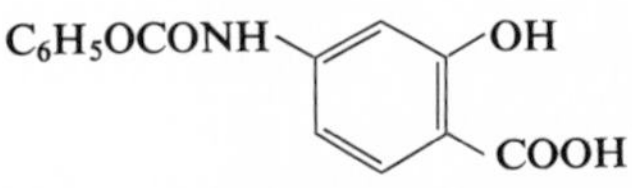

LX

specific for the other isozyme; i.e., **LIX** irreversibly inhibited the skeletal muscle but not heart lactic dehydrogenase (see Table VII). Note that all of these compounds form initial reversible complexes with the enzyme and yet selectivity of irreversible inactivation has been achieved. Since the active site of these two isozymes is probably very similar, it appears that the selectivity of irreversible inhibition has been achieved by taking advantage of differences in the structure of the isozymes outside of the active site, a result which was predicted by Baker.

TABLE VII

SELECTIVE IRREVERSIBLE INHIBITION OF LACTIC DEHYDROGENASE FROM DIFFERENT TISSUES[a]

Compound no.	Skeletal muscle (rabbit)			Heart (beef)		
	K_i (mM)	Rev. EI(%)	Rate of inactivation[c]	K_i (mM)	Rev. EI(%)[b]	Rate of inactivation[d]
LVII	1.7	54	1.0[e]	4.5	3.1	0
LVIII	0.40	83	0.57	2.5	44	1.0[e, f]
LIX	1.5	57	0	1.4	59[g]	0.4[g]
LX	1.1	65	0.8	1.9	51[f]	0[f]

[a] Data taken from B. R. Baker and R. P. Patel, *J. Pharm. Sci.* **53**, 714 (1964) and from Baker (*12*, p. 185).

[b] Percentage of active enzyme in reversible EI complex with 2 mM inhibitor, unless otherwise indicated. Calculated from Eq. (3).

[c] Compared to **LVII** as a standard; relative rate corrected to equal concentration of reversible EI complex.

[d] Compared to **LVIII** as a standard; relative rate corrected to equal concentration of reversible EI complex.

[e] Arbitrary standard that is not the same for two isozymes.

[f] 4 mM inhibitor.

[g] 3 mM inhibitor.

An exciting example of selective irreversible enzyme inhibition is obtained from the research of Baker and his co-workers in the field of cancer chemotherapy (70). In this case, dihydrofolic reductase was isolated from three normal tissues in the mouse (liver, spleen, and intestine) and also from mouse L1210 leukemia. From extensive studies on the mode of binding of reversible inhibitors to these isozymes of dihydrofolic reductase, a number of irreversible inhibitors were prepared which exhibited differential inhibition against these isozymes. The substituted diaminopyrimidine (**LXI**) shows excellent irreversible inhibition of the L1210 dihydrofolic reductase derived from mouse leukemia, whereas **LXI** acts primarily as a reversible inhibitor of the isozymes derived from normal mouse tissues of liver, spleen, and intestines. The theoretical importance of this selective irreversible inhibition of one of the isozymes

LXI

of dihydrofolic reductase cannot be overemphasized. When such selectivity of irreversible inhibition of substrate-identical enzymes can be demonstrated in animal test systems, the day of the rational design of truly selective chemotherapeutic agents will have arrived.

VII. Summary

The rational design of irreversible enzyme inhibitors initially involves the study, by means of reversible inhibitors, of the factors involved in the formation of an EI complex, especially to differentiate binding areas from areas of bulk tolerance. Whereas hydrophobic interactions are generally small when considered on the basis of a single carbon atom, such hydrophobic transfer forces can be significant if the enzyme has a large nonpolar region. For example, if the enzyme has an area that can complex with a hexyl group, the hydrophobic transfer forces for this group alone can amount to a change in free energy of -4.4 kcal which would result in a change in K_i by a factor greater than 1000.

Kinetic studies of irreversible enzyme inactivation by active site-directed inhibitors have demonstrated the importance of both K_i and k_2 for this mechanism. The bridge principle of specificity has been shown to be successful in causing selective irreversible inhibition of a target enzyme while leaving other substrate-identical enzymes functional. Although there are still a number of problems to be solved before useful chemotherapeutics agents are generated by this procedure, it is clear that the first step in the design of agents with truly selective action has now been completed.

ACKNOWLEDGMENT

This manuscript was prepared, in part, during a year that the author spent as a visiting professor at the University of Nijmegen. The generous financial support of the Dutch Organization for Pure Scientific Research is gratefully acknowledged.

REFERENCES

1. L. Michaelis and M. L. Menton, *Biochem. Z.* **49**, 333 (1913).
2. G. G. Hammes, *Accounts Chem. Res.* **1**, 321 (1968).
3. M. Dixon and E. C. Webb, "Enzymes." Academic Press, New York, 1958.
4. J. L. Webb, "Enzyme and Metabolic Inhibitors," Vols. 1, 2, and 3. Academic Press, New York, 1963, 1965, 1966.
5. R. M. Hochster and J. H. Quastel, eds., "Metabolic Inhibitors," Vols. 1 and 2. Academic Press, New York, 1963.
6. J. M. Reiner, "Behavior of Enzyme Systems," p. 151. Burgess, Minneapolis, Minn., 1959.
7. D. W. Woolley, "A Study of Antimetabolites." Wiley, New York, 1952.
8. D. D. Woods, *Brit. J. Exp. Pathol.* **21**, 74 (1940).
9. P. Fildes, *Lancet* **1**, 955 (1940).
10. A. Albert, "Selective Toxicity." Methuen, London, 1968.
11. B. R. Baker, *J. Pharm. Sci.* **53**, 347 (1964).
12. B. R. Baker, "Design of Active-Site-Directed Irreversible Enzyme Inhibitors." Wiley, New York, 1967.
13. L. Wofsy, H. Metzger, and S. J. Singer, *Biochemistry* **1**, 1031 (1962).
14. W. B. Lawson and H. J. Schramm, *J. Amer. Chem. Soc.* **84**, 2017 (1962).
15. W. B. Lawson and H. J. Schramm, *Biochemistry* **4**, 377 (1965).
16. G. Schoellmann and E. Shaw, *Biochem. Biophys. Res. Commun.* **7**, 36 (1962).
17. G. Schoellmann and E. Shaw, *Biochemistry* **2**, 252 (1963).
18. L. L. Bennett, Jr. and J. A. Montgomery, *Methods Cancer Res.* **1**, 549 (1967).
19. D. L. Hill and L. L. Bennett, Jr., *Biochemistry* **8**, 122 (1969).
20. G. B. Elion, S. Callahan, H. Nathan, S. Bieber, R. W. Rundles, and G. H. Hitchings, *Biochem. Pharmacol.* **12**, 85 (1963).
21. G. Elion, A. Kovensky, G. Hitchings, E. Metz, and R. Rundles, *Biochem. Pharmacol.* **15**, 863 (1966).
22. E. M. Wise, Jr. and J. T. Park, *Proc. Nat. Acad. Sci. U.S.* **54**, 75 (1965).
23. D. J. Tipper and J. L. Strominger, *Proc. Nat. Acad. Sci. U.S.* **54**, 1133 (1965).
24. J. L. Strominger, K. Izaki, M. Matsuhashi, and D. J. Tipper, *in* "Topics in Pharmaceutical Sciences" (D. Perlman, ed.) Vol. 1, p. 53. Wiley (Interscience), New York, 1968.
25. G. Kartha, *Accounts Chem. Res.* **1**, 374 (1968).
26. A. Coddington, *Biochim. Biophys. Acta* **99**, 442 (1965).
27. S. Frederiksen, *Arch. Biochem. Biophys.* **113**, 383 (1966).
28. H. P. Baer, G. I. Drummond, and E. L. Duncan, *Mol. Pharmacol.* **2**, 67 (1966).

29. J. L. York and G. H. LePage, *Can. J. Biochem.* **44**, 331 (1966).
30. A. Bloch, M. J. Robins, and J. R. McCarthy, *J. Med. Chem.* **10**, 908 (1967).
31. H. J. Schaeffer, S. Marathe, and V. Alks, *J. Pharm. Sci.* **53**, 1369 (1964).
32. H. J. Schaeffer, K. K. Kaistha, and S. K. Chakraborti, *J. Pharm. Sci.* **53**, 1371 (1964).
33. H. J. Schaeffer, D. D. Godse, and G. Liu, *J. Pharm. Sci.* **53**, 1510 (1964).
34. H. J. Schaeffer and E. Odin, *J. Pharm. Sci.* **54**, 421 (1965).
35. H. J. Schaeffer and P. S. Bhargava, *Biochemistry* **4**, 71 (1965).
36. H. J. Schaeffer and C. F. Schwender, *J. Pharm. Sci.* **56**, 1586 (1967).
37. H. J. Schaeffer and D. Vogel, *J. Med. Chem.* **8**, 507 (1965).
38. B. Belleau and G. Lacasse, *J. Med. Chem.* **7**, 768 (1964).
39. E. J. Cohn and J. T. Edsall, "Proteins, Aminoacids and Peptides," Chapter 9. Reinhold, New York, 1943.
40. J. Iwasa, T. Fujita, and C. Hansch, *J. Med. Chem.* **8**, 150 (1965).
41. H. J. Schaeffer, D. Vogel, and R. Vince, *J. Med. Chem.* **8**, 502 (1965).
42. H. J. Schaeffer and R. Vince, *J. Med. Chem.* **10**, 689 (1967).
43. H. J. Schaeffer and C. F. Schwender, *J. Pharm. Sci.* **56**, 207 (1967).
44. H. J. Schaeffer and C. F. Schwender, *J. Pharm. Sci.* **57**, 1070 (1968).
45. H. J. Schaeffer and C. F. Schwender, unpublished data (1971).
46. B. Belleau, *in* "Physico-Chemical Aspects of Drug Action" (E. J. Ariëns, ed.), Vol. 7, p. 207. Pergamon Press, New York, 1968.
47. D. E. Koshland, Jr., *Proc. 1st Int. Pharmacol. Meet., 1961.* Vol. 7, p. 161 (1962).
48. M. Burr and D. E. Koshland, Jr., *Proc. Nat. Acad. Sci. U.S.* **52**, 1017 (1964).
49. E. Shaw, M. Mares-Guia, and W. Cohen, *Biochemistry* **4**, 2219 (1965).
50. B. R. Baker, W. W. Lee, and E. Tong, *J. Theor. Biol.* **3**, 459 (1962).
51. H. J. Schaeffer, M. A. Schwartz, and E. Odin, *J. Med. Chem.* **10**, 686 (1967).
52. H. J. Schaeffer and E. Odin, *J. Med. Chem.* **9**, 576 (1966).
53. H. J. Schaeffer and R. N. Johnson, *J. Pharm. Sci.* **55**, 929 (1966).
54. H. J. Schaeffer and E. Odin, *J. Med. Chem.* **10**, 181 (1967).
55. H. J. Schaeffer and R. N. Johnson, *J. Med. Chem.* **11**, 21 (1968).
56. A. R. Main and F. Iverson, *Biochem. J.* **100**, 525 (1966).
57. A. R. Main and F. L. Hastings, *Biochem. J.* **101**, 584 (1966).
58. A. M. Gold and D. Fahrney, *Biochemistry* **3**, 783 (1964).
59. L. W. Brox and A. Hampton, *Biochemistry* **7**, 2589 (1968).
60. B. Belleau and H. Tani, *Mol. Pharmacol.* **2**, 411 (1966).
61. B. R. Baker, *Biochem. Pharmacol.* **11**, 1155 (1962); also Baker (*12*, Chapter 9).
62. B. R. Baker, T. J. Schwan, and D. V. Santi, *J. Med. Chem.* **9**, 66 (1966).
63. B. R. Baker and W. Rzestotarski, *J. Med. Chem.* **11**, 639 (1968).
64. B. R. Baker and J. K. Coward, *J. Heterocyclic Chem.* **4**, 202 (1967).
65. B. R. Baker and J. A. Hurlbut, *J. Med. Chem.* **12**, 118 (1996).
66. B. R. Baker and E. H. Erickson, *J. Med. Chem.* **12**, 112 (1969).
67. B. R. Baker and D. V. Santi, *J. Med. Chem.* **10**, 62 (1967).
68. B. R. Baker and J. A. Kozma, *J. Med. Chem.* **11**, 656 (1968).
69. B. R. Baker and J. L. Kelley, *J. Med. Chem.* **11**, 686 (1968).
70. B. R. Baker, G. J. Lourens, R. B. Meyer, Jr., and N. M. J. Vermeulen, *J. Med. Chem.* **12**, 67 (1969).

Chapter 3 The Design of Organophosphate and Carbamate Inhibitors of Cholinesterases

R. D. O'Brien

I. Introduction

This chapter is not designed as a comprehensive review of our knowledge about acetylcholinesterase or organophosphates or carbamates. Several books exist on such topics (*53, 64, 96, 99*).* Instead, I have, after a brief review of relevant "traditional" views, attempted to identify those recent developments which are significant for the design of new inhibitors. This is therefore a biased presentation, and will go into great detail in some areas, while giving scant or no attention to others which might seem more important to many readers. The work from my own laboratory is particularly close to my heart, and of course its relevance will seem especially apparent to me, so I hope that readers will be either equally convinced or (if not) will be tolerant of my over-emphasis.

A few words about terminology. I shall use the term "organophosphate" as a generic one for organic phosphorus compounds; "phosphate" for compounds of the type $(R_1O)(R_2O)P(O)OR_3$; "phosphonate" for (R_1O) $R_2P(O)OR_3$; "phosphorothiolate" for $(R_1O)(R_2O)P(O)SR_3$; "phosphoro-thionate" for $(R_1O)(R_2O)P(S)OR_3$; and "phosphorodithioate" for (R_1O) $(R_2O)P(S)SR_3$.

I shall use "cholinesterase" as a general term to cover the two types which I shall refer to more specifically as "acetylcholinesterase" (sometimes called true cholinesterase or specific cholinesterase) abbreviated as AChE; and "butyrylcholinesterase" (sometimes called pseudocholinesterase or nonspecific cholinesterase or, exasperatingly, cholinesterase) abbreviated as BuChE. The cholinesterases can be quite simply defined as those enzymes which hydrolyze acetylcholine (ACh).

It is now universally agreed that organophosphates and carbamates react with cholinesterase by a mechanism precisely similar to that of true substrates (by which I shall mean compounds whose hydrolysis is briskly catalyzed by one or both of the cholinesterases). In every case there is first complex forma-tion, characterized by a binding constant K_a, which is made up of a forward (k_{+1}) step and a backward (k_{-1}) step; then there is either acylation or phos-phorylation or carbamylation, characterized by a constant k_2; then there is a deacylation or decarbamylation or dephosphorylation step (k_3) giving back original enzyme.

Thus, writing E for the native enzyme bearing its active hydroxyl, and for all compounds writing A as the acylating or phosphorylating or carbamylating

---

* An extensive study (*125*) on the nematocidal activity of over 170 carbamates might interest designers, but is not within the scope of this review.

group, and X as the leaving group (i.e., the rest of the molecule):

$$E + AX \underset{k_{-1}}{\overset{k_{+1}}{\rightleftharpoons}} E \cdot AX \xrightarrow[X]{k_2} EA \xrightarrow[A]{k_3} E \tag{1}$$

Then $K_a = k_{-1}/k_{+1}$; and K_m, that is, as experimentally measured from a Lineweaver-Burk plot, is given (50) by:

$$K_m = \frac{k_3}{k_2 + k_3} \cdot \frac{k_{-1} + k_2}{k_{+1}} \tag{2}$$

Although everyone agrees that reversible binding precedes the k_2 step, not everyone agrees that such binding is experimentally demonstrable. Thus Aldridge, who had pointed out the logical necessity of this binding in the case of organophosphates back in 1953 (7) nevertheless could only demonstrate it kinetically for one rather special organophosphate (9, 112). But Main has demonstrated it for several organophosphates (75, 76, 78, 79). Similarly Winteringham (133, 134) and Reiner and Simeon-Rudolf (113) could not obtain evidence for a complex in carbamate inhibition, but others were able to do so (76, 100, 104) and the failures have been explained as due to inappropriate conditions (100).

In addition, it is possible to obtain for organophosphates and carbamates a parameter by the kinetic procedure of Main (75) [which is essentially similar to that used by Kitz and Wilson (60) for the parallel case of methane sulfonate inhibitors] which he calls the K_a, as defined above; but which I have pointed out (100) is in fact K_y, defined by $K_y = (k_{-1} + k_2)/k_{+1}$, and so called because it derives from the y intercept of a Main plot.* When k_2 is much smaller than k_{-1}, then K_y and K_a are essentially the same; but no facts are available to judge this point.

Finally let us examine the relation of the above parameters to better known constants such as I_{50} (and its negative logarithm, pI_{50}) and the bimolecular rate constant, k_i. Under many conditions, phosphates, and sometimes carbamates, behave *as if* they followed a reaction scheme:

$$E + AX \xrightarrow{k_i} EA + X \tag{3}$$

One can measure an apparent constant k_i. But Main (75) showed that $k_i = k_2/K_a$ for organophosphates, when k_3 can be neglected. This k_i is never a true

---

* That is, a plot of $1/i$ against $t/2.3\Delta \log V$, where i is the inhibitor concentrations, t is the incubation time, and $\Delta \log V$ is the change in logarithm of the velocity of substrate hydrolysis (caused by inhibition).

rate constant, but a ratio of a rate constant to an affinity constant; hence he suggested the term "bimolecular reaction constant." Furthermore, Eq. (3) is only followed when one works with inhibitor concentrations much less than the inhibitor's K_a; this turns out to be a rather common situation, and accounts for the fact that apparent k_i's have been used so successfully for so long.

As for the I_{50} (defined as "the concentration of inhibitor giving 50% inhibition") if the enzyme strictly follows scheme (3) throughout the reaction, and there are no complications, then one can easily show (96) that $k_i = 0.695/I_{50}t$, where t is the time of incubation with inhibitor. Ideally, then, I_{50} is a close measure of k_i; but one should not assume that it measures it until one has proved, for his particular system, that Eq. (3) is in fact followed, i.e., that enzyme reactivity falls off exponentially throughout the reaction. In addition, one must specify t when one reports I_{50}'s or pI_{50}'s.

One of the parameters of maximum interest is K_a, which measures the affinity of compounds for enzyme. Unfortunately it has never been rigorously determined for any substrate or inhibitor of cholinesterase, although K_y is probably quite a good approximation of it. The use of relative "affinities" by Metcalf and Fukuto (85) is not quite correct; they actually compare relative I_{50}'s of carbamates and assume they reflect different affinities; but this assumption is not yet proven, as we shall see.

II. The Structure of the Active Zone of Cholinesterases

A. THE ORIGINAL WILSON MODEL

Largely as a result of the studies of Wilson and collaborators in a period around 1950, there emerged the picture of the active zone* which is most widely accepted today. This was that the active zone contained two sites, as follows.

1. An esteratic site, later shown to involve a serine hydroxyl group, which could become acylated or phosphorylated or carbamylated by appropriate agents. When acylated, a rapid hydrolysis of the acyl enzyme occurrs, so that

---

* The term "active zone" is proposed here in preference to the more usual term "active site," because it is clear that in cholinesterases the total area to which binding of substrates and inhibitors can occur, and within which catalysis of substrates occurs, is rather large. Within it are distinguishable subareas, as will be shown below, and any one subarea (such as the "esteratic site") may well contain at least two groups. We shall therefore reserve the term "site" for distinguishable subareas of the overall "zone," and thus avoid having to use awkward statements such as, "The active site of the enzyme contains two sites."

the overall reaction with, for instance, acetylcholine is a catalytic hydrolysis in accordance with Eq. (1). It is very likely that this same serine hydroxyl can be carbamylated by carbamates and phosphorylated by phosphates; but the k_3 (or regeneration) step which is very fast for acetyl enzyme (half-life about 0.2 msec at 38°C) is rather slow for most carbamates (half-life for methylcarbamates about 15 min) and excessively slow for most phosphates (half-life for diethyl phosphates about 8 hr). As a result, carbamylated enzyme appears to be inhibited, although it recovers activity (if excess carbamate inhibitor is removed) fairly fast; and the phosphorylated enzyme appears

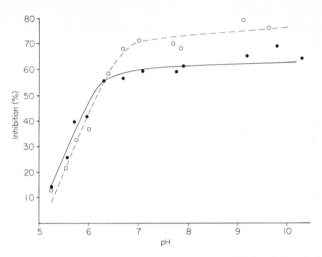

Fig. 1. The pH dependence of inhibition of *Torpedo* AChE by choline (o) and tetra-ethylammonium (●). Redrawn from Bergmann and Shimoni (*18*).

even more convincingly inhibited, because it recovers activity very slowly, even if excess phosphate inhibitor is removed.

2. An anionic site, defined as "a negatively charged structure ... which facilitates enzymic activity by attracting, binding and orienting cationic substrates" (*128*). The evidence for the existence of such a site deserves some review, as will become apparent below. It was originally postulated* simply because the prominent-looking cationic charge on acetylcholine (which in other respects is a rather featureless molecule) seemed to demand it (*126, 129*). The clearest evidence for it (Fig. 1) was that of Bergmann and Shimoni (*18*) who found that inhibition by tetraalkylammoniums shows a marked pH-dependence, being maximal above pH 7 and falling almost to zero at pH 5,

---

* Although in 1943, Zeller and Bissegger had proposed a two-site theory to explain the fact of inhibition of AChE by excess acetylcholine (*138*).

suggesting the involvement of a binding group in the enzyme with a pK_a about 6. Wilson (128) emphasized that "the binding is effectuated by ionic and dispersion forces," which he would undoubtedly rephrase today as "ionic and hydrophobic forces." His evidence for other-than-ionic forces was that addition of more methylenes to alkylammonium gave (within limits) progressively better inhibitors, even though the charge distribution would be unfavorably affected by such additions (128).

B. NEWER VIEWS ON THE CATALYTIC SITE

Wilson's view of the substructure of the catalytic (= esteratic) site was that it must have an acidic and a basic component, for in this way one could account for the fact that a variety of substrates (as well as certain organophosphates which should not react with the anionic site) showed an optimum pH at about 8, compatible with a requirement for two groupings, an acid and a basic, one of which was suboptimal at lower and another suboptimal at higher pH's. He argued that the basic group was involved in the formation of the acyl enzyme, and the acid group was involved in the subsequent cleavage of acyl enzyme (127–129).

Krupka (70) has provided evidence that the catalytic site contains not two, but at least three subsites. One (pK 9.2; active when protonated) which corresponds to one of Wilson's subsites; a second (pK 6.3; active when unprotonated) called B_1, which is involved in deacetylations; and a third (pK 5.5; active when unprotonated) called B_2, which is involved in acetylations.

This very brief statement hardly does justice to the wealth of research involved in this and related studies of Krupka (67–69). The brevity is dictated in part by the fact that the direct relevance to anticholinesterase design is not yet on hand; although it suggests that more than one component within the catalytic site could be a subject for attack. Secondly, most of the conclusions are based upon pH-dependence studies, followed by calculations that assume the dependence reflects participation in catalysis by a group or groups in the active zone which ionize in the range under study. As Reiner and Aldridge point out (112), one must contemplate the alternative possibility, that the conformation of the enzyme changes with pH (as discussed in Section II, E below) and consequently some of the pH-dependent charges may not involve ionization in the active zone itself. And in addition, the binding even of neutral compounds may modify the pK_a of groups in the enzyme, as has been shown recently for chymotrypsin (48). The pK_a shifts varied greatly according to ligand. Consequently apparent new groups (when identified by pK_a) may appear when one compares pH profiles for different substrates, or in the presence and absence of inhibitors.

C. NEWER VIEWS ON THE BINDING SITES

The only binding site in the early Wilson model was the "anionic site" which (as mentioned above) owed much of "its" nature to noncoulombic forces. The Bergmann view of about the same time (17) was that AChE had two such sites whereas BuChE had but one; an argument designed to accommodate the facts that (a) AChE had more affinity for choline than did BuChE, which Adams and Whittaker (2) calculated to imply that AChE bore one ionic site more than BuChE, and (b) that BuChE palpably had one ionic site, as judged by its susceptibility to alkylammonium inhibitors. The Bergmann view has not been widely accepted; and when the Adams and Whittaker data are examined 18 years after their publication, some flaws are apparent.*

More recently, Krupka (70) has added an interesting twist. He argues that the anionic (A) site's apparent pK of 6.3 is an artifact, and that A's true pK_a is 4.3; the pK_a of 6.3 computed for monocation data (such as Fig. 1) is due to the effect of the neighboring group B_1 of the esteratic site (mentioned above) which repels cations when protonated. By this argument he explains two extraordinary phenomena:

1. When a zwitterion, betaine, is used as inhibitor, a strong pH dependence of inhibition is seen even below pH 5 (when a pK 6.3 group would be 95% protonated) and a group in the enzyme which has a pK_a of 4.3 is revealed. Assuming that in the enzyme B_1 is a nitrogen base (pK 6.3) and A is a carboxylic acid (pK 4.3) one would at pH 8 have $\underline{COO^-N}$: which would be optimal for attracting monocations. At pH 5.5 one would have $\underline{COO^-NH^+}$ which would be much poorer for monocations because of the repulsive action of the NH$^+$, but optimal for betaine, $(CH_3)_3N^+CH_2COO^-$, which could now enjoy a double attraction. At pH much less than 4.0 one would have $\underline{COOHNH^+}$ in which the attractive carboxylate ion is lost for betaine.

* The differences computed for K_a for choline for the two enzymes were not due to differences in the inhibitory potency of choline, which is about equipotent for the two enzymes. Instead they were computed differences which rest on assumptions that the K_m of ACh for these enzymes are equal to K_a. Also the K_m values for ACh were taken from different literature references which gave 0.44×10^{-4} for AChE (137) and 14.7×10^{-4} for BuChE [average of Glick (47) and Wright and Sabine (136)], a difference of 33-fold. But this K_m for AChE value is unusually low; other literature values range from 1.9 to 4.5×10^{-4} (94, 114, 116, 128). And of the two values for BuChE, one (47) was done at 25°C and should be discarded in favor of the other, giving $K_m = 11 \times 10^{-4}$. Hence the difference in K_m's for the two enzymes could be as little as 6-fold, and then the difference in K_a for choline would be very small. A quite different objection is that their argument assumes that the only cause for the claimed difference in choline potency is the presence of an extra ionic group in AChE. Since AChE and BuChE differ profoundly in their response to neutral organophosphates (6) the assumption is dubious.

2. Tetraethylammonium (TEA) under acid conditions (pH 5) activates hydrolysis of ACh but not hydrolysis of poor substrates such as phenyl acetate. This is explained if deacetylation is rate-limiting for ACh, and so is determined by the degree of unprotonation of B_1, a deacetylating group; then tetraethylammonium, by binding to the A site, repels protons from the vicinity of B_1 and permits it to remain unprotonated even at low pH. Such an "assist" is of no value to the poor substrates, for which deacetylation is not rate-limiting.

One conclusion is that under acid conditions, the occupation of A by TEA does not hinder ACh hydrolysis (at the deacetylation step) or at least hinders it less than it helps by deprotonation of B_1. Under these conditions, when the enzyme is ACh-saturated the TEA effect is to promote, although when ACh saturation is only partial, the effect is to inhibit; this dual response is due to a combination of an increase in V_{max} coupled with a substantial rise in K_m. Increase of the TEA concentration leads to an increase in the activation of V_{max}, but the effect soon "plateaus," so that 48 mM is no better than 19 mM. Under these conditions one has presumably saturated with TEA. Thus every AChE molecule which is hydrolyzing ACh has a TEA molecule in place; it follows that binding of ACh to the TEA-binding site is not obligatory for ACh hydrolysis, nor does the TEA which is bound obscure the vital parts of the esteratic site.

In the discussion so far the only binding site referred to has been the putative anionic site. And indeed the literature in general has this implication. A priori, the conclusion seems unlikely: the catalytic site must be surrounded by a veritable sea of amino acid residues, and one would expect that each residue (or group of them) would offer a potential binding site for the right compound: all the ionic residues (aspartate, glutamate, arginine, lysine) should offer coulombic sites, all the aromatic ones (tyrosine, phenylalanine, tryptophan) should offer π–π and perhaps charge transfer sites, all the long-alkyl ones (valine, leucine, isoleucine) should offer hydrophobic sites, all the hydroxyl ones (serine, threonine) should offer hydrogen-bonding sites. Considering the inverse argument, we note that a whole galaxy of groups have been attached to simple acyl, phosphoryl, and carbamyl groups, and have given excellent reagents which must indeed bind to some binding site or other—such binding is an absolute prerequisite for good reactivity. Let us therefore look for evidence for a diversity of binding sites, not unlike the multiple sites postulated for chymotrypsin (*38, 57, 117*).

Several pieces of evidence point to the existence of a "hydrophobic patch" of possibly large extent, near the catalytic site. Undoubtedly the progressive and identical increases in inhibitory potency for AChE and BuChE of *n*-alkylammoniums up to eight methylenes long and of bisquaternary ammoniums up to 12 methylenes long, reported by Bergmann (*17*), would be interpreted today as indicating a large hydrophobic patch near the binding site for N^+. A very similar approach has more recently been applied to organophosphates with BuChE by Russian (*1a, 24*) and AChE by American (*21, 22, 23*) workers. The Russians worked with phosphonothiolates [i.e., containing C—P(O)—S—C] and the Americans with phosphates [with P(O)OX] and phosphorothiolates [P(O)SC]. Both employed a variety of "heads" on the alkyl side chain, but both showed that activity increased steadily, in any one series, as one increased the alkyl chain. When a longest chain of six methylenes had been reached, activity abruptly leveled off. It was concluded (*21, 22, 23*) that a hydrophobic patch existed near the esteratic site, large enough to accommodate only six methylenes.

The next complication to be considered arises from the fact that several rather diverse reagents can react with cholinesterases to produce an enzyme which is inhibited with regard to some substrates, but activated with respect to others. Thus AChE can be inhibited irreversibly and severely for ACh but activated for indophenyl acetate (or in some cases inhibited to a minor extent)

by treatment with TDF (*14, 27*) or DPA (*110*) or MCP (*101*). Earlier work had shown that tetraethylammonium can reversibly inhibit ACh hydrolysis by AChE but activate hydrolysis of acetyl fluoride (*91*) and dimethylcarbamyl fluoride (*90*) and inhibition by methylsulfonyl fluoride (*61*). Finally it has been shown (*26*) that CAP inhibits BuChE for ACh hydrolysis while activating it for benzoylcholine hydrolysis.

In the case of the alkylating agent MCP, a fairly detailed exploration of its action was possible (*101*) partly because of its excellent potency, and its convenient property of "autodegradation"—its half-life in water is only 8.5 min at 25°C, and so active material does not need removal before assaying. The fully alkylated enzyme had lost over 99% of its ability to hydrolyze ACh, or to be inhibited by tetraethylammonium or choline or Amiton. Toward indophenyl acetate, its activity was 160% of that of untreated enzyme. For all other compounds (five substrates, five carbamates, five organophosphates) it suffered a modest loss of reactivity, of up to 30-fold. The substrate effects were observed to be all due to changes in k_2, not upon K_m.

There are various ways of interpreting these curious simultaneous inhibitions and activations. My own proposal (*101*) is that they imply three quite separate binding sites, which I shall call α, β, and γ sites. The α site (which has much in common with, and may be the same as, the so-called anionic site) is the site occupied by MCP, DPA, and TDF, and is also an obligatory site for binding of acetylcholine, tetraethylammonium, choline, and Amiton; we may call all seven "α agents." Hence complete treatment with irreversible α agents (most easily accomplished by MCP) virtually abolishes reactivity toward any other α agent. The β site is the binding site of the majority of carbamates and phosphates and also several substrates (phenyl acetate, *p*-nitrophenyl acetate, indoxyl acetate); the reactivity toward β agents is reduced, to varying extents, by treatment with α agents. The γ site is the site for binding of indophenyl acetate, acetyl fluoride, dimethylcarbamyl fluoride, and methylsulfonyl fluoride, i.e., those agents whose reactivity is enhanced by α agents. The fact that β and γ agents are differently affected by α agents is most readily explained (bearing in mind that only their k_2 steps are affected) by assuming that a configurational shift accompanies occupation of the α site, in such a way as to bring the catalytic serine closer to the γ site and further from the β site. I should emphasize that at present this α–β–γ terminology is entirely *operationally* defined; specifically, an α agent is one which suffers total blockade as a result of treatment with MCP or DPA; a β agent is one which does not suffer total blockade but whose k_2 is decreased by prior MCP or DPA treatment; and γ agent is one whose k_2 is increased by MCP or DPA treatment. An α site is defined as the binding site for α agents, and in a parallel way the β and γ sites are defined. The reason I stress the operational aspect is that there may well be separate, noncontiguous sites within each category; in fact I shall argue for two distinct α sites below. The term "α site" would then be a generic one. In other words, those are three *kinds* of binding site, and therefore the number of binding sites per catalytic site is at least three and probably more.

The fact that the β site is occupable by so many diverse reagents implies that it may constitute a large fraction of the area around the catalytic serine. This would also explain the differences in interference by MCP treatment of reactivity for the β agents; thus AChE fully alkylated by MCP is 93 % inhibited for phenyl acetate hydrolysis, but only 22 % for *p*-nitrophenyl acetate hydrolysis. At least a portion of the β site is probably hydrophobic, as judged by the fact that the compound PB72 [$(C_2H_5O)_2P(O)S(CH_2)_5CH(C_2H_5)_2$], which is quite like Amiton but lacks its NH^+ group, and which has been shown to owe virtually all its binding activity to hydrophobic bonding (*23*) binds to the β site, by the above criterion.

Belleau (*14a*) has added many facts about DPA alkylation of red cell

AChE. Two moles of DPA bind per mole of enzyme, and one of the moles is labile at pH 9.5, leaving a mono-DPA enzyme which is 350% activated for indophenyl acetate but cannot hydrolyze ACh. The two alkylatable sites differ markedly. (1) After treatment with ^{14}C-DPA and digestion by the proteolytic preparation, pronase, one can separate out two labeled fragments, one weakly basic and the other strongly basic. (2) When one uses TDF (which is also thought of as "an anionic site agent") to alkylate AChE one obtains an enzyme with 90% of its normal activity for indophenyl acetate and which can now be treated by 10^{-5} M DPA to give an enzyme with 275% of its normal activity for indophenyl acetate. These last two facts show that TDF and DPA can react with two quite different sites, which [simply because both reagents contains the $N^+(CH_3)_3$ group] could perhaps both be "anionic sites." Presumably DPA alone normally attacks both, but it is the alkali-stable site which is involved in the indophenyl acetate-activation phenomenon.

Relatively high concentrations of tubocurarine and flaxedil (so-called "pachycurares") were better inhibitors of mono-DPA enzyme than of bis-DPA (using indophenyl acetate as substrate). Perhaps, Belleau suggests, these pachycurares react with the alkali-labile site.

Let us now examine the bearing of Belleau's findings upon the concept of α, β, and γ binding sites. We may use the term α_1 for the alkali-stable site; it remains true that ACh obligatorily binds to it, since the mono-DPA enzyme (whose α_1 site, according to this new restriction of terminology, is blocked) cannot hydrolyze ACh. We must postulate an α_2 site, defined as the alkali-labile reaction site for DPA. From item (2) above, it seems that TDF, used under Belleau's conditions, reacts with the α_2 site; and that occupation of the α_2 site does not cause activation of indophenyl acetate hydrolysis. Since TDF is [as originally shown by Wofsy and Michaeli (135)] an excellent inhibitor of ACh hydrolysis by AChE, giving 97% inhibition at 10^{-5} M, it seems that the α_2 site must be free (as well as the α_1 site) if ACh hydrolysis is to occur at its full rate. The only alternative explanation would be if under Wofsy and Michaeli's conditions, the α_2 site were selectively alkylated, leaving the α_1 site free. That conditions require rather careful specification (unfortunately not all available at this writing) is shown by the fact that Belleau's conditions of TDF treatment gave enzyme with 90% of its normal activity for indophenyl acetate, whereas Changeux (27) was able to get well over 100% of such activity following TDF treatment.

It seems likely that pachycurares can react with the α_2 site. Whether or not they can react with the α_1 site as well is not clear; it would be interesting to see if they can inhibit AChE which has been treated with TDF under Belleau's conditions.

It will be noted that the postulated α_1 and α_2 sites might correspond to the "two anionic sites" which Bergmann proposed, as described above.

Additional interesting alkylators described by Belleau are as follows: (a) *p*-Methyl-DPA also reacts to give an enzyme that cannot hydrolyze ACh, but is even more activated with respect to indophenyl acetate (500%) than that treated by DPA. With longer *p*-substituents, indophenyl acetate activation is less prominent, and is zero at *p*-pentyl. (b) The quinoline derivative EEDQ also blocks acetylcholine hydrolysis by AChE irreversibly, but allows retention

EEDQ

of 50–60% of its activity for indophenyl acetate (*14c*). There is evidence that (like pachycurares) it is specific for the α_2 site.

Several other recent studies force one to conclude that there are multiple binding sites. Kitz *et al.* (*59a*) found that pachycurares could accelerate the carbamylation and decarbamylation of AChE. Belleau *et al.* (*14b*) found pachycurares protected AChE from inhibition by methanesulfonyl fluoride but not in a competitive way. Chiu and O'Brien found (*30a*) that acetylcholine, phenyl acetate, α-naphthyl acetate, tetraethylammonium, and decamethonium inhibited the hydrolysis of acetylthiocholine by AChE competitively, but the hydrolysis of indophenyl acetate noncompetitively.

Much of the data given above not only indicates that there are multiple binding sites, but also shows that occupation of one binding site increases reactivity at some different site. This undoubtedly involves a configurational change (*91, 101*) perhaps involving a shift of the catalytic serine hydroxyl with respect to the various binding sites (*101*). In that sense, AChE is an allosteric enzyme, and Kitz *et al.* (*59a*) use that terminology. But nobody has reported that the hydrolysis of the normal substrate, ACh, is either inhibited or accelerated by agents acting on a distant site, so a physiological regulatory role, commonly associated with allosteric enzymes, has not yet been demonstrated.

The probable existence of multiple binding sites leads to a serious difficulty in evaluating the forces involved at any one site. For instance, in both early (*129*) and recent (*21*) work, comparisons were made of protonated and un-protonated compounds (i.e., by contrasting ionizable bases at different pH's) or nitrogenous bases and their un-ionized carbon analogs. If it were true that, in such cases, there was but one binding site, then variations in binding to it could give valuable information: by comparing K_a's for an ionized and an isosteric un-ionized compound one could compute the coulombic force involved for the binding of an ionized compound to that site. However, such calculations are impossible if there are (for instance) separate coulombic and hydrophobic binding sites, for the ionic compound would bind to one and the nonionic to the other; the ratio of the K_a's would have no interpretable significance.

D. How Ionic Is the α or "Anionic Site"?

I hope to show that enough doubt exists on the extensive involvement of coulombic forces in binding to this site, that the term α site (or sites) offers advantages. In this discussion, we shall have to speak of "the anionic site" without reference to the possible twofold nature described above (Section II, C) simply because of the novelty of Belleau's data which support that nature.

As mentioned in Section II, A, the best evidence for the existence of an anionic site is that tetraalkylammoniums inhibit AChE (and BuChE) in a pH-dependent way. If coulombic forces were the major ones at work in determining the efficacy of ammoniums, one would expect the smallest ammoniums, with the highest charge density, to be most potent; with the exception that after a certain size was reached, e.g., of R in R_4N^+ compounds, overlapping of the esteratic site would become a factor in addition to blockage of the hypothetical anionic site. In fact, precisely the opposite is true: ammonium is essentially inactive [2 M is required for detectable inhibition (*128*)] and the potency of the R_4N^+ series for eel acetylcholinesterases (*19*) are in the ratio $1:5:100:50$ for R $= CH_3, C_2H_5, C_3H_7$, and C_4H_9. These findings suggest that the importance of hydrophobic and van der Waals' bonding is far greater than that of coulombic binding; and that the contributions of these bondings are maximal with tetrabutylammonium.

In examining the quantitative aspect, let us consider the possibility that all the excellence of ammoniums is due to their alkyl groups, which (if they enjoy the correct steric relations) can bond by van der Waals' or hydrophobic forces to the enzyme surface. Wilson (*128*) has pointed out that because trimethylammonium is only a little better an inhibitor than tetramethylammonium (i.e., 1.2-fold) the fourth methyl group probably cannot bond, presumably because it cannot contact the enzyme. Successive removal of the third and second methylenes diminishes activity 8-fold and 5.8-fold, respectively, corresponding to 1.3 and 1.1 kcal/mole. Removal of the last methylene, if it produced a 1.2 kcal/mole loss, would lead to an I_{50} for ammonium 7.2-fold greater than methylammonium, i.e., 5.1 M. This calculated value is in agreement with Wilson's statement that for ammonium chloride, 2 M is "necessary for inhibition"; presumably by "necessary" he means "in order to see any inhibition." Knowing that the acetylcholine concentration used was 4 mM, and taking the K_m for acetylcholine given as 0.45 mM, and I_{50} for ammonium as 5 M, one can calculate that the K_a for ammonium is 6.33×10^{-1} M, corresponding to a binding energy of 0.31 kcal/mole at 38°C. This represents only 8 % of the binding energy of tetramethylammonium.

Thus at best 8 % of the binding energy of tetramethylammonium, and much less of that of tetraethyl-, tetrapropyl-, and tetrabutylammoniums, is attributable to coulombic forces. The rest must be due to hydrophobic and perhaps van der Waals' bonding. Even this figure of 8 % may be too generous, for it assumes that the coulombic energy is as high in tetramethylammonium as in ammonium. In fact one expects it to be much lower, for the charge is smeared out over a larger sphere, if Thomas and Marlow (120) are right; in fact Belleau and Lacasse (15) claim that "such ions are essentially hydrophobic in nature." It may be that the function of alkylammonium groups in so many effective substrates, inhibitors and reactivators of cholinesterases may be primarily to provide good stereochemistry along with good water solubility.

The other principal line of argument to support the anionic nature of what I call now the α site, was a series of reports that ionized substrates or inhibitors were more reactive with AChE than un-ionized forms or analogs. We shall examine a few cases.

1. 2-Dimethylaminoethyl acetate is hydrolyzed 2.5 times faster* in its protonated than its unprotonated state, as measured by changing pH (129). Even if all this difference was due to a difference in K_a, a 2.5-fold difference would correspond to only 560 cal/mole for the additional binding energy; such an energy is extremely small for an ionic bond, as we shall discuss below.

2. It was shown by Wilson and Bergmann (129) that the inhibition of acetylcholinesterase by the carbamate eserine (a tertiary base) was pH-dependent, and the inhibition by prostigmine (a quaternary salt) was pH-independent. At that time the belief was that carbamates were reversible competitive inhibitors, so the pH independence of prostigmine inhibition occasioned no comment, and all the pH dependence of eserine inhibition was imputed to binding to an anionic site. There is now ample evidence that carbamates carbamylate cholinesterase; in view of the well-known pH dependence of the analogous phosphorylation process, the apparent pH independence of prostigmine is puzzling. Furthermore, it is essential to know the pH dependence of the carbamylation step if one wishes to calculate the role played by "anionic-site binding" of eserine's protonated form as judged by the pH dependence of eserine inhibition.

A recent, very careful, study by Reiner and Aldridge (112) shows an extremely marked pH dependence for inhibition of AChE by 5 carbamates and 2 phosphates. Prostigmine, its N-methyl analog, and its diethyl phosphate analog all showed a bell-shaped pH dependence with a maximum near 8;

* Not 20-fold, as the discussion of Wilson and Bergmann (129) says, but 2.5-fold as Table II in that reference shows.

the data are completely unlike that of Wilson and Bergmann. If this maximum reflects simply the joint effects of two ionizing groups (the assumption commonly made to account for pH optima of substrates), then the data fit the computed curve for two groups of pK_a 6.2 and 10.3. Un-ionized carbamates,

$CH_3NHC(O)O$

Eserine

$(CH_3)_2NC(O)O$ $N(CH_3)_3^+$

Prostigmine

by contrast, show relatively little drop in activity below pH 8; above it, their activity drops off precisely like ionic carbamates.

Now this hypothetical group of pK 6.2 is remarkably similar to the α site, and one could well argue that Reiner and Aldridge's data imply an acid site such as COOH which attracts the N^+ of prostigmine in its COO^- form, and which ionizes with $pK_a = 6.2$; thus the attractiveness falls off on the acid side. Reiner and Aldridge point out that their data could equally well imply the existence of a basic group, such as NH_2, which repels the N^+ of prostigmine in the enzyme's NH_3^+ form, and this repulsiveness increases on the acid side with $pK_a = 6.2$. They prefer this latter interpretation, and point out that it could apply equally well to all the other data which support the "anionic site"; thus such data could as well be interpreted in terms of a "cationic site."

Now these new conclusions do not appear to support my view of the small involvement of coulombic attraction in the α site; they merely invert the ionization. However, close examination of the data (Fig. 2) shows that at

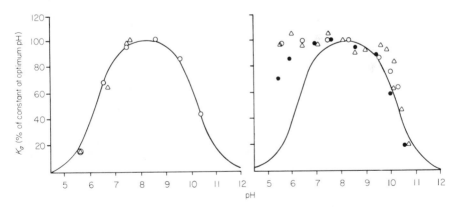

Fig. 2. Inhibition of bovine red cell AChE by ionic carbamates (left) and nonionic (right). Compounds on left: prostigmine (○) and its N-methyl analog (△). On right: 2-isopropoxyphenyl methylcarbamate (○); 3-isopropylphenyl dimethylcarbamate (△) and its N-methyl analog (●). The curves shown are computed on the basis of a joint effect from two groups, with pK_a's of 6.2 and 10.3. Redrawn from Reiner and Aldridge (*112*).

pH 5.5 (the most acid pH tested) the difference between potency of ionized and un-ionized inhibitors, when both are given as %-of-potency-at-optimal-pH, falls between 2-fold and 6.5-fold, depending upon which pair of inhibitors one selects for comparison. If all this difference is due to K_a, the contribution of ionization is quite small; at 25°C it comes to between 540 and 1100 cal/mole. This agrees well with the value of 560 cal/mole given above for the coulombic contribution in ammonium binding.

3. Added evidence against the importance of coulombic binding is the demonstration that some uncharged substrates related to acetylcholine have actually more affinity for the enzyme than does acetylcholine. Thus Wilson's data (128) show the K_m for acetylcholine to be greater than that of acetic anhydride and of dithiolacetic acid $[CH_3C(O)SSC(O)CH_3]$ by factors of 1.1 and 2.3, respectively. These K_m's are made up of K_a (an affinity factor) and k_2 and k_3; since the V_m (which reflects k_2 and k_3;) was much larger for acetylcholine than for these compounds, by factors of 7.7 and 5.6, the affinities of these compounds relative to acetylcholine are presumably even greater than their K_m's suggest, and may well be, respectively, $1.1 \times 7.7 = 8.5$ and $2.3 \times 5.6 = 12.9$.

4. In the case of Amiton and its carbon analog, the K_y values were measured by Main analysis at 25°C; the carbon analog had a K_y 9 times more than

$$(C_2H_5O)_2P(O)SCH_2CH_2NH^+(C_2H_5)_2 \qquad (C_2H_5O)_2P(O)SCH_2CH_2CH(C_2H_5)_2$$
Amiton(protonated form)   Carbon–Amiton

Amiton. Assuming this means a 9-fold difference in K_a, then Amiton enjoys 1.27 kcal/mole of binding energy more than does carbon–Amiton. This represents 18% of Amiton's total binding energy of 6.9 kcal/mole. This figure is probably high, because in fact some of Amiton's superiority is doubtless due to an electronic improvement of k_2 (21).

Conclusion on the α Site

All evidence points to the existence of a modest binding contribution due to the ionization of substrates or inhibitors. The calculated values are typically about 550 cal/mole for ammoniums, representing well under 10% of the total energy of binding. Such a modest contribution is very small for an ionic bond. One may calculate (123, p. 207) that for such a weak force to be involved in two univalent ions of opposite charges, they would be something between 81 and 600 Å apart.* This is absurdly far, and could not be caused by any

---

* The value of 600 Å emerges if one makes the assumption that $D = 1$ where D is the dielectric constant. This impossible-to-test assumption is commonly made in such calculations (123), and assumes interaction in a vacuum. If instead one uses $D = 74.1$ for water at 37.5°C, the charge separation is 81 Å.

site so specifically located as the α site. One must conclude that there is not a true anionic site, that is, a localized anionically charged group within a few angstroms of the esteratic site. There are two plausible alternatives: (1) the α site involves an inducible dipole which gives a contribution in the form of ion-induced dipole interaction and (2) the α site is not at all ionic, but binds through van der Waals' and/or hydrophobic forces, these binding sites being fairly localized and resulting in the specific location of the α site; at some far distance, perhaps up to 600 Å, is an anionic charge which adds a small binding contribution of about 550 cal/mole when the α-binding agent is ionic.

E. ISOENZYMES

All the preceding discussion presupposes that AChE or BuChE represents single entities. Unfortunately this simplifying assumption is probably false. At least seventeen publications [reviewed by LaMotta et al. (71)] show up to seven isoenzymes of BuChE from plasma. There is also increasing evidence that AChE has a subunit structure, and there are various isoenzymes, presumably formed from different combinations of subunits. An early suggestion came in 1963, when two phases were noted in the time-course of heat inactivation of bovine red cell AChE (32). A more detailed study on eel AChE in 1967 showed fast- and slow-sedimenting isoenzymes, using a sucrose gradient technique (49). Adjustment of pH and ionic strength permitted interconversion between these types and (below pH 5) an insoluble form. Two isoenzymes of rat muscle AChE have been shown electrophoretically (31). This situation would not be troublesome for designers of inhibitors, so long as the subunits and their continuations had similar susceptibilities to inhibition. But it seems that such is not the case.

TABLE I

RELATIVE SENSITIVITIES OF AChE AND BuChE ISOENZYMES TO AMITON AT 5°C, pH 7

Isoenzyme	Horse serum BuChE	Bovine erythrocyte AChE
I[a]	100[b]	100[b]
II	4.3	0.45
III	1.1	0.074
IV	0.14	

[a] Isoenzyme I is in each case defined as the most readily phosphorylated one. Data of Main (77).
[b] Arbitrarily assigned.

Entirely kinetic evidence has been produced by Main (77) to show that horse and human serum BuChE and bovine erythrocyte AChE each have several isozymes, which differ markedly in their sensitivity to at least some organophosphates. The isoenzymes were slowly interconvertible (conversion times varying from 5 min to 5 hr) and their constitution varied according to temperature. Table I shows how great were the variations in sensitivity to Amiton of the various isoenzymes. The relative potencies vary with inhibitor. For example, with serum BuChE at 25°C, pH 7.0, isoenzyme I was 43 times more sensitive to Amiton than isoenzyme II, 5.5 times more sensitive to DFP, but only 1.5 times more sensitive to malaoxon.

$$(CH_3O)_2P(O)SCHCOOC_2H_5 \qquad (iso\text{-}C_3H_7O)_2P(O)F$$
$$|$$
$$CH_2COOC_2H_5$$

Malaoxon   DFP

The situation is further complicated by the facts that the isoenzymes interconvert at rather inconvenient rates. Thus when horse serum enzyme at 5°C (principally isoenzyme IV), was rapidly raised to 25°C (principally isoenzyme IV) it took 5 min for the I→IV transition to become complete. For AChE, the transition time at 5°C was between 1 and 7 days. Clearly the practice of using iced enzyme as a stock and bringing it rapidly to the desired temperature, could give large errors.

These findings are too new and too limited to evaluate their full impact. It is clear that their importance varies with different inhibitors. A practical conclusion is that one needs to be particularly careful to assure himself that his inhibition kinetics are truly apparent-first-order (when working with low concentrations of inhibitor—much less than K_a—and with a large excess of inhibitor over enzyme; these are the common conditions). He may then be assured that his mix of isoenzymes does not contain types of greatly varying sensitivity for that particular inhibitor. A second consideration is that when one wishes to extend *in vitro* work on enzyme sensitivity to *in vivo* conditions, he must carefully match the *in vitro* and *in vivo* temperatures.

Of particular importance for those designers of inhibitors who look for physiological effects, is the recent report (36) that two AChE isoenzymes are much more rapidly synthesized than any others studied. Rat retina AChE was explored, and that portion (about 15%) that was soluble in the detergent Myrj 53* was fractionated into 10 isoenzyme bands. When enzyme levels were examined after DFP injection, two of these isoenzymes recovered relatively rapidly; one of them (B_2) was studied further. The recovery could be blocked by acetoxycyloheximide (a blocker of protein synthesis), and other experiments also suggested that resynthesis, rather than reactivation of

* Atlas Chemicals, Indiana.

inhibited enzyme, was involved. A half-life of 3 hr was calculated for B_2, in contrast with 1 or 2 weeks for the eight more stable isoenzymes. The physiological importance of the above findings cannot yet be assessed. If such high-turnover isoenzymes are widespread, and are sufficiently effective to sustain the integrity of cholinergic neurons by themselves, then clearly even long-lasting anticholinesterases will have *in vivo* effects of only an hour or so duration.

F. CHANGES IN ENZYME CONFIGURATION DURING CATALYSIS

The early, somewhat static, views of the interaction of enzymes with substrates and inhibitors envisaged the enzyme surface as a place with a particular topography. By charting it, one could hope to design new agents to interact with it. Since 1959, Koshland's views (for review, see *66*) on enzyme flexibility have modified this view and raised new possibilities. "The assumption that the active site was already formed as a relatively rigid negative of a portion of the substrate molecule was modified to postulate that a fit finally resulted, but the fit occurred only after a change in shape of the enzyme molecule had been induced by the substrate" (*66*).

This wrap-around model does not have as gloomy a set of consequences as one might have anticipated a priori: Baker (*10*) has shown, after years of study with numerous enzymes, that one can add remarkably bulky groups *to certain parts* of substrates, and still have binding and catalysis; in his words, he has shown the degree of "bulk tolerance" in many systems. And there are so many good substrates and inhibitors of cholinesterases, that it is clear that their tolerance for bulk (and for diverse electronic and steric properties) is pretty high.

An unusually interesting follow-through of Koshland's ideas has been that of Belleau and Lavoie (*16*). Working with bovine erythrocyte AChE and a set of 22 competitive inhibitors all of the form $RN^+(CH_3)_3$, they demonstrated the surprising fact that their binding constants (K_a in our terminology) were remarkably similar, so that their ΔF values for inhibition (calculated as $\Delta F = -RT \ln K_a$) averaged -4.2 ± 0.6 cal/mole at 25°C. However, experiments at various temperatures showed that ΔH and ΔS varied greatly: thus the ΔH values ranged from -5.25 to 2.2 kcal/mole. Belleau interprets these findings, by arguments that cannot be entered into here, as implying that all these agents act primarily "to release 'ice-like' water from the binding cleft, a process which is *formally* tantamount to a conformational rearrangement." He subdivides them into classes: those with R as an alkyl group, which expel water from the binding cleft but do not themselves interact with the hypothetical "lattice of hydrogen bonds in the enzyme clefts" (presumably they interact by hydrophobic forces along) and those in which R contains oxygen, π electron compounds, and other suitable groups, which do not only displace, but react with the hydrogen bonds that bond the icelike water.

It thus seems likely that the active zone of AChE is not a rigid two-dimensional structure, but a potentially flexible three-dimensional array. The flexibility may play a different role for different compounds. Thus for alkylammoniums (128) and trialkyl phosphates and phosphorothiolates (23) the replacement of the hydrogen of —$NH(CH_3)_2$ or —$CH(CH_5)_3$ by a methylene gives no improvements in binding, suggesting that the added methylene projects away from the enzyme surface. But Wilson (128) found that when one of the methylenes was removed from the —$N(CH_3)_3$ of acetylcholine, the maximum velocity of hydrolysis is halved and the K_m is doubled, showing that in the binding or, more likely, the k_2 (acylation) step, the enzyme must fold around the $N(CH_3)_3$ group. In 1966 Krupka (70) used two very different arguments* to indicate that the enzyme did indeed change shape in the course of the acylation–deacylation steps. Bracha and O'Brien (23) provide evidence that folding does not occur during phosphorylation of AChE.

III. Design of Organophosphates

We shall discuss here approaches to the design of *in vitro* enzyme inhibitors. It will not be possible in this space (except in rare cases) to examine the more general problem, i.e., what factors permit a good *in vitro* inhibitor to operate successfully *in vivo*, in various organisms.

In the design of organophosphates, it used to be possible to suggest that one had just two factors to examine: a steric aspect, which probably influenced the binding to the enzyme [the K_a step of Eq. (1)], and an electronic aspect, which governed the k_2 or phosphorylation step. The accuracy of this intuitive pair of views has only become testable with the emergence of data upon K_y (which we shall have to accept, for now, as an approximation of K_a) and separately for k_2. Up to now, most of the data have been for k_i, which, as mentioned above, is k_2/K_a, and therefore gives no information about the two steps individually.

A. The Leaving Group

Under usual conditions, all the organophosphates phosphorylate cholinesterase, in accordance with Eq. (1), and hence a group within the organo-

---

* Specifically (1) that the pK_a's of acylation and deacylation differed and so must be accomplished by two different groups; and (2) tetraethylammonium could activate carbamylation by carbamyl fluoride, yet block decarbamylation. Hence the acyl or carbamyl groups must be relocated prior to the hydrolysis step.

phosphate leaves in the course of the reaction. Normally the most acid group is the one with the most "leaving-group character." [We need not consider here such special cases as that of "phosphorylthiocholines" and tertiary analogs in which, at 0°C, all the inhibition was reversible and could be reversed by gel filtration (54).]

Let us begin by examining the accepted picture of the way in which electronic factors influence k_i. The classic work of Aldridge and Davison in 1952 (8) first showed clearly that in a limited series of compounds which were sterically similar (in their case, phenyl-substituted diethyl phenyl phosphates), those substituents which enhanced the susceptibility of the phosphorus to hydroxyl attack (i.e., which enhanced alkaline hydrolyzability) produced a parallel improvement in k_i. This phenomenon, first shown for variously substituted aromatics, has also been demonstrated for alkylphosphonates with various alkyl groups (44). The reason for this correlation between the ability of the inhibitor to react with OH⁻ and with the enzyme is presumably that both involve an electrophilic attack by the phosphorus atom. Consequently, substituents which withdraw electrons from the phosphorus will tend to increase anticholinesterase activity and alkaline hydrolyzability. Simultaneously they will increase the acidity of the leaving group [hence the correlation of such acidity with anticholinesterase activity (58)] and increase the infrared frequency for the P—O leaving group bonds (43). An extremely interesting quantitation of the relation between hydrolyzability and antienzyme activity has been worked out by Ooms (106), who has developed equations for prediction of k_i from hydrolyzability data [reviewed by O'Brien (98)].

By far the best way to express this data is in terms of the correlation of anticholinesterase activity with the σ constant of Hammett or the σ^* constant of Taft. Such a procedure has been used extensively by the Riverside group with good results for aromatic phosphates (13, 43, 84, 87). But poor correlations exist for S-aryl phosphorothiolates (93) and aromatic alkyl phosphonates (45).

If excessively electrophilic substituents are inserted, the compounds become too readily hydrolyzed even under neutral conditions, and their potency therefore drops. Thus addition of one mole of chlorine to one methyl group of schradan increased the anticholinesterase activity 10,000-fold, and reduced its half-life at pH 9 and 15°C from several years to 118 min. But addition of 3 moles of chlorine abolished activity and reduced the half-life to 3 min (118). Thus there is an optimum in addition of electrophilic substituents.

$$[(CH_3)_2N]_2P(O)OP(O)[N(CH_3)_2]_2$$

Schradan

On the basis of the above, one can formulate a tentative rule: electrophilic substituents, when they can affect the electronegative character of the phosphorus, increase anticholinesterase activity, unless the water stability is too far reduced.

A corollary should be that nucleophilic substituents have the opposite effect. This is nearly always true. A well-known example is parathion: if one converts its nitro group to an amino group, anticholinesterase activity is almost abolished (*33*).

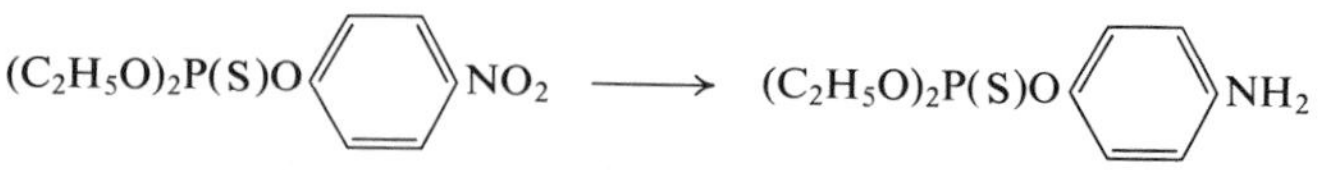

$$(C_2H_5O)_2P(S)O\text{---}\bigcirc\text{---}NO_2 \longrightarrow (C_2H_5O)_2P(S)O\text{---}\bigcirc\text{---}NH_2$$

Parathion   Aminoparathion

Similarly, phosphorus diesters, which are common metabolites of the potent triesters, lack activity because of the huge nucleophilic effect of the anion. Hence dealkylations such as the following constitute detoxification; the average extent [in seven examples studied (*4*)] was 158,000-fold:

$$(CH_3O)_2P(O)OCH\text{=}CCl_2 \longrightarrow \begin{array}{c} {}^-O \\ CH_3O \end{array}\!\!\!\!\!P(O)OCH\text{=}CCl_2$$

Dichlorvos

In certain very special cases, however, phosphorus diesters can have substantial activity: the requirement is that a strategically located basic group, such as —NH$_2$, can form an internal salt with the anion (*4*). Thus the following retains 1/292 of the potency of its triester parent:

$$\begin{array}{c} C_2H_5O \\ {}^-O \end{array}\!\!\!\!\!P(O)SCH_2CH_2N(C_2H_5)_2$$

Deethyl Amiton

The quaternary analog of deethyl Amiton, by contrast, has only 1/80,000 of its parent's potency. Presumably ring formation is hindered in the quaternary compound. The nitrogen is of course obligatory in this phenomenon; dealkylation of "carbon–Amiton" reduces activity 33,000-fold.

$$(C_2H_5O)_2P(O)SCH_2CH_2CH(C_2H_5)_2$$

Carbon–Amiton

It is customary to assume that all those electronic effects are upon the phosphorylation step. Yet it is entirely possible that k_{+1} or k_{-1} steps might involve electronic contributions. It is also rather likely that in the numerous aromatic organophosphates, some charge transfer complex formation can contribute to the binding of appropriate compounds. If so, then ring substituents would have important effects, electrophilic groups being promotional if the organophosphate is acting as the acceptor or adverse if it is acting as the donor. When better ways of studying K_a are available, this possibility would be a rewarding one to study.

Frequently in studies of correlation of k_i with σ constants (or some equivalent measure) it is found that some few compounds are far better inhibitors than one would expect on electronic grounds. In such cases it is argued that the particular substituent has had a substantial effect upon K_a in addition to its predicted effect upon k_2, i.e., that a special binding ability exists. Substituents for which such effects have been shown include the following:

m-Trimethylammonium (ref. *41*)	*m-t*-Butyl (ref. *41*)	ω-*t*-Butyl (ref. *41*) β-Aminoethylthio (ref. *106*)

It is frequently stated that the above substituents are effective because when the phosphorus is adjacent to the esteratic site, these substituents can bind to the anionic site. There are two implications in such statements:

1. There is a rather specific distance from P to the substituent. The most striking case is in the analogous situation of carbamates, for which it was shown (*85*) that of alkylphenyl compounds, the *meta* position was optimal whereas, for alkoxyphenyl compounds, the *ortho* is optimal. In both cases the alkyl portion would then be roughly *meta* to the carbamyl substituent.

Unfortunately the value of this specific-distance consideration cannot yet be confirmed by the enzymological data. For AChE those who argued that there was a single anionic site have produced rather different estimates of the separation of the esteratic and anionic sites in eel AChE, e.g., 5 Å based on pyridinealdoxime reactions (*130*), or less than 2.5 Å based on cyclic quaternary reactions (*40*). Furthermore, there is a suggestion (*97*) that the site separation is greater in houseflies (4.5–5.9 Å) than in mammals (<4.5 Å). Yet the "optimal *meta*" argument has been supported by data from both housefly and bovine AChE. And in addition to this uncertainty (or perhaps as a corollary of this uncertainty) the case for the existence of two anionic sites has been strengthened recently, as discussed above.

2. There is a close match between the shape or charge of the substituent and the anionic site. The uncertainties about the charge status of that site, and its possibly multiple character, were reviewed in Section II, C. The fact that t-butyl- and trimethylammonium groups, in both aromatic and alkyl phosphates, have been highly effective substituents, imply that the isosteric $-\overset{+}{C}(CH_3)_3$ and $-\overset{+}{N}(CH_3)_3$ groupings fit closely into a complementary hole in the enzyme, to give a large binding contribution. But recent work (23) with compounds of the type $(C_2H_2O)_2P(O)OR$ and $(C_2H_5)_2P(O)SR$, where R is a simple branched or unbranched alkyl chain, have refuted this implication. On the contrary, no specific branching of R had "special" binding properties, and all the data conformed with the presence of the simple 6-methylene hydrophobic patch described above.

Next let us consider the effects of manipulating alkyl groups which serve as bridges between the phosphorus and functional groups. Three sorts of effect might be expected a priori. (1) Added methylenes might give a hydrophobic contribution, amounting to a 3-fold improvement in K_a and hence k_i, for each methylene. (2) Suitable alkyl bridges might permit more effective localization of functional groups upon potential binding sites, thus improving K_a. (3) Altering the relation of the functional group to the phosphorus could have an effect on the electronic effect upon the phosphorus, and hence modify k_2. One could imagine that a very short chain could permit inductive effects through the chain; that lengthening the chain would lessen the effect; but that a still longer chain might permit a field effect, i.e., might allow the functional group to appose the phosphorus through ring formation. Just such effects are found upon acidity when one interposes methylene between carboxyls in a dicarboxylic acids (25, p. 626).

Let us consider these effects using malaoxon analogs as examples (Table II). Considering effects upon k_2, the most dramatic drop (100-fold) occurred when both carboethoxy groups were made β, by the interposition of an extra methylene group (compare malaoxon and β-glutarate malaoxon). Probably the worsening of the inductive effect is responsible, and probably the impotence of methyl propoxon derives from the same cause: note that methyl isopropoxon is a good inhibitor, for its carboethoxy is an α type. But although adding-in a second carboethoxy group is helpful (e.g., malonate malaoxon has a k_2 which is 6-fold greater than that of methyl acetoxon), it is surprisingly unimportant for k_2 whether this second group is attached via zero, one, or two methylenes, i.e., in malonate malaoxon, in malaoxon and in α-glutarate malaoxon. K_y is more sensitive to such placement, showing a distinct optimum when the second carboethoxy is α. Indeed, as far as K_y is concerned, a poorly placed second carboethoxy (in malaoxon) is no better than no second carboethoxy at all (in methyl isopropoxon), suggesting that this second carboethoxy

TABLE II

VARIATIONS IN LEAVING GROUPS OF MALAOXON ANALOGS[a]
$(CH_3O)_2P(O)SR$ (all racemic or optically inactive)

R	k_i $(M^{-1} min^{-1})$	k_2 (min^{-1})	K_y (mM)
$-CHCOOC_2H_5$ | $CH_2COOC_2H_5$ Malaoxon	1.4×10^4	52	3.6
$-CHCOOC_2H_5$ | $COOC_2H_5$ Malonate malaoxon	42×10^4	63	0.15
$-CHCOOC_2H_5$ | $CH_2CH_2COOC_2H_5$ α-Glutarate malaoxon	12×10^4	77	0.64
$-CHCH_2COOC_2H_5$ | $CH_2COOC_2H_5$ β-Glutarate malaoxon	0.02×10^4	0.5	2.1
$CH_2COOC_2H_5$ Methyl acetoxon	0.41×10^4	9.9	2.4
$CH_2CH_2COOC_2H_5$ Methyl propoxon	0.0015×10^4	—	—
$CH(CH_3)COOC_2H_5$ Methyl isopropoxon	1.23×10^4	20	1.6

[a] Data from Chiu and Dauterman (29). All pH 7.6, 5°C.

must, for a good K_y, be located rather precisely on a second binding site. Can it be that this second site is the α_2 site, presumably with attachment by hydrogen bonding?

B. ALKYL GROUPS

Of the hundred thousand or so organophosphates reported, the huge majority have bis-*O,O*-ethyl or bis-*O,O*-methyl groups: the variety comes primarily in inventing new leaving groups. Yet some of the highly toxic warfare agents had far more complicated branched alkyl chains, as shown in Fig. 3. When we found (21, 22) that a simple but sufficiently long alkyl chain R could, in compounds of the type $(C_2H_5O)P(O)OR$ or $(C_2H_5O)_2P(O)SR$, give AChE inhibitors almost as potent as paraoxon, we attempted to improve R by suitable branching (23). However, as Fig. 4 demonstrates, the addition of branches to any given straight chain produced only modest improvements in potency. For instance, in compound 3, the pinacolyl group (which is a feature of the very potent soman) was little better than compound 1, which has a simple n-propyl group.

TABLE III

EFFECT OF VARIATIONS IN O,O-DIALKYL GROUPS[a]

R	k_i $(M^{-1} min^{-1})$	k_2 (min^{-1})	K_y (mM)
A. Malaoxon homologs (racemic):			
$(RO)_2P(O)SCH(CH_2COOC_2H_5)COOC_2H_5$			
CH_3	2.8×10^4	67	2.4
C_2H_5	1.4×10^4	52	3.6
n-C_3H_7	1.3×10^4	58	4.5
iso-C_3H_7	0.04×10^4	3.3	8.9
n-C_4H_9	3.8×10^4	25	0.67
B. Paraoxon homologs: $(RO)_2P(O)OC_6H_4NO_2$			
CH_3	5.7×10^4	50	0.89
C_2H_5	12.0×10^4	43	0.36
n-C_3H_7	14.0×10^4	66	0.47
iso-C_3H_3	0.31×10^4	3.2	1.0
n-C_4H_9	24.5×10^4	65	2.7

[a] Data rounded off from Chiu et al. (30). Malaoxons at pH 7.6 and 5°C; paraoxons at pH 7 and 5°C.

Chiu et al. (30) have analyzed the effects of varying the O,O-alkyl groups of malaoxons and paraoxon, as shown in Table III. First let us examine effects upon overall potency (k_i). It is odd that, whereas unbranched chain of C_1 through C_4 are roughly equipotent, the isopropyl substitution gives a pronounced drop in activity. [Such an effect is even more pronounced when bee AChE is examined (35).] It is particularly unexpected that the poor k_i of the isopropyl compound, which for malaoxons (for instance) is 30 times worse than that of the n-propyl isomer, is due more to a drop in k_2 (which is 20 times worse than for n-propyl) then to a rise in K_y (2 times worse than for

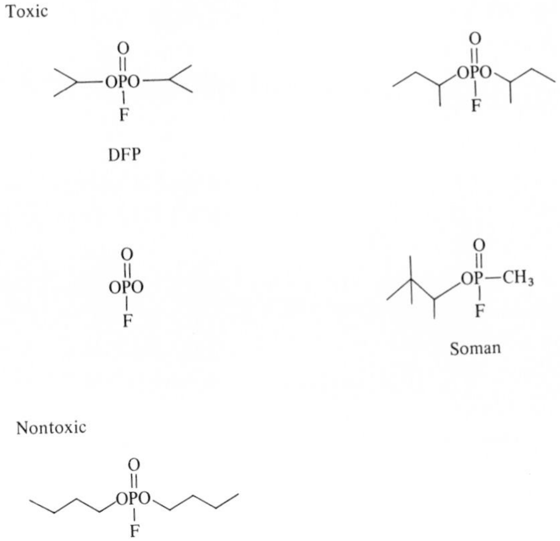

Toxic

DFP

Nontoxic

Fig. 3. Alkyl chains of phosphorofluoridates and phosphonofluoridates. From data of Saunders (*115*).

	log k_i			log k_i
1. 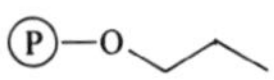	3.2		7. 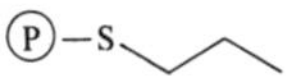	4.0
2. 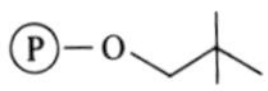	3.2		8. 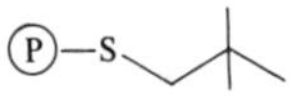	4.0
3. 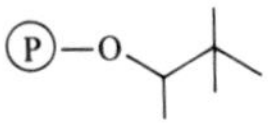	3.4		9. 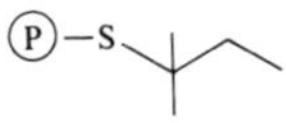	4.6
4. 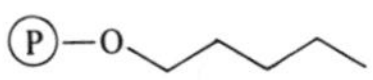	3.9			
5. 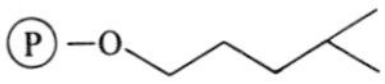	4.3			
6. 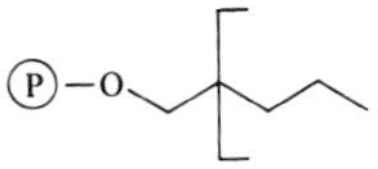	5.2			

Fig. 4. Effect of adding branches to trialkyl organophosphates. k_i is expressed as mole^{-1} min^{-1}. Ⓟ represents $(C_2H_5O)_2P(O)$—. From data of Bracha and O'Brien (*22, 23*).

n-propyl). Precisely the same is true in the paraoxons. This is yet another case (see Section II, F) of a large steric factor in k_2.

Let us now leave aside the isopropoxy effect, and examine Table III for the effects of progressive increases in *linear* alkoxy chains in such compounds. It is at once obvious that potency, k_i and consequently its contributory factors K_a and k_2, are remarkably insensitive to such increases. In malaoxons, the k_i variation is only 3-fold, and in paraoxons only 4-fold. One might have imagined that some hydrophobic bonding would occur, as is discussed above in trialkyl phosphates. If so, each added pair of methylenes would improve K_a and hence k_i 3-fold, and clearly nothing of the sort occurs. The implication is that in these compounds the binding of the leaving group orients the *O,O*-alkoxy groups away from the hydrophobic patch described previously.

The relative insensitivity of k_i to changes in alkyl groups under such orientation conditions emerges also from the work of Becker *et al.* (*11*) in the following phosphonates, with R from C_3H_7 up to $C_{10}H_{21}$:

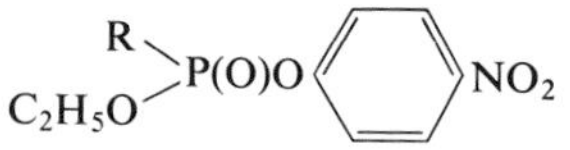

They found that anti-AChE potency decreased rather little (about 10-fold) as one passed from C_3 to C_5, then showed virtually no change. Such behavior was entirely unlike that found for their inhibitory action against chymotrypsin, for which an extremely sharp optimum for C_7 was observed. Becker *et al.* found that in a closely related homologous series:

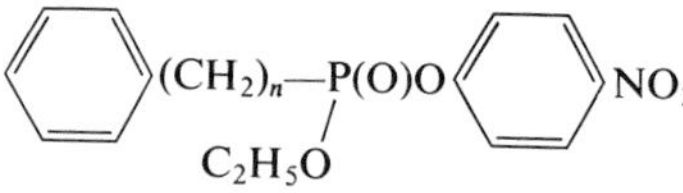

the anticholinesterases activity, which was about equal for $n = 0$ or 1, climbed steadily thereafter so that the compound with the longest chain ($n = 4$) was 25 times more potent than that for $n = 1$. One possibility is that the unsubstituted phenyl group anchored the molecule near the hydrophobic patch, thus permitting an expression of hydrophobic bonding. But one cannot dismiss another possibility: that (as in the malaoxons with different alkyl attachments to the leaving group discussed in Section III, A), the increase of n permitted better positioning of the unsubstituted phenyl group to an aromatic (? π–π) bonding site.

It would seem that, in spite of the work with warfare agents, that adventurous design of the *O,O*-alkyl portions has not often proven very successful, except in some phosphonates. This view is confirmed by the popularity of the use of ethyl and methyl in commercial compounds.

An unexpected class is that (*108*) containing two $ClCH_2CH_2O$ groups, of which the only well-known example is haloxon, an anthelminthic related to the oxygen analog, coroxon, of the older insecticide called coumaphos (formerly Co-ral).

$(C_2H_5O)_2P(O)O$ [structure] Cl

$(ClC_2H_4O)_2P(O)O$ [structure] Cl

Coroxon   Haloxon

Haloxon was much less toxic to rats (LD_{50} 896 mg/kg) than was coumaphos (LD_{50} 56 mg/kg) and even less than was coroxon (LD_{50} 9.8 mg/kg). Since coroxon is the active inhibitor derived metabolically from coumaphos, it provides a more suitable comparison. Although precise data were not provided, there is no reason to believe that the inhibitory potency k_i is very different for chloroethoxy than for ethoxy compounds. But other parameters are unusual, notably the spontaneous reactivation rate [the k_3 step of Eq. (1)]. Thus enzyme (calf erythrocyte AChE) inhibited with coroxon showed no spontaneous recovery, whereas that inhibited by haloxon recovered 50% in 30 min.

Haloxon has a remarkable species selectivity which seems to relate to differences in brain AChE (*73*). Thus the relative potency for geese:ducks:hens is about 200:20:1. The insensitivity of the hen is apparently due to its very fast k_3 (reactivation) rate: in 30 min there is about 60% recovery of its activity. The relative k_3 rates for geese:ducks:hens is 0:0.2:1. In addition there are effects upon the induced reversibility by 2-pyridine aldoxime, but these need not concern us here.

Next let us turn to alkyl additions to functional groups within the leaving group. Main and Hastings (*78*) performed a classic study in 1966 on the relative effects upon phosphorylation and alkylation. They compared the effects of malaoxon analogs upon phosphorylation and acylation, i.e., they compared malaoxon analogs as inhibitors with the corresponding butyryl esters as substrates.

$(CH_3O)_2P(O)SCHCOOR$ $CH_3CH_2CH_2COOR$ $HS—CHCOOR$
$\qquad\qquad\quad |$ $|$
$\qquad\qquad CH_2COOR$ CH_2COOR

Malaoxon analogs   Butyryl esters   Thiomalate esters

They showed that when R was methyl, ethyl, *n*-propyl, isopropyl, or *n*-butyl, the acidity of the thiomalates varied little (pK_a from 6.68 to 6.97) and so, as expected, k_2 of the malaoxon analogs varied relatively little (2.6 for isopropyl; others between 6.6 and 22.6 min^{-1}). The catalytic hydrolysis of the butyryl esters also varied only modestly, from 1.17 to 13.6 min^{-1}. But the K_y for the malaoxons and the K_m for the esters varied greatly, and in parallel fashion. Assuming that both reflected primarily differences in affinity, we can say that affinity for the two kinds of compound changed in a remarkably parallel way, the relative affinities from C_1 through C_4 being $1:3:24:30$ for the malaoxons, and $1:6:18:31$ for the esters. Assuming (as the authors do) that only one of the two alkyl groups in each malaoxon binds to the active site, then we may calculate the average binding energy per added methylene as 690 cal/mole at 25°C. This value is in excellent agreement with the theoretical value of 730 cal/mole for the hydrophobic contribution of a methylene group. Undoubtedly, then, the R groups are binding to the hydrophobic patch near the catalytic site.

C. The Thiono Effect

It is well established that phosphorothionates are very much worse anti-cholinesterases than their corresponding phosphates* [reviewed by Heath (53) and O'Brien (96)]. Only part of this difference is due to the poorer electrophilic character of the S than of the O; for instance, the alkaline hydrolyzabilities of parathion and paraoxon differ only 10-fold but their anti-AChE activities differ 10^5-fold. Heath (53) suggests that (quite apart from electrophilic considerations) the O is necessary for hydrogen bonding.

TABLE IV

The Thiono Effect in

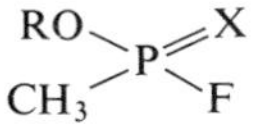

$$\begin{array}{c} RO \\ CH_3 \end{array} P \begin{array}{c} X \\ F \end{array}$$

WHERE X IS S OR O[a]

| | k_i (25°C, pH 7.7) | | |
R	P(O) type	P(S) type	Ratio
Isopropyl	1.4×10^7	7.6×10^4	184
Cyclohexyl	3.3×10^8	1×10^5	3300
1,3,3-Trimethylpropyl	6×10^7	2×10^7	3
1,3-Dimethylbutyl	2×10^8	9.6×10^6	21

[a] Data of Boter and Ooms (20). Values are for faster enantiomorph.

* A single exception that has been reported [Lovell, quoted by O'Brien (99, p. 63)] is:

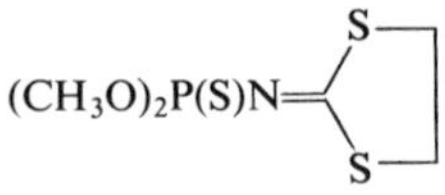

$$(CH_3O)_2P(S)N = \begin{array}{c} S \\ S \end{array}$$

Table IV shows that the extent of the thiono effect can vary greatly with the alkyl substituent. It shows that, contrary to what we have all come to expect, the thiono effect can be extremely small in some cases. Clearly we need more facts to account in full for the thiono effect *in vitro*.

It has been pointed out (*95*) that if different organisms have different abilities to degrade a class of organophosphate, and hence enjoy a measure of protection, then this effect would have an even greater opportunity of showing itself in P(S) than in P(O) compounds, because of the time lag necessary while the P(S) is converted to R(O) metabolically. This is the "opportunity factor" enjoyed by P(S) compounds. An attempt was made (*103*) to convert three nonselective phosphates into more selective compounds, by making their thiono analogs. The following compounds were prepared, but their selectivity for houseflies as compared to mice was little better than their phosphate parents.

$(iso\text{-}C_3H_7O)_2P(S)F$ $[(CH_3)_2N]_2P(S)F$ $(iso\text{-}C_3H_7NH)_2P(S)F$

Thiono-DFP   Thiono-dimefox   Thiono-mipafox

D. The Thiolo Effect

It has been frequently observed, especially in organophosphates whose leaving groups resemble choline, that the phosphates are virtually inactive whereas the phosphorothiolates are highly active. This phenomenon has been called "the thiolo effect" (*21*). Typically, compounds such as the following (of which nine examples exist) have about 10,000-fold less anticholinesterase activity than their thiolo analogs (*102, 119*).

$$\begin{matrix} CH_3 \\ \diagdown \\ C_2H_5O \diagup \end{matrix} P(O)OCH_2CH_2\overset{+}{N}(CH_3)_3 \qquad\qquad (C_2H_5O)_2P(O)OCH_2CH_2\overset{+}{N}(CH_3)_3$$

$$(C_2H_5O)_2P(O)OCH_2CH_2N(CH_3)_2 \qquad\qquad (C_2H_5O)_2P(O)OCH_2CH_2N(C_2H_5)_2$$

On such evidence, it might seem reasonable to argue that a large thiolo effect is usual in such compounds, whose leaving groups lack very potent electrophilic effects upon the phosphorus. However, a more extensive set of studies (*21–23*) has unexpectedly shown that in simple trialkyl phosphates (whose leaving group also have exceptionally small electrophilic character) the thiolo effect is usually very small. Table V shows examples selected from 19 pairs of compounds of which only 3 showed a large thiolo effect, and one which showed a negative effect. It follows that what was thought to be a general situation turns out to be a special case. The commonest case, a small thiolo effect of 3- to 6-fold, is compatible with the report that thiolo compounds are attacked by OH⁻ at about 17 times the rate of their P—O—C analogs (72). It is the unusual, large thiolo effect that requires a special explanation.

An examination of the data from which these "thiolo effect" ratios are drawn suggests that the primary oddity is that when the longest chain in the compound is C_4, the phosphate is unusually inactive. One possibility is that such a compound can bind to the enzyme in a way which forbids its subsequent phosphorylation; such "adverse binding" is familiar in chymotrypsin (56, 117). Presumably the phosphorothiolates cannot bind adversely* because of the different bond angle of P—S—C (100°C) as compared with P—O—C (109°C).

TABLE V

THE THIOLO EFFECT IN $(C_2H_5O)_2P(O)XR$ WHERE X IS O OR S[a]

R	Ratio (k_i for X = S)/(k_i for X = O)
—C_2H_5	710
—C_3H_7	6.4
—C_4H_9	33.0
—C_5H_{11}	3.4
—$C_{10}H_{21}$	0.13
—$CH(C_2H_5)_2$	78
—$CH_2CH(C_2H_5)_2$	1,780
—$(CH_2)CH(C_2H_5)_2$	3.2
$(CH_2)_3CH(C_2H_5)_2$	4.5
$(CH_2)_2N(C_2H_5)_2$	20,400

[a] Data selected from Bracha and O'Brien (21, 22).

In summary of the thiolo effect, a designer should expect that thiolo compounds will frequently be about 5-fold better as anticholinesterases than their oxy analogs (assuming that one can tolerate the decreased aqueous stability of the thiolo compound); in certain special cases, the thiolo will be enormously better than its oxy analog—but primarily because the oxy analog is unexpectedly poor.

E. PHOSPHONATES AND S-PHENYL COMPOUNDS

Although there has been (42, 44) extensive synthesis of phosphonates (i.e., compounds with one alkyl or aryl group bonded directly to the phosphorus), they have not been actively used commercially, with the somewhat odd

* In fact the dip in activity at C_4 is shown to a modest extent in phosphorothiolates also (21, 22) and in one of the two series of phosphonothiolates studied (24).

EPN

exception of EPN. Nevertheless, in 1965 is was reported (*82*) that several phosphonodithioates showed substantial advantages in potency and in effectiveness in control of resistant houseflies, as compared with their phosphorodithioate analogs. Extremely high anticholinesterase potency (I_{50} for human plasma BuChE: 7×10^{-8} M) was noted in the presumed metabolite of a phosphonodithioate.

Presumably the absence of electronegative ring substituents in this compound is compensated by the fact that there is a thiophenol leaving group. Thioacids are much stronger acids than oxyacids, especially in aromatics; thiophenol is 1000 times more acid than phenol (*5*). One might therefore expect that the corresponding phosphorothiolate would be active also; but the authors suggest that there is often unexpected potency in phosphonates without electrophilic substituents, and promise further reports along this line. But very recently it has been reported that $(CH_3O)_2P(O)S$-phenyl and $(C_2H_5O)_2P(O)S$-phenyl are potent inhibitors, the I_{50} values being, respectively, 2×10^{-6} M and 2.8×10^{-7} M (*93*). Such compounds become still better upon adding electrophilic substituents, improving about 100-fold with p-chloro or p-bromo substitution. These facts argue against any unusual properties of P—C as compared with their P—O—C analogs.

Murdock and Hopkins point out the small spread of anticholinesterase potency in response to aromatic substitution in the S-phenyl compounds (*93*): the spread was only 20-fold, as compared with 1000-fold in various O-phenyl compounds (*43*). It seems plausible to argue that the unsubstituted S-phenyl parent lies fairly close to the optimum for electronegativity of the phosphorus; it is improved only 30-fold by inserting a p-nitro group.

F. STEREOSPECIFICITY

There are well-documented cases which show that, as expected, cholinesterases react preferentially with one or other form of enantiomorphic inhibitors. Two kinds of asymmetry have been explored: around the phosphorus, and around the carbon of a substituent. We will discuss the former first.

The effects upon k_i are moderately large, and differ somewhat with the enzyme type and source. Thus with $(C_2H_5O)(C_2H_5)P(O)SCH_2CH_2SC_2H_5$, Aaron *et al.* (*1*) isolated enantiomorphs and found the *l* form to be 18-fold more potent than the *d* form for eel AChE, 20-fold for horse serum BuChE and 10-fold for human erythrocyte AChE. With phosphonates synthesized by usual routes, one of course produces *dl* mixtures, and kinetic studies on inhibition of cholinesterase reveal two components, as shown for instance by Michel (*92*) for sarin.

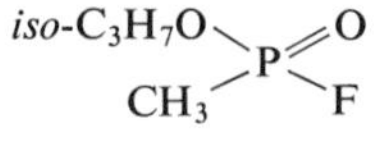

$$iso\text{-}C_3H_7O \diagdown \!\! \underset{CH_3 \diagup}{P} \!\! \diagup\!\!\!\!\diagup^{O}_{\diagdown F}$$

Sarin

It has seemed natural to conclude that when stereospecificity is found, it is due to specificity in the binding step. Such a conclusion implies that steric factors control the binding step and electronic factors control the catalytic steps. Unhappily this simple picture is probably incorrect, just as it has proved incorrect for chymotrypsin, for which the stereospecificity "is exercised in catalytic rather than binding steps" (*57*). Table VI shows clearly that the enantiomorphs of ethyl malaoxon differ substantially in anticholinesterase potency; but (more surprisingly) that the 4.5-fold difference in k_i is due about equally to differences in phosphorylating potency and in binding; the k_2's differ 2.0-fold and the K_y's 2.1-fold. Clearly, then, there is a steric involvement in the phosphorylation (k_2) step. Similarly, (Table VI) in a pair of geometrical

TABLE VI

Steric Factors in Carboethoxy Phosphates[a]

	k_i (M^{-1} min^{-1})	k_2 (min^{-1})	K_y (mM)
A. Enantiomorphs of malaoxon: $(CH_3O)_2P(O)SCH(CH_2COOC_2H_5)COOC_2H_5$			
d form	2.8×10^4	63	2.3
l form	0.63×10^4	31	4.9
B. *cis-trans* Isomers of mevinphos: $(CH_3O)_2P(O)OC(CH_3)=CHCOOCH_3$			
cis	3.5×10^4	59	1.7
trans	0.18×10^4	5.6	3.2

[a] From Chiu and Dauterman (*28*). All pH 7.6, 5°C.

isomers in which electronic differences should be small; the *cis* form owes most of its 20-fold superiority in k_i to a 10-fold superiority in k_2, when compared to the *trans* isomers. Again the k_2 step has a steric requirement.

G. SELECTIVE INHIBITION *in Vitro* BY ORGANOPHOSPHATES

It is well established, and we do not need to dwell long upon it, that AChE and BuChE have some substantial differences in their sensitivity. The data from several sources have been tabulated [Tables 3.7 and 3.8 of O'Brien (*96*) and 6.12 and 6.13 of Heath (*53*)]. It is clear that some compounds show a distinct preference for one or other enzyme: thus *iso*-OMPA, $[(CH_3)_2CHNHP(O)]_2O$, is 13,200-fold more effective against dog red cell AChE than against dog serum BuChE (*6*). These preferences vary greatly with species, being 11,300-fold for horse, 530-fold for rat, but only 56-fold for man. It is interesting that in the majority of cases the BuChE is the more sensitive; only methyl paraoxon $(CH_3O)_2P(O)C_6H_4NO_2$ is better for AChE, and the extent varies from 170-fold in rat (*37*) to 2-fold in horse (*6*). Unfortunately it is hard to construct an explanation for these differences, although Aldridge (*6*) has made some attempt to match substrate specificity to organophosphate specificity.

Of more interest to those who design organophosphates for selective toxicants, is the extent to which organisms differ in the sensitivity of their AChE, since it is this enzyme which appears to be the usual target. That species variations exist is shown by the data in the previous paragraph, as well as by extensive studies upon substrate preferences of AChE from rat, spider mite, and housefly, using 17 acetylcholine analogs whose primary differences were in configuration about the N^+ (*34, 80, 81*).

Organophosphates have frequently demonstrated species specificity. Dichlorvos is 501 times and ruelene is 794 times more effective against housefly AChE than against human erythrocyte enzyme; this enzyme selectivity parallels selective toxicity for these organisms (*99*, p. 283). Similarly diisopropyl paraoxon is 40 times better against housefly than against bee AChE, and

$(CH_3O)_2P(O)OCH{=}CCl_2$

Dichlorvos

$(iso\text{-}C_3H_7O)_2P(O)O$ —◯— NO_2

Diisopropyl paraoxon

correspondingly 22 times more toxic to flies than bees. But unhappily, a more extensive exploration showed that in other closely related compounds, the enzyme selectivity failed to correspond to selective toxicity. Thus diethyl and dibutyl paraoxon were more potent (1.6 and 2.0 times, respectively) against fly then against bee enzyme, yet more toxic (10 and 17 times) against bees than against flies (*35*; see also *83*). Other noncorrespondences involve compounds which are *not* selectively toxic but are selective anticholinesterases. In at least one case, famoxon, this phenomenon was clearly shown to be due to a compensating difference in rates of degradation in the organisms involved, i.e., mice and milkweed bugs (*105*). Nevertheless, cases do exist where a fairly thorough examination of all the factors has led to the conclusion that AChE sensitivity determines toxicity. One case involves the unusually high sensitivity of housefly AChE to dimethoxon (*121*) and the other, the unusually low sensitivity of frog brain AChE to paraoxon (*109*). Frog brain AChE has also been known since 1946 to be unusually insensitive to the carbamate, eserine (*52*). Finally we may mention an odd case of species specificity of BuChE:

$(CH_3O)_2P(O)O$⟨⟩$SO_2N(CH_3)_2$ $(CH_3O)_2P(O)SCH_2C(O)NHCH_3$

                                                                          Dimethoxon

Famoxon

that of plaice muscle is extremely sensitive to DFP, with a pI_{50} (under unstated conditions) of 9.3 (*74*).

In summary of this section, it is clear that marked differences in enzyme sensitivity occur between species. In several cases, this leads to selective toxicity; but not infrequently, other variations in metabolism or penetration (for instance) outweigh the expected effect.

IV. Design of Carbamates

A. THE REACTION OF CARBAMATES WITH CHOLINESTERASES

The knowledge in this field is far less orderly than in the field of organophosphate design. For every proposal in the literature one gets the feeling that an equal but opposite proposal also exists. Fortunately the uncertainties about overall mechanism [uncertainties which have been reviewed at length (*99*)] have now been resolved, and laboratories which in 1965 (*85*) and 1966 (*39*) still had hesitations, had agreed by 1967 (*86*) that Eq. (1) represents the facts. Expressed verbally, carbamates are substrates for cholinesterases, which they carbamylate. They have very low turnover numbers (in the order of 0.05/min) due to their small k_3 (decarbamylation) rate. They are competitive inhibitors in that they compete with substrate for the active site, so that high concentrations of substrate offer protection. They appear as if they were reversible inhibitors, i.e., washing or dialysis for a few hours reverses the inhibition; but in fact this is not due to reversal of the inhibitory step, but due to completion of the reaction of Eq. (1); thus enzyme is indeed regenerated, but the original carbamate is not, for it is hydrolyzed in the process. They are therefore not reversible inhibitors (because the inhibitor is not recovered), nor irreversible (because the enzyme can recover if excess inhibitor is removed) but might be called "ongoing inhibitors."

Two crucial observations which leave little doubt that the carbamylation mechanism of Eq. (1) is followed, were (1) enzyme inhibited by a variety of carbamates recovers at a rate solely dictated by its N-substituents; thus all N-methyl carbamates give an enzyme which recovers with a half-life of about 39 min at 25°C (*131, 132*). The implication is that the remainder of the carbamate left before the recovery step, and is therefore a true leaving group. (2) The direct demonstration with a tritiated carbamate that the putative leaving group did indeed come off, and the rate it came off was the same as the rate of recovery of the enzyme (*104*).

Next let us state the evidence that complex formation does indeed precede carbamylation. One can only "see" such complex formation experimentally when one works with carbamate concentrations close to K_a; this means a much higher concentration than is usually used, and leads to a very rapid inhibition, so that procedures have to be employed that permit following a complete reaction within a minute or two. Under such circumstances one can show (*76, 100, 104*) that the so-called Main equation (see Section I) is followed; consequently, even infinite inhibitor concentration does not give total inhibition in a short time. There is thus a saturation phenomenon. Hellebrand (*55*) has produced precisely comparable evidence for complex formation, but using the kinetic treatment of Wilson. Consequently, there must be a complex formation as in Eq. (1) and it cannot be that:

$$AX + E \rightarrow AE + X \tag{4}$$

Other researchers (*113, 133, 134*) have suggested that Eq. (4) is experimentally followed under all practical conditions, but the arguments against their views have been presented (*100*).

The second piece of evidence for complex formation is the experimental demonstration (*100*) that when one adds carbamate to an ongoing reaction of AChE and substrate, one sees a prompt reaction attributable to complex formation, followed by a slower reaction attributable to carbamylation. The K_y and k_2 values were obtained from this kind of experiment agree well with those from a Main plot.

B. Effect of Substituents

The fact that the huge majority of carbamates are aromatic (rather unlike the situation in organophosphates) suggests that $\pi-\pi$ interactions can be important in binding them to the enzyme. For instance, compound **I** below is about 1000 times less potent that compound **II** (*86*).

I   II

This finding could be interpreted in terms of the much better leaving-group character (acidity) of a phenol than a cyclohexanol, were it not for the fact that acid character bears no such simple relationship to anticholinesterase activity in methyl carbamates, as we shall see.

The early work (65, 84, 87) from Riverside suggested that (again unlike the situation in organophosphates) electron-withdrawing substituents worsened inhibitory potency in aromatic carbamates. Three groups of compounds were involved: m- and p-substituted phenyl methylcarbamates and xylenyl methylcarbamates. In two studies (65, 87) a direct plot of potency* against σ was prepared; but the curves were rather flat, indicating a not-very-sensitive dependence on σ.

However, although up to 1965 (85) the Riverside work had shown a negative dependence of k_i upon σ, more recent work from their and our laboratory (86, 104) has suggested that in phenyl methylcarbamates, k_i is unrelated to σ. In phenyl dimethylcarbamates, our work (104) shows a fairly steep dependence of k_i upon σ, but in a positive way; the correlation of k_i was rather better with alkaline hydrolyzability (correlation coefficient $r = 0.87$) than with σ ($r = 0.78$). Thus these aromatic dimethylcarbamates had an electron dependence like that of organophosphates.

In harmony with the view that in methylcarbamates, acidity of the leaving group is unimportant (a proposition which is the corollary of the statement that high σ substituents of aromatic leaving groups are not helpful) are the reports from several sources on potency of oxime carbamates (3, 86, 124). Some examples are (3, 124):

Methylcarbamate of cyclohexanone oxime

CH_3—S—$C(CH_3)_2$CH=NOC(O)NHCH$_3$

Temik

2-Methylcarbamoyloximino-1,3-dithiolane

* The K_i values in Kolbezen *et al.* (65) are not k_i values, but were calculated on the basis of the then-prevalent view that carbamates were true reversible inhibitors with a simple dissociation constant, K_i.

The oximes from which these carbamates derive have very little acidity; thus the pK_a of the dithiolane oxime is 10.7, and of cyclohexanone oxime is over 12, compared with phenol 9.8 (*3*).

The Riverside group has for several years stressed the fact that steric factors predominated over electronic factors in determining potency, suggesting that a good fit upon the enzyme surface was the primary objective in designing carbamates. An especially convincing demonstration was that in a dozen halo-substituted phenyl methylcarbamates, inhibitory activity was entirely unrelated to electron-withdrawing potency and excellently correlated with the radius of the halogen atom (*89*). The special excellence of *m*-alkyl or *o*-alkoxy substituents has been commented upon in Section III, A. In papers dating from 1954 this group has prepared many dozens of compounds, especially phenyl methylcarbamates (*65, 86, 88*). One of their most interesting suggestions is additivity of the logarithms of what they call "affinity" *A*. It is important to note that these "affinities" are *not* true relative affinities, i.e., simple functions of K_a. Instead they are relative potencies, based on comparisons of I_{50} values of the substituted with the unsubstituted carbamate. The only justification for calling them "affinities" is if *all* the variation in potency were due to variation in K_a.

For example, in the methylcarbamates, the 3-chlorophenyl has log $A = 4$, from which one can calculate log A for 3,5-dichlorophenyl as $\log(4 + 4) = 0.9$; one finds log A experimentally as 1.23. The values for log A in other 3,5-substituted phenylcarbamates are as follows: $C(CH_3)_3$ calc. 3.0, found 3.4; $(CH_3)_2N$ calc. 1.7, found 1.9; CH_3O calc. 1.3, found 1.4; $CH(CH_3)_2$ calc. 3.1, found 3.8; CH_3 calc. 1.45, found 1.5. A discrepancy of 1 in the calculated as compared with the found indicates a 10-fold discrepancy in the "affinities" themselves.

It will be noted that in every case the observed effects are less then the predicted, by factors up to 8-fold. Nevertheless, in all the above cases, the disubstituted are better than the monosubstituted, by factors varying between 2 and 10. A factor of 2-fold is attributable to improved probability of the *m*-substituent attaching to a favored location, but larger factors must imply that the added substituents contribute separately to the binding (or to the carbamylation). The simplest hypothesis would be that the whole ring binds to a hydrophobic area (or the ring could react by $\pi-\pi$ bonding near such an area) and that additional hydrophobic ring substituents contribute to hydrophobic bonding. Assuming each methylene contributes 730 cal at 37°C, then it should improve K_a about 3-fold. An added isopropyl should thus improve K_a about 9-fold and in fact A is 10.3 times higher for the 3,5-diisopropyl (compound 9) then for the 3-isopropyl. Similarly, compound 10 should be 3-fold better then the 3-isopropyl; the observed difference is 6-fold. And compound 6 should be 9 times better than compound 1; actually it is 2.6 times

TABLE VII

HIGHLY INHIBITORY SUBSTITUTED PHENYL METHYLCARBAMATES,
ROC(O)NHCH$_3$[a]

No.	R	A[b]	No.	R	A[b]
1.		11,000	9.		6,060
2.		1,250	10.		3,570 or 3,850
3.		1,100	11.		2,560
4.		1,420	12.		1,180
5.		1,250	13.		2,560
6.		28,500	14.		2,777
7.		40,000	15.		1,670
8.		20,000	16.		18,200

[a] Data of Metcalf and Fukuto (85, 86). The methylcarbamyl group is attached to R at the bottom bond.   [b] A = Potency relative to phenyl methylcarbamate.

better. The hydrophobic argument is thus helpful, but not convincing all by itself.

In some cases double substitution is worse than single. Thus the 2,6-dichloro compound is 270-fold less potent than the 2-chloro, perhaps because of hydrolytic instability or perhaps because of hindered ring rotation. (There is nothing inherently bad about 6-halo substitution; indeed addition of a 6-chloro improves the inhibitory activity of the already potent 3-isopropylphenyl methyl-carbamate by over 4-fold.) And while the 3-trimethylammonium compound is one of the very best, with $A = 11,000$, yet the 3,5-bistrimethylammonium analog is 6 times worse; probably it is very unstable hydrolytically, for which theory Metcalf and Fukuto provide evidence (86).

Let us now examine the question, is there truly something special about *meta* substitution; and if so, what character is most important for the sub-stituent? Of the more than one hundred substituted phenyl methylcarbamates compounds summarized in Metcalf and Fukuto (85, 86), a handful stand out as being over 1000 times more inhibitory than their parent (Table VII). Let us first comment on compounds *not* good enough to appear in the table: these include most *p*-substituted compounds, and most *ortho* compound with the exception of O-alkoxy and O-alkylthio compounds; as pointed out before, the latter (because of the bond angles of O and S) may be roughly equivalent spatially to *m*-alkyl compounds.

Excellent inhibitors commonly have $CH(CH_3)_2$ or $N^+(CH_3)_3$ in the *meta* position. It is hard to escape the conclusion that *meta* substituents can inter-act with a site (the α site?) which can accept all these groups, and cannot therefore be entirely anionic in character. Examining analogs of $N^+(CH_3)_3$ compounds in which one quaternary group is replaced by $N(CH_3)_2$ (the formula shown being that anticipated at neutral pH*) shows them to be weaker inhibitors by factors of 70 for compound 15; 25 for compound 7; 21 for compound 6; and an amazing 440 for compound 1. A part of this variability is due to the fact that for $N^+(CH_3)_3$ or $CH(CH_3)_2$, the *meta* position is optimal, whereas for $N(CH_3)_2$ the *ortho* position is optimal. [This difference in optimum is surprising in view of the fact that $CH(CH_3)_2$ and $N(CH_3)_2$ are very nearly isosteric.] If one compares o-$N(CH_3)_2$ with m-$CH(CH_3)_2$, their A values differ only 6-fold. In this series of substituents, then, the $N^+(CH_3)_3$ is clearly superior to $N(CH_3)_2$. But this superiority is probably not due to the effect of the charge, since $N^+(CH_3)_3$ is not consistently superior to $C(CH_3)_3$ (compound 1 is 20 times more potent than its isosteric uncharged m-t-butylphenyl analog; yet compound 15 is rather worse than 11). One is driven to question whether all the variability is truly due to K_a variation; perhaps k_2 (carbamylating)

---

* The pK_a of dimethylaniline is 5.1 (5, 122). The carbamyl substituent would probably weaken the basicity a little. At neutral pH the $N(CH_3)_2$ would be about 99% in the un-protonated form.

variation occurs, accounting for the excellence of compound 1; and we shall see below that indeed k_2 variation might be significant in *meta*-substituted compounds.

A comparison of *t*-butyl with the isopropyl analogs shows the latter to be better by factors of 3 (compounds 10 and 12) or 2 (compounds 9 and 11) or 1.2 (comparing *m*-isopropyl phenyl- with *m*-*t*-butylphenyl methylcarbamates). Presumably the extra methyl, far from reacting with the enzyme surface, renders the group too bulky to fit optimally in a cavity; but the effect is slight.

Finally, it is apparent that there is a small group of supercarbamates, which are multisubstituted, and have A values greater than 10,000. In the very best case (compound 7) the effects are almost precisely additive: log A calculated as before is 4.5 and log A found is 4.6. The additivity of compound 7 implies

TABLE VIII

Effect of Substituents in Aromatic Carbamates[a]

	N-Methyl phenylcarbamates		N,N-Dimethyl phenylcarbamates	
	k_2 (min^{-1})	K_a (mM)	k_2 (min^{-1})	K_a (mM)
Unsubstituted	6.8	23.7	0.24	10.3
m-Isopropyl	80.7	0.18	6.3	2.5
m-Nitro	0.45	0.7	0.15	0.92

[a] Data from Hastings *et al.* (*51*). pH 7.6, 25°C.

that two bondings can occur fully independently, without interaction. The implication is that there are two centers: perhaps one in the *para* position is coulombic, the other near the *meta* or *ortho* position is hydrophobic. If one examines, by contrast, the next best supercarbamate, compound 6, the effects are less than additive: the calculated log A is 6.8, but the observed is 5.5. Presumably one or other substituents [probably the $(CH_3)_3N^+$, for by itself in that position, i.e., in compound 1, it is very potent] binds the ring in a location which does not permit an optimal contribution of binding by the isopropyl group.

It is rather startling to find that these supercarbamates come close to obeying the rather lightheartedly held "Kilsheimer rule" (*59*) which suggested that good carbamates had about 15 atoms (excluding hydrogen). Compound 6, 7, and 8 have 18 atoms.

The above view that potency was primarily a function of good fit plus ample hydrophobic bonding, seemed to find confirmation when analysis of k_2 and K_y became possible; again we must assume for discussion that K_y

approximates K_a. In the 13 carbamates we studied (104) virtually all the variation was in K_y rather than in k_2: the K_y values varied from 0.007 to 73 mM, whereas the k_2 values only varied from 0.13 to 3.0 min^{-1}; for the ten methylcarbamates, the k_2 range was only from 1.05 to 3.0. But more recent work by Hastings *et al.* (51) has concentrated on *m*-substituted compounds [our work (104) had dealt primarily with *p*-substituted compounds]. As Table VIII shows, in these *m*-compounds there was much variation in the k_2 values, which ranged from 0.15 to 81 min^{-1}.

Hansch and Deutsch (50a) have used their $\sigma-\pi$ analysis to explore the extent to which purely hydrophobic factors account for the variation in potency of methylcarbamates. σ represents the Hammett constant, which measures the ability of a particular substituent to withdraw electrons, and π is the Hansch constant, which measures the hydrophobic contribution of substituents. It is defined by $\pi = \log P_x - \log P_H$, where P_H is the partition coefficient in octanol–water for a parent compound and P_x that of a derivative.

They found with 53 phenyl methylcarbamates, a fairly good correlation of potency (measured by I_{50}) with π (correlation coefficient $r = 0.77$) and little correlation with σ. Taking π and σ together accounted for most of the variation in I_{50} ($r = 0.84$). These values were about the same for the 23 *para* and the 30 *meta* compounds. One would expect that these quite good correlations would owe some of their imperfections to the fact that they involved I_{50} and hence had both K_a and k_2 terms in them. This view is confirmed by Hansch's finding (private communication) that with eight phenyl methylcarbamates whose K_y values we had published (104) most of the variability was attributable to π variation and a little to σ variation. When both π and σ were taken into account, the correlation coefficient $r = 0.95$. By contrast, the k_2 values for methylcarbamates showed no such correlation; and for dimethylcarbamates, neither K_y nor k_2 showed a correlation.

An interesting anomaly in the importance-of-fit argument is that, although (as expected) the alkoxy compound below differs (6-fold) in the anticholinesterase potency of its d and l isomers, the alkylthio analog shows very little difference between d and l isomers (46).

OC(O)NHCH$_3$ OC(O)NHCH$_3$

—OCHC$_2$H$_5$ —SCHC$_2$H$_5$
 CH$_3$ CH$_3$

I_{50}: d form 6 × 10^{-6} M I_{50}: d form 8 × 10^{-8} M
 l form 1 × 10^{-6} M l form 12 × 10^{-8} M

If it turns out that indeed "fit" far outweighs carbamylating activity in determining anticholinesterase activity, one should note that our present theoretical view will need modification. At first thought one might imagine he could say simply "carbamylation is not the rate-determining factor." But this is incorrect. The concept of a rate-determining step is only valid in a sequence of irreversible steps; thus if the sequence were

$$AX + E \xrightarrow{k_1} AXE \xrightarrow{k_2} AE + X$$

instead of Eq. (1), then the slower of k_1 or k_2 would indeed determine production of AE; consequently if k_1 were by far the slower, then doubling k_1 would double AE production, whereas doubling k_2 would have no effect. But since, instead, Eq. (1) is true, the production of AE under usual conditions is determined by $k_i = k_2/K_a$, as Main has shown (75). Consequently, whatever the relative magnitudes of k_2 or K_a, anything that doubles the effectiveness of k_2 or K_a will double k_i. Therefore, if Eq. (1) is precisely followed, the unimportance of σ cannot be explained away by saying "K_a is rate-limiting and k_2 is not." Rather it is that k_2 is insensitive to electrophilic substituents.

One should note that in phosphates k_2 is very sensitive to electrophilic substituents and in this way parallels the sensitivity of k_{OH} (the alkaline hydrolysis rate); in carbamates, k_2 is insensitive but k_{OH} is highly sensitive in the expected direction (65, 104). Thus the precise analogy between attack on OH^- and on AChE is true for phosphates, not for carbamates. A possible way out of the dilemma has been indicated (104) by referring to the similar case of insensitivity of k_{OH} to substituents in acetanilides. In that case (12) it was suggested that a hydroxylated intermediate was formed in the reaction, and that those substituents which improved formation of the intermediate also improved its breakdown. A specific pathway could be (where EOH is AChE with its serine hydroxyl)

$$\begin{array}{ccc}
\underset{\displaystyle \overset{|}{OR}}{\overset{\displaystyle \overset{O}{\parallel}}{EOH \cdot C-NHCH_3}} & \underset{k_{-2a}}{\overset{k_{+2a}}{\rightleftharpoons}} & \underset{\displaystyle \overset{|}{OR}}{\overset{\displaystyle \overset{OH}{|}}{E-O-C-NHCH_3}} \\
\text{Complex} & & \downarrow k_{2b} \\
& & \overset{\displaystyle \overset{O}{\parallel}}{E-O-C-NHCH_3 + ROH}
\end{array}$$

If, as was true in acetanilides, k_{+2a} had a positive dependence on σ, and $(k_{-2a} + k_{2b})$ had a negative dependance on σ, the overall reaction constant k_2 could be independent of σ.

Little can be said about an aspect of great potential interest: the nature of the N-substituent. Only N-methyl- and N-dimethylcarbamates are commonly employed in medicinal or insecticidal compounds. The dimethyl compounds are somewhat worse inhibitors than the corresponding methyl compounds to an extent of about 5-fold (*85*, *104*). A variety of *N*-ethyl, *N*-benzyl, NH$_2$, and *N*-phenylcarbamates had little or no inhibitory (or toxic) effectiveness (*39*, *65*). The deuterated compound, 3-isopropylphenyl *d,d,d*-methylcarbamate, had potency identical to its undeuterated analog (*39*).

The Riverside group has also explored some more exotic *N*-substituents, including a trifluoromethyl group, a trimethylsilyl group and an aziridinyl group. None was a good inhibitor (*39*). Their failure to find new and interesting *N*-substituents explains why only the majority of commercial compounds are *N*-methyl or *N*-dimethyl. The apparent exception of Mecarbam (*107*) is probably misleading, since it most likely acts as a phosphorylating rather than a carbamylating agent.

$$(C_2H_5O)_2P(S)SCH_2C(O)N(CH_3)COOC_2H_5$$

Mecarbam

Three other commercial compounds comprise the *N*-acetyl, *N*-propionyl, and *N*-butyryl derivatives of 3-isopropylphenyl methylcarbamate. Their inhibitory potencies were about one-thousandth of their unacylated parent, yet their (synergized) potency against houseflies or mosquitoes was better than that parent (*39*). Probably, as Fahmy *et al.* suggest, they undergo deacylation *in vivo*, so that their parent is the actual toxicant.

C. The Inapplicability of Organophosphate Data to Carbamate Design

Since designers of organophosphate inhibitors would often be happy to be able to design a carbamate inhibitor, it is very sad that the wealth of data from study of the former problem is surprisingly useless in study of the latter. We will first document this contention, then discuss its significance.

We have seen that in the organophosphates a suitable (acid) leaving-group character is essential; in aromatics, this can be achieved by electrophilic ring substituents or by an unsubstituted thiophenol. In carbamates we have noted that this is not true. Only in one or two cases can this failure be attributed to the excessive instability to hydrolysis, e.g., *p*-nitrophenyl methylcarbamate. Most dimethylcarbamates have ample stability (*104*).

One might hope that in those organophosphates which are potent inhibitors in spite of poor acidity of their leaving group, their leaving groups must compensate by having high affinity for the enzyme surface. Such leaving groups should be excellent candidates for attachment to methylcarbamyl groups. But in at least two such cases, the attempt has not been highly successful. One was the case of analogs of carbon–Amiton type compounds; we made

$CH_3NHC(O)O(CH_2)_nCH(C_2H_5)_2$ with $n = 1$ and 2; but both were devoid of activity (21). Similarly, a variety of compounds were prepared based on quinolinols and hydroxystilbazoles (62). Compounds such as the following were exceptionally potent reversible inhibition of AChE.

Eight ethyl phosphoryl derivatives and 10 methylcarbamate derivatives were prepared from these and the related isoquinolinium compounds. Only the methylcarbamates need be discussed here. The authors suggested a relation existed between the K_i for the reversible inhibitors and the k_i for the corresponding carbamates. As Fig. 5 shows, the relation is not a close one; for four quinoliniums with k_i about $10^{-5.5}$ one can get carbamates whose potency varies 100-fold. Nevertheless, it is true that the most and the least potent quinolines gave rise to (respectively) the most and the least potent methylcarbamate.

The lack of correlation between potencies of related phosphates and carbamates has two possible implications. Firstly, it should be noted that there is no direct evidence that the *catalytic site* is the same for both classes. More specifically, serine has been shown to be the catalytic site for organophosphates; but the group which becomes carbamylated by carbamates has never been identified. It is entirely plausible that different groups could be involved. If both were normally a part of the overall substrate–catalysis scheme, then purely kinetic data would not reveal a difference; one would need to employ product analysis as in the case of the organophosphates.

Secondly, one must consider the possibility that carbamates utilize different *binding sites* than organophosphates and substrates. The results of analysis by the MCP technique (Section II, C) indicate that both most commonly use a β site; but within that site there may be subsites which favor one or the other class. The favoritism would not be on grounds of difference in affinity for leaving group per se; instead it may be that a binding site that in an organophosphate successfully apposes the P(O) to the organophosphate's catalytic site cannot successfully appose the C(O) of the analogous carbamate to its own catalytic site.

V. Future Approaches to Design of Anticholinesterases

The above heading was cast in general terms, to remind the reader that, although the organophosphates and carbamates are the best known anti-

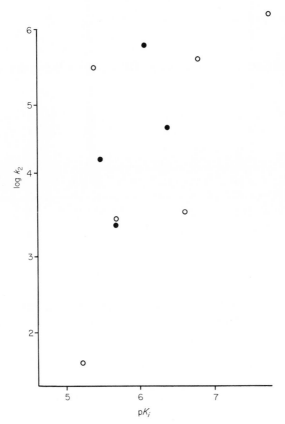

Fig. 5. Correlation of K_i, the dissociation constant for quinolinium and isoquino-liniums acting as reversible inhibitors, and k_2 for the derived dimethylcarbamates acting as ongoing inhibitors. Data includes diquaternary (●) and monoquaternary (○) compounds. Plotted from data of Kitz and Ginsburg (62).

cholinesterases (and the only ones whose design we shall discuss) yet many other alkylating and acylating possibilities exist, and deserve exploration.

It is apparent that we have a long way to go in exploring the topography of the elusive active zone. My proposal that there are at least four binding sites, and Krupka's suggestions of multiplicity within the catalytic site, may seem an alarming escalation to some. Yet my guess is that there may be numerous other binding sites yet undescribed. As the exploration of isoenzymes continues, we may find as many categories of binding site as there are orders of enzyme structure. We may anticipate that binding sites juxtaposed to the catalytic site by primary and secondary structure will be relatively fixed and ever-present. Other sites juxtaposed by tertiary folding may be shifted by changes in such folding (induced, e.g., by urea) too far to act as useful binding sites (i.e., useful for subsequent reaction with the catalytic site). Perhaps such a change is induced by reagents such as DPA and MCP. Finally, it is possible that the different quaternary structures, which presumably characterize the different isoenzymes, may give new possibilities for useful bindings; if so, we would expect to find inhibitors which can selectively inhibit certain isoenzymes.

A phenomenon related to the above suggestions is that the conformation of AChE (as explored by optical rotatory dispersion) is modified by reaction with diethyl phosphoric anhydride [tepp; $(C_2H_5O)_2P(O)OP(O)(OC_2H_5)_2$] (63).

It follows from these considerations that one line of research in inhibitor design would be to explore the effects of changes in tertiary and quaternary structure upon sensitivity to various inhibitors. Such studies, and parallel ones on changes in catalytic activity similar to those described above (Section II, C), should give fuller knowledge on topography that may lead to new types of inhibitor.

Another line of research is to explore systematically the binding character of those sites which have already been indicated. The γ site is particularly attractive in this regard. Presumably one would begin with substrates or inhibitors known to have suitable specificity, and prepare series of analogs designed to modify (separately) shape and electronic and hydrophobic character.

In principle, such studies should be equally useful for carbamate or organophosphate design. But we need assurance that the same component of the catalytic site is carbamylated by carbamates and phosphorylated by organophosphates. Should that not be the case, it is entirely possible that the two classes of inhibitor employ quite different (although possibly overlapping) types of binding site. Such a line of research may help clear up the puzzle of the uncertain role of electronic factors in determining reactivity of carbamates for AChE.

A pleasant aspect of the concept of multiple binding sites is that we need not feel that we are eternally reworking old approaches and old structures. We have every reason to hope that new anticholinesterases of outstanding potency and selectivity can be prepared.

REFERENCES

1. H. S. Aaron, H. O. Michel, B. Witten, and J. I. Miller, *J. Amer. Chem. Soc.* **80**, 456 (1958).
1a. A. A. Abdubakhabov, N. N. Godovikov, M. I. Kabachnik, S. S. Mikhailov, V. I. Rozengart, and R. V. Sitkevich, *Izv. Akad. Nauk SSSR Ser. Khim.* No. 4, 744 (1968).

2. D. H. Adams and V. P. Whittaker, *Biochim. Biophys. Acta* **4**, 543 (1950).
3. R. W. Addor, *J. Agr. Food Chem.* **13**, 207 (1965).
4. A. H. Aharoni and R. D. O'Brien, *Biochemistry* **7**, 1538 (1968).
5. A. Albert and E. P. Serjeant, "Ionization Constants of Acids and Bases." Methuen, London, 1962.
6. W. N. Aldridge, *Biochem. J.* **53**, 62 (1953).
7. W. N. Aldridge, *Biochem. J.* **54**, 601 (1953).
8. W. N. Aldridge and A. N. Davison, *Biochem. J.* **52**, 663 (1952).
9. W. N. Aldridge and E. Reiner, *in* "Structure and Reactions of DFP-Sensitive Enzymes" (E. Heilbronn, ed.), p. 125. Forsvarets Forskningsanstalt, Stockholm, 1967.
10. B. R. Baker, "Design of Active-site Directed Irreversible Inhibitors." Wiley, New York, 1967.
11. E. L. Becker, T. R. Fukuto, D. C. Canham, and E. Boger, *Biochemistry* **2**, 72 (1963).
12. M. L. Bender and R. J. Thomas, *J. Amer. Chem. Soc.* **83**, 4183 (1961).
13. E. Benjamini, R. L. Metcalf, and T. R. Fukuto, *J. Econ. Entomol.* **52**, 94 (1959).
14. B. Belleau, *in* "Fundamental Aspects of the Reaction of Drug-Receptor Interactions" (J. F. Danielli, J. F. Moran, and D. J. Triggle, eds.), p. 121. Buffalo, New York, 1968.
14a. B. Belleau, private communication (1969).
14b. B. Belleau, V. Di Tullio, and Y.-H. Tsai, *Mol. Pharmacol.* **6**, 41 (1970).
14c. B. Belleau, V. Di Tullio, and D. Godin, *Biochem. Pharmacol.* **18**, 1039 (1969).
15. B. Belleau and G. Lacasse, *J. Med. Chem.* **7**, 768 (1964).
16. B. Belleau and J. L. Lavoie, *Can. J. Biochem.* **46**, 1397 (1968).
17. F. Bergmann, *Discuss. Faraday Soc.* **20**, 126 (1955).
18. F. Bergmann and A. Shimoni, *Biochim. Biophys. Acta* **9**, 473 (1952).
19. F. Bergmann and M. Wurzel, *Biochim. Biophys. Acta* **11**, 440 (1953).
20. H. L. Boter and A. J. J. Ooms, *Rec. Trav. Chim. Pays-Bas* **85**, 21 (1966).
21. P. Bracha and R. D. O'Brien, *Biochemistry* **7**, 1545 (1968).
22. P. Bracha and R. D. O'Brien, *Biochemistry* **7**, 1555 (1968).
23. P. Bracha and R. D. O'Brien, *Biochemistry* **9**, 741 (1970).
24. A. P. Brestkin, N. N. Godovikov, E. I. Godyna, M. I. Kabachnik, M. Y. Mikhelson, E. V. Rozengart, and V. A. Yakovlev *Dokl. Akad. Nauk SSSR* **158**, 880 (1964).
25. H. C. Brown, D. H. McDaniel, and O. Hafliger, *in* "Determination of Organic Structures by Physical Methods" (E. A. Braude and F. C. Nachod, eds.), p. 567. Academic Press, New York, 1955.
26. J. A. Castro, *Biochem. Pharmacol.* **17**, 295 (1968).
27. J.-P. Changeux, T. Podleski, and J.-C. Meunier, *in* "Membrane Proteins," p. 225. Little, Brown, Boston, 1969.
28. Y. C. Chiu and W. C. Dauterman, *Biochem. Pharmacol.* **18**, 359 (1969).
29. Y. C. Chiu and W. C. Dauterman, *Biochem. Pharmacol.* **18**, 1665 (1969).
30. Y. C. Chiu, A. R. Main, and W. C. Dauterman, *Biochem. Pharmacol.* **18**, 2171 (1969).
30a. Y. C. Chiu and R. D. O'Brien, *Pesticide Biochem. Physiol.* (in press) (1971).
31. N. Christoff, P. J. Anderson, P. Slotwiner, and S. K. Song, *Ann. N.Y. Acad. Sci.* **135**, 150 (1966).
32. M. H. Coleman and D. D. Eley, *Biochim. Biophys. Acta* **67**, 646 (1963).
33. J. W. Cook, *J. Agr. Food Chem.* **5**, 859 (1957).
34. W. C. Dauterman and K. N. Mekrota, *J. Insect Physiol.* **9**, 257 (1963).
35. W. C. Dauterman and R. D. O'Brien, *J. Agr. Food Chem.* **12**, 318 (1964).
36. G. A. Davis and B. W. Agranoff, *Nature (London)* **220**, 227 (1968).
37. A. N. Davison, *Biochem. J.* **60**, 339 (1955).
38. B. F. Erlanger, *Proc. Nat. Acad. Sci. U.S.* **58**, 703 (1967).

39. M. A. H. Fahmy, R. L. Metcalf, T. R. Fukuto, and D. J. Hennessy, *J. Agr. Food Chem.* **14**, 79 (1966).
40. S. L. Friess and H. D. Baldridge, *J. Amer. Chem. Soc.* **78**, 2482 (1956).
41. T. R. Fukuto, *Advan. Pest Contr. Res.* **1**, 147 (1957).
42. T. R. Fukuto, *Annu. Rev. Entomol.* **6**, 313 (1961).
43. T. R. Fukuto and R. L. Metcalf, *J. Agr. Food Chem.* **4**, 930 (1956).
44. T. R. Fukuto and R. L. Metcalf, *J. Amer. Chem. Soc.* **8**, 372 (1959).
45. T. R. Fukuto, R. L. Metcalf, and M. Y. Winton, *J. Econ. Entomol.* **52**, 1121 (1959).
46. T. R. Fukuto, R. L. Metcalf, and M. Y. Winton, *J. Econ. Entomol.* **57**, 10 (1964).
47. D. Glick, *Biochem. J.* **31**, 521 (1937).
48. D. M. Glick, *Biochemistry* **7**, 3391 (1968).
49. M. A. Grafius and D. B. Miller, *Biochemistry* **6**, 349 (1967).
50. H. Gutfreund and B. R. Hammond, *Biochem. J.* **73**, 526 (1959).
50a. C. Hansch and E. W. Deutsch, *Biochim. Biophys. Acta* **126**, 117 (1966).
51. F. L. Hastings, A. R. Main, and F. Iverson, *J. Agr. Food Chem.* **18**, 497 (1970).
52. R. D. Hawkins and B. Mendel, *J. Cell. Comp. Physiol.* **27**, 69 (1946).
53. D. F. Heath, "Organophosphorus Poisons." Pergamon Press, Oxford, 1961.
54. E. Heilbronn-Wikstrom, *Sv. Kem. Tidskr.* **77**, 3 (1965).
55. K. Hellenbrand, *J. Agr. Food Chem.* **15**, 825 (1967).
56. H. T. Haung and C. Niemann, *J. Amer. Chem. Soc.* **74**, 59 (1952).
57. D. W. Ingles and J. R. Knowles, *Biochem. J.* **108**, 561 (1968).
58. J. A. A. Ketelaar, *Trans. 9th Int. Congr. Entomol.*, *1951*, Vol. 2, p. 318 (1953).
59. J. R. Kilsheimer and H. H. Moorefield, *139th Nat. Meet. Amer. Chem. Soc.* (1961).
59a. R. J. Kitz, L. M. Braswell, and S. Ginsburg, *Mol. Pharmacol.* **6**, 108 (1970).
60. R. Kitz and I. B. Wilson, *J. Biol. Chem.* **237**, 3245 (1962).
61. R. Kitz and I. B. Wilson, *J. Biol. Chem.* **238**, 745 (1963).
62. R. J. Kitz and S. Ginsburg, *Biochem. Pharmacol.* **17**, 525 (1968).
63. R. J. Kitz and L. T. Kremzner, *Mol. Pharmacol.* **4**, 104 (1968).
64. G. B. Koelle, "Cholinesterases and Anticholinesterase Agents." Springer, Berlin, 1963.
65. M. J. Kolbezen, R. L. Metcalf, and T. R. Fukuto, *J. Agr. Food Chem.* **2**, 865 (1954).
66. D. E. Koshland, *Cold Spring Harbor Symp. Quant. Biol.* **28**, 473 (1963).
67. R. M. Krupka, *Biochemistry* **2**, 76 (1963).
68. R. M. Krupka, *Biochemistry* **3**, 1749 (1964).
69. R. M. Krupka, *Biochemistry* **5**, 1983 (1966).
70. R. M. Krupka, *Biochemistry* **5**, 1988 (1966).
71. R. V. LaMotta, R. B. McComb, C. R. Noll, H. J. Wetstone, and R. F. Reinfrank, *Arch. Biochem. Biophys.* **124**, 299 (1968).
72. L. Larsson, *Sv. Kem. Tidskr.* **70**, 405 (1958).
73. R. M. Lee and W. R. Pickering, *Biochem. Pharmacol.* **16**, 941 (1967).
74. J. Lundin, *in* "Structure and Reactions of DFP Sensitive Enzymes" (E. Heilbronn, ed.), p. 13. Forsvarets Forskningsanstalt, Stockholm, 1967.
75. A. R. Main, *Science* **144**, 992 (1964).
76. A. R. Main, *in* "Structure and Reactions of DFP-Sensitive Enzymes" (E. Heilbronn, ed.), p. 129. Forsvarets Forskningsanstalt, Stockholm, 1967.
77. A. R. Main, *J. Biol. Chem.* **244**, 829 (1969).
78. A. R. Main and F. L. Hastings, *Biochem. J.* **101**, 584 (1966).
79. A. R. Main and F. Iverson, *Biochem. J.* **100**, 525 (1966).
80. K. N. Mehrotra and W. C. Dauterman, *J. Insect. Physiol.* **9**, 293 (1963).
81. K. N. Mehrotra and W. C. Dauterman, *J. Neurochem.* **10**, 119 (1963).
82. J. J. Menn and K. Szabo, *J. Econ. Entomol.* **58**, 734 (1965).

83. R. L. Metcalf and M. Frederickson, *J. Econ. Entomol.* **58**, 143 (1965).
84. R. L. Metcalf and T. R. Fukuto, *J. Econ. Entomol.* **55**, 340 (1962).
85. R. L. Metcalf and T. R. Fukuto, *J. Agr. Food Chem.* **13**, 220 (1965).
86. R. L. Metcalf and T. R. Fukuto, *J. Agr. Food Chem.* **15**, 1022 (1967).
87. R. L. Metcalf, T. R. Fukuto, and M. Frederickson, *J. Agr. Food Chem.* **12**, 231 (1964).
88. R. L. Metcalf, T. R. Fukuto, and M. Y. Winton, *J. Econ. Entomol.* **53**, 828 (1960).
89. R. L. Metcalf, T. R. Fukuto, and M. Y. Winton, *J. Econ. Entomol.* **55**, 889 (1962).
90. H. P. Metzger and I. B. Wilson, *J. Biol. Chem.* **238**, 3432 (1963).
91. H. P. Metzger and I. B. Wilson, *Biochem. Biophys. Res. Commun.* **28**, 263 (1967).
92. H. O. Michel, *Proc. Fed. Amer. Soc. Exp. Biol.* **14**, 255 (1955).
93. L. L. Murdock and T. L. Hopkins, *J. Agr. Food Chem.* **16**, 954 (1968).
94. D. Nachmansohn and I. B. Wilson, *Advan. Enzymol.* **12**, 259 (1951).
95. R. D. O'Brien, *Can. J. Biochem. Physiol.* **37**, 1113 (1959).
96. R. D. O'Brien, "Toxic Phosphorus Esters." Academic Press, New York, 1960.
97. R. D. O'Brien, *J. Agr. Food Chem.* **11**, 163 (1963).
98. R. D. O'Brien, *Annu. Rev. Entomol.* **11**, 369 (1966).
99. R. D. O'Brien, "Insecticides: Action and Metabolism." Academic Press, New York, 1967.
100. R. D. O'Brien, *Mol. Pharmacol.* **4**, 121 (1968).
101. R. D. O'Brien, *Biochem. J.* **113**, 713 (1969).
102. R. D. O'Brien and B. D. Hilton, *J. Agr. Food Chem.* **12**, 53 (1964).
103. R. D. O'Brien and B. D. Hilton, *J. Agr. Food Chem.* **13**, 381 (1965).
104. R. D. O'Brien, B. D. Hilton, and L. P. Gilmour, *Mol. Pharmacol.* **2**, 593 (1966).
105. R. D. O'Brien, E. C. Kimmel, and P. R. Sferra, *J. Agr. Food Chem.* **13**, 366 (1965).
106. A. J. J. Ooms, Ph.D. Thesis, University of Leiden, The Netherlands (1961).
107. M. Pianka, *Chem. Ind. (London)* p. 324 (1961).
108. W. R. Pickering and J. C. Malone, *Biochem. Pharmacol.* **16**, 1183 (1967).
109. J. L. Potter and R. D. O'Brien, *Entoml. Exp. Appl.* **6**, 319 (1963).
110. J. E. Purdie and R. A. McIvor, *Biochem. Biophys. Acta* **128**, 590 (1966).
111. J. R. Rapp, C. Niemann, and G. E. Hein, *Biochemistry* **5**, 4100 (1966).
112. E. Reiner and W. N. Aldridge, *Biochem. J.* **105**, 171 (1967).
113. E. Reiner and V. Simeon-Rudolf, *Biochem. J.* **98**, 501 (1966).
114. J. C. Sabine, *Blood* **6**, 151 (1951).
115. B. C. Saunders, "Some Aspects of the Chemistry and Toxic Action of Organic Compounds Containing Phosphorus and Fluorine." Cambridge Univ. Press, London and New York, 1957.
116. R. Shukuya, *J. Biochem. (Tokyo)* **38**, 225 (1951).
117. D. S. Sigman and E. R. Blout, *J. Amer. Chem. Soc.* **89**, 1747 (1967).
118. E. Y. Spencer and R. D. O'Brien, *J. Agr. Food Chem.* **1**, 716 (1953).
119. L. E. Tammelin, *Acta Chem. Scand.* **11**, 1340 (1957).
120. J. Thomas and W. Marlow, *J. Med. Pharm. Chem.* **6**, 107 (1963).
121. T. Uchida, H. S. Rahmati, and R. D. O'Brien, *J. Econ. Entomol.* **58**, 831 (1965).
122. R. C. Weast, "Handbook of Chemistry and Physics," 45th ed. Chem. Rubber Publ. Co., Cleveland, Ohio, 1964.
123. J. L. Webb, "Enzyme and Metabolic Inhibitors," Vol. 1. Academic Press, New York, 1963.
124. M. M. J. Weiden, H. H. Moorefield, and L. L. Payne, *J. Econ. Entomol.* **58**, 154 (1965).
125. H. B. A. Welle, Ph.D. Thesis, University of Utrecht, The Netherlands (1964).
126. V. P. Whittaker, *Physiol. Rev.* **31**, 312 (1951).
127. I. B. Wilson, *Biochim. Biophys. Acta* **7**, 466 (1951).

128. I. B. Wilson, *J. Biol. Chem.* **197**, 215 (1952).
129. I. B. Wilson and F. Bergmann, *J. Biol. Chem.* **185**, 479 (1950).
130. I. B. Wilson and C. Quan, *Arch. Biochem. Biophys.* **73**, 131 (1958).
131. I. B. Wilson, M. A. Harrison, and S. Ginsburg, *J. Biol. Chem.* **236**, 1498 (1961).
132. I. B. Wilson, M. A. Hatch, and S. Ginsburg, *J. Biol. Chem.* **235**, 2312 (1960).
133. F. P. W. Winteringham, *Nature (London)* **212**, 1368 (1966).
134. F. P. W. Winteringham and K. S. Fowler, *Biochem. J.* **101**, 127 (1966).
135. L. Wofsy and D. Michaeli, *Proc. Nat. Acad. Sci. U.S.* **58**, 2296 (1967).
136. C. I. Wright and J. C. Sabine, *J. Pharmacol. Exp. Ther.* **78**, 375 (1943).
137. C. I. Wright and J. C. Sabine, *J. Pharmacol. Exp. Ther.* **93**, 230 (1948).
138. E. A. Zeller and A. Bissegger, *Helv. Chim. Acta* **26**, 1619 (1943).

Chapter 4 The Design of Reactivators for Irreversibly Blocked Acetylcholinesterase

I. B. Wilson and Harry C. Froede

We present here a brief discussion of the principles involved in the reactivation of acetylcholinesterase that has been inhibited by irreversible organophosphate anticholinesterases. These anticholinesterases are phosphate triesters or phosphonate diesters containing a good leaving group. The conjugate acid corresponding to the leaving group must usually be fairly acidic (*1, 2*) and therefore this linkage might better be described as an anhydride bond rather than an ester bond. Thus typical inhibitors have the structure:

$$RO\diagdown \underset{\underset{R'}{\diagup}}{\overset{\overset{O}{\|}}{P}}-X$$

where X is a leaving group corresponding to acids such as diethylphosphoric acid, hydrofluoric acid, *p*-nitrophenol, hydrocyanic acid, and thiocholine. There are, however, cases in which the leaving group is a rather hydrophobic alcohol (*2a*). The group R may be an alkyl or aryl group and R′ may be an alkyl, aryl, alkyloxy, aroyloxy, or sometimes an ammonium group. There are evidently a wide variety of permutations and combinations of basic structures possible.

The presence of a good leaving group marks these compounds as phosphorylating agents and many chemists assumed from the start that inhibition of the enzyme involved phosphorylation of the protein structure. There were various kinds of evidence in support of this assumption. There was, first of all, a marked distinction between these inhibitors and reversible inhibitors in that the former required measurable times to produce inhibition when the concentration of the inhibitor was in absolute terms quite low but still high enough to produce complete inhibition (3). The rate constant for this inhibition showed a large temperature coefficient, again in distinction to reversible inhibitors, and this served to support the contention that a covalent reaction was involved. Similarly, the second-order rate constant for inhibition paralleled the second-order rate constant for the reaction of the inhibitor with hydroxide ion (4–8). Also, inhibition of the enzyme was not generally reversed by dilution nor by dialysis of the protein.

More direct evidence that hydrolytic enzymes were phosphorylated by these compounds came from the reaction of [^{32}P]DFP (diisopropylfluorophosphate-32), with large quantities of chymotrypsin, in which it was shown that ^{32}P remained with the protein and more important that fluoride in approximately equivalent amounts appeared in the solution (9).

At this point it is best to review the theory of enzymic hydrolysis (10). In Scheme 1 E is the enzyme, S is acetylcholine, E' is the acetyl enzyme, P$_1$

$$E + S \underset{k_2}{\overset{k_1}{\rightleftharpoons}} E \cdot S \xrightarrow{k_3} E' + P_1$$

$$\downarrow \quad H_2O, k_4$$

$$E + P_2$$

Scheme 1

is choline, and P$_2$ is acetic acid. In this scheme the enzyme acts as a nucleophile and choline as a leaving group. The acetylation of the enzyme must be reversible. It is written as irreversible for the usual case where the choline concentration is effectively zero. The scheme thus involves the transient formation of a covalent intermediate, the acetyl enzyme. The identity of the group that is acetylated was originally left unspecified, although a possible role of histidine was implied. However, subsequent events indicated that the hydroxyl group of serine is very probably the site of acetylation. The role of imidazole appears to be that of a general base promoting the nucleophilicity of serine (11, 12). The value of k_4 is thought to be rather smaller than k_3 so that deacetylation is rate-controlling (13, 14). A pictorial presentation of the enzyme–substrate

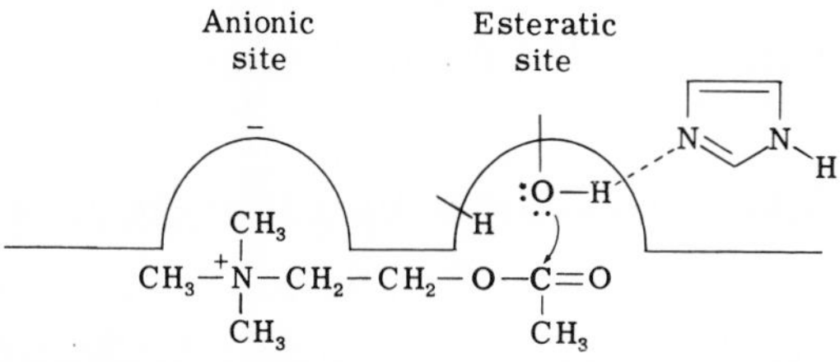

Fig. 1. Representation of the active site of acetylcholinesterase and the enzyme–substrate complex with acetylcholine.

complex is shown in Fig. 1; this immediately suggests that the organophosphates may react in a similar way as a substrate but producing a phosphoryl enzyme rather than an acetyl enzyme (*8, 15*). The inhibition rate does in fact show a pH dependence similar to the pH dependence of acetylcholine hydrolysis (*16, 17*). In sharp contrast to the acetyl enzyme which hydrolyzes in 0.1 msec, the phosphoryl enzyme reacts with water only very slowly (*37*). The dimethylphosphoryl enzyme requires 1.0–15 hr, the diethylphosphoryl enzyme, 3–60 hr depending on salt concentration, pH, and temperature (*18–26*). The diisopropylphosphoryl enzyme hardly hydrolyzes at all because another more rapid phenomenon called aging intervenes (*5, 21, 23–26*).

   The important point is that the organophosphate reacts in a similar manner as a substrate and that the same serine that normally is acetylated is in this instance phosphorylated and perhaps by the very same mechanism. In Scheme 2 we have written the phosphorylation step as reversible to emphasize its reversible nature, although in actual practice the inhibition of the enzyme would be conducted without adding HX or X⁻ and would proceed therefore in the presence of only negligible concentrations of these substances produced as a result of the inhibition reaction itself. Evidently this scheme might be applicable to other types of compounds and it does indeed hold for carbamates

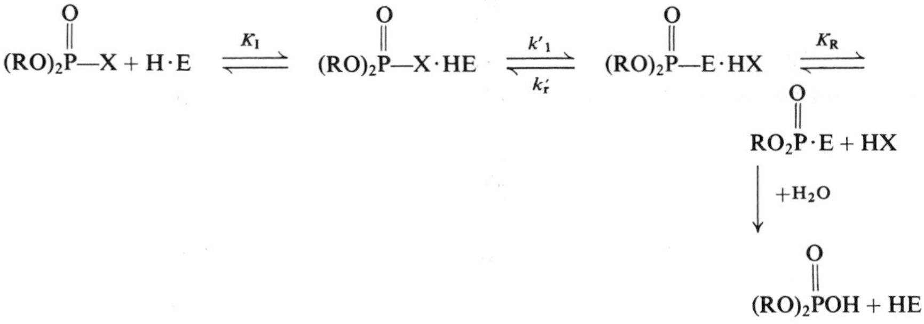

Scheme 2

and methane sulfonates (27–34). The formation of the reversible addition complex or Michaelis complex

$$(RO)_2\overset{\overset{\textstyle O}{\|}}{P}—X\cdot HE$$

is not easy to demonstrate because good inhibitors react so rapidly that inhibition occurs "instantaneously" at concentrations where the concentration of this complex is sufficiently large to affect the kinetics. Nonetheless it has been shown to exist in reactions with some methane sulfonates and organophosphates (32, 35, 36).

Scheme 2 suggests that the restoration of enzyme activity or reactivation of the inhibited enzyme can be accomplished by dephosphorylation of the phosphorylated enzyme. Many nucleophiles do in fact reactivate the inhibited enzyme. Reactivators include pyridine, imidazole, guanidines, amidines, hydroxylamine, hydroxamic acids, oximes, amino acids, fluoride thiocholine, and choline (15, 23, 37–39). Even water reactivates the enzyme slowly (18–20, 37).

From Scheme 2 the rate of inhibition of enzyme, when the enzyme concentration is much lower than the inhibitor concentration, is pseudo-first-order with the rate constant given by

$$k_i = k_i'/[1 + (K_I/[I])]$$

When $[I] \ll K_I$, which is usually the case in experiments with good inhibitors, the rate becomes:

$$k_i = (k_i' \cdot [I])/K_I$$

Similarly the pseudo-first-order rate constant for reactivation is

$$k_r = k_r'/[1 + (K_R/[R])]$$

which becomes

$$k_r = (k_r' \cdot [R])/K_R \qquad R = HX$$

when $R \ll K_R$. However, this latter condition is often not applicable. The inhibition and reactivation at low [I] and low [R] can be represented

$$E + I \underset{k_r}{\overset{k_i}{\rightleftarrows}} E' + R$$

It is therefore apparent that for every inhibitor there is a conjugate reactivator and that the ratio

$$k_i/k_r = K_I$$

is the equilibrium constant for the inhibition reaction with the particular inhibitor.* This equilibrium constant is related to the equilibrium constant (K_3) for the hydrolysis of the inhibitor, and the equilibrium constant (K_2) for the hydrolysis of the phosphoryl enzyme, thus:

$$(EtO)_2POX + HE \xrightleftharpoons{K_1} (EtO)_2POE + HX$$

$$(EtO)_2POE + H_2O \xrightleftharpoons{K_2} (EtO)_2POOH + HE$$

$$(EtO)_2POX + H_2O \xrightleftharpoons{K_3} (EtO)_2POOH + HX$$

$$K_1 K_2 = K_3$$
$$\therefore k_i/k_r = K_3/K_2$$

If, for convenience, we now restrict the discussion to diethylphosphoric acid derivatives, K_2 is a constant. If diethylphosphoryl fluoride is the inhibitor, fluoride is the conjugate reactivator. Reactivation is easily observed with fluoride and the ratio k_i/k_r was determined as 2.3×10^4 at pH 7.0, 25°C (40). If now K_3 were known, K_2 could be evaluated. However, K_3 is not known. The calculation was made nonetheless by assuming that K_3 in acid solution had a similar value as the equilibrium constant for the hydrolysis of fluorophosphoric acid. This seems very reasonable but recent studies indicate that this assumption is surprisingly wrong and that the equilibrium constant for the hydrolysis of diethylphosphoryl fluoride is much larger than the equilibrium constant for the hydrolysis of fluorophosphoric acid—about 10^4 times as large. On this newer basis it appears that K_2 has a value in the order of magnitude of 5×10^{10} at pH 7.0 and 25°C (41).

The value of K_2 depends upon the enzyme and preliminary indications are that diethylphosphorylacetylcholinesterase is far less stable than the corresponding derivatives of butyrylcholinesterase and chymotrypsin (41). The relative ease of reactivating acetylcholinesterase is due in a large measure to the instability of the diethylphosphoryl enzyme derivative. K_3 is a property of the inhibitor, K_2 of the enzyme, and these together fix the ratio of k_i and k_r. Thus the ratio is fixed by thermodynamics but the level of k_i and k_r is fixed by the kinetic interaction of the reactants with the enzyme.

Both choline and thiocholine reactivate the diethylphosphoryl enzyme at easily measured rates. However, the conjugate inhibitor of choline (O-diethylphosphorylcholine) does not inhibit at a discernable rate, whereas the conjugate inhibitor of thiocholine is a potent inhibitor (42, 43). The difference

---

* Equilibrium constants are considered here for expressions written in terms of analytical concentrations and therefore are pH-dependent.

in rates of inhibition must result from grossly different values of K_3. It would thus appear that the P—S linkage is a "high energy bond." The importance of an acidic leaving group for inhibition is easily understood since this tends to make K_3 large even without considering the ionization of the product.

There may be another related reason why O-diethylphosphorylcholine is not an inhibitor; the value of K_3/K_2 may be so low ($\sim 10^{-6}$) that given 0.01 % choline as an impurity in the preparation, no discernible inhibition would exist at equilibrium. Thus, although O-diethylphosphorylcholine would appear to have the structural requirements for good kinetic interaction with the enzyme, its failure to inhibit the enzyme can be understood in thermodynamic terms, i.e., a value of K_3 that is too low.

As already mentioned, reactivation can be realized with numerous nucleophiles. In many instances the anion of the reactivator is the more potent nucleophile and it is generally regarded to be the actual reactivator. There then comes about a balance between opposing effects related to the pK_a of the compound. A relatively low pK_a will ensure a good supply of anion but will indicate a relatively poor nucleophile. This can be put in quantitative terms using a Brønsted type equation as indicated later.

Since reactivation is a nucleophilic displacement reaction, it is pertinent to briefly summarize (if in somewhat oversimplified fashion) some of the factors that determine nucleophilicity (44).

Basicity and Polarizability. The basicity, which is the nucleophilicity toward hydrogen ions, can be assigned a numerical value, the pK_a of the conjugate acid. The basicity is usually taken as the reference point for the discussion of the nucleophilicity toward other electrophilic centers. Studies of the nucleophilic displacement reaction with compounds such as sarin

$$\text{Pr}_i\text{O} \diagdown \overset{\displaystyle O-}{\underset{\displaystyle CH_3 \diagup}{\overset{\displaystyle |}{P^+}}}\!\!-F$$

indicate that basicity is very important and that polarizability is unimportant (44a).

α-Effect. The α-effect refers to enhanced nucleophilicity over what would be expected from the basicity of the nucleophile that occurs when the nucleophile contains an atom with unshared electrons next to the nucleophilic center. Thus hydroxylamine, hydroxamic acids, and oximes are α nucleophiles. The α-effect is important in reactions with tetravalent phosphorus.

Charge Effect. The charge effect refers to enhanced nucleophilicity compared to the basicity that is found in nucleophiles that contain a cationic structure such as a quaternary ammonium function. (An example of such a compound is 3-hydroxyphenyltrimethylammonium.) The explanation offered for this effect is that the cationic charge as a field weakens the basicity toward hydrogen ion but does not have this weakening effect on nucleophilicity toward electrically neutral substrates (45).

Hydrogen Bonding. The charge effect is either unimportant with α nucleophiles (45) or relatively small (45a). If the nucleophile contains, in addition to the nucleophilic center, a functional group capable of forming a hydrogen bond as in catechols, the formation of hydrogen bonds between nucleophile and substrate may contribute to nucleophilicity. This effect is not believed to be important in hydroxamic acids.

The reaction of sarin with nucleophiles follows the Brønsted law; the reaction with hydroxamic acids for example is given by:

$$\log k_N = 0.80\,pK_a - 3.87$$

and for aldoximes by:

$$\log k_N = 0.619\,pK_a - 3.95$$

where k_N is the second-order rate constant for the anion, which is believed to be the actual nucleophile. For ketoximes the constants are 0.642 and -3.25. It is important to emphasize that hydroxamic acids do not show a charge effect and oximes only a very small charge effect (45, 45a, 46).

Fluoride ion is found to be a good nucleophile for phosphorus despite its low basicity and poor nucleophilicity toward carbon (47, 48) and compounds in which the nucleophilic center resides on sulfur, despite their good nucleophilicity toward carbon, are extremely poor nucleophiles toward phosphorus. Thiocholine, however, is a good nucleophile toward the inhibited enzyme.

Returning now to the reactivation reaction, it is apparent that if the same simple relationships were to hold when the inhibited enzyme is the target of the nucleophile as when the target is a simple compound, we could write

$$\log k_N = \beta pK_a + \log A$$

where k_N is the second-order rate constant for the actual nucleophilic species. For example, in the case of a hydroxamic acid, the actual nucleophile is the hydroxamate anion and k_N is calculated from the observed rate constant and the calculated concentration of anion. Now, if the nucleophile is the anion, the fractional concentration of anion is given by $[1 + (H^+/K_a)]^{-1}$, and the actual observed second-order rate constant k_{obs} at any pH corresponding to the analytical concentration of the nucleophile is given by

$$k_{obs} = AK_a^{-\beta}/[1 + (H^+/K_a)]$$

The maximum value depends upon K_a since β is fixed and we must select H^+ to correspond to a physiological pH, say, pH 7.2, if we are interested in using these compounds as drugs. The optimum K_a is obtained by setting the derivative of k_{obs} with respect to $K_a = 0$. In this way we get

$$pK_a(\text{optimum}) = -\log\left[(1/\beta) - 1\right] + pH$$

Thus if $\beta = 0.5$ the optimum pK_a is the same as the pH at which the reactivation will be run; let us say pH 7.2. A more probable value of β is 0.7. In this case the optimum pK_a is 7.6. The change is not great. In fact changing β from 0.2 to 0.9 changes the optimum pK_a only from 6.4 to 8.2 (19).

Suppose the optimum pK_a for reactivation at pH 7.2 is 7.8, ($\beta = 0.80$) how bad will it be to use a reactivator of the same series with a pK_a of 11. The rate of reaction will be reduced only by a factor of 4. If the pK_a of the reactivator is 5.0, the effect will be somewhat larger: the rate will be reduced by a factor of 25.

Thus we see that if the Brønsted-type equation holds for enzyme reactivation, we will get a range of observed rates of reactivation for reactivators of a particular type (say hydroxamic acids) that is determined only by selecting the wrong pK_a and this range is rather small. In fact in the above example if we restrict our pK_a values to 6–11, the range is only a factor of 4. Thus if such a relationship were to hold, there would be very little that we could do in terms of drug design.

It is quite clear that there is much to be learned from this kind of treatment yet at the same time it is evident that this treatment based upon studies with simpler systems does not envisage the possibilities of widely different capabilities for reactivating enzymes, capabilities that do indeed vary by as much as 10^6-fold for reasonably similar nucleophiles.

This difference comes about because the inhibited enzyme, say the diethylphosphoryl enzyme, is on the one hand a phosphate triester but yet retains much of its enzyme properties. It is able to bind substances and discriminate between different structures. Moreoever, the catalytic machinery which is involved normally in deacetylation may be available for dephosphorylation.

Before going into these matters it is reasonable to inquire into where the rate of reactivation of the diethylphosphoryl enzyme lies relative to the rate with which simpler compounds (such as sarin) undergo nucleophilic substitution. Although there is no single answer to this question because the rate of dephosphorylation of the enzyme depends so much upon the particular nucleophile, some simple examples will help to set a reference level of reactivity. The half time for the hydrolysis of sarin is about 50 hr and for the diethylphosphoryl enzyme from electric eel about 48 hr. Similarly the rate constant for sarin with hydroxylamine is 1.3 liters $mole^{-1}$ min^{-1} and for diethylphosphoryl enzyme (eel) about 0.2 liters $mole^{-1}$ min^{-1}. Thus the inhibited enzyme reacts with nucleophiles about as rapidly as sarin (perhaps somewhat slower) in the absence of any special features in the nucleophile. For further comparison we note that tetraethylpyrophosphate reacts about five times less rapidly with anionic nucleophiles than does sarin. Thus, broadly speaking, the rates of enzyme reactivation are also about the same as the rates of reaction of TEPP with simple nucleophiles. Inhibited enzyme from human red cells reacts somewhat slower perhaps by a factor of 4 or 5. Thus we see that the enzyme is a reasonably good leaving group.

The inhibited enzyme can be reactivated with choline. Now choline can not be regarded as an important nucleophile in neutral aqueous solution and its marked activity would therefore seem to be associated with the special relationship which choline has toward this enzyme. The rate of reactivation when plotted as a function of choline concentration shows a saturation effect, i.e., approaches a constant value and indicates that choline is bound to the inhibited enzyme prior to the reactivation reaction. Evidently the binding of choline by the inhibited enzyme serves to promote its nucleophilicity. As already mentioned, sulfur compounds do not show nucleophilicity toward phosphorus, yet thiocholine is a good reactivator. Again it would appear that binding of thiocholine promotes the nucleophilicity of this compound.

There is another very big difference in reactivation as opposed to nucleophilic displacement in simpler compounds. Reactivation has a pH dependence in the form of a bell-shaped curve (*19*, *25*), whereas nucleophilic displacement in simpler compounds increases with pH in accord with the dissociation of the conjugate acid of the nucleophile. If the nucleophile in reactivation is the conjugate base of the reactivator, then the bell-shaped curve indicates that some acidic group in the inhibited enzyme is also necessary for reactivation. This kind of scheme may be appropriate when the conjugate base of the reactivator is available in good supply, yet the bell-shaped curve does not demand such a mechanism. A bell-shaped curve would also be observed if the conjugate acid and a basic enzyme site were necessary. The first seems the more probable when the reactivator is a good nucleophile with a reasonably low pK_a.

In the case of choline it is quite possible that reactivation follows a somewhat different course. It is possible that the very low concentration of conjugate base (choline dipolar ion) at neutral pH coupled with the lesser binding that this species would have to the inhibited enzyme would make reactivation by this route negligibly slow. On the other hand, it is possible that the nucleophilicity of the choline hydroxyl group is promoted by hydrogen bonding with some basic group such as imidazole. This mechanism would be similar to the role envisaged for the histidine imidazole group in promoting the nucleophilicity of the serine hydroxyl group during the normal functioning of the enzyme with substrates. In Scheme 2 the reactivator is represented as HX.

This arises from the necessity of writing either HX or X⁻. In the text it is
indicated that most investigators consider X^- to be the nucleophile but the
authors think this is not necessarily so and that in some special cases such as
choline, HX may be the reactivating species.

Whatever the detailed mechanism may be, the rationale in seeking highly
effective reactivators has been to incorporate quaternary ammonium structures
into a molecule containing a nucleophilic center (49–51). The thought has
been to exploit the hydrophobic and coulombic binding features of the anionic
site (16, 25) so as to produce binding of the nucleophile at very low concentrations. If now the mode of binding should be such that the nucleophilic
center would be suitably disposed relative to the phosphorus atom and other
enzymic functional groups that might be involved, the adduct of nucleophile
and inhibited enzyme would react rapidly to yield the dephosphorylated
enzyme. Such a compound would be described in modern popular terminology as a site-directed reactivator.

We have tacitly assumed that the phosphorylation occurs at the esteratic
site and that the same group that is normally acetylated is phosphorylated.
This conclusion arises from the enzyme theory. It is supported by the reactivation with choline and thiocholine. It is also supported by the observation that
simple substituted ammonium ions, such as tetramethylammonium ion, that
reversibly inhibit the enzyme prevent reactivation by nucleophiles—and also
prevent inhibition of the enzyme by organophosphates (15, 53–56).

In the inhibition reaction the enzyme serves as a nucleophile but again the
reaction is not simple for the pH dependence is a bell-shaped curve (16, 17).
This curve is similar to the pH curve for the enzymic hydrolysis of acetylcholine but does differ distinctly from it. Acetylcholine hydrolysis is not,
however, the proper reference. We would like to compare phosphorylation
with acetylation and in the hydrolysis of acetylcholine the slower step at least
at neutral pH is deacetylation. Acetylation is rate controlling with much poorer
substrates such as β-bromoethylacetate and therefore this substrate is more
suitable for the comparison of pH effects. In this comparison the bell-shaped
curves for inhibition and hydrolysis are identical (16, 57, 58).

These arguments and others not recorded here serve to substantiate the
fundamental idea that the enzyme site that is phosphorylated is the same as
the enzyme site that is acetylated and that the mechanisms of the two reactions
are similar, if not identical. It should be noted, however, that the rate constants for phosphorylation which depend upon the inhibitor are typically
about 10^5 liters mole^{-1} min^{-1} and may run as high as 10^8, whereas the second-
order rate constant for acetylation is about 10^{10} liters mole^{-1} min^{-1} when
acetylcholine is the substrate.

The correctness of the idea of a site-directed reactivator is illustrated in
Table I where the first four compounds of the structure (19)

$$\underset{N}{\bigcirc}-\underset{O}{\overset{O}{\underset{\parallel}{C}}}-CH{=}NOH \quad and \quad \underset{\underset{CH_3}{\overset{+}{N}}}{\bigcirc}-\underset{O}{\overset{O}{\underset{\parallel}{C}}}CH{=}NOH$$

TABLE I

Compound[a]	pK_a	Second-order rate constant (liter mole^{-1} min^{-1})	pH
Nicotinoyl formaldoxime	7.8	8.0×10	7.9
Nicotinoyl formaldoxime methiodide	7.2	2.5×10^3	7.9
Isonicotinoyl formaldoxime	7.8	2.2×10	7.9
Isonicotinoyl formaldoxime methiodide	7.1	2.3×10^3	7.9
Pyridine-2-aldoxime	10.4	1.8×10^{-1}	7.0
Pyridine-2-aldoxime methiodide	8.0	1.4×10^4	7.0
Pyridine-4-aldoxime	10.2	5.0×10^{-1}	7.0
Pyridine-4-aldoxime methiodide	8.6	3.0×10^2	7.0
Pyridine-3-aldoxime	10.2	1.6×10^{-1}	7.0
Pyridine-3-aldoxime methiodide	9.2	1.0×10^{-2}	7.0

[a] The first four entries are at 0.03 M NaCl, pH 7.9 and the remainder at 0.1 M NaCl, pH 7.0.

are compared as reactivators. We recall that oximes as nucleophiles do not show a charge effect and we note also that the pK_a values of the tertiary compounds are slightly higher than the pK_a values of the quaternary compounds and closer to the optimal pK_a for reactivation at pH 8.0. The tertiary compounds are therefore slightly better nucleophiles than the quaternary compounds yet the quaternary compounds are far better reactivators. The superiority of the quaternary compounds, 30- to 100-fold, is in a range that could be explained by better binding. It should be noted that the two tertiary compounds reactivate the inhibited enzyme slightly faster than predicted from their nucleophilicity toward sarin.

Another interesting comparison is the tertiary pyridine-2-aldoxime and the quaternary pyridinium-2-aldoxime (2-PAM) as well as the corresponding 3 and 4 derivatives. Tertiary pyridine-2-aldoxime reactivates the inhibited enzyme at a rate which is very close to what is expected from its nucleophilicity toward sarin. This is also true of the tertiary 3 and 4 derivatives. On the other hand, the quaternary compound 2-PAM reactivates the inhibited enzyme 2×10^4 times more rapidly than would be expected from its pK_a. This rate enhancement is far greater than can be accounted for by binding alone and implies some sort of special orientation or a different mechanism than occurs with those reactivators whose activities conform to their pK_a values. The quaternary 4 derivatives are also especially active, although considerably less active than the 2 derivative. Here we run into a difficulty.

If we propose to explain the high activity of the 4 derivatives in terms of noncovalent interactions with the inhibited enzyme which bring about a special orientation of the nucleophile, we would expect this possibility to depend very much upon the structure of the compound. These pyridine

syn 4-PAM   anti 4-PAM

aldoximes are planar molecules. It is therefore surprising that the *syn* and *anti* 4-PAM's are comparably active, for it we should fix the quaternary nitrogen at the anionic site and also fix the orientation of the ring, the oxygen atoms would fall in different locations and also in a different location from the oxygen of *syn* 2-PAM. In this regard it is not quite certain which atom, N or O, is the nucleophilic center in oximes. It is known that both N and O of hydroxylamine can react as nucleophilic centers with carboxylic esters (*59*). However, it was shown that only the oxygen can serve as a nucleophilic center in the reaction of hydroxamic acids with sarin (*45*). There are many compounds already noted, such as pyridine, in which only N can be the nucleophilic center. It is therefore possible that both N and O can serve as nucleophilic centers in oximes and if this possibility is allowed, the extra freedom so arising might provide an explanation of the high activity of these compounds. The extra freedom might also be obtained if the ring position is not fixed and two or more different orientations are allowable. Such explanations would not be compelling, although they might well be correct.

Since all of these reactivators that contain a cationic ammonium function are bound by the free enzyme and probably most of them are bound also by the inhibited enzyme, it is apparent that binding alone cannot be important. Indeed one would not expect binding alone to be significant but rather the question is whether the more stable configurations in the complex of reactivator and inhibited enzymes, places the nucleophilic center in a position relative to the phosphorus atom from which facile reaction can occur. The anionic site of the enzyme can be taken as the origin of coordinates and the location of the phosphorus atom can be located with reasonable probability by reference to the structure of neostigmine. Neostigmine, a carbamate, is a very effective inhibitor of this enzyme. Carbamate inhibitors carbamylate the enzyme and, unlike phosphate inhibitors, the rate is not greatly influenced by the pK_a of the conjugate acid of the leaving group (*60*). Since there are very wide differences in the effectiveness of carbamate inhibitors (*29, 30*), it can be concluded that molecular complementarity is a very important consideration in determining activity (*24, 25, 49*). Neostigmine has a planar structure

(except for the methyl groups of the quaternary function and the methyl group hydrogen atoms of the carbamate function). The carbonyl atom is evidently in a good position (coordinates: 3.4, 3.3, 0 Å) to react with the nucleophilic center of the enzyme. This same position would also be a probable position in which to find the carbonyl carbon atom in the resulting carbamyl enzyme. This same position then should also be a probable position for the phosphorus atom in the diethylphosphoryl enzyme. There may also be other stable positions. It turns out that if 2-PAM is superposed upon this coordinate system the nucleophilic oxygen will point toward the phosphorus atom and fall one bond length from it, if the configuration of the oxime is *anti*. Thus we can account for the very high activity of 2-PAM if its configuration were *anti*. Similarly *anti* 4-PAM would superpose well, Wilson *et al.* had previously advanced this theory (*19*). However, it is now known that the 2-PAM that has been made and which is extremely active is the *syn* compound (the *anti* compound has not been made) and that *syn* 4-PAM is more active than *anti* 4-PAM (*61, 62*). Although a priori the coordinate system defined by neostigmine would seem to be a good basis for relating activity to molecular complimentarity, as explained above, it does not lead to an explanation of the relative activities of the pyridine oximes and we have no simple explanation at present.

A further advance in attaining reactivators of great potency involves the incorporation of a second cationic center in the reactivator (*63–67*). This is most easily accomplished in the bis compounds based on 4-PAM. Thus trimethylene bis 4-PAM, which is the most active of these compounds, is

500 times more active than 4-PAM (*65*) and about 5 to 50 times more active than 2-PAM in reactivating TEPP-inhibited acetylcholinesterase (*64, 65*). Whereas most bis 4-PAM compounds are considerably more active than 4-PAM, this is not true for the bis 2-PAM compounds. Only those compounds with short bridges of 3, 4, or 5 bond lengths are more active than 2-PAM (*65*). Pentamethylene bis 2-PAM is only three times more potent than 2-PAM.

The second pyridine oxime is not an essential feature of the bis compounds since a diquaternary compound in which one cationic group is a trimethylammonium function or a pyridine function has the same activity (*65*). Similarly, the nature of the bridge does not seem to be especially important since compounds with bridges that contain oxygen as well as carbon are effective (*66, 67*).

The rationale for synthesizing the bis reactivators was based upon the knowledge that bis quaternary compounds are more effective reversible inhibitors of acetylcholine esterase than the simpler monoquaternary compounds from which they are derived by about 1 order of magnitude (*68, 69*). However, the effect on reactivation is greater than could be anticipated since the activities of the diquaternary reactivators of the 4-PAM series are more than 2 orders of magnitude greater than the monoquaternary compound. The effect is even more pronounced with diquaternaries based upon 2 and 4 benzolypyridine ketoximes (*70*). The rate is enhanced in this case by more than 3 orders of magnitude; the resulting compounds are about as active as the bis 4-PAM's. In this case the effect was observed with both the *syn* and *anti* oximes so that this very large effect is not dependent upon the oxime configuration.

The relative reactivation rates observed with the various isomers of the quaternary benzoylpyridine ketoximes (monoquaternary compounds) are also of some interest although they are considerably less active than the quaternary pyridine aldoximes. The *syn* 4* is about five times more active than the *anti* 4 just as in the aldoxime series. But in contrast to the aldoximes the 2 *syn* compound is less active than the 4 *syn* derivative. The 2 *syn* compound is also far less active than the 2 *anti* compound. These results suggest that the 2 *anti* derivative of PAM might be far more active than the presently available 2 *syn* derivative.

In summary, although the inhibited enzyme is a phosphate triester in which the enzyme can serve as a good leaving group, its reactivity toward nucleophiles is very different from the reactivity of simpler compounds, such as sarin, with nucleophiles. The reactivity of the inhibited enzyme is not determined solely by the pK_a of the nucleophile within a given class of compounds. There are abundant possibilities of enormous enhancement in reactivity

---

* In naming these compounds, *syn* or *anti*, the benzene ring plays the role of hydrogen in the pyridine aldoximes. Thus the relationship between the oxime OH and the pyridine rings are the same in these similarly identified aldoximes and ketoximes.

resulting from the binding of the nucleophile and the concept of a site-directed reactivator is real and highly appropriate. However, we cannot at present explain all the experimental observations in terms of a single simple geometric relationship between nucleophile and inhibited enzyme.

In regard to the design of a drug that might serve as an antidote to the organophosphate anticholinesterases, we have considered only the *in vitro* reactivation of the enzyme by the drug. We have not discussed such important matters as distribution of the drug in the animal body and toxicity of the drug. In this particular case these matters do not immediately arise because one of the very best reactivators 2-PAM turned out to be effective as an antidote (*71–79*) toward anticholinesterases that produce inactive acetylcholinesterase derivatives which can be readily reactivated in solution. The toxicity of 2-PAM is surprisingly low but TMB_4 is rather more toxic. For this reason 2-PAM is preferred. Evidently 2-PAM is distributed to those regions of the animal body where the inhibition of acetylcholinesterase is critical. One attempt to change the distribution of the oxime in the animal body by modifying 2-PAM so as to alter the lipid solubility of the compound seems to have been successful (*80*).

REFERENCES

1. L. Larsson, *Sv. Kem. Tidskr., Diss.* **70**, 405 (1958).
2. R. J. Kitz, S. Ginsburg, and I. B. Wilson, *Mol. Pharmacol.* **3**, 225 (1967).
2a. P. Bracha and R. D. O'Brien, *Biochemistry* **9**, 741 (1970).
3. K. B. Augustinsson and D. Nachmansohn, *J. Biol. Chem.* **179**, 543 (1949).
4. W. N. Aldridge, *Biochem. J.* **46**, 451 (1950).
5. B. J. Jandorf, H. O. Michel, N. K. Schaffer, P. Egan, and W. H. Summerson, *Discuss. Faraday Soc.* **20**, 134 (1955).
6. W. N. Aldridge and A. Davison, *Biochem. J.* **51**, 62 (1952).
7. W. N. Aldridge, *Chem. Ind. (London)* p. 473 (1950).
8. W. N. Aldridge, *Biochem. J.* **54**, 422 (1953).
9. E. F. Jansen, M. D. F. Nutting, R. Jang, and A. K. Balls, *J. Biol. Chem.* **185**, 209 (1950).
10. I. B. Wilson, F. Bergmann, and D. Nachmansohn, *J. Biol. Chem.* **186**, 781 (1950).
11. L. W. Cunningham, *Science* **125**, 1145 (1957).
12. F. H. Westheimer, *Proc. Nat. Acad. Sci. U.S.* **43**, 969 (1957).
13. I. B. Wilson and E. Cabib, *J. Amer. Chem. Soc.* **78**, 202 (1956).
14. R. M. Krupka, *Biochemistry* **3**, 1749 (1964).
15. I. B. Wilson, *J. Biol. Chem.* **199**, 113 (1952).
16. I. B. Wilson and F. Bergmann, *J. Biol. Chem.* **185**, 479 (1950).
17. K. B. Augustinsson, *Ark. Kemi* **6**, 331 (1953).
18. W. N. Aldridge, *Biochem. J.* **55**, 763 (1953).
19. I. B. Wilson, S. Ginsburg, and C. Quan, *Arch. Biochem. Biophys.* **77**, 286 (1958).
20. F. Hobbiger, *Brit. J. Pharmacol.* **6,** 21 (1951).
21. H. S. Jansz, D. Brons, and M. G. P. J. Warringa, *Biochim. Biophys. Acta* **34**, 573 (1959).
22. W. Aldridge and A. Davison, *Biochem. J.* **55**, 763 (1953).
23. D. R. Davies and A. L. Green, *Biochem. J.* **63**, 529 (1956).
24. I. B. Wilson, S. Ginsburg, and E. K. Meislich, *J. Amer. Chem. Soc.* **77**, 4286 (1955).

25. I. B. Wilson, *Discuss. Faraday Soc.* **20**, 119 (1955).
26. F. W. Hobbiger, *Brit. J. Pharmacol.* **11**, 295 (1956).
27. D. K. Myers, and A. Kemp, *Nature (London)* **173**, 33 (1954).
28. D. K. Myers, *Biochem. J.* **62**, 557 (1956).
29. I. B. Wilson, M. A. Hatch, and S. Ginsburg, *J. Biol. Chem.* **235**, 2312 (1960).
30. I. B. Wilson, M. A. Harrison, and S. Ginsburg, *J. Biol. Chem.* **236**, 1498 (1961).
31. F. Iverson and A. R. Main, *Biochemistry* **8**, 1889 (1969).
32. R. Kitz and I. B. Wilson, *J. Biol. Chem.* **237**, 3245 (1962).
33. P. Turini, S. Kurooka, M. Steer, A. N. Corbascio, and T. P. Singer, *J. Pharmacol. Exp. Ther.* **167**, 98 (1969).
34. J. F. Ryan, S. Ginsburg, and R. J. Kitz, *Biochem. Pharmacol.* **18**, 269 (1969).
35. A. R. Main and F. Iverson, *Biochem. J.* **100**, 525 (1966).
36. P. E. Braid and M. Nix, *Can. J. Biochem.* **47**, 1 (1969).
37. I. B. Wilson, *J. Biol. Chem.* **190**, 111 (1951).
38. G. Gilbert, T. Wagner-Jauregg, and G. M. Steinberg, *Arch. Biochem. Biophys.* **93**, 469 (1961).
39. E. Heilbronn, *Acta Chem. Scand.* **18**, 2410 (1964).
40. I. B. Wilson and R. A. Rio, *Mol. Pharmacol.* **1**, 60 (1965).
41. H. C. Froede and I. B. Wilson, Unpublished observations (1970).
42. L. E. Tammelin, *Acta Chem. Scand.* **11**, 1340 (1957).
43. L. E. Tammelin, *Ark. Kemi* **12**, 287 (1958).
44. J. O. Edwards, *J. Chem. Educ.* **45**, 387 (1968).
44a. J. O. Edwards and R. G. Pearson, *J. Amer. Chem. Soc.* **84**, 16 (1962).
45. J. Epstein, P. L. Cannon, Jr., H. O. Michel, B. E. Hackley, Jr., and W. A. Mosher, *J. Amer. Chem. Soc.* **89**, 2937 (1967).
45a. Y. Ashani, Ph.D. Thesis, Hebrew Univ. (1970).
46. G. M. Steinberg and R. Swidler, *J. Org. Chem.* **30**, 2362 (1965).
47. I. Dostrovsky and M. Halmann, *J. Chem. Soc.* p. 508 (1953).
48. G. DiSabato and W. P. Jencks, *J. Amer. Chem. Soc.* **83**, 4393 (1961).
49. I. B. Wilson and E. K. Meislich, *J. Amer. Chem. Soc.* **75**, 4628 (1953).
50. I. B. Wilson and S. Ginsburg, *Biochim. Biophys. Acta* **18**, 168 (1955).
51. D. R. Davies and A. L. Green, *Discuss. Faraday Soc.* **20**, 269 (1955).
52. I. B. Wilson, *J. Biol. Chem.* **197**, 215 (1952).
53. G. B. Koelle, *J. Pharmacol. Exp. Ther.* **88**, 232 (1946).
54. K. B. Augustinsson, *Acta Chem. Scand.* **4**, 1149 (1950).
55. K. B. Augustinsson and M. Grahn, *Acta Physiol. Scand.* **27**, 10 (1952).
56. F. Bergmann and A. Shimoni, *Biochim. Biophys. Acta* **8**, 520 (1952).
57. F. Bergmann, R. Segal, A. Shimoni, and M. Wurzel, *Biochem. J.* **63**, 684 (1956).
58. D. F. Heath, *Int. Ser. Monogr. Pure Appl. Biol.* **13**, 156 (1961).
59. W. P. Jenks and J. Carrinolo, *J. Amer. Chem. Soc.* **82**, 1778 (1960).
60. R. J. Kitz, S. Ginsburg, and I. B. Wilson, *Biochem. Pharmacol.* **16**, 2201 (1967).
61. D. Carlström, *Acta Chem. Scand.* **20**, 1240 (1966).
62. E. J. Poziomek, D. N. Kramer, W. A. Mosher, and H. O. Michel, *J. Amer. Chem. Soc.* **83**, 3916 (1961).
63. E. J. Poziomek, B. E. Hackley, Jr., and G. M. Steinberg, *J. Org. Chem.* **23**, 714 (1958).
64. F. Hobbiger and P. W. Sadler, *Nature (London)* **182**, 1672 (1958).
65. I. B. Wilson and S. Ginsberg, *Biochem. Pharmacol.* **1**, 200 (1959).
66. F. Hobbiger and V. Vojodic, *Biochem. Pharmacol.* **15**, 1677 (1966).
67. A. Luettringhaus and I. Hagedorn, *Arzneim.-Forsch.* **14**, 1 (1964).
68. F. Bergmann and R. Segal, *Biochem. J.* **58**, 692 (1954).

69. A. Funke, J. Bagot, and F. Depierre, *C. R. Acad. Sci.* **239**, 329 (1954).
70. R. J. Kitz, S. Ginsburg, and I. B. Wilson, *Biochem. Pharmacol.* **14**, 1471 (1965).
71. H. Kewitz and I. B. Wilson, *Arch. Biochem. Biophys.* **60**, 261 (1956).
72. H. Kewitz, I. B. Wilson, and D. Nachmansohn, *Arch. Biochem. Biophys.* **64**, 456 (1956).
73. F. Hobbiger, *Brit. J. Pharmacol.* **12**, 438 (1957).
74. I. B. Wilson and F. Sondheimer, *Arch. Biochem. Biophys.* **69**, 468 (1957).
75. H. Edery and G. Schatzberg-Porath, *Science* **128**, 1137 (1958).
76. T. O. King and E. Poulsen, *Arch. Int. Pharmacodyn.* **114**, 118 (1958).
77. T. Namba and K. Hiraki, *J. Amer. Med. Assoc.* **166**, 1834 (1958).
78. D. Grob and R. J. Johns, *Amer. J. Med.* **24**, 497 (1958).
79. J. H. Wills, A. M. Kunkel, R. V. Brown, and G. E. Groblewski, *Science* **125**, 743 (1957).
80. I. B. Wilson, *Biochim. Biophys. Acta* **27**, 196 (1958).

Chapter 5 Inhibition of Protein Biosynthesis: Its Significance in Drug Design

Arthur P. Grollman

I. Introduction

Many established antimicrobial and antitumor drugs exert their therapeutic effects by inhibiting some phase of protein biosynthesis, and the enzymic mechanisms that are sensitive to the action of these compounds represent potential targets for the design of chemotherapeutic agents. This chapter will consider drug design based on the inhibition of protein synthesis in the context of susceptible enzymic reactions. Since the biochemistry of protein synthesis has been extensively reviewed (1–3), only those biosynthetic reactions that appear to be most suitable for the desired spectrum of therapeutic activity will be considered. In certain cases, structure–activity relationships that establish a basis for the design of potentially useful drugs will be described.

A frequently overlooked benefit of considering biochemical events in drug design is that it sometimes allows one to predict limits on the chemotherapeutic potential of a given group of agents. Accordingly, the molecular basis of toxicity, as it relates to protein synthesis, will also be considered.

II. Protein Biosynthesis

This section outlines the principal events in protein biosynthesis as they are currently understood. The original literature is reviewed in references 1–3.

The biosynthesis of proteins takes place on ribosomes which can be classified according to size. Ribosomes found in the cytoplasm of cells from animals, higher plants, fungi, yeasts, and protozoa, have an approximate sedimentation coefficient of 80 S, whereas the ribosomes found in bacteria, blue-green algae, and chloroplasts have a sedimentation coefficient of 70 S. The ribosomes of the 70 S type differ from the 80 S variety in chemical composition and in sensitivity to various antibiotics.

Protein synthesis involves a precisely controlled polymerization of amino acids on the polynucleotide template of messenger RNA (mRNA). The sequence of nucleotides in mRNA determines the sequence of amino acids found in proteins. The pairing of a trinucleotide codon in aminoacyl transfer RNA (tRNA) to a complementary sequence of nucleotides in mRNA brings the proper amino acid to the physical site of protein synthesis.

Translation of mRNA consists of three phases: initiation, elongation, and termination of the peptide chain (cf. Fig. 1). In *E. coli*, the first stage involves the formation of a complex between 30 S ribosomal subunits and mRNA and requires the presence of a specific protein factor. The peptide chain is initiated by a molecule of formylmethionyl-tRNA$_{fMet}$ which binds to an AUG codon in mRNA (**I**). GTP and additional protein factors function in this binding of formylmethionyl-tRNA$_{fMet}$ to the mRNA–30 S ribosomal subunit complex. A 50 S subunit adds to this initiation complex to form a mRNA–70 S ribosome complex (**II**) and formylmethionyl-tRNA is translocated from the A (aminoacyl) site to the P (peptidyl) site on the ribosome (**III**). One molecule of GTP is cleaved to GDP and inorganic phosphate during this final step of the initiation process.

Elongation of the peptide chain begins with the binding of a second molecule of aminoacyl-tRNA to the trinucleotide codon located in the A site on the

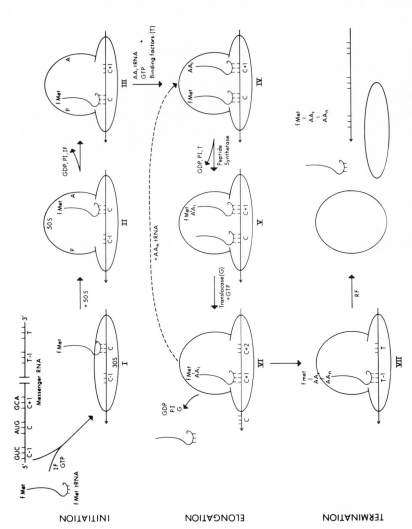

Fig. 1. Schematic representation of the reactions involved in protein synthesis. Abbreviations used: IF, initiation factors; RF, release factors; fMet, formylmethionyl; tRNA, transfer RNA; C, initiation codon; T, termination codon; PI, inorganic phosphate; AA, amino acid residue; P, peptidyl (or donor) site; A, aminoacyl (or acceptor) site.

ribosome (IV). Binding of aminoacyl-tRNA to ribosomes requires GTP, magnesium, and the "T" factor, which is a complex of two proteins, T_u and T_s. The subsequent formation of the first peptide bond in the chain occurs by transfer of formylmethionine to the N-terminal amino group of the aminoacyl-tRNA located at the aminoacyl site (V). This reaction is catalyzed by an enzyme (peptide synthetase) which appears to be an integral part of the 50 S ribosomal subunit. Another translocation follows in which free $tRNA_{fMet}$ is released from the ribosome and the second molecule of tRNA, containing the nascent peptide chain, moves from the A to the P site on the ribosome (VI). Translocation requires the "G" factor and GTP and involves a movement of the ribosome relative to mRNA. Elongation of the chain occurs by a repetition of the preceding steps until the peptide chain is completed upon reading of a specific "termination" codon (VII). Peptide release is also catalyzed by specific protein factors.

Protein synthesis in animal cells (4, 5) has been studied primarily in extracts prepared from rat liver or rabbit reticulocytes. Methionyl-tRNA (5a) has been identified as an initiator of protein synthesis in animal cells and globin mRNA (6) and a possible protein initiation factor for globin synthesis (7, 7a) have recently been reported. Two transfer factors, TF-I and TF-II, which seem to correspond to T and G factors, respectively, have been isolated and purified from rat liver and from rabbit reticulocytes. TF-I requires GTP for binding of aminoacyl-tRNA to the mRNA–ribosome complex. Purified TF-I shows GTPase activity but hydrolysis of GTP is not required for binding of tRNA. TF-II catalyzes the translocation reaction; its activity is associated with the hydrolysis of one molecule of GTP.

Yeast, fungi, amoeba, and higher plants appear to share most of the features of protein synthesis in animal cells but the specific enzymes involved have only been isolated and characterized in the case of certain species of yeast (8, 9).

III. Inhibitors of Protein Synthesis

A number of antibiotics inhibit specific reactions in protein synthesis in bacteria (10, 11), including puromycin, which serves as a chain-terminating analog of aminoacyl-tRNA (12); sparsomycin, which selectively inhibits the activity of the peptide synthetase (13); tetracycline, which prevents the binding of aminoacyl-tRNA to ribosomes (14); and fusidic acid, which inhibits G factor (15). Chloramphenicol also inhibits peptide synthetase (16) and competes with lincomycin and other antibiotics for binding sites on the 50 S ribosomal subunit (11). Streptomycin and related aminoglycoside antibiotics interact with a specific protein of the 30 S subunit, inhibiting protein synthesis or causing misreading of mRNA by interfering with the binding of aminoacyl-tRNA and peptidyl-tRNA (17, 18). Aurintricarboxylic acid (19, 19a) and pactamycin (20) inhibit initiation of protein synthesis under certain experimental conditions. Many additional antibiotics interfere with protein synthesis in bacteria but their precise mode of action has not been completely clarified (cf. 21).

Certain antibiotics, as well as other agents, inhibit protein synthesis in animal cells. The actions of puromycin and sparsomycin are similar to those observed in bacteria while fusidic acid inhibits both translocation and the associated GTPase activity (22). Aurintricarboxylic acid (23) and pactamycin (24) are active inhibitors of protein synthesis in animal cells. Diphtheria toxin irreversibly inactivates transferase activity, apparently by catalyzing the transfer of the ADP-ribose moiety of NAD to TF-II (25).

Cycloheximide (26), emetine (27, 28), and anisomycin (29) inhibit protein synthesis in animal cells, yeast, and higher plants but have no effect on bacteria. The effects of cycloheximide have been interpreted in several ways. Schweet and his colleagues (30) reported that cycloheximide prevents the attachment of peptide synthetase to the ribosome, while the experiments of Munro et al. (31) and of McKeehan and Hardesty (32) suggest that cycloheximide inhibits the activity of TF-II. Emetine also inhibits TF-II (32a) while anisomycin acts on the peptide synthetase (32a, 32b).

Inhibitors of protein synthesis have also been classified according to their specificity toward ribosomes (11). Antibiotics of the chloramphenicol, macrolide, lincomycin, streptogramin A, and streptogramin B groups act on 70 S but not on 80 S ribosomes. Tenuazonic acid, pactamycin, emetine, anisomycin, tylocrebrine, cycloheximide, and the glutarimide antibiotics act on 80 S but not on 70 S ribosomes. On the other hand, amicetin, gougerotin, sparsomycin, edeine, and antibiotics of the tetracycline and puromycin groups affect both 70 S and 80 S ribosomes. Although streptomycin is specific for 70 S ribosomes, some reports have suggested that neomycin is active on 80 S, as well as 70 S, ribosomes, and certain other antibiotics in this group have only been tested with 70 S ribosomes.

IV. Design of Antibacterial Agents

Although formerly considered to be quite different, the mechanism of protein synthesis in bacteria and in animal cells now appears to be similar in many respects. One important difference lies in the specificity of the transfer enzymes which participate in chain elongation. When prepared from bacteria, these enzymes do not catalyze protein synthesis on isolated mammalian ribosomes;

conversely, the analogous enzymes prepared from animal cells do not act on bacterial ribosomes but do so on 80 S ribosomes prepared from yeast or plant sources (33). This specificity for ribosomes may be related to the selective inhibition of protein synthesis in bacteria by certain antibiotics and by cycloheximide, emetine, tylocrebrine, and anisomycin in animal cells, yeast and plants. Mitochondrial protein synthesis in yeast and animal cells, which bears many similarities to bacterial protein synthesis, is inhibited by chloramphenicol but not by cycloheximide (34) or emetine (34a).

The usefulness of chloramphenicol as a chemotherapeutic agent is clearly established but its therapeutic application has been restricted by the toxic action of the drug on bone marrow. There is no convincing evidence that the toxicity of chloramphenicol derives from an ability to inhibit protein synthesis and, in fact, the available data suggest that chloramphenicol does not inhibit protein synthesis to a significant degree in animal cells (35). The enzymic reaction in bacterial protein synthesis (possibly the peptide synthetase) that is sensitive to the action of chloramphenicol is, therefore, an ideal target for antimicrobial agents. A drug could profitably be sought which inhibits this reaction by the same mechanism as chloramphenicol but which is less toxic to man. The activity of this enzyme would provide a convenient screening assay to identify new compounds that are unrelated structurally to chloramphenicol but which act in the same manner as this drug. The enzyme seems to be similar in all bacteria, and its inhibition has lethal effects on bacteria at concentrations which do not affect the same process in animal cells.

The structural components of the ribosome may also offer useful information for drug design. For example, streptomycin is known to bind to a specific ribosomal protein in those bacteria which are sensitive to the effects of this drug (36, 37). Other antibiotics which bind to ribosomes may also act on specific protein or RNA components of the ribosome. Techniques are available for the isolation of these antibiotic-specific components. Rapid and convenient assays for the binding of aminoacyl-tRNA (38) or antibiotics (39) to ribosomes have been described which provide additional screening procedures to detect new agents acting specifically on these reactions.

V. Design of Amebicidal Agents

Emetine (27, 28), cycloheximide (26), and anisomycin (29) are directly acting amebicides that inhibit the elongation of the polypeptide chain subsequent to the transfer of aminoacyl-tRNA to the polyribosome. At concentrations of 10^{-6} to 10^{-8} M, these compounds inhibit protein synthesis by 98% in *Entamoeba histolytica*, intact HeLa cells, rabbit reticulocytes, and in cell-free extracts prepared from certain animal cells or *Saccharomyces fragilis*. The analogous reactions in extracts of *E. coli* are unaffected by 10^{-4} *M* concentrations of these compounds. This spectrum of inhibition is consistent with the known specificity of the enzymes responsible for chain elongation

TABLE I

SPECIFICITY OF IPECAC ALKALOIDS AND OTHER COMPOUNDS
AS AMEBICIDES AND AS INHIBITORS OF PROTEIN BIOSYNTHESIS[a]

Inhibitor	Amebicidal activity[b]	Inhibition[c]	
		Intact cells $(\mu M)^d$	Cell-free $(\mu M)^e$
Ipecac alkaloids			
(−)-Emetine	1000	0.7	3
(−)-Dehydroemetine	1000	0.4	4
(−)-Noremetine	200	20	30
(+)-*O*-Methylpsychotrine	<10	300	800
(−)-*N*-Methylemetine	<10	100	700
(−)-Isoemetine	<10	12	200
(±)-Trisdehydroemetine	<10	>1000	650
Other compounds			
Tubulosine	400	0.15	1.2
Anisomycin	1000	0.15	0.3
Cryptopleurine	—	0.15	0.7
Tylocrebrine	1000	0.3	0.8

[a] The data in this table are taken, in part, from unpublished studies of Jarkovsky and Grollman (*41a*).

[b] Adapted from reported values in the literature (*42, 42a*) as determined relative to emetine in growing cultures of *E. histolytica*. Certain assays were performed by Dr. Nathan Entner, using published techniques (*42b*).

[c] Concentration of inhibitor required for 50% inhibition of protein synthesis.

[d] Determined in rabbit reticulocytes (*29*).

[e] Determined in cell-free lysate prepared from rabbit reticulocytes (*41a*).

in bacteria for bacterial ribosomes (*40*) and the interchangeability of the analogous enzymes isolated from yeast, plant, and animal cells for ribosomes from these sources (*33*). DNA synthesis in HeLa cells is partially inhibited by emetine, cycloheximide, and anisomycin, a secondary activity common to all known inhibitors of protein synthesis in animal cells, while RNA synthesis is only minimally affected. Activation of amino acids, chain initiation, and release of completed polypeptides are not inhibited. If these inhibitors are added after protein synthesis is initiated, the nascent peptide remains firmly attached to the polyribosome structure. This response differs from that induced by puromycin which results in the disaggregation of polyribosomes and the release of polypeptides (41). Inhibition of protein synthesis is as rapid and effective in the preformed ribosome–mRNA–enzyme complexes of crude preparations of reticulocytes and rat liver microsomes as it is in partially purified systems to which the peptide chain-elongation enzymes are added separately.

TABLE II

EFFECTS OF AMEBICIDAL AGENTS ON PROTEIN BIOSYNTHESIS IN *E. histolytica*

Drug	LD_{100} $(\mu M)^a$	Inhibitory capacity $(\mu M)^b$
Emetine	2.0	2.0
Cycloheximide	0.2	0.2
Paromomycin	10	$> 100^c$
Fumagillin	0.1	$> 80^c$
Mantomide	100	$> 100^c$
Acriflavine	200	400
Diodohydroxyquin	50	50
Carbarsone	20	200
Tubulosine	5	5

[a] Expressed as the concentration of emetine required for 100% killing of *E. histolytica* (42b).
[b] Expressed as the concentration of emetine required for 50% inhibition of protein biosynthesis in *E. histolytica* (42c).
[c] Highest concentration tested. Inhibition less than 50%.

The amebicidal properties of the compounds mentioned above reflect their mode of action as demonstrated by comparing their structure–activity relationships with their amebicidal potency and capacity to inhibit protein synthesis. The capacity of various ipecac alkaloids to inhibit protein synthesis in intact rabbit reticulocytes and cellfree extracts has been compared to their amebicidal activity (Table I). With the exception of certain *N*-substituted derivatives, such as *N*-(3-oxo-*n*-butyl) emetine, the relative efficacy of the alkaloids tested as inhibitors of protein synthesis in intact reticulocytes corresponds closely to their comparative ED_{50} in inhibiting protein synthesis in cell-free preparations and to their *in vitro* toxicity against cultures of *E. histolytica*. The inactivity of *N*-substituted derivatives in the cell-free preparations suggested that enzymic hydrolysis of the substituent group was occurring in HeLa cells and in *E. histolytica*, a reaction which has been confirmed experimentally.

Other evidence supports the concept that inhibition of protein synthesis represents a potent mechanism of amebicidal action. Entner and Grollman have studied the effects of direct-acting amebicides on protein synthesis in *E. histolytica* (Table II) (*42b, 42c*). Emetine, cycloheximide, anisomycin, puromycin, tubulosine, acriflavine, diodoquin, and paromomycin, quickly inhibit protein synthesis by more than 50 % at the concentration of drug which eventually causes 100 % killing of amoeba. The observed inhibition of protein synthesis could be secondary to primary effects on associated metabolic pathways; however, the first five of the aforementioned drugs are known to act directly on protein synthesis in other organisms. Conversely, several established amebicides, the most potent being fumigillin, are toxic to intact *E. histolytica* at concentrations which do not affect protein synthesis in this organism.

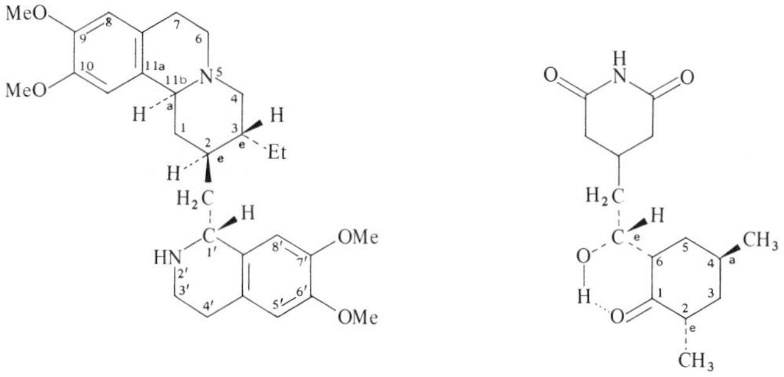

Fig. 2. Structural formulas of emetine and cycloheximide.

The availability of many stereoisomers and derivatives of emetine (cf. *43*, *49*) has made it possible to demarcate precisely the structure–activity requirements for the inhibition of protein synthesis by members of this series (*27*). The (R) configuration at C-1' and the secondary nitrogen atom at the 2'-position are essential requirements for activity (see Fig. 2 and Table I). These conclusions are based, in part, on the inactivity of the epimer with the (S) configuration at C-1' (isoemetine) and the loss of activity by unsaturation at the 1',2'-position (O-methylpsychotrine) or by substitution of the secondary nitrogen (N-methylemetine). Unsaturation at the 2,3-position (dehydro-emetine) destroys the asymmetry at carbons 2 and 3 without loss of biological activity, but further oxidation to 1,2,3,4,5,11b-trisdehydroemetine creates a positive charge at the tertiary nitrogen atom and results in inactivation of the compound. The presence of a *cis*-ethyl side chain results in optimal activity but this group is not essential since noremetine, N-propylemetine, and even deethylemetine retain some biological activity. If the ethyl side chain is present as the 2,3-*trans*-isomer, activity is markedly reduced. Similarly, inactivity of the 11b-epimer of dehydroemetine is most probably a result of steric influences.

Siegel, Sisler, and Johnson have tested various glutarimide antibiotic isomers of cycloheximide (Fig. 2) for their capacity to inhibit protein synthesis (*45*). Replacement of the imide hydrogen of cycloheximide by a methyl group, esterification of the hydroxyl with acetate or conversion of the ketone to an oxime, results in great diminution or complete loss of biological activity, suggesting that the keto, hydroxyl, and imide groups are involved in a three-point attachment of the glutarimide antibiotics to their receptor. Since epicycloheximide was not available, the probable importance of the correct configuration of the carbon bearing the hydroxyl could not be demonstrated directly. Any modification of the spatial position of this hydroxyl group in relation to the cyclohexanone ring, however, as in neocycloheximide (which has an axially oriented side chain) or inactone (in which C-5 to C-6 is unsaturated) results in loss of biological activity. Available data also offer evidence for a hydrogen-bonded conformation in the biologically active forms. β-Dihydrocycloheximide in which intramolecular hydrogen bonding is sterically prevented is inactive, while α-dihydrocycloheximide in which stronger hydrogen bonding is demonstrable has some activity. The active compound, streptimidone, which has an open chain in place of the cyclohexanone ring, would still assume the conformation of cycloheximide if stabilized by intramolecular hydrogen bonding.

The most significant conclusion to be drawn from the results of Siegel, Sisler, and Johnson (*45*) and the structure–activity data in Table I is that the essential positions for biological activity in the glutarimide antibiotics have corresponding positions in the ipecac alkaloids (*27*). In addition, there are topochemical resemblances between cycloheximide and the part of the emetine molecule containing the essential positions for biological activity (Fig. 3).

Interpretations of a necessarily tentative character may be useful in defining the possible interactions of these inhibitors with their biological receptor (enzyme). One postulated receptor site would presumably bind the hydroxyl of cycloheximide or the secondary nitrogen of emetine. The loss of activity which accompanies the replacement of the hydrogens at these positions with methyl or acetyl groups is consistent with the view that these positions are involved in hydrogen bonding to the receptor. Although an intramolecularly hydrogen-bonded conformation appears to be favored in cycloheximide, preferential bonding of the hydroxyl hydrogen to a receptor site is not precluded.

Additional testing of analogous compounds will be required to define fully the receptor site corresponding to the tertiary nitrogen of emetine or the imide nitrogen of cycloheximide. The imide grouping of cycloheximide is rendered inactive by *N*-methylation. This observation implies that the hydrogen atom on the imide nitrogen is involved in bonding since the two adjacent carbonyl groups effectively prevent bonding through the π electrons. If the tertiary nitrogen of emetine is hydrogen-bonded in a similar manner, the hydrogen atom must be supplied via the receptor. A bifunctional site in the receptor that could protonate as well as accommodate a hydrogen atom, such as a hydroxyl or an imidazole group, would satisfy these requirements. In-

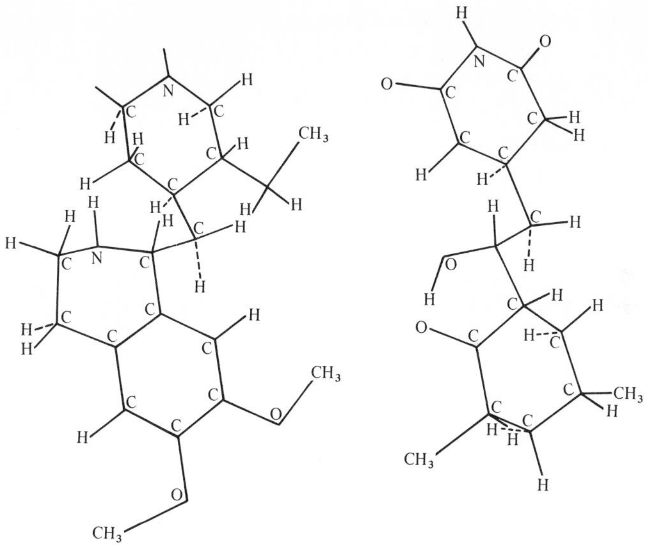

Fig. 3. Tracing of Dreiding models of cycloheximide (right) and part of emetine (left). In the conformation shown, cycloheximide is superimposable over the corresponding portion of the emetine molecule.

activity of trisdehydroemetine may result from repulsion by the positively charged nitrogen atom or from the effective removal of free electrons at this position. Steric effects also seem to be involved in the area of this nitrogen atom since reversal of configuration at the adjacent 11b position [(+)-dehydro-isoemetine] creates significant hindrance at the lower face of the molecule and is associated with a corresponding decrease in biological activity (*42*).

Although C-1′ of emetine and the asymmetric carbon of the side chain of cycloheximide may be involved in binding to the receptor, it is probable that they serve instead to fix the spatial position of the secondary nitrogen atom of emetine and the hydroxyl group of cycloheximide. The asymmetric carbon at C-6 of cycloheximide would fulfill a similar function since, in order for the quasi ring of cycloheximide to correspond to the ring of emetine, the configuration at C-6 must be such that the side chain is equatorial to the cyclohexanone ring.

Cycloheximide acts reversibly in the above biochemical reactions while the effects of emetine are irreversible (Fig. 4). Among the glutarimide antibiotics and ipecac alkaloids, where extensive structure–activity relationships can be established, reversibility is associated with the presence of an oxygen atom at a position other than those involved in the inhibition of protein synthesis. The action of streptovitacin A and acetoxycycloheximide, which differ from cycloheximide only in having an equatorial hydroxyl or acetoxy substitution

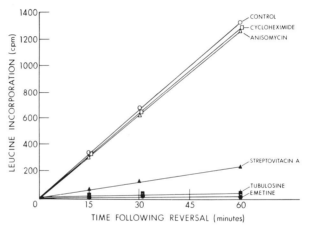

Fig. 4. Reversibility of the effects of various inhibitors on protein synthesis. Suspension cultures of HeLa cells were exposed to the indicated inhibitor for 2 min. The cells were collected by centrifugation, washed and resuspended in fresh medium containing ^{14}C-leucine. Protein synthesis was measured by the incorporation of leucine into trichloroacetic acid-insoluble material.

at the C-4 position, closely resembles emetine in being partially or totally irreversible (Fig. 4). It appears that the property of irreversibility may be conferred by a secondary binding site which is not essential for inhibition of protein synthesis.

The usefulness of the foregoing analysis of structure–function relationships in drug design is illustrated by the degree to which biological activity can be predicted on the basis of structure in nonanalogous series. Two examples may be cited: the postulated structure common to the glutarimide antibiotics and ipecac alkaloids (**I**, Fig. 5) which is found in the indole alkaloid, tubulosine; and structure **II** (Fig. 6), relating anisomycin and the pyrrolidine antibiotics to the phenanthrene alkaloids.

Although biological activity had not been reported for tubulosine (Fig. 5), it contained the topochemical requirements of structure **I**. Biochemical studies (46) established that the action of tubulosine is: (1) species-specific, being active against certain mammalian cells, protozoa and yeast but inactive against preparations of bacteria; (2) structurally specific, requiring a secondary nitrogen atom at the 2′-position and the (R) configuration at the 1′-carbon for activity; (3) selective, as RNA synthesis is unaffected at concentrations of tubulosine which totally inhibit protein synthesis; and (4) exerted during the elongation of the peptide chain. Subsequent studies showed that tubulosine was equal to emetine in amebicidal activity against several strains of *Entamoeba histolytica* (46).

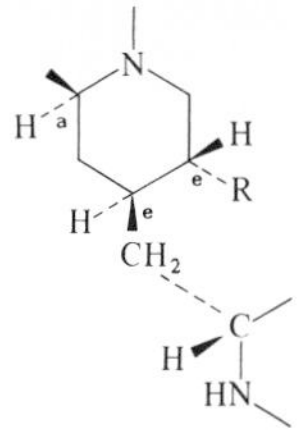

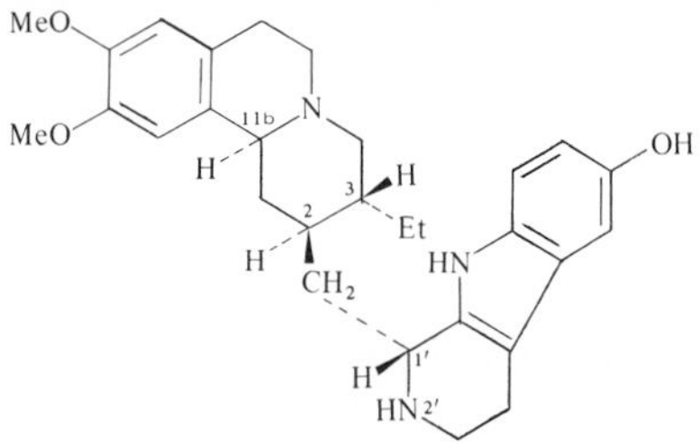

Tubulosine

Fig. 5. Structural formulas of tubulosine and of I, which contains the topochemical requirements for inhibition of protein synthesis based on an analogy between the ipecac alkaloids and the glutarimide antibiotics (27).

Similarly, cryptopleurine, tylocrebrine, and structurally related alkaloids (47) that were discovered in screening for antitumor compounds contain structure **II** (Fig. 6) in common with anisomycin and other pyrrolidine antibiotics. Based on these conformational resemblances, cryptopleurine and tylocrebrine were found to possess amebicidal activity and to inhibit protein synthesis (Table I). The overall effects of these alkaloids on protein synthesis (48) resemble those reported for anisomycin (29); however, this particular analogy must be considered tentative until similar sites of action and comparative structure–activity relationships for these compounds are established.

Determination of the precise structural requirements for inhibition of the translocase reaction in protein biosynthesis has practical implications for drug design. Structure of natural products and antibiotics are often complex and their chemical synthesis is difficult. Furthermore, it is difficult to modify these compounds chemically to obtain less toxic derivatives. An alternative approach for developing pharmaceutically active compounds in this series would utilize structures **III**, **IV**, or **V** (Fig. 7) as models for the synthesis of related compounds (27). Analogs based on these models are relatively easy to prepare, requiring only a site for hydrogen binding adjacent to an asymmetric carbon of the (R) configuration linked through a methylene group to a sterically unhindered six-membered ring. Procedures have been developed for the measurement of protein biosynthesis which permit rapid assay of inhibitory activity. The more active compounds could then be tested in animals to determine if more favorable therapeutic ratios might be discovered.

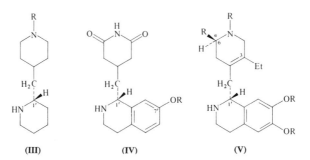

Fig. 6. Structural formulas of cryptopleurine, anisomycin and **II**, which is common to all phenanthrene alkaloids and pyrrolidine antibiotics.

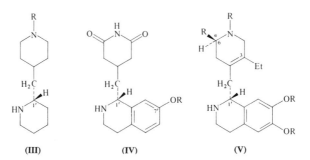

Fig. 7. Representative model compounds containing the essential structural features for the inhibition of protein synthesis.

The assumption that the spatial position of the two nitrogen atoms of emetine was the critical determinant of biological activity led to the preparation of a number of diamines, some of which have many times the amebicidal activity of emetine *in vitro* (49, 50). As the stereochemistry of the carbon corresponding to C-1′ of emetine was ignored in formulating the structure–activity relationships of these compounds, their inactivity as inhibitors of protein synthesis is not surprising.

A further practical application of drug design derives from the ability to relate toxicity of drugs to their therapeutic activity based on their mode of action. The most important adverse effect limiting the clinical use of emetine is its cardiotoxic action. This observation is remarkable considering that the turnover of protein in cardiac muscle is slow. However, two established cardiotoxins encountered in clinical practice, emetine and diphtheria toxin, are inhibitors of protein biosynthesis in animal cells. Like emetine, diphtheria toxin has been shown to inhibit protein synthesis (51) by acting on chain-elongation reactions (25). Despite the low overall rate of protein synthesis in cardiac muscle (52), some important protein necessary for cardiac function is clearly being turned over at a sufficiently rapid rate to be affected by these agents.

As described above, the effects of these compounds on protein synthesis correlate quantitatively and qualitatively with their effects on *E. histolytica*. It can therefore be predicted with some confidence that further increase in biological activity will be accompanied by increased toxicity. Nevertheless, despite its relative toxicity, emetine has been successfully used for over 300 years in the treatment of amebiasis and, more recently, for the treatment of granulomatous diseases (53). This margin of selective toxicity for emetine could be exploited and selectivity might be increased by finding related agents which distribute themselves differently in human tissues.

VI. Design of Antitumor Agents

All of the inhibitors of protein synthesis described in the previous section possess some degree of antitumor activity *in vivo*. Among the ipecac alkaloids, the structural requirements for the inhibition of protein synthesis also correspond to cytotoxicity. In contrast to amebiasis, where short-term treatment is sufficient to eradicate the causative agent, tumor chemotherapy is frequently continued over extended periods of time. The chemotherapeutic usefulness of inhibitors of protein synthesis has always been limited by their general cytotoxic activity. This is not surprising in light of their general effects on all types of protein synthesis in animal cells. However, they do not have suppressive effects on the bone marrow and may prove useful in conjunction with other antitumor drugs.

A different type of inhibition of protein synthesis is manifested by depletion of asparagine in animals cells. The finding that certain leukemias and other tumors have a specific nutritional requirement for L-asparagine (54) constitutes the only established instance of a specific metabolic difference between neoplastic cells and normal cells. The suppression of such leukemias by L-asparaginase (55) constitutes the only specific therapy known at present for any type of cancer. Leukemic cells resistant to the effects of asparaginase exhibit

substantial asparagine synthetase activity (56). It thus appears that aspara-
ginase-sensitive tumors have a "metabolic error," i.e., they lack asparagine
synthetase (56). The presence or absence of this metabolic error can be pre-
determined *in vitro* by determining the L-asparagine requirements of cell
suspensions prepared from lymphomatous nodes, the bone marrow, or the
buffy coat of the peripheral blood (55). Chemotherapy with asparaginase has
been limited by the small available supply of this enzyme and by hypersensitivity
reactions reported with crude enzyme preparations (55), although the latter
problem might be overcome by adding the enzyme to the dialysis bath during
hemodialysis. The qualitative biochemical difference in the metabolism of
asparagine observed in neoplastic and normal tissues suggests other therapeutic approaches. For example, drugs should be sought that selectively
inhibit the utilization and biosynthesis of asparagine in tumors (56).

It is apparent that an effective rationale for cancer chemotherapy awaits
further elucidation of the biology of neoplastic tissues at the molecular level.
It has been suggested that neoplasia is a decrease of cell differentiation expressed
as an alteration in the control of cellular metabolism and function (57, 58).
If certain tumors do arise as potentially reversible aberrations in differentiation,
this fact would have important implications for the design of antineoplastic
agents. Rather than the conventional emphasis on cytotoxic drugs, regulatory
agents should be sought which might favor redifferentiation of the tumor.
Instead of designing inhibitory agents, one should seek drugs that modify
protein synthesis by affecting the translation of mRNA. The concentration
of tRNA and the activity of the translocase have both been shown experimentally to control this process. This approach is not without precedent if
one considers the action of corticosteroids in cancer chemotherapy. There is
increasing evidence that these and other hormones exert their primary effects
at the level of gene transcription and possibly gene translation (59).

VII. Design of Emetic Agents

Emetine, in the form of ipecac, is widely used as an emetic agent in the
therapy of croup and for acute poisonings. The emetic properties of the drug
and its isomers are not contingent upon their capacity to inhibit protein
synthesis (59a). Since the adverse effects, including the cardiotoxic properties,
derive from the latter activity, it should be possible to use biologically inactive
analogs of emetine, such as *o*-methylpsychotrine or isoemetine as potent and
safe emetic agents.

VIII. Design of Antiviral Agents

All inhibitors of protein biosynthesis in animal cells prevent viral replication but in order to have a significant effect on virus replication, sufficient antibiotic must be used to inhibit protein synthesis in the host cell. Some of these compounds, such as emetine, have been shown to have activity against viral infection *in vitro* (*28*) and in experimental animals (*60*). This type of inhibition may prove only of limited value in the development of useful antiviral agents due to its cytotoxic effects on the host cell.

All viral RNA attaches to host cell ribosomes at some stage in the replicative pathway. The molecular basis for the action of interferon appears to be an altered ability of host cell ribosomes to bind viral mRNA (*61–63*), suggesting a novel mode for the design of antiviral agents, as described elsewhere (*23*). Interference with the binding of mRNA results in the inhibition of viral protein synthesis. A model system was devised that would distinguish compounds that inhibit the binding and subsequent function of viral mRNA while only affecting slightly the function of host cell mRNA (*23*). Several triphenylmethane dyes, including aurintricarboxylic acid, showed this selective inhibition which may be a promising approach for the development of novel antiviral agents (*19*; cf. Chapter 6).

IX. Conclusions

It is apparent that a study of the mechanism of action of compounds inhibiting protein biosynthesis offers a rational and practical approach in the search for chemotherapeutic and other potentially useful drugs. Examples of the application of these concepts have been cited and promising new approaches to the design of antimicrobial, amebicidal, antitumor, antiviral, and emetic agents suggested.

ACKNOWLEDGMENT

The preparation of this chapter and some of the experimental studies described herein were supported by research grants from the National Cancer Institute and the American Cancer Society.

REFERENCES

1. P. Lengyel and D. Soll, *Bacteriol. Rev.* **33**, 264 (1969).
2. F. Lipmann, *Science* **164**, 1024 (1969).
3. S. Ochoa, *Naturwissenschaften* **55**, 505 (1968).
4. K. Moldave, *Annu. Rev. Biochem.* **34**, 419 (1965).
5. R. Schweet and R. Heintz, *Annu. Rev. Biochem.* **35**, 723 (1966).
5a. A. E. Smith and K. A. Marcker, *Nature* **226**, 607 (1970).
6. F. Labrie, *Nature (London)* **221**, 1217 (1969).
7. R. L. Miller and R. Schweet, *Arch. Biochem. Biophys.* **125**, 632 (1968).
7a. P. M. Pritchard, J. M. Gilbert, D. A. Shafritz, and W. F. Anderson, *Nature* **226**, 511 (1970).
8. D. Richter, H. Hameister, H. G. Petersen, and F. Klink, *Biochemistry* **7**, 3753 (1968).
9. M. S. Ayuso and C. F. Heredia, *Biochim. Biophys. Acta* **145**, 199 (1967).
10. B. Weisblum and J. Davies, *Bacteriol. Rev.* **32**, 493 (1968).
11. D. Vazquez and R. E. Monro, *Wiss. Berlin, Kl. Med.* p. 569 (1968).
12. D. Nathans, *Proc. Nat. Acad. Sci. U.S.* **51**, 585 (1964).
13. I. H. Goldberg and K. Mitsugi, *Biochemistry* **6**, 383 (1967).
14. G. Suarez and D. Nathans, *Biochem. Biophys. Res. Commun.* **18**, 743 (1965).
15. N. Tanaka, T. Kinoshita, and H. Masukawa, *J. Biochem. (Tokyo)* **65**, 459 (1969).
16. F. E. Hahn, *in* "Antibiotics. I. Mechanism of Action" (D. Gottlieb and P. D. Shaw, eds.), p. 308. Springer, Berlin, 1967.
17. B. D. Davis, *Asian Med. J.* **11**, 78 (1968).
18. J. Modolell and B. D. Davis, *Proc. Nat. Acad. Sci. U.S.* **67**, 1148 (1970).
19. A. P. Grollman and M. L. Stewart, *Proc. Nat. Acad. Sci. U.S.* **61**, 719 (1968).
19a. M. L. Stewart, A. P. Grollman, and M. T. Huang, *Proc. Nat. Acad. Sci. U.S.* **68**, 97 (1971).
20. L. B. Cohen, A. E. Herner, and I. H. Goldberg, *Biochemistry* **8**, 1312 (1969).
21. D. Gottlieb and P. D. Shaw, eds., "Antibiotics. I. Mechanism of Action." Springer, Berlin, 1967.
22. M. Malkin and F. Lipmann, *Science* **164**, 71 (1969).
23. A. P. Grollman, *Antimicrob. Ag. Chemother.* p. 36 (1969).
24. B. Colombo, L. Felicetti, and C. Baglioni, *Biochim. Biophys. Acta* **119**, 109 (1966).
25. T. Honjo, Y. Nishizuka, O. Hayaishi, and I. Kato, *J. Biol. Chem.* **243**, 3553 (1968).
26. H. D. Sisler and M. R. Siegel, *in* "Antibiotics. I. Mechanism of Action" (D. Gottlieb and P. D. Shaw, eds.), p. 283. Springer, Berlin, 1967.
27. A. P. Grollman, *Proc. Nat. Acad. Sci. U.S.* **56**, 1867 (1966).
28. A. P. Grollman, *J. Biol. Chem.* **243**, 4089 (1968).
29. A. P. Grollman, *J. Biol. Chem.* **242**, 3226 (1967).
30. R. L. Heintz, M. L. Salas, and R. S. Schweet, *Arch. Biochem. Biophys.* **125**, 488 (1968).
31. H. N. Munro, B. S. Baliga, and A. W. Pronczuk, *Nature (London)* **219**, 944 (1968).
32. W. McKeehan and B. Hardesty, *Biochem. Biophys. Res. Commun.* **36**, 625 (1969).
32a. M. T. Huang and A. P. Grollman, *Federation Proc.* **29**, 609 (1970).
32b. D. Vazquez, E. Battaner, R. Neth, G. Heller, and R. E. Monro, *Cold Spring Harbor Symp. Quant. Biol.* **24**, 369 (1969).
33. B. Parisi, G. Milanesi, J. L. Van Etten, A. Perani, and O. Ciferri, *J. Mol. Biol.* **28**, 295 (1967).
34. G. D. Clark-Walker and A. W. Linnane, *J. Cell Biol.* **34**, 1 (1967).

34a. S. Perlman and S. Penman, *Biochem. Biophys. Res. Commun.* **40**, 941 (1970).
35. M. Ochoa, Jr. and I. B. Weinstein, *J. Biol. Chem.* **239**, 3834 (1964).
36. P. Traub, K. Hosokawa, and M. Nomura, *J. Mol. Biol.* **19**, 211 (1966).
37. T. Staehelin and M. Meselson, *J. Mol. Biol.* **19**, 207 (1966).
38. M. Nirenberg and P. Leder, *Science* **145**, 1399 (1965).
39. D. Vazquez, *Biochim. Biophys. Acta* **114**, 277 (1966).
40. R. Rendi and S. Ochoa, *J. Biol. Chem.* **237**, 3711 (1966).
41. S. Villa-Trevino, E. Farber, T. Staehelin, F. O. Wettstein, and H. Noll, *J. Biol. Chem.* **239**, 3826 (1964).
41a. Z. Jarkovsky and A. P. Grollman, unpublished studies (1970).
42. A. Brossi, M. Baumann, F. Burkhardt, R. Richie, and J. R. Frey, *Helv. Chim. Acta* **45**, 2219 (1962).
42a. C. Dobell and P. P. Laidlaw, *Parisitology* **18**, 206 (1926).
42b. N. Entner, *J. Protozool.* **8**, 131 (1961).
42c. N. Entner and A. P. Grollman, unpublished results (1970).
43. H. T. Openshaw, N. C. Robson, and N. Whittaker, *J. Chem. Soc.* p. 101 (1969) (see also preceding papers in this series).
44. S. Teitel and A. Brossi, *J. Amer. Chem. Soc.* **88**, 4068 (1966) (see also preceding papers in this series).
45. M. R. Siegel, H. D. Sisler, and F. Johnson, *Biochem. Pharmacol.* **15**, 1213 (1966).
46. A. P. Grollman, *Science* **157**, 84 (1967).
47. E. Gellert, T. R. Govindachari, M. V. Lakshmikantham, I. S. Ragade, R. Rudzats, and N. Viswanathan, *J. Chem. Soc.* p. 1008 (1962).
48. G. R. Donaldson, M. R. Atkinson, and A. W. Murray, *Biochem. Biophys. Res. Commun.* **31**, 104 (1968).
49. D. M. Hall, S. Mahboob, and E. E. Turner, *J. Chem. Soc.* p. 1842 (1950).
50. D. A. Berberian, R. G. Slighter, and A. R. Surrey, *Antibiot. Chemother. (Washington, D.C.)* **11**, 245 (1961).
51. R. S. Goor and A. M. Pappenheimer, Jr., *J. Exp. Med.* **126**, 899 (1967).
52. B. M. Beller, *Circ. Res.* **22**, 501 (1968).
53. A. I. Grollman, *Surg., Gynecol. Obstet.* **120**, 792 (1965).
54. J. D. Broome, *J. Exp. Med.* **118**, 99 (1963).
55. H. F. Oettgen, L. J. Old, E. A. Boyse, H. A. Campbell, F. S. Philips, B. D. Clarkson, L. Tallal, R. D. Leeper, M. K. Schwartz, and J. H. Kim, *Cancer Res.* **27**, 2619 (1967).
56. B. Horowitz, B. K. Madras, A. Meister, L. J. Old, E. A. Boyse, and E. Stockert, *Science* **160**, 533 (1968).
57. C. L. Markert, *Cancer Res.* **28**, 1908 (1968).
58. H. C. Pitot, *Cancer Res.* **28**, 1880 (1968).
59. G. M. Tompkins, E. B. Thompson, S. Hayashi, T. Gelehrter, D. Granner, and B. Peterkofsky, *Cold Spring Harbor Symp. Quant. Biol.* **31**, 349 (1966).
59a. S. C. Wang, personal communication (1968).
60. E. Grunberg and H. N. Prince, *Antimicrob. Ag. Chemother.* p. 527 (1967).
61. W. K. Joklik and T. C. Merigan, *Proc. Nat. Acad. Sci. U.S.* **56**, 558 (1966).
62. H. B. Levy and W. A. Carter, *J. Mol. Biol.* **31**, 561 (1968).
63. P. I. Marcus and J. M. Salb, *Virology* **30**, 502 (1966).

Chapter 6   Enzymes and Their Synthesis as a Target for Antibiotic Action

M. H. Richmond

I. Introduction

If a compound is to be an effective antibacterial agent, it must act as a potent and specific inhibitor of one of the many biochemical processes involved in cell duplication. Only if such processes can be blocked completely will the growth of a bacterial culture be inhibited sufficiently to ensure that there is no slow residual growth leading to a chronic rather than to an acute infection. Although a number of different types of molecular target, such as nucleic acid biosynthesis, ribosome action, and the like, are available to antibacterial agents (*1*) many of these compounds rely for their effect on interference with the function of an essential enzyme; and certainly when considering the design of new antibacterial substances the active center of some key enzyme is often the target chosen for attack. Yet the majority of inhibitors are only transient in their effect. Often the treated culture starts to grow again after only a relatively short delay, and in many cases (particularly in laboratory cultures) it is difficult to distinguish the inhibited from the uninhibited culture after overnight growth. In this article some of the reasons underlying this comparatively transient effect of most inhibitory compounds will be examined together with reasons for believing that covalent linkages between an inhibitor and a key enzyme is the only effective way of blocking growth. Previously discussion has been confined largely to the physiological considerations (*1*); here we are concerned mainly with genetic effects.

II. Competitive Inhibitors of Enzymes

It has long been known (*2*) that certain chemical compounds that bear a close structural analogy to the natural substrate of an enzyme can interfere with the action of that enzyme against its natural substrate even when both the substrate and the inhibitor are present at the same time. This phenomenon is normally studied with pure preparations *in vitro* and indeed it is only under these conditions that the effect is really striking. A typical example is the action of malonate. *In vitro*, this compound is an effective competitive inhibitor of succinic dehydrogenase, an essential enzyme of the tricarboxylic acid cycle in both mammalian and bacterial cells. Yet despite the undoubted fact that malonate is an effective inhibitor of this enzyme *in vitro*, the compound is completely inactive as an overall growth inhibitor of both mammalian and bacterial cells.

The reason that competitive inhibitors are not more effective *in vivo* appears to be twofold. First, the effect of such inhibitors may easily be reversed if the natural substrate accumulates in sufficient quantity. This is particularly so when the affinity of the inhibitor for the enzyme is of the same order or lower than that of the natural substrate, as is often the case. Normally, when enzymes are examined for their sensitivity to competitive inhibitors *in vitro*, they alone are present in the test and the inhibitor and substrate are added in carefully controlled amounts. But when the enzymes are examined in the cell, they exist as part of a functioning biosynthetic pathway and any action that blocks such an enzyme immediately leads to the accumulation of the natural precursor of the inhibited enzyme; and this is precisely the step that will reduce the effectiveness of the inhibitor by a straight competitive effect.

The second reason for the short duration of the effect of many inhibitors is due to the appearance and selection of mutants. In this case mutation in the gene responsible for the synthesis of the target enzyme leads to the formation of an altered gene product that is less sensitive than before to the action of the inhibitor. Since this route to a resistant culture involves the selection of what is initially only a single cell in the population, this type of response is slower to develop than the phenotypic resistance caused by the accumulation of the natural substrate. However, the process is ultimately no less effective.

The mutation of an enzyme so that it is less sensitive to inhibitor action may be based on two types of change; but both are due to an alteration in the primary amino acid sequence of the enzyme and cause exchange of a single amino acid residue for another at some point. (Whether this really occurs has only been established in very few cases.) In some cases, the mutation makes the enzyme very much less sensitive to the inhibitor without altering the affinity of the enzyme for the natural substrate to any great extent. A good example of this type of mutant is provided by the altered pteroic acid synthetase enzyme in sulfonamide-resistant pneumococci (Table I) (3). In this case the

TABLE I

AFFINITY CONSTANTS FOR p-AMINOBENZOIC ACID AND FOR
SULFONAMIDE AS EXHIBITED BY WILD-TYPE AND MUTANT
VARIANTS OF TETRAHYDROPTEROIC ACID SYNTHETASE[a]

	Affinity constant ($M \times 10^{-3}$)	
	Wild-type	Mutant
p-Aminobenzoic acid	0.1	0.06
Sulfonamide	0.5	65

[a] Data from Wolf and Hotchkiss (3).

wild-type version of the target enzyme has twice the affinity for sulfonamide as it has for p-aminobenzoic acid, the normal substrate of the enzyme. However, the enzyme from mutated cells has a 1000-fold lower sensitivity of sulfonamide, whereas the affinity for p-aminobenzoic acid is scarcely affected. Thus, in physiological terms, in a growing culture, the mutant enzyme is entirely resistant to sulfonamide because it is impossible to transport sufficient of the compound into a cell to inhibit the enzyme however much inhibitor is added to the growth medium. However, the enzyme is still able to handle p-amino-benzoic acid for folic acid biosynthesis and consequently the sulfonamide-resistant mutation is not lethal.

The other type of mutant that appears to emerge under these circumstances is one in which the interaction of the enzyme with *both* the inhibitor *and* the natural substrate is impaired to the same extent. This type of mutation only produces viable resistant cultures when the affinity of the unmutated enzyme for the inhibitor is initially lower than the affinity for the natural substrate. If this is so, than a fall in affinity for the natural substrate following mutation may reduce the efficiency of the enzyme to some extent without making it completely inactive. But an equal fall in affinity for the inhibitor, starting from an initial point of lower affinity anyway, can often yield an enzyme that is now effectively resistant to inhibitor action solely because it is impracticable to achieve a high enough inhibitor concentration in the cells. A good example of this situation is provided by the effect of mutation on the sensitivity to histidine and to 2-thiazole alanine of the enzyme synthesizing compound III in the histidine biosynthetic pathway in *E. coli* (Table II). In this case histidine

TABLE II

INHIBITION OF THE SYNTHESIS OF "COMPOUND III" BY HISTIDINE AND BY 2-THIAZOLE ALANINE IN WILD-TYPE *Escherichia coli* AND IN A MUTANT RESISTANT TO 2-THIAZOLE ALANINE[a]

	Concentration of inhibitor (M)	Compound III synthesis (% inhibition)	
		Wild-type	Mutant
Histidine	Nil	0	0
	5×10^{-5}	25	8
	7×10^{-5}	55	8
	10^{-4}		35
	2.5×10^{-4}		55
2-Thiazolealanine	Nil	0	0
	10^{-3}	45	0
	2×10^{-3}	58	35
	8×10^{-3}	85	50

[a] Data from Moyed (*4*).

and 2-thiazole alanine are not substrates to these enzymes but feedback inhibitors acting at the *allosteric*, rather than the *active*, center of the enzyme (*4*). However, for the purposes of our argument, the comparative interaction of these two compounds at this site is entirely analogous to the action of a substrate at an active center. The unmutated enzyme is half inhibited by a concentration of 7×10^{-5} *M* histidine or by 1.5×10^{-3} *M* 2-thiazole alanine; but after mutation 2-thiazole alanine must be present at a concentration of about 10^{-2} *M* to be effective, and this is an impossible concentration to achieve inside the cell. The mutation also reduces sensitivity to histidine, but with 50% inhibition achieved at a histidine concentration of 2×10^{-4} *M* some regulatory effect of this compound can still take place even though it is somewhat less effective than in the unmutated culture.

Basically, therefore, competitive inhibitors of enzymes are poor potential inhibitors of the growth of bacterial cultures because their effect is liable to reversal either phenotypically by the accumulation of the natural competitor or genotypically by the appearance of mutant cells in the population in which sensitivity to the inhibitor is so reduced that the compound can never be supplied in sufficient quantities to be effective. Even inhibitors that have a higher affinity for the target enzyme than the normal substrate (such as sulfonamide, for example) are susceptible to challenge by the second of these two routes.

III. Irreversible Inhibitors or Enzymes as Antibacterial Agents

Against this background of a rapidly acquired phenotypic or genotypic resistance to simple competitive inhibitors, any irreversible (noncompetitive) inhibitor will show up as an altogether more effective proposition as an inhibitor of bacterial growth. If a compound is drawn to the active center of an enzyme by a structural analogy to the natural substrate but then interacts chemically to form a stable linkage with the enzyme, it is clear that however high the accumulation of the natural substrate, and it certainly will accumulate, little displacement of the blocking compound is likely to occur. As a consequence, therefore, a physiological resistance to this type of inhibitor is most unlikely to arise.

Although it is impossible to be completely dogmatic on the matter, it is also most unlikely that mutation of the target enzyme can lead to an effective

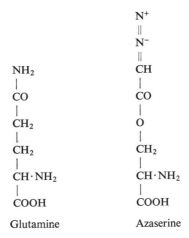

Fig. 1. The structural formulas of glutamine and azaserine.

mutant version of the enzyme protein. The reasons underlying this point can be demonstrated quite well by reference to the case of azaserine, a structural analog of glutamine (Fig. 1) that inhibits purine biosynthesis, in both mammalian and bacterial cells, by blocking the formation of formylglycinamidine ribotide from formylglycinamide and glutamine (Fig. 2) (5, 6). In the normal biosynthetic reaction glutamine acts as a source of an —NH— group to convert the amide residue to an amidine, but azaserine, if present, inhibits the enzyme irreversibly by being drawn to the active center by its structural similarity to glutamine. Unlike glutamine, however, whose reaction with the enzyme active center is transient, and only involves a very labile bond, azaserine is bound covalently by a firm covalent link.

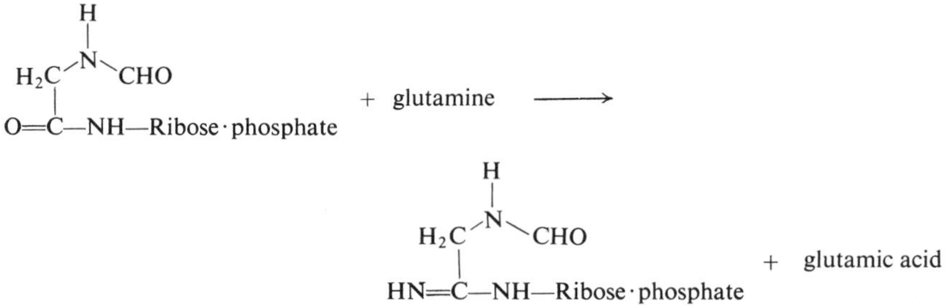

$$
\begin{array}{c}
\text{H} \\
| \\
\text{H}_2\text{C} \overset{\text{N}}{\diagdown} \text{CHO} \\
| \\
\text{O}{=}\text{C}\text{—NH—Ribose}\cdot\text{phosphate}
\end{array}
\quad + \text{ glutamine} \quad \longrightarrow
$$

$$
\begin{array}{c}
\text{H} \\
| \\
\text{H}_2\text{C} \overset{\text{N}}{\diagdown} \text{CHO} \\
| \\
\text{HN}{=}\text{C}\text{—NH—Ribose}\cdot\text{phosphate}
\end{array}
\quad + \text{ glutamic acid}
$$

Fig. 2. Formation of formyl glycinamide ribotide from formyl glycinamide + glutamine, a step in the biosynthesis of purines in bacterial and mammalian cells.

The target enzyme in this situation has been shown to have a cysteine residue in its active center and this residue has been implicated in the transfer of the —NH— residue (7). In the presence of azaserine, however, and regardless of whether glutamine is present or not, the —SH group is acylated according to the reaction:

$$
\begin{aligned}
\text{ENZ—SH} + \text{N}_2\cdot\text{CH}\cdot\text{CO}\cdot\text{O}\cdot\text{CH}_2\cdot\text{CH(NH}_2)\cdot\text{COOH} \rightarrow \\
\text{ENZ—S}\cdot\text{CH}_2\cdot\text{CO}\cdot\text{O}\cdot\text{CH}_2\cdot\text{CH(NH}_2)\cdot\text{COOH} + \text{N}_2
\end{aligned}
$$

The outcome of this step is that the cysteine residue at the active center is now substituted and in the form of an —S$\cdot$CH$_2\cdot$CO$\cdot$O$\cdot$CH$_2\cdot$CH(NH$_2$)$\cdot$COOH derivative; and in practice this bond is so stable that it will withstand all the chemical manipulations involved in purifying the enzyme and isolating a peptide from the enzyme following trypsin digestion and "fingerprinting" of the azaserine-inhibited enzyme (7). In contrast, the complex between the enzyme and glutamine is so labile that the complex does not survive purification of the enzyme.

The reason why mutation cannot provide a means of escape from the action of azaserine—and the same is true of any irreversible inhibitor in which there is a strong covalent bond formed between the inhibitor and the enzyme active center—is inherent in the possible types of amino acid that can be incorporated into the protein structure, and in the nature of the genetic code. Take, for example, the case of the enzyme inhibited by azaserine. The two possible RNA codons that can code for cysteine are UGU and UGC, and this implies that the part of the gene specifying the active center cysteine in this enzyme will be either $\frac{ACA}{(TGT)}$ or $\frac{ACG}{(TGC)}$. On the assumption that the gene structure is $\frac{ACA}{(TGT)}$, mutation in the first base of the codon can give CCA and $\frac{G}{T}$ this will lead, ultimately, to the replacement of cysteine at the active center by arginine, glycine, or serine depending on the precise nature of the initial mutation. Similarly, mutation in the second position of the codon leads to the possibilities $A\overset{A}{G}A$ and the consequent amino acids substitution of cystine $\overset{}{\underset{T}{}}$ by phenylalanine, serine, or tyrosine. Finally, mutation in the last base gives $AC\overset{G}{C}$ and the possible amino acid substitution of cysteine by tryptophan. In $\overset{}{\underset{T}{}}$ short, therefore, if the DNA codon for cysteine is $\frac{ACA}{(TGT)}$, the only possible replacements of cysteine in the protein are arginine, glycine, serine, phenylalanine, tyrosine, or tryptophan. Similarly, if the DNA codon involved is not $\frac{ACA}{(TGT)}$ but $\frac{ACG}{(TGC)}$ a similar line of argument gives the amino acid replacements of cysteine to be the same as when the DNA codon is $\frac{ACG}{(TGC)}$. The arguments underlying these interconversions are shown diagrammatically in Fig. 3.

The overall effect of mutation in this enzyme system therefore will certainly allow the replacement of cysteine in the active center by some other amino acid that will now not react with azaserine, but the mutated enzyme will not interact with glutamine either since cysteine is necessary for this process in the unmutated enzyme. Thus mutation to resistance to azaserine can only be achieved at the expense of loss of the catalytic ability to use glutamine as a source of —NH— groups for purine synthesis, and since purine synthesis is essential for growth, such mutants will be lethal.

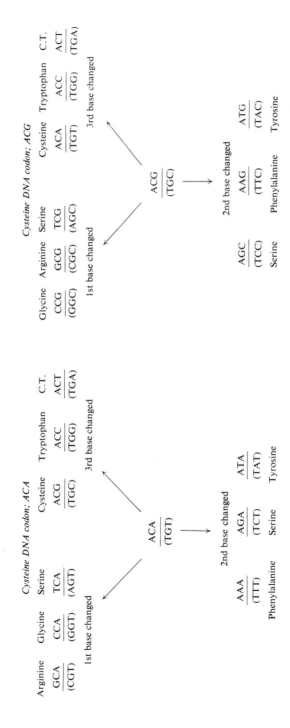

Fig. 3. The potential molecular interconversions of a cysteine residue at the active center of an enzyme on the basis of point mutation in its structural gene.

IV. Conclusion

The arguments produced above largely reinforce the views on inhibitor action expressed by others concerned mostly with the fields of pharmacology (8) and cancer chemotherapy (9); namely that noncompetitive inhibitors that form irreversible complexes with the active center of an enzyme are enormously more effective than are straightforward competitive inhibitors [for example, see the effect of DFP (8)]. The considerations are, however, particularly important in the field of antibacterial chemotherapy since the high growth rate and mutational flexibility of bacterial cultures makes them particularly effective at altering their properties rapidly, particularly where the behavior of populations rather than individual cells is important.

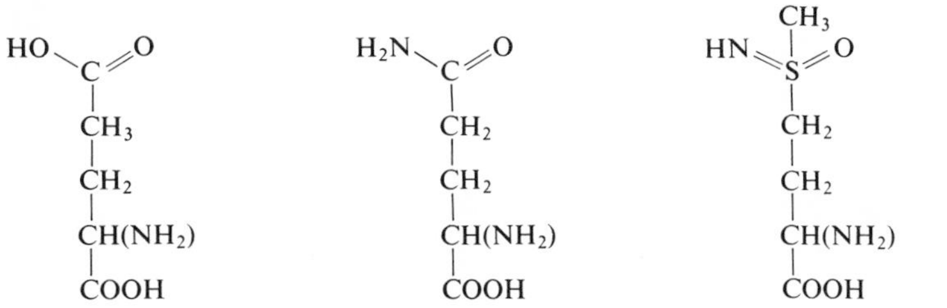

$$
\begin{array}{ccc}
\mathrm{HO}_{\diagdown}\underset{\mathrm{C}}{{}}{\diagup}^{\mathrm{O}} & \mathrm{H_2N}_{\diagdown}\underset{\mathrm{C}}{{}}{\diagup}^{\mathrm{O}} & \overset{\mathrm{CH_3}}{\underset{\mathrm{HN}_{\diagdown}}{{}}}\underset{\mathrm{S}}{{}}{\diagup}^{\mathrm{O}} \\
| & | & | \\
\mathrm{CH_3} & \mathrm{CH_2} & \mathrm{CH_2} \\
| & | & | \\
\mathrm{CH_2} & \mathrm{CH_2} & \mathrm{CH_2} \\
| & | & | \\
\mathrm{CH(NH_2)} & \mathrm{CH(NH_2)} & \mathrm{CH(NH_2)} \\
| & | & | \\
\mathrm{COOH} & \mathrm{COOH} & \mathrm{COOH} \\
\text{Glutamic acid} & \text{Glutamine} & \text{Methionine sulfoximine}
\end{array}
$$

Fig. 4. Structural analogy of glutamic acid, glutamine, and methionine sulfoximine.

The crucial inflexibility of bacterial cells to noncompetitive inhibitors, particularly if they interact with amino acid residues in an enzyme active center, derives from the exigencies of the genetic code and from the limited range of different types of amino acid that can be introduced into proteins by living cells. This ensures that it is impossible to remove by mutation a residue sensitive to attack by an inhibitor without inactivating the enzyme against its normal substrate at the same time. Furthermore, since a mutational event of this type will almost certainly be lethal as far as the cell is concerned, there will be no opportunity for a second mutation to take the molecular refashioning of the enzyme a stage further.

The corollary of these arguments, therefore, is that attempts to design antibacterial compounds in the laboratory, as opposed to attempts to develop or modify compounds already developed in living organisms by the effect of natural selection, should incorporate some chemical grouping in the molecule capable of forming a stable complex with an amino acid residue at the active center of the target enzyme. Such groups are few and far between, particularly since structural analogy with the normal substrate must always be borne in mind. Nor are they always obvious: thus methionine sulfoximine (Fig. 4) is also a structural analog of glutamine that binds irreversibly to the glutamine synthetase enzyme (*10*). In this case the

$$-S\overset{\displaystyle O}{\underset{\displaystyle \underset{H}{N}}{{}}}$$

group of the inhibitor seems to be responsible for the reactive properties of the molecule. Perhaps it is for this reason the chemically unexpected groupings of the —CH=N⁻=N⁺ in azaserine and of

$$\begin{array}{c} -CH-CH- \\ | \quad\;\; | \\ C\;-\;N- \\ O \end{array}$$

in penicillin are necessary for effective activity in these antibiotics.

REFERENCES

1. M. H. Richmond, *Symp. Soc. Gen. Microbiol.* **16**, 301 (1966).
2. J. B. Quastel and W. R. Wooldridge, *Biochem. J.* **22**, 689 (1928).
3. B. Wolf and R. D. Hotchkiss, *Biochemistry*, **2**, 145 (1963).
4. H. S. Moyed, *J. Biol. Chem.* **235**, 1098 (1961).
5. S. C. Hartman, B. Levenberg, and J. M. Buchanan, *J. Amer. Chem. Soc.* **77**, 501 (1955)
6. J. M. Buchanan, B. Levenberg, I. Melnick, and S. C. Hartman, *in* "The Leukemias: Etiology, Pathophysiology and Treatment" (J. W. Rebuck and R. W. Monto, eds.), p. 523. Academic Press, New York, 1957.
7. T. C. French, I. B. Dawid, and J. M. Buchanan, *J. Biol. Chem.* **238**, 2186 (1963).
8. I. B. Wilson, *Fed. Proc., Fed. Amer. Soc. Exp. Biol.* **18**, 752 (1959).
9. B. R. Baker, *Cancer Chemother. Rep.* **4**, 1 (1959).
10. A. Meister, *Advan. Enzymol.* **31**, 183 (1968).

Chapter 7   The Rational Design of Antiviral Agents

Arthur P. Grollman and Susan B. Horwitz

I. Introduction

Virus replication involves numerous biochemical mechanisms which might profitably be utilized in the rational design of antiviral agents. This chapter will review the molecular biology of virus replication with special reference

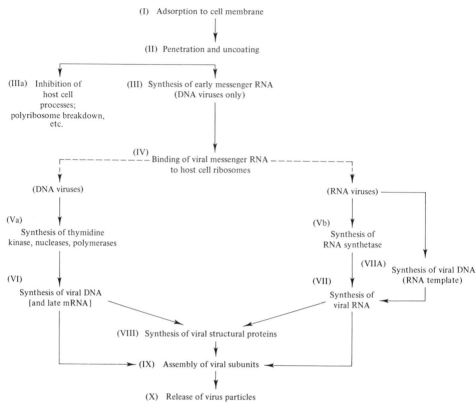

Fig. 1. General scheme for viral replication showing probable sites of action of established antiviral agents. (I) Neuraminidase (RDE); (II) adamantadine; (III) actinomycin; (IV) aurintricarboxylic acid, interferon; (VA) and (VB) cycloheximide, emetine, fluorophenyl-alanine, puromycin, and other inhibitors of protein synthesis; (VI) bromodeoxyuridine and other halogenated nucleosides, cytosine arabinoside; (VII) acetylaranotin, sporodesmins, gliotoxin, and related compounds containing the epidithiapiperazinedione moiety; (VI) and (VII) isatin-β-thiosemicarbazide, hydroxybenzylbenzimidazole and guanidine; (VIII) in-hibitors listed under VA and VB, rifampicin; (IX) quinomycin A, *p*-fluorophenylalanine; (X) substituted dihydroisoquinolines (UK 2054) and related inhibitors of neuraminidase.

to approaches which seem promising for the development of new antiviral agents.

   Although the replicative cycle may vary from one given virus–host cell combination to another, the process generally includes (1) adsorption, (2) penetration and uncoating, (3) *de novo* synthesis of messenger RNA (mRNA) (by DNA viruses only), (4) binding of viral mRNA to ribosomes, (5) synthesis of viral enzymes, including the viral RNA polymerase, (6) synthesis of viral nucleic acids and structural proteins, (7) assembly of subunits, and (8) release of virus particles. Some of these steps are unique for viruses, thereby representing potential sites of action for antiviral agents. Certain drugs with antiviral activity have already been shown to be inhibitors of these processes (cf. Fig. 1).

The genetic material of a given virus may be single- or double-stranded DNA, or single- or double-stranded RNA, and the nature of this viral genome determines the sequence of replication. Viruses also differ in size and in the complexity of the protein encapsulating their nucleic acid. Many viruses replicate in the cytoplasm of their host cells, while others replicate, at least partly, in the nucleus.

A. Adsorption and Penetration

Viruses are adsorbed on specific receptor sites on the cell membrane of the host cell. In primates, for example, poliovirus is adsorbed to brain, spinal, and intestinal cells but not to cells of the heart, lung, and skeletal muscle (1, 2). Following its adsorption, the genetic material, along with additional parts of the virus, enter the cytoplasm of the cell.

Other viruses, such as vaccinia virus, are initially engulfed by a segment of the host cell membrane in a process resembling phagocytosis. The phospholipid coat of the virus is removed and the viral genetic material is released into the cytoplasm of the host cell. The uncoating process requires the synthesis of RNA and protein (3), and it is presently believed that vaccinia virus is capable of directing its own uncoating (4).

The coat protein of the virus participates in the adsorption of the virus to the host cell (5–7). The initial step in the adsorption process proceeds at 0°C and most likely represents a reversible noncovalent type of binding while the subsequent steps are temperature-dependent and irreversible (8). Poliovirus is known to be chemically altered by adsorption, as evidenced by a change in its antigenic specificity (9).

B. Inhibition of Host Cell Functions

After penetration of certain viruses, the synthetic facilities of the host cell are directed toward viral replication, and there is a reduction in the synthesis of nucleic acid and proteins in the host cell (10, 11). These metabolic processes are probably inhibited by protein(s) whose synthesis is directed by the viral genome. Host cell mRNA is degraded, and the polysomes are disaggregated to a functionally intact pool of single ribosomes and subunits which are later utilized in the biosynthesis of viral proteins.

C. ATTACHMENT AND FUNCTION OF VIRAL mRNA

In DNA viruses, mRNA is first transcribed from the viral genome, while the RNA of RNA viruses functions as its own messenger. mRNA associates with a number of smaller ribosomal subunits derived from the host cell and is subsequently joined by the larger subunits to form the viral polyribosome which serves as the functional unit of protein synthesis for the virus.

Newly synthesized ("early") mRNA, transcribed from parental DNA, appears in the cytoplasm of the infected cell shortly after infection with vaccinia virus. Within 2 min after synthesis, this form of mRNA is found in polyribosome complexes where it serves as a template for the synthesis of such viral enzymes as thymidine kinase, deoxyribonuclease, and DNA polymerase (12–15).

The synthesis of "early" enzymes continues for 3–4 hr following infection with vaccinia virus. At this time, a "switch-off" protein inactivates "early" mRNA so that these enzymes are no longer produced (16–17). The "switch-off" protein is coded for by mRNA that is produced later in the replicative cycle from progeny DNA. "Late" mRNA appears to code principally for structural viral proteins and also controls the translation of certain "early" mRNA's.

The chemical basis for the attachment of mRNA to ribosomes has been established using bacteriophage RNA and synthetic polynucleotides as mRNA with ribosomes prepared from E. coli. These studies indicate that (1) mRNA attaches to a specific site on the ribosome, (2) specific protein factors are involved in the binding process (18), (3) approximately 30 nucleotides of mRNA are involved in the messenger binding site (19), (4) base-pairing is not required (20), and (5) divalent cations are required to neutralize the charge on the phosphate groups of RNA or, possibly, to serve as a bridge between mRNA and the ribosome (21).

D. BIOSYNTHESIS OF VIRAL NUCLEIC ACIDS

In uninfected cells, both RNA and DNA are synthesized on templates composed of DNA. In cells infected with DNA viruses, viral DNA serves as a template for its own replication and for the synthesis of viral specific mRNA. The enzymic synthesis of viral DNA may be catalyzed by either the DNA polymerase of the host cell or of the virus (22). It seems likely that a viral RNA polymerase transcribes viral DNA into viral-specific mRNA (23, 24), but the participation of the analogous enzyme in the host cell has not been excluded (25).

RNA acts as template for its own replication as well as for the synthesis of viral specific proteins in RNA viruses (cf. *26*). A completely new enzyme, variously termed RNA synthetase, replicase or viral polymerase, is required to form progeny RNA from parental RNA (*27*). The enzyme catalyzes the copying of the parental (plus) strand into its complementary (minus) strand, and the synthesis of new plus strands. The replicative form of RNA, which is partly double-stranded and resistant to ribonuclease, is found in the cytoplasm of cells infected with single-stranded RNA viruses (*28*).

Viral RNA polymerase was first isolated and purified from bacteriophage (*29*), and much of our knowledge of the specificity of RNA replication derives from its study. This enzyme can detect differences between the RNA of closely related species of virus (*30*) and catalyzes the net synthesis of biologically intact infectious RNA (*31*). The RNA polymerase of bacteriophage requires homologous RNA as template (*30*) and similar specificity may obtain for the RNA polymerase of animal viruses. Since viral RNA polymerase differs in substrate specificity from the RNA polymerase of the host cell, it presents an ideal target for the design of antiviral drugs.

RNA tumor viruses, including Rous sarcoma, feline leukemia, mammary tumor, and Rauscher murine leukemia, contain a DNA polymerase that uses viral RNA as a template (*31a,b,c*). The discovery of this enzyme activity represents the first report of the biosynthesis of DNA on an RNA template. RNA tumor viruses introduce other unique enzyme activities into the host cell, including a DNA-dependent DNA polymerase, an endonuclease and, possibly, a ligase (*31d,e,f*). The product of the RNA-dependent DNA polymerase is a double-stranded DNA–RNA hybrid, whose DNA strand is complementary to the viral RNA (*31c*). Formation of this hybrid appears to be the first step in the biosynthesis of double-stranded DNA, the second step being catalyzed by the DNA-dependent DNA polymerase. DNA formed by these viral enzymes may be integrated into the host genome, thus accounting for the phenomena of transformation. The endonuclease and ligase found in virus-infected cells may participate in this process.

E. Biosynthesis of Viral Proteins

The mechanism for the biosynthesis of viral coat protein resembles the synthesis of normal cell proteins on polyribosomes (cf. Chapter 5 in this volume). Viral RNA acts as messenger for this synthetic process which requires ribosomes, binding enzyme, peptide synthetase, translocase, and possibly initiation and termination factors derived from the host cell. Some viral messengers are polycistronic and, in the case of bacteriophage, these cistrons are translated in a sequential fashion (*32*). After completion of synthesis, viral proteins are released from the ribosome.

Formation of structural proteins by cleavage of viral polypeptides has been found to occur during replication of poliovirus (*32a,b,c*), other small RNA viruses (*32c*), and certain DNA viruses (*32d*). Such viral polypeptides may arise from a few, or perhaps a single, large polypeptide.

II. Approaches to the Design of Antiviral Agents

Traditional screening procedures test the effects of potential antiviral compounds on virus-infected cells in tissue culture or on experimentally infected animals. When active compounds are detected, structure–activity relationships are established but studies of their mode of action usually follow only as an academic afterthought. An alternative approach to the design of antiviral compounds (*33*) reverses this experimental sequence by (1) first selecting biochemical steps in virus replication that would theoretically be susceptible to drug-induced inhibition; (2) identifying inhibitors for these reactions; (3) determining the structure–activity relationships of related compounds, and (4) using the structural requirements so determined as a chemical basis for the design of additional compounds to be tested for antiviral activity. This approach to rational drug design depends, in large measure, on the judicious selection of the biochemical pathway to be inhibited (*34*). Some aspects of viral replication described in the preceding section will be considered as a basis for the design of antiviral agents.

A. Inhibition of Attachment

The structure of receptors on cell membranes should prove useful in designing inhibitors of virus attachment. The action of neuraminidase on human erythrocytes prevents the attachment of certain myxoviruses, including influenza virus (*35, 36*). Oligosaccharides containing neuraminic acid could be tested for their capacity to inhibit the binding of viruses to cell membranes and the structure of these molecules used as a starting point for the synthesis of chemically defined inhibitors of attachment.

B. Inhibition of Penetration

Adamantadine has been shown to prevent the penetration of certain strains of RNA viruses into animal cells (*37*). Once the virus has penetrated the cell membrane, this drug shows no further effect on viral replication. As the processes of attachment and penetration are highly specific, it is not surprising that adamantadine is effective only against certain viruses (*38*). Some of the clinical trials (cf. *39, 40*) of adamantadine have not been particularly encouraging, and it might be argued that inhibition of penetration is not a profitable lead to the design of antiviral agents. Nevertheless, adamatadine effects a relatively nontoxic selective inhibition of virus replication *in vivo*, and final judgment of the effectiveness of this mode of action should be reserved until chemically unrelated compounds that inhibit by this mechanism have been tested.

The mode of action of adamantadine has recently been reexamined (*70*). These studies suggest that adamantadine inhibits uncoating of virus in the cells and that inhibition of penetration does not seem to play a significant role in the antiviral action of the drug.

C. INHIBITION OF THE BINDING OF mRNA

A strand of viral mRNA binds to the ribosomes of the host cell and serves as template for the synthesis of viral proteins and enzymes. Inhibition of viral mRNA attachment to ribosomes is an attractive mechanism for the design

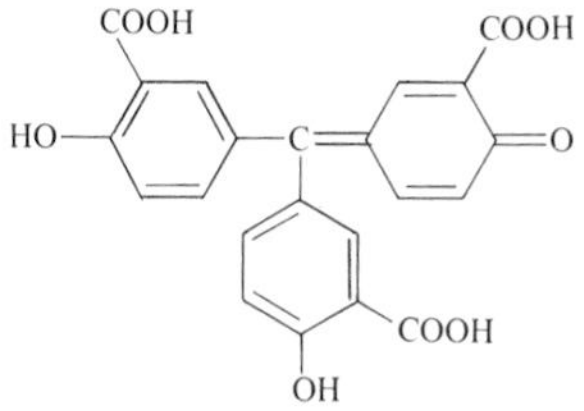

Aurintricarboxylic acid (ATA)

Fig. 2. Structural formula of aurintricarboxylic acid.

of potential antiviral agents if this could be achieved without affecting the analogous process in the host cell. The functional effect of this selective inhibition would be to prevent the initiation of viral protein synthesis without interfering with the translation of mRNA by the host cell. Interferon may act in this manner (*41–43*), and chemical agents with such properties were found by screening organic compounds for their capacity to inhibit protein synthesis in cell-free systems that use bacteriophage RNA as mRNA (*44*). Such preparations allow the observer to compare the effects of inhibitors on protein synthesis directed by endogenous mRNA with that directed by bacteriophage mRNA.

Using extracts prepared from *E. coli*, it was found that aurintricarboxylic acid (ATA) (Fig. 2) and related triphenylmethane dyes were active inhibitors of the initiation of protein synthesis (45, 46). It was also established that ATA was bound to the 30 S subunit of the bacterial ribosome and thus prevented the attachment of bacteriophage RNA (45). If this type of mRNA was allowed to attach to the ribosome before adding the dye, protein synthesis continued, but rebinding of mRNA to free ribosomes was inhibited (44, 44a). Further studies have shown that ATA has identical effects on the binding of mRNA to ribosomes prepared from animal cells (33, 46).

A structure–activity study revealed that the quinoid form of the triphenyl-methane moiety, containing o-salicyl or o-catechol functions in two of the aromatic nuclei and a single carboxylic or sulfonic acid function in the third ring, was required for biological activity. These structural assignments suggest the design of other compounds which act in the same manner.

The preceding observations follow the proposed sequence for drug design described in the initial paragraph of this section. Although ATA and related biologically active dyes do not readily penetrate animal cell membranes, several synthetic methods are available to overcome these problems of drug transport. Acetylation of the polar groups allows penetration of the dye through the cell membrane of cells in suspension culture. These protective groups are subsequently cleaved by intracellular esterases to yield the active compound (47). An alternative approach would superimpose the functional groups required for biological activity on relatively nonpolar structures such as steroids and alkaloids.

D. INDUCERS OF INTERFERON

The biochemistry of interferon, as discussed in recent symposia (48, 49) and reviews (50–52), suggests several possibilities for the rational design of antiviral agents. Progress is being made toward the use of human interferon as a therapeutic agent (cf. 53). Another approach derives from the observation that interferon production is stimulated by virus infection or by the administration of polynucleotides or a variety of chemical compounds. Some of those appear promising, although side effects have been reported (54–56).

Reovirus RNA and the replicative form of RNA isolated from E. coli infected with MS2 coliphage induce resistance to virus infection in vitro and in vivo. As Hilleman and his co-workers have demonstrated (57, 58), the administration of these RNA's stimulates the production of interferon. The broad-spectrum protection against viral infection induced in this way suggested the use of synthetic polynucleotides, including polyriboinosinic–polyribo-cytidylic acid (59), which possess a double-stranded conformation. Chemically modified RNA's (60), and even single-stranded RNA's (61), may also induce the production of interferon. Among polynucleotides, secondary structure appears to be an important determinant of biological activity.

Other chemically defined macromolecular stimulators of interferon production include synthetic polymers derived from ethylene maleic anhydride or polyacrylic acid (62). These anionic copolymers are active *in vivo* in mice against Friend leukemia virus (63) and stimulate the production of interferon in man (64). The structural requirements for the activity of these polymers appear to be a molecular weight of 17,000, or greater, and a saturated aliphatic carbon chain with carboxylated groups in alternate or adjacent positions, on two out of every four or five carbons (65).

The only synthetic compound of low molecular weight that has, so far, been shown to stimulate the production of interferon is tilorone (65a). This agent, effective orally against a broad spectrum of DNA and RNA viruses, suggests that a search for other small molecules that stimulate interferon production may be fruitful.

E. INHIBITION OF VIRAL RNA POLYMERASE

Many organic compounds have been screened for their inhibitory activity against the RNA replicase of bacteriophage Qβ (66). Several of these agents possess the desired specificity, i.e., inhibiting the viral enzyme at concentrations

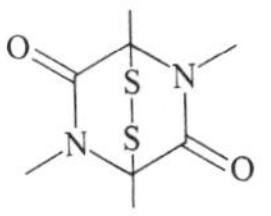

Epidithiapiperazinedione

Fig. 3. Structural formula of the epidithiapiperazinedione nucleus found in gliotoxin and related compounds with antiviral activity.

which do not affect the DNA-dependent RNA polymerase of the host cell (66, 68). In animal cells, gliotoxin (71), acetylaranotin, (LL-s88α) (72), chetomin, and the sporidesmins (73) affect the replication of RNA viruses by inhibiting the synthesis of viral RNA. A simple compound, containing the epidithiapiperazinedione nucleus (Fig. 3), common to all of these compounds, inhibits the multiplication of RNA viruses (75) and could serve as a starting point for chemical modification. Selenocystine (67, 69) and α-amanitin (69a, 69b) have also been reported to be selective inhibitors of influenza virus-induced RNA polymerase.

The preceding group of inhibitors appears to be specific for a protein component of the viral RNA polymerase rather than for the template. This type of interaction is more likely to result in selective inhibition of the viral enzyme, considering the lack of specificity of antibiotics which interact with DNA. The viral RNA polymerase, itself, is clearly different from the enzyme in the host cell.

An interesting approach for subverting the specificity of viral RNA polymerase has been suggested by the experiments of Spiegelman and his associates (76). They have demonstrated that the RNA of mutant bacteriophage are replicated more rapidly than the wild type (77). By superinfecting with appropriately chosen defective mutants, it is possible to "cure" a cell infected with bacteriophage since these mutants replicate but fail to produce viable progeny. A similar approach is theoretically feasible in the therapy of infections caused by animal viruses.

F. Inhibition of Viral Nucleic Acid Synthesis

Halogenated nucleosides, such as bromodeoxyuridine, are effective inhibitors of viral replication by virtue of their incorporation into viral nucleic acid (cf. 78). Other nucleoside analogs, such as cytosine arabinoside (ara C) (79, 80), inhibit the same process but are incorporated only to a limited extent. All of these agents inhibit nucleic acid metabolism in the host cell and must depend on kinetic differences or species specificity between the virus and the host cell for selective toxicity (81). If virus-specific nucleic acids (82) were ultimately discovered, analogs of these molecules would offer a better approach to the design of antiviral agents since they should prove more selective than analogs of common nucleosides. The antiviral agents isatin-β-thiosemi-carbazone (IBT) (83, 84), hydroxybenzylbenzimidazole (HBB) (85) and guanidine (86) appear to interfere selectively with some phase of viral nucleic acid synthesis, but their mechanism of action has not been established precisely.

The RNA-dependent DNA polymerase of RNA tumor viruses and other enzymes involved in viral DNA synthesis represent potential sites of action for antiviral compounds (provided that similar enzymes are not subsequently discovered in uninfected cells). Indeed, inhibition of replication of these viruses by actinomycin was an important early clue to the existence of DNA-dependent DNA polymerase (86a). Drugs, such as actinomycin, that inhibit virus replication by virtue of interacting with DNA templates would be of less practical value than those which might interact with viral RNA in a specific manner. Even greater specificity might be found in compounds that inhibit enzyme activity by virtue of an interaction with the protein component of the enzyme. N-Demethylrifampicin may be such a compound (100).

Transformed cells have the capacity to revert to normal; furthermore, there are mutant strains of RNA tumor viruses that do not cause transformation (86b). These findings imply that continued expression of viral genes is necessary to maintain the transformed state, suggesting that antiviral agents might prevent malignant transformation of the host cell. This property would assume additional importance if the product of the viral gene responsible for transforming a normal cell were present in a covert (inactive) form. It has been suggested that viruses in such a state can be activated by carcinogens, irradiation or even the normal aging process (86c). Thus, drugs that interfere with the expression of viral information might prove prophylactic against a number of forms of viral-induced cancer. After integration of the viral genome into the nucleic acid of the host cell, chemotherapy by any mechanism may well prove ineffective.

G. INHIBITION OF PROTEIN SYNTHESIS

Inhibitors of protein synthesis in animal cells, such as emetine (87, 88) and anisomycin (89), have been shown to manifest antiviral activity in cell culture and in experimental animals (90). The function of enzymes utilized by the virus in synthesizing viral protein are inhibited by the administration of the drugs. The effects on protein synthesis are their only known direct mode of action, and it is presumed that the antiviral effect of those compounds is mediated by the same mechanism. Although the demonstrated activity indicates that selective antiviral effects can be obtained *in vivo*, protein synthesis in the host cell is affected by the concentration of drug required to inhibit virus replication. Accordingly, their therapeutic use may be associated with considerable toxicity.

Certain viral proteins, including structural peptides formed from high molecular weight precursors, are formed at a relatively late stage in the replicative process. The synthesis of these proteins is prevented by inhibitors of protein synthesis and, possibly, by rifampicin. Rifampicin inhibits the increase of particulate RNA polymerase activity in cells infected with vaccinia virus (90a), as well as the synthesis of a polypeptide required for the formation of viral cores (32d). Rifampicin treatment results in a failure of virus assembly (*viz. infra*), manifested by an accumulation of incomplete viral envelopes (90b). Rifampicin and the structurally related streptovaricins (90c) have significant antiviral activity at concentrations which do not apparently affect host-cell metabolism. Thus, this selective inhibitory mechanism seems preferable to the nonspecific inhibition of protein synthesis. Antiviral activity of rifampicin has been attributed to the hydrazone side chain of the antibiotic (90d).

H. INHIBITION OF tRNA FUNCTION

Bacteriophage infection is associated with changes in tRNA (91). The biochemistry of tRNA could be exploited for antiviral therapy if it proves to be essential for the translation of viral mRNA and not of host mRNA in animal cells. For example, several unusual "minor" bases occur in tRNA (92). Most of these are synthesized by secondary modification of bases previously incorporated into a polynucleotide strand. Since the minor bases are critical for the function of certain tRNA's, it is possible that a new type of drug might be developed which interferes selectively with the enzymes responsible for their synthesis, thus modifying the function of the tRNA.

I. INHIBITION OF VIRUS ASSEMBLY AND RELEASE

It has been suggested that it is possible to inhibit the assembly of viral subunits into mature virus in the intact cell. Low doses of p-fluorophenyl-alanine, an analog of phenylalanine, inhibit the assembly of poliovirus (93) and adenovirus (94). Recent observations with quinomycin A (95) have shown that it inhibits the multiplication of phage T_2 progency without interfering measurably with the synthesis of phage DNA, RNA, or protein. In addition, if an enzyme were required for the assembly of viral subunits (96), this would provide a specific step the inhibition of which would prevent the production of mature virus.

The neuraminidase found on the surface of myxoviruses is thought to facilitate their release from the host cell (97, 98). Specific inhibitors of this enzyme have been sought, and a number of substituted dihydroisoquinolines were found to have a direct inactivating effect on the influenza virus particle (99).

III. Conclusions

Despite wide interest in the chemotherapy of viral diseases, no effective broad-spectrum antiviral drug has been discovered by empirical screening procedures. A rational approach to the design of antiviral agents depends on a judicious selection of biochemical pathways that are susceptible to the effects of chemical agents. The most apparent mechanisms are those which are specific for virus replication and are not required for host-cell metabolism. Elucidation of the mode of action of the available antiviral agents and recent advances in the molecular biology of virus replication suggest susceptible mechanisms to be exploited in the search for new antiviral drugs.

ACKNOWLEDGMENTS

The preparation of this chapter and some of the experimental studies described herein were supported by Public Health Service Research Grant No. CA-10666 from the National Cancer Institute. We are grateful to Dr. Marshall Horwitz and Dr. Donald Summers for critically reviewing the manuscript.

REFERENCES

1. L. C. McLaren, J. J. Holland, and J. T. Syverton, *J. Exp. Med.* **109**, 475 (1959).
2. J. J. Holland, *Virology* **15**, 312 (1961).
3. W. K. Joklik, *J. Mol. Biol.* **8**, 277 (1964).
4. B. Woodson, *Bacteriol. Rev.* **32**, 127 (1968).
5. J. J. Holland, L. C. McLaren, and J. T. Syverton, *J. Exp. Med.* **110**, 65 (1959).
6. P. DeSomer, A. Prinzie, and E. Schonne, *Nature (London)* **184**, 652 (1959).
7. I. M. Mountain and H. E. Alexander, *Fed. Proc., Fed. Amer. Soc. Exp. Biol.* **18**, 587 (1959).
8. J. J. Holland and B. H. Hoyer, *Cold Spring Harbor Symp. Quant. Biol.* **27**, 101 (1962).
9. L. Philipson and S. Bengtsson, *Virology* **18**, 457 (1962).
10. E. F. Zimmerman, M. Heeter, and J. E. Darnell, *Virology* **19**, 400 (1963).
11. S. Penman and D. Summers, *Virology* **27**, 614 (1965).
12. Y. Becker and W. K. Joklik, *Proc. Nat. Acad. Sci. U.S.* **51**, 577 (1964).
13. C. Jungwirth and W. K. Joklik, *Virology* **27**, 80 (1965).
14. B. R. McAuslan, *Biochem. Biophys. Res. Commun.* **19**, 15 (1965).
15. S. Kit and D. R. Dubbs, *Virology* **26**, 16 (1965).
16. B. R. McAuslan, *Virology* **21**, 383 (1963).
17. B. R. McAuslan, *Virology* **20**, 162 (1963).
18. M. Revel, M. Herzberg, A. Becarevic, and F. Gross, *J. Mol. Biol.* **33**, 231 (1968).
19. M. Takanami, Y. Yan, and T. H. Jukes, *J. Mol. Biol.* **12**, 761 (1965).
20. P. B. Moore, *J. Mol. Biol.* **22**, 21 (1966).
21. J. D. Watson, *Bull. Soc. Chim. Biol.* **46**, 1399 (1964).
22. M. Green, *Cold Spring Harbor Symp. Quant. Biol.* **27**, 219 (1962).
23. J. R. Kates and B. R. McAuslan, *Proc. Nat. Acad. Sci. U.S.* **57**, 314 (1967).
24. J. R. Kates and B. R. McAuslan, *Proc. Nat. Acad. Sci. U.S.* **58**, 134 (1967).
25. H. S. Ginsberg, L. J. Bello, and A. J. Levine, *in* "The Molecular Biology of Viruses" (J. S. Colter and W. Paranchych, eds.), p. 547. Academic Press, New York, 1967.
26. P. H. Höfschneider and P. Häusen, *in* "Molecular Basis of Virology" (H. Fraenkel-Conrat, ed.), p. 169. Reinhold, New York, 1968.
27. D. Baltimore, H. J. Eggers, R. M. Franklin, and I. Tamm, *Proc. Nat. Acad. Sci. U.S.* **49**, 843 (1963).
28. D. Baltimore, *Proc. Nat. Acad. Sci. U.S.* **51**, 450 (1964).
29. I. Haruna, K. Nozu, Y. Ohtaka, and S. Spiegelman, *Proc. Nat. Acad. Sci. U.S.* **50**, 905 (1963).
30. I. Haruna and S. Spiegelman, *Proc. Nat. Acad. Sci. U.S.* **54**, 579 (1965).
31. S. Spiegelman, I. Haruna, I. B. Holland, G. Beaudreau, and D. Mills, *Proc. Nat. Acad. Sci. U.S.* **54**, 919 (1965).
31a. G. M. Temin and S. Mizutani, *Nature* **226**, 1211 (1970).
31b. D. Baltimore, *Nature* **226**, 1209 (1970).
31c. S. Spiegelman, A. Burny, M. R. Das, J. Keydar, J. Schlom, M. Travnicek, and K. Watson, *Nature* **228**, 430 (1970).
31d. S. Mizutani, D. Boettiger, and H. M. Temin, *Nature* **228**, 424 (1970).
31e. J. Riman and G. S. Beaudreau, *Nature* **228**, 427 (1970).
31f. S. Spiegelman, A. Burny, M. R. Das, J. Keydar, J. Schlom, M. Travnicek, and K. Watson, *Nature* **227**, 1029 (1970).
32. K. Eggen and D. Nathans, *J. Mol. Biol.* **39**, 293 (1969).

32a. M. F. Jacobson and D. Baltimore, *J. Mol. Biol.* **33**, 369 (1968).
32b. D. F. Summers and J. V. Maizel, Jr., *Proc. Nat. Acad. Sci. U.S.* **59**, 966 (1968).
32c. J. J. Holland and E. D. Kiehn, *Proc. Nat. Acad. Sci. U.S.* **60**, 1015 (1968).
32d. E. Katz and B. Moss, *Proc. Nat. Acad. Sci. U.S.* **66**, 677 (1970).
33. A. P. Grollman, *Antimicrob. Ag. Chemother 1968.* p. 36 (1969).
34. A. P. Grollman, *Annu. Rep. Med. Chem.* p. 218 (1969).
35. G. K. Hirst, *in* "Viral and Rickettsial Diseases of Man" (F. L. Horsfall and I. Tamm, eds.), p. 216. Lippincott, Philadelphia, Pennsylvania, 1965.
36. P. I. Marcus, *Bacteriol. Rev.* **23**, 232 (1959).
37. F. J. Stanfield, R. F. Haff, and R. C. Stewart, *Bacteriol. Proc.* p. 114 (1966).
38. E. M. Neumayer, R. F. Haff, and C. E. Hoffmann, *Proc. Soc. Exp. Biol. Med.* **119**, 393 (1965).
39. H. A. Wendel, M. T. Snyder, and S. Pell, *Clin. Pharmacol. Ther.* **7**, 38 (1966).
40. A. A. Smorodintsev, G. I. Karpuchin, A. M. Malysheva, E. G. Shvetsova, S. A. Burov, L. M. Chramtsova, D. M. Zlydnikov, S. A. Romanov, L. Yu. Taros, Yu. G. Ivannikov, and S. D. Novoselov, *Ann. N.Y. Acad. Sci.* **173**, 44 (1970).
41. W. K. Joklik and T. C. Merigan, *Proc. Nat. Acad. Sci. U.S.* **56**, 558 (1966).
42. H. B. Levy and W. A. Carter, *J. Mol. Biol.* **31**, 561 (1968).
43. P. I. Marcus and J. M. Salb, *Virology* **30**, 502 (1966).
44. A. P. Grollman and M. L. Stewart, *Proc. Nat. Acad. Sci. U.S.* **61**, 719 (1968).
44a. R. E. Webster and N. D. Zinder, *J. Mol. Biol.* **42**, 425 (1969).
45. A. P. Grollman and M. L. Stewart, *Fed. Proc., Fed. Amer. Soc. Exp. Biol.* **28**, 725 (1969).
46. M. L. Stewart, A. P. Grollman, and M. T. Huang, *Proc. Nat. Acad. Sci. U.S.* **68**, 97 (1971).
47. B. Rotman and B. W. Papermaster, *Proc. Nat. Acad. Sci. U.S.* **55**, 134 (1965).
48. G. Rita, ed., "The Interferons." Academic Press, New York, 1968.
49. "Interferon," *J. Gen. Physiol.* **56**, Suppl. (1970).
50. M. S. Finkelstein and T. C. Merigan, *Calif. Med.* **109**, 24 (1968).
51. M. R. Hilleman, *J. Cell. Physiol.* **71**, 43 (1968).
52. C. E. Hoffmann, *Annu. Rep. Med. Chem.* p. 117 (1969).
53. A. J. Beale, *Ann. N.Y. Acad. Sci.* **173**, 770 (1970).
54. M. Absher and W. R. Stinebring, *Nature (London)* **223**, 715 (1969).
55. H. L. Lindsay, P. W. Trown, J. Brandt, and M. Forbes, *Nature (London)* **223**, 717 (1969).
56. R. H. Adamson and S. Fabro, *Nature (London)* **223**, 718 (1969).
57. A. A. Tytell, G. P. Lampson, A. K. Field, and M. R. Hilleman, *Proc. Nat. Acad. Sci. U.S.* **58**, 1719 (1967).
58. A. K. Field, G. P. Lampson, A. A. Tytell, M. M. Nemes, and M. R. Hilleman, *Proc. Nat. Acad. Sci. U.S.* **58**, 2102 (1967).
59. A. K. Field, A. A. Tytell, G. P. Lampson, and M. R. Hilleman, *Proc. Nat. Acad. Sci. U.S.* **61**, 340 (1968).
60. J. P. Ebel, J. H. Weil, G. Beck, C. Bollack, L. Colobert, and P. Louisot, *Biochem. Biophys. Res. Commun.* **30**, 148 (1968).
61. S. Baron, N. N. Bogomolova, A. Billian, H. B. Levy, C. E. Buckler, R. Stern, and R. Naylor, *Proc. Nat. Acad. Sci. U.S.* **64**, 67 (1969).
62. T. C. Merigan, *Nature (London)* **214**, 416 (1967).
63. W. Regelson, *Advan. Chemother.* **3**, 303 (1968).
64. T. C. Merigan and W. Regelson, *N. Engl. J. Med.* **277**, 1283 (1967).
65. T. C. Merigan, *in* "Ciba Foundation Symposium on Interferon" (G. E. W. Wolstenholme and M. O'Connor, eds.), p. 50. Little, Brown, Boston, Massachusetts, 1967.
65a. G. D. Mayer and R. F. Krueger, *Science* **169**, 1214 (1970).

66. I. Watanabe, I. Haruna, Y. Yamada, K. Nagaoka, and S. Seki, *Proc. Jap. Acad.* **44**, 1038 (1968).
67. P. P. K. Ho, C. P. Walters, F. Streightoff, L. A. Baker, and D. C. DeLong, *Antimicrob. Ag. Chemother. 1967*, p. 636 (1968).
68. I. Haruna, I. Watanabe, Y. Hamada, and K. Nogoaka, *Ann. N.Y. Acad. Sci.* **173**, 404 (1970).
69. P. P. K. Ho and C. P. Walters, *Ann. N.Y. Acad. Sci.* **173**, 438 (1970).
69a. Th. Wieland, *Science* **159**, 946 (1968).
69b. R. Rott and C. Scholtissek, *Nature (London)* **228**, 56 (1970).
70. N. Kato and H. J. Eggers, *Virology* **37**, 632 (1969).
71. P. A. Miller, K. P. Milstrey, and P. W. Trown, *Science* **159**, 431 (1968).
72. P. W. Trown, H. F. Lindh, K. P. Milstrey, V. M. Gallo, B. R. Mayberry, H. L. Lindsay, and P. A. Miller, *Antimicrob. Ag. Chemother. 1968*, p. 225 (1969).
73. A. Taylor, *in* "Biochemistry of Some Foodborne Microbial Toxins" (R. I. Mateles and G. N. Wogan, eds.), p. 69. M.I.T. Press, Cambridge, Massachusetts, 1967.
74. D. Brewer, D. E. Hannah, and A. Taylor, *Can. J. Microbiol.* **12**, 1187 (1966).
75. P. W. Trown, *Biochem. Biophys. Res. Commun.* **33**, 402 (1968).
76. S. J. Spiegelman, *Harvey Lect.* **64**, 1 (1969).
77. D. R. Mills, R. L. Peterson, and S. Spiegelman, *Proc. Nat. Acad. Sci. U.S.* **58**, 217 (1967).
78. W. H. Prusoff, *Pharmacol. Rev.* **19**, 209 (1967).
79. S. S. Cohen, *Progr. Nucl. Acid. Res. Mol. Biol.* **5**, 1 (1966).
80. C. G. Smith, *in* "The Control of Growth Processes by Chemical Agents" (A. D. Welch, ed.), p. 33. Pergamon Press, Oxford, 1968.
81. A. S. Kaplan and T. Ben-Porat, *Ann. N.Y. Acad. Sci.* **173**, 346 (1970).
82. L. V. Crawford, *Advan. Virus Res.* **14**, 89 (1969).
83. D. J. Bauer, *Ann. N.Y. Acad. Sci.* **130**, 110 (1965).
84. B. Woodson and W. K. Joklik, *Proc. Nat. Acad. Sci. U.S.* **54**, 946 (1965).
85. H. J. Eggers and I. Tamm, *J. Exp. Med.* **113**, 657 (1961).
86. D. Crowther and J. Melnick, *Virology* **15**, 65 (1961).
86a. H. M. Temin, *Nat. Cancer Inst. Monog.* **17**, 557 (1964).
86b. G. S. Martin, *Nature* **227**, 1021 (1970).
86c. R. J. Huebner and G. T. Todaro, *Proc. Nat. Acad. Sci. U.S.* **64**, 1087 (1969).
87. A. P. Grollman, *Proc. Nat. Acad. Sci. U.S.* **56**, 1867 (1966).
88. A. P. Grollman, *J. Biol. Chem.* **243**, 4089 (1968).
89. A. P. Grollman, *J. Biol. Chem.* **242**, 3226 (1967).
90. E. Grunberg and H. N. Prince, *Antimicrob. Ag. Chemother. 1966*, p. 257 (1967).
90a. B. R. McAuslan, *Biochem. Biophys. Res. Commun.* **37**, 289 (1969).
90b. P. M. Grimley, E. N. Rosenblum, S. J. Mims, and B. Moss, *J. Virol.* **6**, 519 (1970).
90c. N. A. Quintrell and B. R. McAuslan, *J. Virol.* **6**, 485 (1970).
90d. Z. Zakay-Rones and Y. Becker, *Nature* **226**, 1162 (1970).
91. N. Sueoka, T. Kano-Sueoka, and W. J. Gartland, *Cold Spring Harbor Symp. Quant. Biol.* **31**, 571 (1966).
92. K. Miura, *Progr. Nucl. Acid. Res. Mol. Biol.* **6**, 39 (1967).
93. M. D. Scharff, D. F. Summers, and L. Levintow, *Ann. N.Y. Acad. Sci.* **130**, 282 (1965).
94. M. S. Horwitz and M. D. Scharff, *Abstr. Soc. Pediat. Res.*, p. 99 (April, 1969).
95. K. Sato, Y. Niinomi, K. Katagiri, A. Matsukage, and T. Minagawa, *Biochim. Biophys. Acta* **174**, 230 (1969).
96. W. B. Wood, R. S. Edgar, J. King, I. Lielausis, and M. Henninger, *Fed. Proc., Fed. Amer. Soc. Exp. Biol.* **27**, 1160 (1968).

97. B. L. Padgett and D. L. Walker, *J. Bacteriol.* **87**, 363 (1964).
98. W. W. Ackermann and H. F. Maassab, *J. Exp. Med.* **100**, 329 (1954).
99. J. D. Coombes, K. W. Brammer, N. M. Larin, C. R. McDonald, M. S. Tute, and G. M. Williamson, *Ann. N.Y. Acad. Sci.* **173**, 462 (1970).
100. G. Smith, S. Yang, F. Herrera, J. Whang-Peng, and R. Gallo, *J. Clin. Invest.* **50**, 86a (1971).

Chapter 8　Design of Penicillins

A. E. Bird and J. H. C. Nayler

I. Introduction

For almost twenty years following Sir Alexander Fleming's historic observation of their antibacterial properties penicillins were obtainable only by culturing a suitable mold on a nutrient medium and extracting the antibiotic so produced. In this way, a small number of penicillins (**I**) containing different side chains (R in **I**) were characterized, but it was not until the later 1940's that means were found of preparing certain penicillins containing R groups not found in nature. These novel penicillins were obtained by adding carboxylic acids RCO_2H, or related structures, to the fermentation brew, whereupon in favorable instances the "precursor" was utilized by the mold and its acyl radical incorporated into the side chain of a new penicillin. The scope of this procedure proved to be strictly limited, only certain types of monosubstituted acetic acids being acceptable to the mold, but it nevertheless represented the first possibility of deliberately designing a new penicillin.

$$ \underset{\text{I}}{\begin{array}{c} \text{RCONHCH—HC} \overset{S}{\diagup}\diagdown \text{CMe}_2 \\ | \qquad\qquad | \qquad\quad | \\ \text{CO——N——CHCOOH} \end{array}} \qquad \underset{\text{II}}{\begin{array}{c} \text{H}_2\text{NCH—HC} \overset{S}{\diagup}\diagdown \text{CMe}_2 \\ | \qquad\quad | \qquad\quad | \\ \text{CO——N——CHCOOH} \end{array}} $$

Another early approach to new penicillins involved the preparation by fermentation, either with or without a side chain precursor, of a penicillin containing a reactive functional group in its side chain which could then be further modified by chemical means. However, only a few penicillins were amenable to such treatment, while the majority had chemically inert side chains which could not be expected to undergo chemical reactions under conditions which the sensitive nucleus (i.e., the fused β-lactam–thiazolidine ring system) would withstand.

Penicillins containing a wider variety of R groups were, of course, potentially accessible by total chemical synthesis, but in practice this proved unexpectedly difficult. A total synthesis was reported by Sheehan and Henery-Logan (*98a*) in 1957 but it was lengthy and inefficient, and consequently only a very few penicillins have been prepared in this way.

The advance which finally made possible the preparation of large numbers of penicillins with many different side chains was made in the Beecham Laboratories in 1957 (*7*). It stemmed from the observation that cultures of *Penicillium chrysogenum* grown in the absence of side chain precursor produced, in addition to the expected low yield of "natural" penicillins, a further β-lactam-containing substance which had previously escaped notice because of its virtual lack of antibiotic activity. The new substance proved to be 6-aminopenicillanic acid (**II**), conveniently abbreviated to 6-APA. Soon afterward a second and still more convenient route to 6-APA was developed, namely the enzymic removal of the acyl side chain of benzylpenicillin or other penicillin produced by fermentation. The great value of 6-APA lies in the fact that its amino group may be acylated by chemical means to introduce an unlimited number and variety of side chain structures. In the last ten years thousands of such "semisynthetic" penicillins have been produced all over the world. The structures and approved names of the currently available marketed penicillins are given in Table I. All of these, except penicillins G and V, are made by acylation of 6-APA.

For a general account of the chemistry of 6-APA and the penicillins the reader is referred to a review by Doyle and Nayler (*31*) which covers the literature up to 1963, while an admirable survey of the therapeutic aspects has been produced by Lynn (*70*).

The present review treats the subject in a more specialized way. It is concerned with the relationship of structure to biological properties, and the use or potential use of such relationships in the design of clinically effective penicillins. Since the biological properties of any substance must of necessity be a consequence of its chemical and physicochemical characteristics a brief account of the latter is appropriate.

The most important chemical properties of penicillins result from the great reactivity of the strained amide bond in the fused β-lactam of the nucleus. Thus penicillins are slowly hydrolyzed to the biologically inactive penicilloic acids (**III**), hydrolysis being catalyzed by heavy metal salts, acids, and particularly by bases. Simple opening of the β-lactam ring is also brought about by other nucleophiles; for example, reaction with ammonia or primary amines gives monoamides of penicilloic acids. Another important degradation of penicillins occurs in acid solution and results in complex structural rearrangements involving the side chain amide group as well as the β-lactam ring.

$$
\begin{array}{cc}
\text{RCONHCH—HC}^{\diagup S\diagdown}\text{CMe}_2 & \text{PhCHCONHCH—HC}^{\diagup S\diagdown}\text{CMe}_2 \\
\quad\;|\qquad\qquad\quad| & \qquad|\qquad\qquad\qquad\quad| \\
\text{CO}_2\text{H} \;\; \text{NH—CHCOOH} & \text{NH}_3^+ \quad\;\; \text{CO—N—CHCOO}^- \\
\textbf{III} & \textbf{IV}
\end{array}
$$

Since the various penicillins differ only with respect to the nature of the side chain, which is remote from the carboxyl group, they would not be expected to differ significantly in acid strength. Measurement in fact shows that all penicillins are relatively strong acids with pK_a values of 2.65 ± 0.1 (*54a, 85*). When the side chain contains a basic group the molecule tends to exist as a zwitterion, as exemplified by ampicillin (**IV**) which has a pK_a of 7.24 for the amino group. For therapeutic purposes most penicillins are administered as sodium, potassium, or other salts which are usually freely soluble in water and sparingly soluble in organic solvents. By contrast the free acids tend to be readily soluble in organic solvents and sparingly soluble in water.

The penicillin structure (**I**) contains three asymmetric centers and hence is theoretically capable of existing in eight optically active forms. In practice however, penicillins are derived, directly or indirectly, from natural sources

TABLE I

STRUCTURES AND APPROVED NAMES OF COMMERCIALLY
AVAILABLE PENICILLINS

Approved name	Side chain structure	
	R in **I**	Stereochemistry
Benzylpenicillin (penicillin G)	PhCH$_2$—	—
Phenoxymethylpenicillin (penicillin V)	PhOCH$_2$—	—
Phenethicillin	PhOCH— | Me	Mixed epimers
Propicillin	PhOCH— | Et	Mixed epimers
Phenbenicillin	PhOCH— | Ph	Mixed epimers
Methicillin	[benzene ring with OMe, OMe substituents]	—
Nafcillin	[naphthalene ring with OEt substituent]	—
Oxacillin	[isoxazole ring: Ph, Me]	—
Cloxacillin	[chlorophenyl isoxazole ring: Cl, Me]	—
Dicloxacillin	[dichlorophenyl isoxazole ring: Cl, Cl, Me]	—
Ampicillin	PhCH— | NH$_2$	D
Carbenicillin	PhCH— | COOH	Mixed epimers

and represent only one of the eight possible structures. The natural isomer has the stereochemistry shown in **V**, and there is no reason to suppose that any other isomer would be biologically active. On the other hand, some penicillins contain one or more additional asymmetric centers in the side chain, a case in point being ampicillin (**IV**). Penicillins with the nucleus as in **V** but with different stereochemistry in the side chain are all biologically active, but not necessarily to the same degree.

V

Attempts to relate the chemical structure of molecules to their biological effects may be either qualitative or quantitative. In practice the approach used to develop new penicillins, as with most other drugs, has been largely qualitative. Thus, many different side chains have been introduced, initially in rather random fashion, and the products examined for useful properties. When desirable properties were observed in a particular structure further analogs of that structure were prepared and examined. Ideas of structure–activity relationships were thus developed on semiempirical lines, and these served as a guide in planning the synthesis of further analogs. In some cases, and particularly when stereochemical considerations are dominant, there is at present no convenient way of expressing such relationships in quantitative terms. On the other hand, when charge distribution and lipid–water partition are important, it is possible to make use of substituent constants which can be handled mathematically. This approach has been extensively developed by Hansch and his co-workers in the past seven years (*44, 45, 45a*). Partition coefficients, which reflect the ability of compounds to pass through lipid membranes or to form noncovalent hydrophobic bonds, are used to define a new substituent constant, $\pi = \log(P_X/P_H)$, where P_X is the partition coefficient of a derivative and P_H is that of a parent compound. In the model system used by Hansch the partition coefficients are measured between *n*-octanol and water. The π or $\log P$ values may be used with other substituent constants, such as the Hammett and Taft σ or E_s values, in multiparameter regression analysis, to obtain equations relating biological effect to the physical properties of the compounds. Application of this procedure is helped by the discovery that many π or $\log P$ values can be calculated from a few measured values, because of the additive nature of the constants.

The introduction of this type of quantitative treatment has probably come too late to have a major influence in the design of semisynthetic penicillins.

However, it is interesting to attempt to rationalize measurements of anti-bacterial activity and serum binding in this way, and some results are described in Sections II,A and II,C. In this work we have relied almost entirely on calculation of π values for the penicillin side chain (R in **I**) from Hansch's published π values, with penicillin itself (**I**, R = H) being regarded as the parent of the series. Examples of the calculation of side chain π values are given by Bird and Marshall (*13*). Subsequent to acceptance of that paper for publication, Hansch and Anderson published (*46*) a new set of π values for substituents in aliphatic compounds. These values are more appropriate for calculation of the side chain π values of penicillins without an aromatic ring than are the earlier values (*55*) derived from measurements on *n*-propyl-benzene and its ω-substituted derivatives. Consequently, these later π values (*46*) were used where appropriate to calculate the side chain π values used in the work reported here. Also an inadvertent error in several of the values used in reference *13* was corrected by deduction of 0.2 π unit for a tertiary carbon and 0.32 π unit for a quaternary carbon (*49*).

In addition to this quantitative treatment of antibacterial activity and serum binding, we give a qualitative description of the relationship of side chain structure to hydrolysis by β-lactamase and to various properties which affect the behavior of penicillins *in vivo*.

II. Effect of Penicillins on Bacteria

A. CORRELATIONS OF STRUCTURE WITH MIC VALUES

It is noteworthy that nearly all of the thousands of penicillins which have been made since 6-APA became available show significant antibiotic activity. Retention of activity while varying a structural feature within such wide limits is unusual, and obviously indicates the great importance of the nucleus in the antibiotic properties of penicillins. This is further emphasized by the complete or near complete loss of activity which often occurs when the nucleus is chemically modified (*31, 83*). However, the minimum inhibitory concentra-tions (MIC's) and the spectrum of activity often show marked changes when the side chain structure is altered. Until quite recently attempts to correlate these changes with side chain structure were of a qualitative rather than a quantitative nature, and the basis for them was purely empirical. Thus it was soon found that most penicillins, irrespective of the nature of the side chain, have considerable activity against most Gram-positive cocci. The chief exception to this generalization is the resistance of β-lactamase producing strains of staphylococci to many penicillins. This is a special phenomenon which is considered in detail in Section II,B. Since good activity against sensitive Gram-positive organisms is widespread, the selection of new compounds for clinical use in this area has tended in recent years to be governed more by factors such as suitability for oral administration.

Good activity against Gram-negative bacteria is much less common among penicillins and when it does occur it is usually found that only certain organisms are susceptible. Penicillins with useful activity against some Gram-negative bacteria often have rather simple side chains such as a straight alkyl chain of up to about 6 carbon atoms, an alkylthioalkyl chain of similar size, a benzyl group, or its heterocyclic equivalents such as pyridylmethyl or thienylmethyl. Introduction of hydrophobic substituents such as alkyl or halogen into the α-position of the side chain markedly reduces activity against Gram-negative organisms. Conversely, hydrophilic α-substituents such as amino, hydroxy, or carboxy may enhance activity against such organisms.

The first major impact of these findings on clinical chemotherapy was the introduction of D-α-aminobenzylpenicillin (ampicillin) as a broad spectrum antibiotic effective against many strains of *E. coli*, *Salmonella*, *Proteus*, *Shigella*, and *Haemophilus* as well as the Gram-positive streptococci and staphylococci. The D-configuration of the side chain in ampicillin is important because the L-epimer is markedly less active against the Gram-negative organisms. A similar difference occurs between the epimers of α-hydroxybenzylpenicillin, which is intermediate between benzylpenicillin and ampicillin in broad spectrum activity. A relatively recent development in the field of broad spectrum penicillins is the introduction of α-carboxybenzylpenicillin (carbenicillin). This compound retains the activity of ampicillin except that it is rather less active against Gram-positive bacteria, and has the additional advantage of useful activity against *Pseudomonas* and certain strains of *Proteus* which were resistant to all previously known penicillins as well as to many other antibiotics.

The above findings are summarized in Table II, which also indicates the magnitude of the various activities. In particular these figures show how a typical Gram-positive organism such as *Staphylococcus aureus* is much more sensitive to penicillins in general than are Gram-negative bacteria.

Some attempts have been made at a more quantitative rationalization of MIC's for certain penicillins using the π/σ regression analysis technique outlined in Section I. Hansch and his co-workers (*47, 48*) applied the method to the MIC values of two sets of penicillins with side chain structures **VI** and **VII**. Regression of the MIC's against two strains of *Staphylococcus aureus* for set **VI** gave poor results for the MIC's measured in the absence of serum, but good results for those measured in the presence of serum. The difference between MIC's in the presence and absence of serum is due to the binding of the penicillin to serum protein, and the better correlation with π

TABLE II

ACTIVITY OF SOME REPRESENTATIVE PENICILLINS
AGAINST VARIOUS BACTERIA *in Vitro*

Side chain (R in **I**)	Minimum inhibitory concentration (μg/ml)			
	S. aureus Oxford	*E. coli*	*S. typhi*	*Ps. aeruginosa*
H	1	20	10	>400
CH_3CH_2	0.12	13	7	>200
$CH_3(CH_2)_4$	0.008	36	4	>200
$CH_3(CH_2)_8$	<0.004	170	80	>200
$CH_3CH_2SCH_2$	0.02	12	12	>400
$PhOCH_2$	0.02	140	63	>200
$PhCH_2$	0.01	35	1.8	>500
PhCH— (DL) $\mid$ Cl	0.02	125	25	>500
PhCH— (DL) $\mid$ Me	0.04	100	20	>400
PhCH— (D) $\mid$ NH_2	0.05	4	0.4	>200
PhCH— (L) $\mid$ NH_2	0.1	12	2.5	>200
PhCH— (D) $\mid$ OH	0.04	4	1	>400
PhCH— (L) $\mid$ OH	0.1	20	4	>400
PhCH— (DL) $\mid$ COOH	1.25	5	5	50
Ph	0.1	>200	180	>200
(2,6-dimethoxyphenyl, OMe / OMe)	0.5	>200	500	>200

CH$_3$(CH$_2$)$_n$CH—
           |
           O

[structure VI: benzene ring with —X substituent]

VI

[structure VII: benzene ring with OX$_1$ top, OX$_1$ bottom, X$_2$ left]

OX$_1$

X$_2$

OX$_1$

VII

that was found for the MIC in the presence of serum appears to reflect the good correlation that exists between π and the extent of serum binding (see Section III,C). MIC values measured in serum were the only ones available for set **VII** and these also gave a good correlation with π. In our work described below we are solely concerned with MIC's measured in the absence of serum.

We have applied regression analysis to the MIC values of three sets of penicillins with structurally related side chains (see Table III). Their MIC's against four organisms, two Gram-negative (*Escherichia coli* and *Salmonella typhi*) and two Gram-positive (*Streptococcus faecalis* and a nonpenicillinase-producing strain of *Staphylococcus aureus*) were used. The regression analysis was carried out using the Hansch equation, Eq. (1), as the mathematical model, and with simpler equations obtained from Eq. (1) by omission of one or more terms. In Eq. (1),

$$\log(1/C) = A\pi^2 + B\pi + Cx + D \tag{1}$$

C is the MIC in mmoles/liter, π and x apply to the penicillin side chain and x is either the Hammett σ value or the Taft σ^* or E_s value. A, B, C, and D are the regression coefficients. The validity of the equations was tested statistically by consideration of the correlation coefficient, r, the residual variance, s^2, and the significance level of the regression coefficients determined by Student's t test. When both the π^2 and π terms are statistically significant, and the π^2 term has a negative coefficient, a π value for optimum activity (π_0) can be calculated (44).

The π values were calculated as outlined in Section I. Hammett σ values were taken from the compilation by Jaffé (57). Taft σ^* values (105) were calculated from values given by Barlin and Perrin (6) and by Charton (20). The E_s values were from Taft (105) and were corrected to E_s^c by the method of Hancock (43) in accordance with Hansch's recommendation (45).

MIC values are usually measured by a twofold dilution technique, so the precision is not very high. Calculation from multiple determinations of the MIC's of six penicillins against a variety of organisms gave a variance for $\log(1/C)$ ranging from 0.01 to 0.06, with a mean of 0.034. Thus, if the residual variance, s^2, in a regression approaches 0.03 the regression can be regarded as complete with data of the accuracy used here, because we do not expect to correlate the error variance. Obviously, it is also necessary for a complete

TABLE III

CHARACTERISTICS OF THREE SETS OF PENICILLINS USED
FOR STRUCTURE–ACTIVITY REGRESSIONS

Set	Side chain (R in I)	Range of side chain π values	Range of σ^* or σ values	Range of log $(1/C)$ values[a]
A Alkylpenicillins	C_nH_{2n+1} $n = 1$ to 10 and 15, chain straight or branched	0.5 to 4.68 and 7.5	-0.39 to 0^b	E. coli 0.32–1.16 S. typhi 0.62–2.23 S. aureus 3.15–5.05 S. faecalis 1.46–3.10
B Ring substituted α-aminobenzyl-penicillins[c,e]	X $-\overset{*}{C}H-$ NH_2 X = halogen, NH_2, OH, Me, OMe	-0.55 to 2.27	-0.66 to 0.71^d	E. coli 0.92–2.31 S. typhi 1.62–2.36 S. aureus 3.10–4.02 S. faecalis 1.77–2.58
C Monosubstituted methylpenicillins	$R'CH_2-$ R' = alkyl or aryl, with or without a functional group such as halogen, ether, thioether, amide, ester, NH_2, NO_2	-0.34 to 4.5 and $-0.75, -1.96$	-0.13 to 1.3^b	E. coli 0.02–1.75 S. typhi 0.31–2.61 S. aureus 2.77–5.33 S. faecalis 1.10–3.33

[a] Where C is the MIC in mmoles/liter.
[b] σ^* values for the whole side chain.
[c] Mostly m- and p-substituents, o-substituted compounds were omitted from correlations including σ.
[d] σ values for X.
[e] * Asymmetric center. MIC's for set B are for the mixture of epimers.

regression, if it is to be meaningful, to "explain" a high proportion of the variance in the data, i.e., to have a high value of the correlation coefficient, r. The MIC values were taken from measurements made at different times over a period of some years, so that some changes in the sensitivities of the strains

TABLE IV

Equations Correlating the MIC Values of Penicillins with π and σ or σ^*

Bacterium	Penicillin set[a]	Equation $\log(1/C) =$	n [b]	r [c]	s^2 [d]	Eq.
E. coli	A	$-0.163\,\pi + 2.301\,\sigma^* +$ 1.558	13	0.849	0.037	(2)
	B	$-0.507\,\pi + 2.065$	15	0.905	0.034	(3)
	C	$-0.127\,\pi - 0.343\,\sigma^* +$ 1.267	38	0.485	0.099	(4)
S. typhi	A	$-0.358\,\pi^2 + 1.690\,\pi +$ $6.924\,\sigma^* + 0.979$	13	0.920	0.062	(5)
	B	$-0.144\,\pi - 0.289\,\sigma +$ 2.225	12	0.831	0.025	(6)
	C	$-0.129\,\pi - 0.757\,\sigma^* +$ 2.046	45	0.453	0.345	(7)
S. aureus	A	$-0.187\,\pi^2 + 1.602\,\pi +$ $4.922\,\sigma^* + 2.455$	12	0.880	0.091	(8)
	B	$0.229\,\pi + 3.411$	14	0.587	0.065	(9)
	C	$0.464\,\pi + 3.358$	41	0.789	0.215	(10)
S. faecalis	A	$-0.085\,\pi^2 + 0.812\,\pi +$ $3.052\,\sigma^* + 1.360$	16	0.867	0.051	(11)
	B	$0.361\,\pi - 0.485\,\sigma +$ 1.888	13	0.684	0.061	(12)
	C	$0.273\,\pi + 1.711$	45	0.735	0.118	(13)

[a] See Table III.
[b] Number of points used to calculate the equation.
[c] Correlation coefficient.
[d] Residual variance.

used may have occurred. This is an additional possible source of random error in the data, but we doubt if it would be large relative to the experimental variance discussed above.

The equations obtained for the three sets of penicillins are presented in Table IV. All the terms in these equations are justified at the 90% level by a t test on the regression coefficients. The residual variance of Eqs. (2), (3), and (6) is close enough to the mean error variance of 0.034, referred to above, for these regressions to be regarded as complete. These equations also give fairly high correlation coefficients, with 72, 83, and 69 %, respectively, of the variance in the data "explained" by the regression (i.e., $r^2 = 0.72$, etc.). Five other equations, Eqs. (5), (8), (9), (11), and (12), have a combination of a fairly low residual variance and a high or fairly high correlation coefficient. These eight reasonably satisfactory regressions all apply to penicillin sets A and B, that is, the alkyl- and the ring-substituted α-aminobenzylpenicillins, in which the structural variations are slight. The regressions for set C, where greater changes in structure occur, are incomplete in terms of residual variance and the correlation coefficients are rather low, although they are all significant at the 99 % level. These incomplete regressions strongly suggest that a property (or properties) other than those described by π and σ or σ^* is important in determining the activity of penicillins in general. The satisfactory regressions for sets A and B then imply that this additional property does not vary sufficiently to be of major importance in determining the relative activities of the penicillins used to calculate these equations. Consequently the equations for sets A and B should be regarded as valid only for the type of side chain for which they were derived. On the other hand, the equations for set C are applicable to a wider range of structures, but the incomplete nature of the regressions means that MIC values predicted from them are unlikely to be accurate. Thus we must conclude that although the equations quoted represent adequate correlations from the mathematical standpoint, their usefulness in predicting the activities of new penicillins is severely limited. However, some interesting information can be derived from them concerning optimum π values.

Equations (2)–(4), (6), (7), (9), (10), (12), and (13) all have a linear π term with a positive or negative slope, which implies that MIC increases indefinitely as π is increased or decreased, respectively, outside the range used for calculation of the equation. This improbable conclusion illustrates the fact that the regression equations are applicable only for π and σ or σ^* values within or near the range of those used to calculate them. If we assume [cf. Eq. (1)] that the relationship between $\log(1/C)$ and π should be represented by a parabola with a negative π^2 term, then a linear relation with π implies that the range of π values studied is inadequate to define the apex of the parabola, i.e., the π value for optimum activity (π_0). In this case a negative slope for the linear relationship shows that the π values used to calculate the equation are mostly above π_0 and a positive slope means that they are mainly below π_0. The signs of the slopes in our linear equations are remarkably consistent. In all cases a positive slope is obtained for regression of the MIC's against Gram-positive bacteria and a negative slope is found for the Gram-negative bacteria in qualitative agreement with recent results of Biagi et al. (*11a*). This implies that the π_0 values will be near or above 4 for the Gram-positive bacteria and near or below zero for the Gram-negative organisms (cf. the ranges of π values in Table III). Definite π_0 values can be calculated for the alkylpenicillins from Eqs. (5), (8), and (11). Equations (8) and (11) give values of 4.27 and 4.28, respectively, for activity against *S. aureus* and *S. faecalis*. These values are consistent with the value near or above 4 deduced from the linear equations for Gram-positive organisms. However, Eq. (5) gives a π_0 value of 2.35 for activity against *S. typhi*, which conflicts with the value near or below zero deduced from the linear equations for Gram-negative bacteria. This conflict might partly arise as follows. The low slope associated with π in all the linear equations except Eq. (3) shows that MIC values are not highly dependent on π. Consequently an optimum π within the range of π values covered by the penicillins might be fairly easily obscured by experimental error in the MIC measurements. This explanation could apply to the regressions represented by Eqs. (2), (4), and (7). However, it is not applicable to the regressions for penicillin set B, because the maximum π value in this set is 2.27. Thus if π_0 is near 2 most of the π values are below the optimum and this should give a positive slope for the linear π term and not the negative one that is found in Eqs. (3) and (6). Consequently we must conclude that either π_0 for the action of penicillins on *E. coli* and *S. typhi* differs with the type of side chain structure, or the value of 2.35 from Eq. (5) is spurious.

It is interesting to note that the higher π_0 found for the action of penicillins on Gram-positive organisms than on Gram-negative ones agrees with the findings of Lien *et al.* (*69*) for several sets of antibacterial substances with a variety of structures. They found that the π_0 values fall into two roughly constant groups, with the average value for Gram-positive bacteria about 2 units greater than that for Gram-negative organisms. They attributed this difference to the greater lipid content of the cell wall in Gram-negative than in Gram-positive bacteria. This high lipid content presumably tends to prevent or slow down passage of lipophilic compounds through the wall by absorption effects, so that the more hydrophobic a compound is, the greater difficulty it experiences in reaching the site of action. Some support for the applicability of this hypothesis to penicillins comes from some results of Strominger and his co-workers (*100*). They measured the concentration of three penicillins required to inhibit the cell free transpeptidase enzyme from *E. coli*, which is postulated to be the ultimate site of action of penicillins. Comparison of these concentrations with those required to inhibit growth of the bacterium suggests that benzylpenicillin reaches the site of action less easily than the less hydrophobic penicillins, ampicillin and methicillin. This is in qualitative agreement with our finding of a negative slope for the π terms in regressions for *E. coli*.

The above discussion has ignored the role of steric effects of the penicillin side chain on penicillin activity. The different MIC's which are often found (*34, 41*, and Table II) for epimeric penicillins when the side chain contains an asymmetric center show that such effects can be important. Effects of this type cannot be rationalized by π/σ analysis because the calculated π and σ values of stereoisomers are identical. The implication from the regressions of set C that a factor other than π and σ is important in determining penicillin activity led us to investigate the inclusion in regressions of the Taft E_s parameter as a measure of the steric effects of side chain substituents. Unfortunately E_s is not an additive constant and values are available for only a limited number of groups, so we were unable to include E_s in regressions for all the penicillins of set C. However, E_s values were available for the side chain groups of 23 penicillins and were included, in the corrected form E_s^c, in regressions with π and σ^*. The side chain structures were alkyl- and simple-substituted alkyl or aralkyl groups. Two equations, (14) and (15), were obtained in which the E_s^c term was statistically significant. Equation (14) described activity against *E. coli* and is significant at only the 90% level. Addition of a π term gives a

$$\log(1/C) = 0.174\ E_s^c + 1.112 \tag{14}$$

$$
\begin{array}{ccc}
n & r & s^2 \\
20 & 0.440 & 0.073
\end{array}
$$

$$\log(1/C) = 0.317\ \pi + 0.140\ E_s^c + 1.662 \tag{15}$$

$$
\begin{array}{ccc}
n & r & s^2 \\
23 & 0.804 & 0.070
\end{array}
$$

nonsignificant regression. However, the variance in the *E. coli* MIC's is very small and this may not be a fair test of the E_s^c parameter. Equation (15) correlates activity against *S. faecalis*. Here the E_s^c term is significant at the 95% level and this regression indicates that the steric parameter can sometimes be important in correlating the activity of penicillins. However, no significant regressions were obtained for the MIC's of this set of penicillins against *S. typhi* and *S. aureus*, although the variance in the MIC's was quite high. Very similar results were obtained with the uncorrected, E_s, parameter.

Steric effects assume even greater significance in rationalizing the activity of penicillins against bacteria which secrete a penicillin-destroying enzyme. This presents a special problem of great practical importance which is dealt with in Section II,B.

B. THE ROLE OF β-LACTAMASE

It has been recognized since 1940 that some bacteria produce an enzyme which catalyzes the hydrolysis of penicillins to antibacterially inactive products (3). Once the structure of penicillin had been established the reaction product was identified as the corresponding penicilloic acid (2). The enzyme was originally called penicillinase, but nowadays the term β-lactamase is preferred. This term also embraces enzymes which act in a similar fashion on the β-lactam ring of cephalosporins. The β-lactamases from different bacteria are not identical; differences in the relative rates of hydrolysis of penicillins are quite common, and those enzymes which have been purified show different amino acid content and different physical properties. A general review of β-lactamases has been given by Citri and Pollock (21).

β-Lactamase activity is of great clinical significance because it can severely limit the therapeutic efficacy of β-lactam antibiotics. Certain strains of both Gram-positive and Gram-negative pathogenic bacteria produce β-lactamases, the most troublesome being strains of *Staphylococcus aureus*. Such strains of staphylococci were originally rare, but widespread use of penicillin has led to their selective proliferation. Thus in many parts of the world, and particularly in hospitals, a large proportion of staphylococci are now β-lactamase producing "resistant" strains. Consequently, the development of semisynthetic penicillins which resist inactivation by β-lactamase, and especially by staphylococcal β-lactamase, is very important.

All penicillins known prior to 1957 were inactivated by all forms of β-lactamase, although there were differences in the rates of hydrolysis (8). Consequently, when it became possible to prepare semisynthetic penicillins, high priority was given to a search for compounds which would be stable to β-lactamase and also retain antibacterial activity. However, in the absence of detailed knowledge of the chemistry of β-lactamases, there could be no question of designing a resistant penicillin by a theoretical approach. The approach adopted was the empirical one of preparing as many different types of penicillin as possible and testing for the desired property. In this section we describe how this approach met with success and how the initial empiricism has been supplemented by rational interpretation and systematic exploitation. The following discussion should be read in conjunction with Table V, which gives MIC values for various penicillins against a sensitive and a resistant strain of *S. aureus*. Those penicillins which are stable to β-lactamase show only a small difference between these two MIC's, while those which are hydrolyzed show large or very large MIC's against the resistant strain.

Benzylpenicillin and phenoxymethylpenicillin were probably the most active and clinically effective of the older (β-lactamase-susceptible) penicillins, so it was natural that many of the newer compounds studied were variants of these structures. Replacement of one or both of the α-hydrogen atoms of the side chain by other groups was prominent among these variations.

Derivatives of phenoxymethylpenicillin obtained by introduction of alkyl or aryl groups on the α-carbon show a similar antibacterial spectrum to that of the parent compound; that is, very little activity against Gram-negative organisms and high activity toward Gram-positive bacteria. However, some

TABLE V

MINIMUM INHIBITORY CONCENTRATIONS OF PENICILLINS AGAINST
A SENSITIVE AND A RESISTANT STRAIN OF *Staphylococcus aureus*

Side chain structure (R in I)		MIC (μg/ml)	
		Sensitive	Resistant [a]
PhOCH—	X = H	0.02	250
$\mid$	Me	0.05	125
X	Et	0.05	125
	Ph	0.1	50
	X = H	0.01	500
	NH$_2$	0.1	>500
PhCH—	COOH	1.25	50
$\mid$	NHC$\underset{NH_2}{\overset{NH}{<}}$	0.25	1.25
X			
	Ph	0.05	175
Ph$_3$C—		0.15	0.3
	X = Y = OMe	0.5	2.5
	X = H Y = COOH	5	12.5
	H Ph	0.25	1.25
	H I	0.25	125
		0.25	0.5
		6.25	25
		2.5	6.25

TABLE V—*continued*

Side chain structure (R in I)		MIC (μg/ml)	
		Sensitive	Resistant [a]
(quinoxaline structure) ...COOH		0.5	1.25
(isoxazole structure) X, N-O, Y	X = Y = Me	0.25	>250
	X = Ph Y = H	0.1	250
	Ph Me	0.25	1.25
	o-ClC$_6$H$_4$ Me	0.1	0.5
	2,6-Cl$_2$C$_6$H$_3$ Me	0.1	0.25

[a] Values determined with a large inoculum. Penicillins which are hydrolyzed by β-lactamase would probably give smaller MIC's with smaller inocula.

of these penicillins are rather more resistant to staphylococcal β-lactamase than is phenoxymethylpenicillin itself. Thus it has been reported (*39*) that propicillin, α-phenoxyisopropylpenicillin and α-phenoxyisobutylpenicillin, show quite low MIC values against β-lactamase-producing *S. aureus* when tested with a small inoculum. However, the MIC's were considerably higher when a large inoculum was used. This effect of inoculum size is not observed with the much more resistant penicillins such as methicillin. Consequently the phenoxymethylpenicillin derivatives are unsuitable for treatment of infection caused by "highly resistant" staphylococci which produce large quantities of β-lactamase, although they may be used against "mildly resistant" staphylococcal infections where only small quantities of enzyme are produced.

Analogs of benzylpenicillin in which one of the α-hydrogen atoms has been replaced include the α-amino and α-carboxyderivatives (ampicillin and carbenicillin, respectively). These penicillins, and many similar structures, show a considerable degree of resistance to the β-lactamases of some Gram-negative bacteria (*102*), but they are susceptible to inactivation by staphylococcal β-lactamase. The only mono-α-substituted benzylpenicillin which has been reported (*106*) to show a high degree of resistance to staphylococcal β-lactamase is the α-guanidino compound. The activity of this penicillin against β-lactamase producing staphylococci *in vitro* suggests that it might be of clinical value against such infections, but so far it does not seem to have been applied in this way.

Historically the first penicillin to show high resistance to staphylococcal β-lactamase was an αα-disubstituted benzylpenicillin prepared (15) in the Beecham Laboratories in 1958. This compound was triphenylmethylpenicillin, and it quickly became apparent that resistance to β-lactamase was associated with the presence of three bulky substituents on the α-carbon atom of the side chain. Analogs in which two of the three phenyl groups were replaced by ethyl or methyl were less resistant to the enzyme, while diphenylmethyl- and βββ-triphenylethylpenicillins were essentially sensitive to it. Triphenylmethylpenicillin and several of its close analogs had good activity against Gram-positive bacteria, including β-lactamase-producing staphylococci, in vitro. However, they had little or no activity in vivo. This is now thought to be largely due to extensive binding of these very hydrophobic compounds to serum albumin and to other body proteins and fatty tissues.

Results such as those outlined above suggested that a promising way to render penicillins resistant to β-lactamase was to introduce steric hindrance around the side chain amide group. The first penicillin of clinical value against highly resistant β-lactamase-producing staphylococci was developed in the Beecham Laboratories in 1959 by following up this concept of steric hindrance. Benzoic acids substituted in both ortho positions constitute one of the classic examples of steric hindrance (74), and hence a series of penicillins was prepared (29) by condensing such acids with 6-APA. The first such compound to be prepared was 2,6-dimethoxyphenylpenicillin, which proved to be highly resistant to staphylococcal β-lactamase and to have useful activity against resistant staphylococci both in vitro and in vivo. It has been in clinical use since 1960 under the approved name of methicillin.

Many other 2,6-disubstituted phenylpenicillins, either with or without additional substituents elsewhere in the benzene ring, were also prepared. All were essentially stable toward β-lactamase, but none was more active than methicillin. Analogs with only one ortho substituent were also examined, but small groups such as methyl and methoxy, or halogen atoms, failed to confer adequate resistance to β-lactamase. By contrast, introduction of a single phenyl or other aryl group (54), or of a carboxyl group or amides derived therefrom (82) into the ortho position conferred considerable stability toward the enzyme.

All the substituted phenylpenicillins suffer from the disadvantage that their activity against Gram-positive bacteria is of a relatively modest order, while that against Gram-negative bacteria is virtually nonexistent. This seems to stem from a fundamentally unfavorable molecular structure, the parent (unhindered) phenylpenicillin being considerably less active than benzylpenicillin (see Table II). α-Naphthylpenicillin is at least as active as phenylpenicillin against sensitive (i.e., non-β-lactamase-producing) Gram-positive bacteria, and this fact suggested that 2-substituted 1-naphthylpenicillins might have useful activity against resistant staphylococci. With these structures both the 2-substituent and the residue of the fused benzene ring would contribute to the steric effect and consequent resistance to β-lactamase. A series of 2-alkoxy-1-naphthylpenicillins in fact showed excellent stability toward staphylococcal β-lactamase and greater activity than methicillin against both sensitive and resistant staphylococci (16, 94). One of the series, 2-ethoxy-1-naphthylpenicillin (nafcillin), is in clinical use in the United States.

Since resistance to β-lactamase seemed to be largely due to steric factors, it was expected to be retained when a benzene ring in the side chain was replaced by a 6-membered heteroaromatic ring. Various 2,4-disubstituted 3-pyridylpenicillins and 4,6-disubstituted 5-pyrimidylpenicillins were found to be comparable to methicillin in stability toward staphylococcal β-lactamase, but unfortunately their inherent antibacterial activity was relatively weak. Replacement of the naphthalene ring in nafcillin and its homologs by a quinoline ring also results in retention of activity against β-lactamase-producing staphylococci (16). Further evidence of the efficacy of a single judiciously placed carboxyl group in conferring resistance to β-lactamase is provided by 3-carboxy-2-quinoxalinylpenicillin (quinacillin). This compound has good activity against all staphylococci, but has little activity against bacteria of other species (86).

Penicillins derived from 5-membered heterocyclic acids have also been studied extensively. The isoxazole ring system has received particularly thorough attention (27, 28, 30, 50) since the inherent antibacterial activity of 4-isoxazolylpenicillins is considerable and several convenient syntheses of 3,5-disubstituted isoxazole-4-carboxylic acids are available. The external bond angles are of course wider in a 5-membered than in a 6-membered ring, so bulkier *ortho* substituents are required to produce a similar steric effect. It was therefore not surprising to find that 3,5-dimethyl-4-isoxazolylpenicillin was less stable than methicillin toward staphylococcal β-lactamase, while both 3-phenyl- and 5-phenyl-4-isoxazolylpenicillins were less stable than *o*-biphenylylpenicillin. In order to obtain adequate β-lactamase resistance in the 4-isoxazolyl series it was found necessary to have two *ortho* substituents, at least one of which was relatively bulky. The requirements of good stability toward the enzyme combined with good antistaphylococcal activity were met when the 3-substituent was phenyl or substituted phenyl and the 5-substituent was methyl or another lower alkyl group. The isomeric 3-alkyl-5-aryl-4-isoxazolyl penicillins were equally stable but slightly less active. Activity against resistant staphylococci at least as great as that of nafcillin, and several times better than that of methicillin, was found in a number of 3-aryl-5-methyl-4-isoxazolylpenicillins. Three members of this series (oxacillin, cloxacillin, and dicloxacillin) are at present in clinical use and, unlike methicillin, they are well absorbed when given by mouth. As with other penicillins derived from highly hindered side chain acids, their activity is restricted to Gram-positive bacteria.

Replacement of the isoxazole ring in the above penicillins by other 5-membered heterocycles appears to confer no advantages. In the 2,4-disubstituted 3-furyl series (51), as well as among the 3,5-disubstituted 4-isothiazolylpenicillins (75), the most effective combinations of substituents appear to be very similar to those found in the isoxazole series.

It is apparent from the above discussion that a considerable range of semisynthetic penicillins having good activity against β-lactamase-producing staphylococci is now available. Methicillin, oxacillin, and cloxacillin are the most widely used of these penicillins and many workers (24, 26, 40, 42, 60, 78, 81, 95, 99) have shown that they are hydrolyzed much more slowly than benzylpenicillin by all forms of β-lactamase which have been tested. However, comparison of hydrolysis rates alone is not an adequate guide to the stability of these penicillins at clinical concentrations. The affinity of methicillin and oxacillin for staphylococcal β-lactamase, as indicated by their Michaelis constants (40, 78), is very low, so that maximum hydrolysis rates are achieved only at high substrate concentrations. Novick (78) calculated the half-lives of some penicillins in the presence of staphylococcal β-lactamase at penicillin concentrations adequate to inhibit growth of penicillin-sensitive staphylococci. Under these conditions the half-life of methicillin was 5×10^5 times that of benzylpenicillin, although their maximum hydrolysis rates differ by a factor of only 30.

In addition to solving a clinical problem, the advent of β-lactamase-stable penicillins has led to a deeper understanding of the behavior of the enzyme. Several studies, which are reviewed by Citri and Pollock (21), have led to the conclusion that the active site of β-lactamases is flexible and that alignment between enzyme and substrate involves a change in the conformation of the site. The structure of the penicillin side chain is decisive in determining the conformation adopted by the enzyme (22). Thus some side chain structures induce a catalytically active conformation of the enzyme, while other penicillins are stable to the enzyme because they induce a conformation which is unfavorable for hydrolysis.

It is clear that steric properties of the side chain are of primary importance in inducing a noncatalytic enzyme conformation. Steric hindrance near the side chain amide group may prevent this group from binding the penicillin at the active site of the β-lactamase. The fact that the hindered penicillins are only weakly bound to the enzyme is indicated by their low affinity constants. However, it seems unlikely that this effect alone could induce a noncatalytic enzyme conformation. An alternative (or perhaps an additional) way in which a steric effect could operate is by restriction of rotation about the single bond between the side chain and the amide carbonyl group. Such a restriction could constrain the penicillin molecule into a configuration not readily accommodated at the active site of the enzyme. Depue *et al.* (*26*) have explained the effect of methicillin on the conformation and reactivity of β-lactamase in this way.

It is obvious that any attempt at quantitative correlation of the β-lactamase stability of a wide range of penicillins would have to allow for steric effects. Unfortunately, Taft E_s values are not available for any of the important side chain structures. In the circumstances it was not surprising to find (*12*) that no statistically significant correlations were obtained in attempted regression analysis of the Michaelis constants and maximum hydrolysis rates of two groups of penicillins (*26*, *40*) using side chain π values and either σ^* values or the pK_a's of the side chain acids.

C. Mode of Action as a Basis for the Design of Penicillins and Penicillin Analogs

Penicillins belong to the group of antibiotics which inhibit the growth of sensitive bacteria by interfering with the completion of the wall structure in dividing cells (*73*, *80*). It should perhaps be explained that the wall is an essential feature of bacterial cells which has no counterpart in animal cells. It is a rigid but permeable structure, located on the outside of the cytoplasmic membrane, which gives the cell its mechanical strength. Serious impairment of the wall structure causes the cell to burst under its own internal osmotic pressure. In recent years a great deal has been learned about the chemical structure of bacterial cell walls. Major components of all walls studied include teichoic acids, which are polymers composed for the most part of glycerol or ribitol phosphates, and a highly crosslinked mucopeptide structure for which the names murein and peptidoglycan have been proposed. Other components, found most abundantly in Gram-negative bacteria where the wall is less clearly differentiated from the underlying cytoplasmic membrane than is the case in Gram-positive cocci, include additional amino acids and lipids.

In the present context the relevant portion of the wall structure is the murein. The whole of the murein of a single cell can be regarded as a bag-shaped molecule with a molecular weight of billions. Its three-dimensional structure consists of a series of "backbone" chains of acetylated amino sugars, with alternate hexosamine units carrying D-lactic acid linked as an ether. The carboxyl group of the lactic acid is itself linked as an amide to a peptide chain, and crosslinking of different peptide chains completes the structure. The crosslinking reaction involves the elimination of one molecule of D-alanine and is brought about by a transpeptidase enzyme. The energy of the broken peptide bond appears to be utilized in forming the new bond, a significant consideration in a process occurring outside the cytoplasmic membrane where there is presumably no pool of ATP available. Recently a cellfree preparation of the transpeptidase has been obtained from *E. coli* (*56, 100*). It is inhibited by penicillins, thus confirming an earlier hypothesis (*113*) that it represents the site of action of the antibiotics.

The discussion thus far has been concerned with the general features common to all bacteria. Actually the broad outline of the murein structure appears to be similar in all bacteria, but differences of detail have been observed. In staphylococci the sequence of four amino acids linked to the carboxyl group of lactic acid is L-Ala-D-Glu-L-Lys-D-Ala, and this same sequence appears to persist in most pathogens except that in many Gram-negative organisms the lysine is replaced by the closely related α,ϵ-diaminopimelic acid. The glutamic acid is linked to lysine via the γ-carboxyl group, the α-carboxyl group being present as the simple amide in staphylococci but possibly in other forms in other bacteria. The crosslinkage is formed between the carboxyl group of D-alanine and the ϵ-amino group of lysine (or diaminopimelic acid) in a neighboring chain. The linkage may be direct or may be made by means of a further short peptide chain, e.g., in staphylococci there is a "bridge" of five glycine units. Thus the general crosslinking reaction may be represented as follows, X and Y representing the residues of different peptide chains:

$$
\begin{array}{ccccc}
\text{X} & & & \text{X} & \\
| & & & | & \\
\text{L-Lys} & \quad \text{Y} & \xrightarrow{\text{enzyme}} & \text{L-Lys} & + \quad \text{D-Ala} \\
| & + \quad | & & | & \\
\text{D-Ala} & \quad \text{NH}_2 & & \text{D-Ala—NH—Y} & \\
| & & & & \\
\text{D-Ala} & & & & \\
\end{array}
$$

VIII

Various investigators (*31, 108, 113*) have suggested that penicillin may inhibit the enzymic reaction by reason of a structural resemblance to some portion of the peptide **VIII**. The hypothesis is attractive because penicillin itself is an acyldipeptide of a peculiarly modified kind, the bicyclic nucleus being derived from L-cysteine and D-valine. The most cogently advocated of several possible analogies is that which regards the penicillin nucleus as simulating the terminal D-Ala-D-Ala of **VIII**, in which case the penicillin side chain would occupy a position corresponding to lysine in **VIII**.

The above reasoning led Strominger (*108*) to suggest that coupling the carboxyl group of lysine to the amino group of 6-APA would give a semi-synthetic penicillin with a particularly close structural resemblance to **VIII** and which might exhibit advantageous antibacterial properties. The lysyl derivative of 6-APA was in fact prepared in these laboratories at an early stage of our work, but while both it and the *N,N'*-dibenzyloxycarbonyl intermediate had antibacterial activity this was of a quite unexceptional order and considerably less than that of the therapeutically useful penicillins. This result is not really surprising since experience shows that when a group of drugs is believed to act by competing with a natural substrate the most active members are usually not those with the most obvious structural similarity to that substrate, e.g., the most active sulfonamides are rather distantly related to *p*-aminobenzoic acid. Possibly the most effective drugs contain structural features which enable them to combine at the site of action by additional mechanisms of van der Waals or hydrogen bonding not available to the natural substrate.

In the case of penicillins it may well be that benzene or other planar rings in various positions in the side chain facilitate combination at the site of action. While such benzene rings are not essential for activity, the usual empirical variation of side chain structures generally reveals that the most active penicillins in any given series contain one or more benzene rings. The isosteric thiophene ring can generally be substituted for benzene with little effect on activity. It can hardly be a coincidence that every one of the dozen or more penicillins currently marketed in various parts of the world contains one or more benzene rings (see Table I), while the marketed cephalosporins contain either benzene or thiophene rings. The advantage of the aromatic compounds could certainly not be predicted by examination of the murein structure, which itself contains no aromatic rings of any kind.

Penicillins are known to combine irreversibly with bacteria by opening of the β-lactam ring, resulting in the formation of covalently attached penicilloyl radicals (*23*). The active site of the transpeptidase involved in crosslinking the cell-wall mucopeptide, or some immediately adjacent functional group in the enzyme, may well be among the sites acylated by penicillin in this way. The enzyme would of course be irreversibly inhibited by such acylation, and cell-wall synthesis would be blocked. Furthermore, such a site might be particularly vulnerable to penicilloylation since the penicillin molecule could be accommodated there initially by noncovalent bonds as a result of a structural resemblance to the natural peptide substrate of the enzyme, and would then be ideally placed for covalent bond formation to occur (*31*).

If these ideas correctly represent the mode of action of penicillin at the molecular level, it might be possible to design synthetic molecules which would not themselves be penicillins, but which would act in a similar fashion. Penicillin may be regarded as an acyldipeptide structure in which the peptide bond is "activated" by incorporation in the strained fused-ring β-lactam–thiazolidine nucleus, the nonplanarity of which is considered to suppress normal amide resonance. There is, however, no reason to believe that the fused ring structure is an absolute requirement for activity, since activation of the peptide bond could in principle be achieved in various other ways.

One attempt to design a synthetic antibacterial substance along the above lines was made by Henery-Logan and Limburg (*53*), who based their approach on the great reactivity of *N*-acylaziridines compared with unstrained amides.

They accordingly synthesized 1-(phenylacetamidoacetyl)aziridine-2-carboxylic acid (**IX**), but unfortunately it showed only a very low order of antistaphylococcal activity.

Nayler and co-workers (*72, 76*) based their approach on the enhanced reactivity of diacylimides compared with simple amides. Three series of compounds were synthesized wherein a second carbonyl group was bound to the peptide nitrogen of an acyldipeptide. The first two series consisted of α-(acylaminosuccinimido)carboxylic acids (**X**) (*72*), and *N*-(acylglycyl)-α-oxopyrrolidine-2-carboxylic acids (**XI**) (*76*). In the third series the structural

resemblance to penicillins was increased by incorporating the sulfur atom and *gem*-dimethyl groups to give various *N*-(acylglycyl)-5,5-dimethyl-2-oxothiazolidine-4-carboxylic acids (**XII**) (*76*). None of these compounds showed more than very slight antibacterial activity. The failure of these early attempts to design molecules simulating the antibacterial activity of penicillins is disappointing but, in our present incomplete state of knowledge, not surprising.

III. Behavior of Penicillins *in Vivo*

If an antibiotic is to be effective it must obviously be capable of reaching the site of infection in sufficient concentration to inhibit growth of the pathogen. The drug is usually carried to the site of infection in the blood, from which it diffuses into the infected tissue. It is, therefore, of fundamental importance that the drug, however administered, be capable of attaining a significant concentration in the blood. Penicillin blood levels, like those of any drug, depend on the interplay of many factors, which will be considered in the following sections.

A. ACID STABILITY

The acid stability of penicillins is important in consideration of their behavior *in vivo* because a stable compound is much more likely to be absorbed efficiently into the bloodstream after oral administration than is a labile analog which may be extensively inactivated at the acid pH of the stomach. A qualitative indication of the acid stability of clinically important penicillins is given in Table VI.

TABLE VI

ACID STABILITY OF CLINICALLY USED PENICILLINS

Poor stability	Moderate stability	High stability
Benzylpenicillin	Nafcillin	All α-phenoxyalkyl-penicillins
Methicillin	Carbenicillin	All 4-isoxazolyl-penicillins
		Ampicillin

The two main products of acid decomposition of a penicillin are the corresponding penicillenic (**XIII**) and penillic (**XIV**) acids (*31*). Their formation

must directly involve the side chain amide group, and is probably initiated (*59*) by the electronic displacements indicated in **XV**. Consequently the nature of the side chain (R) would be expected to have a considerable effect on the course of the reaction. In particular the inductive effect of an electron-attracting group in the side chain should tend to inhibit the electronic displacements shown in **XV** and so increase stability to acid degradation.

The importance of an electron-attracting group in the side chain was first suggested by Abraham (*1*) to explain the enhanced acid stability of phenoxy-methylpenicillin compared with benzylpenicillin. Subsequently work with semisynthetic penicillins has shown (*32, 33*) the existence of a correlation between the acid stability and the inductive effect on their side chains, as measured by the pK_a's of the side chain acids (RCOOH). Unfortunately data

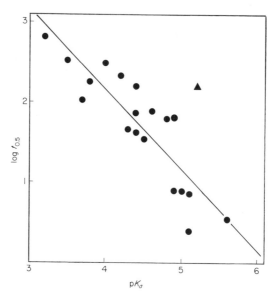

Fig. 1. Logarithm of the half-life of penicillins in 50% EtOH/H$_2$O at pH 1.3 and 35°C plotted against the pK_a of the side chain acids in 50% EtOH/H$_2$O. (●) Data from Doyle *et al.* (*32, 33*). (▲) Cloxacillin.

are available for only a very limited number of types of side chain structure. The data for 19 penicillins given by Doyle *et al.* (*32, 33*), together with pre-viously unpublished data for cloxacillin, are plotted in Fig. 1. With the exception of cloxacillin, a reasonable correlation is found between $\log t_{0.5}$ and pK_a, where $t_{0.5}$ is the half-life of the penicillin in 50% aqueous ethanol at pH 1.3 and 35°C. The pK_a values were measured for the side chain acids dissolved in 50% aqueous ethanol. The line in Fig. 1 is the best straight line through 19 points (omitting cloxacillin), and it has Eq. (16).

$$\log t_{0.5} = -0.995 \text{ p}K_a + 6.125 \qquad \begin{array}{ccc} n & r & s^2 \\ 19 & 0.876 & 0.120 \end{array} \qquad (16)$$

The scatter about this line is almost certainly due to the fact that 14 of the penicillins have an *ortho*-substituted phenyl or naphthyl side chain. The difficulty of applying extrathermodynamic relations to *ortho*-substituted compounds is well known (*67*). Equation (17) was obtained for the five penicillins without an *ortho*-substituent (these are phenoxymethyl-, benzyl-, and α-amino-, α-methoxy-, and α-chlorobenzylpenicillins).

$$\log t_{0.5} = -0.961\ pK_a + 6.177 \qquad \begin{array}{ccc} n & r & s^2 \\ 5 & 0.959 & 0.082 \end{array} \qquad (17)$$

The correlation coefficient shows that 92% of the variance in the data is accounted for. The measurements were not highly accurate, so some experimental error variance is to be expected and the correlation seems to be nearly perfect.

The acid stability of cloxacillin ($t_{0.5} = 160$ min) is much greater than would be predicted from the pK_a of its side chain acid. This may be due to the weak, but definite, basicity of the isoxazole ring (*84*). Under the conditions of the acid stability test a significant proportion of the cloxacillin molecules may be stabilized by protonation of the isoxazole nitrogen atom. The pK_a of the side chain acid as measured by titration with alkali would then not be entirely appropriate for the correlation, since it would only reflect the situation pertaining in the unprotonated species. Similar considerations are likely to apply to other isoxazolylpenicillins, and indeed to any penicillin containing a very weakly basic group close to or conjugated with the side chain amide link. They will not apply when the substituent is more strongly basic, as in ampicillin, since then the measurements of penicillin half-life and side chain pK_a will both apply essentially to the *N*-protonated species.

Confirmation of the importance of electron-attracting groups in the side chain in enhancing acid stability has recently been provided by Panarin *et al.* (*79, 79a*). They obtained near perfect linear correlations between the logarithm of the decomposition rate of several substituted phenyl and phenoxymethyl penicillins at low pH and the Hammett σ values of the substituents.

It should be pointed out that while considerable stability in acid is highly desirable in a penicillin intended for oral use, it does not in itself ensure that the drug will be absorbed into the bloodstream. The most acid-stable penicillin will be useless for the oral treatment of systemic infections if it is unable to pass through the wall of the gastrointestinal tract. Conversely, a penicillin of only modest acid stability which is well absorbed in the stomach or intestine may give useful blood levels after oral administration. Thus although the acid-labile benzylpenicillin is preferably given by injection, the lower and erratic blood levels obtained by the oral route are still sufficient to have a therapeutic effect against sensitive staphylococci or streptococci. On the other hand, carbenicillin is more acid stable than benzylpenicillin and yet gives no significant blood levels after oral administration in man (*62*). Again, nafcillin has only modest acid stability and yet is used as an oral drug, whereas its highly acid-stable isostere, 3-ethoxy-4-quinolylpenicillin, gives no detectable blood levels by the oral route.

B. Absorption from the Gastrointestinal Tract

Absorption of many drugs from the gut is believed to depend mainly on their ionization state and lipid–water partition characteristics (*17, 96*). The pK_a values of most penicillins are close to 2.7 (*85*), so the proportion of lipid-soluble un-ionized compound will be high at the acid pH of the stomach, but will become progressively smaller as the penicillin passes into the near neutral environment of the intestine. Thus if penicillins are absorbed by passive diffusion through a lipid membrane, absorption seems likely to take place mainly in the stomach and the first part of the duodenum. Since the pK_a values of different penicillins are very similar the proportion ionized at a particular pH will be essentially constant for different penicillins. Consequently if the pH-partition hypothesis applies to absorption of penicillins, then their rates of absorption should be related only to their partition coefficients. Confirmation of this postulate requires either measurement of absorption rates for several penicillins or an estimate of the proportion of an oral dose which is absorbed into the bloodstream.

Measurement of absorption rates is difficult and there seem to be no figures available for penicillins. The proportion of a dose excreted in the urine after oral administration is often regarded as a measure of the extent of absorption. This view has been criticized by Kunin (*65*), who pointed out that the urinary recovery does not reflect absorption alone, but also depends on the amount inactivated and excreted by nonrenal mechanisms. There is some evidence that nonrenal excretion of penicillins occurs via the liver and that the rate varies considerably with different penicillins (*18, 66, 93, 109*). Thus comparison of urinary recoveries after oral administration of penicillins will not necessarily indicate the relative extent of absorption. However, the ratio of urinary recovery after oral and intramuscular administration of the same compound should distinguish differences in absorption from the other factors (*65*). Comparison of such ratios for different penicillins should then indicate the relative extent of absorption. Results obtained (*65*) in this way for oxacillin and dicloxacillin show a considerably greater extent of absorption for the more hydrophobic compound, dicloxacillin. Unfortunately the amount of data of this type is very limited and it is impossible to decide if the absorption of penicillins in general is in accordance with the pH-partition hypothesis. Moreover, it seems improbable that an amphoteric penicillin such as ampicillin would be absorbed by this mechanism. At the acid pH of the stomach, ampicillin will exist largely as the cation (**XVI**) with some zwitterion (**IV**), while in the neutral environment of the intestine the forms present will be **IV** and the anion **XVII**. Thus throughout the entire pH range of the gut the lipid solubility

$$\begin{array}{ccc}
& \overset{S}{\diagup}\diagdown & \\
\text{PhCHCONHCH—CH} & & \text{CMe}_2 \\
| & | & | \\
\text{NH}_3{}^+ & \text{CO—N} & \text{—CHCOOH}
\end{array}$$

XVI

$$\begin{array}{ccc}
& \overset{S}{\diagup}\diagdown & \\
\text{PhCHCONHCH—CH} & & \text{CMe}_2 \\
| & | & | \\
\text{NH}_2 & \text{CO—N} & \text{—CHCOO}^-
\end{array}$$

XVII

of ampicillin seems likely to be negligible, yet urinary recoveries after oral and intramuscular administration (*65*) suggest that about 30% of the oral dose is absorbed.

The *p*-hydroxy derivative of ampicillin (*23a*), but not the *m*-hydroxy isomer, is very much better absorbed than ampicillin itself. The most efficiently absorbed of all amino-substituted penicillins so far reported appears to be 1-aminocyclohexylpenicillin (cyclacillin) (*54a, 94a*), although its antibacterial activity *in vitro* is relatively modest. Ampicillin and these other α-amino penicillins may be absorbed by a special mechanism, possibly one which normally handles amino acids or small peptides. By contrast, β-amino-α-phenylethylpenicillin is reported (*4*) not to give significant blood levels after oral administration in man, although it is acid-stable.

C. SERUM BINDING

It is well known that penicillins, in common with many other drugs, combine reversibly with the albumin fraction of serum. This reaction is important for the design of penicillins because of its effect on antibacterial activity, and because variation of the penicillin side chain can produce very large changes in the extent of binding, e.g., at clinical concentrations ampicillin is 18% and cloxacillin 94% bound to human serum (*91*).

There is good evidence (*64, 89*) to show that in the presence of serum only the free fraction of an antibiotic is antibacterially active, so that the MIC against any one organism is often greater in the presence of serum than in its absence. Also, it is only the free fraction which can diffuse from the bloodstream into tissues where the site of infection is likely to be located. However, the bound antibiotic is not "lost," because binding is a reversible equilibrium and removal of free antibiotic from the blood stream causes dissociation of some of the protein–antibiotic complex. The rate of this dissociation is so fast that it is unlikely to be a limiting factor in removal of free antibiotic from the serum (*107*).

The clinical significance of the situation outlined above has been the subject of some dispute in the literature, which has recently been discussed by Rolinson (89) and by Warren (111). Rolinson concluded that "The significance of the protein binding of an antibiotic can only be judged in relation to the serum concentrations obtained with a given dosage and the activity of the antibiotic against the pathogen in question. Protein binding is likely to preclude therapeutic effect only if the extent is such that the level of free drug in serum, and at the site of infection, is reduced to a subinhibitory level. Examination of data concerning antibiotics known to be clinically effective suggests that a therapeutic effect is attainable with serum levels of unbound drug only slightly higher than the inhibitory concentration for the pathogen, provided such concentrations are maintained for an adequate period of time." Warren's study led him to suggest that it may not be essential to maintain the serum level of an antimicrobial agent above the inhibitory concentration and he concluded that "perhaps ... our present knowledge is inadequate to interpret the meaning of penicillin serum levels and protein binding."

Several authors (10, 14, 64, 91, 97) have shown the existence of wide variations between the extent of serum binding of different penicillins, but there has generally been little attempt to relate these differences to the penicillin structures. An exception to this was the work of Scholtan (97), who showed that the different extents of binding of six penicillins are qualitatively correlated with the hydrophobic character of their side chains. This led Scholtan to suggest that penicillins are bound to albumin primarily by hydrophobic bonding of the side chain. Scholtan's work also established the fact that configurational differences in the side chain do not affect the extent of binding, thus the D- and L-epimers of α-aminobenzylpenicillin and of α-phenoxy-n-propylpenicillin are each bound to the same extent.

Further evidence that penicillins are bound to albumin by their side chain has been obtained by Kunin (63) and Fischer and Jardetsky (35). Kunin, in a detailed study of the inhibition of binding of benzylpenicillin, phenoxymethylpenicillin, and o-biphenylylpenicillin, found that high concentrations of the corresponding side chain acids were effective inhibitors, but the nucleus, 6-APA, had little or no effect. Fischer and Jardetsky observed marked differences between the NMR spectra of benzylpenicillin in the presence and absence of bovine serum albumin, and these differences pointed to the benzene ring as the main binding site.

The capacity of albumin to bind penicillins is naturally not unlimited, so the proportion of bound drug (B) decreases at high concentrations. However, at the concentrations of penicillin encountered in clinical use (i.e., below $\sim 10^{-4}$ M) a given volume of serum will contain considerably more albumin molecules than penicillin molecules, and under these conditions B is almost independent of concentration (63, 91) and can be regarded as a constant characteristic of the particular penicillin. B values quoted here were measured at suitably low concentrations using an ultrafiltration technique.

Scholtan (98) determined the association constants for the binding of eight penicillins in human serum and showed them to be proportional to partition coefficients measured in isobutanol and pH 7.4 aqueous buffer. A direct relationship between the extent of binding and partition coefficients can also be demonstrated without calculating association constants, since the ratio B/F serves the same purpose (B and F being the proportions of bound and free penicillin, respectively).

Table VII shows the relation between B values and the measured partition coefficients between n-octanol and water for ten penicillins. It represents an extension of data reported by Bird and Marshall (13), who included only the first seven penicillins. Equation (18) was calculated from these figures. The calculated B values in Table VII and the fairly high correlation coefficient show that this is a reasonably good regression. The figures in parentheses are the 90% confidence limits on the slope, n is the number of points used to

$$\log(B/F) = 0.675 \, (\pm 0.221) \log P - 0.789 \qquad (18)$$

n	r	s^2
10	0.896	0.060

calculate the equation, r is the correlation coefficient, and s^2 is the residual variance.

For predictive purposes it is obviously desirable to use π values rather than measured partition coefficients. Bird and Marshall (13) obtained Eq. (19) to correlate the binding of 79 penicillins of diverse structural type.

$$\log(B/F) = 0.504 \, \pi - 0.665 \qquad (19)$$

n	r	s^2
79	0.924	0.066

$$\log(B/F) = 0.555 \, (\pm 0.046) \, \pi - 0.753 \qquad (20)$$

n	r	s^2
79	0.908	0.080

Equation (19) has subsequently been amended to Eq. (20) as a result of re-calculation of π values (see Section I).

A general equation for penicillins of diverse structure can only be obtained when π can be calculated for the complete penicillin side chain. Consequently penicillins with an isoxazole ring in the side chain were omitted from the above regression because no π value was available for this heterocycle. This was unfortunate in view of the therapeutic importance of isoxazolylpenicillins.

In such circumstances it is possible to use a new parent member of the series and to calculate π values (designated π^* to avoid confusion) for its substituted derivatives. In Table VIII data are presented for a series of oxacillin derivatives substituted in the benzene ring, oxacillin itself being regarded as the parent of the series. The π^* values were calculated from values measured for nitrobenzene derivatives (12, 37). This seems a logical choice because a 3-isoxazolyl radical attached to a benzene ring is *meta*-directing.

TABLE VII

LOG P AND OBSERVED AND CALCULATED B VALUES, WHERE P IS THE PARTITION COEFFICIENT OF THE PENICILLIN FREE ACID BETWEEN n-OCTANOL AND WATER, AND B IS PERCENT BOUND TO HUMAN SERUM

Penicillin	Log P [a]	Observed B (%)	Calculated B [b] (%)
Methicillin	1.13	49	48.5
α-Hydroxybenzyl	1.31	53.2	55.5
Benzyl	1.76	60.7	71.5
Phenoxymethyl	2.01	79.5	78.7
Phenethicillin	2.19	81.5	83
Propicillin	2.58	86.1	89.9
α-Phenoxyisopropyl	2.68	92.5	91.3
n-Heptyl	3.32	92.4	96.5
Cloxacillin	2.44	94	87.8
Dicloxacillin	2.83	97	93

[a] The log P values for the first seven penicillins differ systematically from those originally published (13). The values given here are calculated with the concentration in both phases expressed as w/v, the earlier values were with the concentration in the octanol phase expressed as w/w.
[b] Calculated from Eq. (18).

Equation (21) represents the data in Table VIII in a reasonably satisfactory regression. The residual variance is quite low and the rather low correlation coefficient is partly due to the low variance of the data; the B values range from only 79 to 99%.

$$\log(B/F) = 0.676\ (\pm 0.135)\ \pi^* + 0.946 \tag{21}$$

$$\begin{array}{ccc} n & r & s^2 \\ 23 & 0.815 & 0.044 \end{array}$$

The very different intercept in Eqs. (20) and (21) is due to the use of π in the first and π^* in the second.

TABLE VIII

π^* Values and Observed and Calculated B Values for Oxacillin
Derivatives, Where π^* Is for the Substituent X and B is Percent
Bound to Human Serum

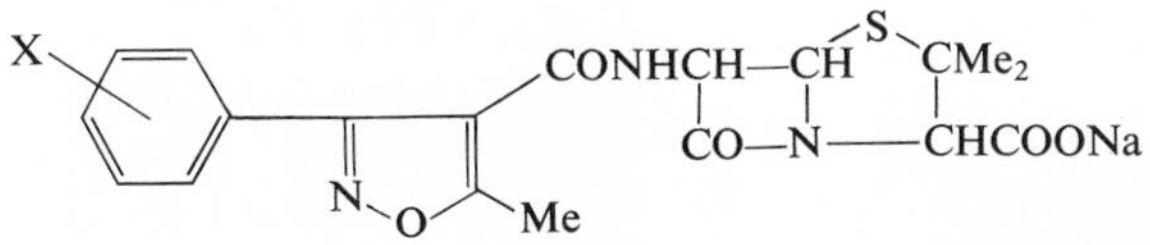

X	$\pi^{* a}$	Observed B (%)	Calculated B^b (%)
H	0	93	89.7
2-F	−0.14	91	87.7
2,6-F$_2$	−0.28	91.5	85.2
2-Cl	0.41	94	94.4
3-Cl	0.61	97	95.8
4-Cl	0.54	96	95.1
2,6-Cl$_2$	0.82	97	97.0
3,5-Cl$_2$	1.22	99	98.2
2-Br	0.58	94	95.6
4-Br	0.60	95.2	95.7
2-Cl, 6-F	0.27	94.7	93.2
2-Br, 6-F	0.44	93	94.5
2-Br, 6-Cl	0.99	96	97.6
2-Cl, 3-OH	0.56	93.6	95.4
2-Cl, 4-OH	0.52	96.5	95.2
2-Cl, 5-OH	0.56	89	95.4
2-Cl, 4-NO$_2$	0.02	81.5	90.1
2-Cl, 5-NO$_2$	0.05	80	90.5
4-OH	0.11	94.7	91.3
3-NH$_2$	−0.48	81	80.7
4-NH$_2$	−0.46	86	81.2
3-NO$_2$	−0.36	89.5	83.5
4-NO$_2$	−0.39	79	82.8

[a] π values from Bird and Marshall (12) and Fujita et al. (37) for the nitrobenzene series.
[b] Calculated from Eq. (21).

Superior regressions to the general Eq. (20) can sometimes be derived for sets of penicillins of more restricted structural type. Thus it was found that 56 penicillins containing a functional group (amine, amide, ether, or halogen) α- to the side chain amide gave Eq. (22), with a higher correlation coefficient and lower residual variance than Eq. (20). It is interesting that the slopes of

$$\log (B/F) = 0.628 \ (\pm 0.041) \ \pi - 0.807 \tag{22}$$

$$
\begin{array}{ccc}
n & r & s^2 \\
56 & 0.959 & 0.040
\end{array}
$$

Eqs. (18), (21), and (22) are similar to those found by Hansch (45) for the binding of phenols (0.681 ± 0.08), barbiturates (0.582 ± 0.35), and carboxylic acids (0.594 ± 0.22) to bovine serum albumin. However, Eq. (23), with a significantly different slope, was obtained for a set of penicillins with a hydrocarbon side chain or an aryl side chain directly linked to the amide group. The lower slope of Eq. (23) indicates that the serum binding of these penicillins

$$\log (B/F) = 0.438 \ (\pm 0.086) \ \pi - 0.693 \tag{23}$$

$$
\begin{array}{ccc}
n & r & s^2 \\
19 & 0.901 & 0.068
\end{array}
$$

does not increase with the introduction of hydrophobic substituents as steeply as the general equation (20) would predict. The explanation of this difference in slope is not apparent, but anomalies are sometimes seen with other penicillin structures. One such example is provided by 3,5-diisopropyl-4-isoxazolylpenicillin, which is not appreciably more bound than the 3,5-dimethyl analog (57 and 56%, respectively), although the former has a considerably higher π value. In spite of such occasional anomalies, the general conclusion must be that the extent of serum binding of most penicillins increases with hydrophobic character.

D. METABOLISM

Antibacterially active metabolites of several penicillins have been detected (14, 90, 92) by chromatography of urine, and the presence of a metabolite of cloxacillin in the blood has been established (90). It is probable that the penicillanic acid nucleus remains intact and the metabolic change is in the side chain. However, a definite structure has been assigned only to a metabolite of phenoxymethylpenicillin, which is reported (110) to be the p-hydroxy derivative. The metabolites are less hydrophobic than the parent penicillins, as indicated by their R_f values on paper chromatography, but it is not known whether this results in any significant pharmacological effects, such as faster excretion.

No accurate quantitative data is available for the extent of metabolite formation, but there appears to be a general tendency for it to increase with increasing partition coefficient. Thus the least hydrophobic of the penicillins tested (90), ampicillin, benzylpenicillin, and methicillin, show very little or no metabolite formation, the more hydrophobic compounds such as phenethicillin and the isoxazolyl penicillins form moderate amounts of metabolite, while the most hydrophobic compound tested, phenbenicillin, gave relatively large amounts of two different metabolites.

Such evidence as is available (*90*) suggests that the antibacterial spectrum and MIC values of these metabolites are similar to those of the parent penicillins. Consequently, metabolite formation is probably not a major factor in the efficacy of penicillins *in vivo*.

E. EXCRETION

Penicillins are excreted by both the liver and the kidney (*66*). The rate of excretion in normal individuals is quite rapid and this causes a relatively short duration of significant blood levels after administration of a single dose.

The relation of penicillin structure to excretion rates has received very little study. Kirby and his co-workers (*18, 93, 109*) have investigated the excretion of several intravenously administered penicillins in both normal individuals and those with renal failure. The results (*93*) show plasma half-lives for nonrenal excretion in the order oxacillin < cloxacillin < dicloxacillin, i.e., the more hydrophobic the compound, the slower is it excreted by the liver. However, this relation does not hold for other penicillins, because methicillin was found (*18*) to give much slower nonrenal excretion than the more hydrophobic penicillin, oxacillin.

Excretion of penicillins by the kidney involves two processes, glomerular filtration and tubular secretion, which operate by quite different mechanisms. In view of this it is not possible to relate the renal clearance values of Kirby *et al.* (*18, 93, 109*) to the penicillin structures.

The glomerular membrane is a porous structure which permits passage of low molecular weight compounds, but retains large molecules such as protein, so that drug molecules bound to protein cannot be excreted by this mechanism. Consequently, the rate of excretion of penicillins by glomerular filtration should be inversely proportional to the extent of serum binding, and so should be related to the partition coefficients of the penicillins. However, glomerular filtration appears to be less important than tubular secretion for the excretion of penicillins (*89*). One indication of this is the increased and prolonged blood levels which are obtained when the tubular secretion blocking drug probenecid, is administered with penicillins (*11, 88*). Tubular secretion is believed to involve "active transport" of the penicillins as their anions, by a general process for excretion of anions (*112*). The rate of excretion by such a mechanism will probably not be proportional to the concentration of unbound penicillin in serum, at least once this level exceeds an unknown threshold value corresponding to the capacity of the active transport mechanism. As unbound drug is removed in this way it will rapidly be replenished by dissociation of the protein complex (*38, 107*). A high level of serum binding will thus be much less of a hindrance to tubular secretion than to glomerular filtration (*89*).

The blood levels of some drugs (e.g., sulfonamides) are prolonged by reabsorption of excreted material from the concentrated urine into the bloodstream through the kidney tubules. This process probably involves passive diffusion of the un-ionized drug molecules through the lipid membrane wall of the tubules (*112*). Reabsorption seems unlikely to be important for penicillins because the aqueous phase from which it occurs will be at pH 6 or above. At this pH penicillins exist almost entirely as the lipid insoluble anions.

F. The Relation of Side Chain Structure to Blood Levels

The preceding sections have surveyed various factors which are important in determining the blood levels of penicillins. Unfortunately, the amount of data available for most penicillins is quite inadequate to enable the relative importance of these various factors to be assessed. In the circumstances it is not surprising that no general relationship between blood levels and side chain structure has been discerned. Nevertheless, some logical patterns do emerge for penicillins of restricted structural types. Thus for the four α-phenoxyalkylpenicillins which have been used clinically, the serum levels following oral administration are in the sequence phenoxymethyl $< \alpha$-phenoxyethyl $< \alpha$-phenoxypropyl $< \alpha$-phenoxybenzyl (*70*), which is also the order of increasing hydrophobic character. In the isoxazole series a similar sequence (i.e., oxacillin $<$ cloxacillin $<$ dicloxacillin) is found for both intravenous (*93*) and oral (*9, 61, 77*) administration. In these series increasing hydrophobic character probably facilitates absorption from the gut and this is one likely cause of the blood level sequence. However, the results (*93*) for intravenously administered isoxazole penicillins suggest that the rates of excretion of these compounds also differ in such a way as to produce the observed blood level sequence. It is not known whether there is any mechanistic relation between these differing excretion rates and the hydrophobic character of the penicillins. It should be pointed out that from the therapeutic viewpoint the high total blood levels found in the more hydrophobic members of these series do not represent pure gain, because the more hydrophobic compounds are also the more serum bound (see Tables VII and VIII). It is the unbound penicillin which is antibacterially active, and the concentration of this does not necessarily parallel the total blood levels.

IV. Derivatives Which Liberate Penicillins *in Vivo*

Various attempts have been made to overcome the problem of the rapid elimination of benzylpenicillin from the body following injection of the readily water-soluble sodium or potassium salts. Many sparingly soluble salts have been prepared from benzylpenicillin and organic bases, and two which have been widely employed clinically are the procaine salt (*101*) and the *N,N'*-dibenzylethylenediamine salt (*104*). When suspensions of these salts are injected intramuscularly soluble penicillin is only slowly released and hence is found in the bloodstream over a prolonged period. With such preparations only infrequent injections are required, but it must be stressed that the longer duration of the blood levels is only achieved at the cost of a much lower concentration at any one time. Such preparations can therefore only be recommended for therapeutic use when the infecting organism is very sensitive to penicillin.

Another type of derivative which achieves the same purpose as the above sparingly soluble salts, though with rather less prolongation of the blood levels, consists of certain penicillin esters which undergo particularly ready hydrolysis with liberation of the active drug. The first of these to achieve popularity was the 2-diethylaminoethyl ester of benzylpenicillin, generally injected as the sparingly water-soluble hydroiodide (*36, 58*). A more recent introduction is the acetoxymethyl ester of benzylpenicillin (penamecillin), which is moderately well absorbed in animals and man after oral administration (*5, 25*). An enzyme in the blood apparently hydrolyzes penamecillin to acetic acid, formaldehyde, and free benzylpenicillin. Various acyloxymethyl esters of ampicillin (**IV**) are also readily hydrolyzed in blood, and exceptionally high serum levels of ampicillin are observed following oral administration of the pivaloyloxymethyl ester (pivampicin) (*23b*). It is unlikely that the above esters have any significant antibacterial activity per se, since simple esters which do not hydrolyze readily are relatively inactive.

An example of modification of a different part of the molecule is provided by hetacillin, an interesting cyclic structure (**XVIII**) prepared by condensation of ampicillin (**IV**) with acetone (*52*). Here again it is doubtful whether hetacillin has significant antibacterial activity per se since in other penicillins activity usually requires an unsubstituted amide nitrogen in the side chain [e.g., *N*-alkyl derivatives of phenoxymethylpenicillin are essentially inactive (*68*)].

$$\text{PhCH—CO}$$
$$\text{HN}\diagdown\begin{array}{c}|\\ \text{CMe}_2\end{array}\diagup\text{N—CH—CH}\diagup^{S}\diagdown\text{CMe}_2$$
$$\text{CO—N——CHCOOH}$$

XVIII

However, the reaction between ampicillin and acetone is readily reversible so that in neutral dilute aqueous solution hetacillin undergoes rapid hydrolysis with liberation of ampicillin, and the apparent antibacterial activities of the two compounds are identical.

In view of these properties it is hardly to be expected that hetacillin given by injection would act any differently from ampicillin. On the other hand, hydrolysis of hetacillin to ampicillin occurs much more slowly at acid than at neutral pH, so it is conceivable that a substantial proportion of an oral dose of hetacillin could be absorbed as such and only liberate ampicillin in the bloodstream. If this occurred the blood level picture would not necessarily be the same as that following oral administration of ampicillin. Unfortunately, the comparative blood levels following oral administration of hetacillin and ampicillin are subject to conflicting reports. American laboratories report hetacillin peak levels equal to or greater than those of ampicillin (*19, 109*), but European studies indicate that ampicillin gives a substantially higher peak (*71, 87, 103*). It seems to be agreed that the peak occurs later with hetacillin than with ampicillin and that the blood levels 6–8 hr after dosing are higher with hetacillin, but by this time the levels of both drugs are so low that only the most sensitive bacteria could be expected to respond.

V. Concluding Remarks

An entirely rational approach to the design of clinically useful penicillins remains a distant goal, although some success has been achieved in relating structure to particular biological properties. The quantitative regressions of MIC values presented in Section I,A are of strictly limited predictive value, and it seems that a parameter other than π, σ or E_s would be necessary to obtain more generally applicable regressions. The relative positions in space of the various functional groups in the molecule may be important, but it is not obvious how this could be expressed in a mathematical parameter. The successful use of the qualitative concept of steric hindrance near the side chain amide group in designing penicillins which resist hydrolysis by β-lactamase illustrates the importance of steric factors.

Much progress has been made in elucidating the mode of action of penicillins on the bacterial cell, but this has not as yet proved helpful in designing improved pencillins.

The stability or instability of penicillins in acid has been correlated with the inductive effect of side chain substituents. This has enabled acid-stable penicillins to be designed, many of which are suitable for oral administration. The blood levels of penicillins, as of other drugs, are a resultant of many interacting factors and no general relationship to side chain structure has been demonstrated. Nevertheless, the good correlation found between π and the extent of serum binding represents a useful first step toward predicting the behavior of penicillins *in vivo*.

ACKNOWLEDGMENT

The authors are indebted to numerous colleagues who prepared and tested many of the penicillins discussed, and particularly to Dr. G. N. Rolinson and Mr. R. Sutherland for measurements of serum binding and MIC values and to Mr. A. C. Marshall for his major contribution to the regression analyses.

REFERENCES

1. E. P. Abraham, *G. Microbiol.* **2**, 102 (1956).
2. E. P. Abraham, W. Baker, W. R. Boon, C. T. Calam, H. C. Carrington, E. Chain, H. W. Florey, G. G. Freeman, R. Robinson, and A. G. Sanders, *in* "The Chemistry of Penicillin" (H. T. Clarke, J. R. Johnson, and R. Robinson, eds.), Chapter 2, p. 10. Princeton Univ. Press, Princeton, New Jersey, 1949.
3. E. P. Abraham and E. Chain, *Nature (London)* **146**, 837 (1940).
4. G. Acocella, G. C. Baroni, and F. B. Nicolis, *Curr. Ther. Res., Clin. Exp.* **7**, 226 (1965).
5. H. P. K. Agersborg, A. Batchelor, G. W. Cambridge, and A. W. Rule, *Brit. J. Pharmacol.* **26**, 649 (1966).
6. G. B. Barlin and D. D. Perrin, *Quart. Rev. Chem. Soc.* **20**, 75 (1966).
7. F. R. Batchelor, F. P. Doyle, J. H. C. Nayler, and G. N. Rolinson, *Nature (London)* **183**, 257 (1959).
8. O. K. Behrens and M. J. Kingkade, *J. Biol. Chem.* **176**, 1047 (1948).
9. J. V. Bennett, C. F. Gravenkemper, J. L. Brodie, and W. M. M. Kirby, *Antimicrob. Ag. Chemother.* p. 257 (1965).
10. J. V. Bennett and W. M. M. Kirby, *J. Lab. Clin. Med.* **66**, 721 (1965).
11. K. H. Beyer, H. F. Russo, E. K. Tillson, A. K. Miller, W. F. Verwey, and S. R. Grass, *Amer. J. Physiol.* **166**, 625 (1951).
11a. G. L. Biagi, M. C. Guerra, A. M. Barbaro, and M. F. Gamba, *J. Med. Chem.* **13**, 511 (1970).
12. A. E. Bird and A. C. Marshall, unpublished work (1968).
13. A. E. Bird and A. C. Marshall, *Biochem. Pharmacol.* **16**, 2275 (1967).
14. J. M. Bond, M. Barber, J. W. Lightbown, and P. M. Waterworth, *Brit. Med. J.* **2**, 956 (1963).
15. E. G. Brain, F. P. Doyle, K. Hardy, A. A. W. Long, M. D. Mehta, D. Miller, J. H. C. Nayler, M. J. Soulal, E. R. Stove, and G. R. Thomas, *J. Chem. Soc.* p. 1445 (1962).
16. E. G. Brain, F. P. Doyle, M. D. Mehta, D. Miller, J. H. C. Nayler, and E. R. Stove, *J. Chem. Soc.* p. 491 (1963).
17. B. B. Brodie, *in* "Absorption and Distribution of Drugs" (T. B. Binns, ed.), p. 16. Livingstone, Edinburgh and London, 1964.

18. R. J. Bulger, D. D. Lindholm, J. S. Murray, and W. M. M. Kirby, *J. Amer. Med. Ass.* **187**, 319 (1964).
19. P. A. Bunn, S. Milicich, and J. S. Lunn, *Antimicrob. Ag. Chemother.* p. 947 (1966).
20. M. Charton, *J. Org. Chem.* **29**, 1222 (1964).
21. N. Citri and M. R. Pollock, *Advan. Enzymol.* **28**, 237 (1966).
22. N. Citri and N. Zyk, *Biochim. Biophys. Acta* **99**, 427 (1965).
23. P. D. Cooper, *Bacteriol. Rev.* **20**, 28 (1956).
23a. E. A. P. Croydon and R. Sutherland, *Antimicrob. Ag. Chemother.* (in press) (1970).
23b. W. V. Daehne, E. Frederiksen, E. Gundersen, F. Lund, P. Mørch, H. J. Petersen, K. Rohort, L. Tybring, and W. O. Godtfredsen, *J. Med. Chem.* **13**, 607 (1970).
24. N. Datta and M. H. Richmond, *Biochem. J.* **98**, 204 (1966).
25. J. Demonty, *Rev. Med. Liege* **20**, 168 (1965).
26. R. H. Depue, A. G. Moat, and A. Bondi, *Arch. Biochem. Biophys.* **107**, 374 (1964).
27. F. P. Doyle, J. C. Hanson, A. A. W. Long, and J. H. C. Nayler, *J. Chem. Soc.* p. 5845 (1963).
28. F. P. Doyle, J. C. Hanson, A. A. W. Long, J. H. C. Nayler, and E. R. Stove, *J. Chem. Soc.* p. 5838 (1963).
29. F. P. Doyle, K. Hardy, J. H. C. Nayler, M. J. Soulal, E. R. Stove, and H. R. J. Waddington, *J. Chem. Soc.* p. 1453 (1962).
30. F. P. Doyle, A. A. W. Long, J. H. C. Nayler, and E. R. Stove, *Nature (London)* **192**, 1183 (1961).
31. F. P. Doyle and J. H. C. Nayler, *Advan. Drug Res.* **1**, 1 (1964).
32. F. P. Doyle, J. H. C. Nayler, H. Smith, and E. R. Stove, *Nature (London)* **191**, 1091 (1961).
33. F. P. Doyle, J. H. C. Nayler, H. R. J. Waddington, J. C. Hanson, and G. R. Thomas, *J. Chem. Soc.* p. 497 (1963).
34. A. R. English and T. J. McBride, *Antimicrob. Ag. Chemother.* p. 636 (1962).
35. J. J. Fischer and O. Jardetsky, *J. Amer. Chem. Soc.* **87**, 3237 (1965).
36. H. F. Flippin, W. V. Matteucci, N. H. Schimmel, L. E. Bartholomew, and W. P. Boger, *Antibiot. Chemother. (Washington, D.C.)* **2**, 208 (1952).
37. T. Fujita, J. Iwasa, and C. Hansch, *J. Amer. Chem. Soc.* **86**, 5175 (1964).
38. A. Goldstein, *Pharmacol. Rev.* **1**, 102 (1949).
39. A. Gourevitch, G. A. Hunt, J. J. Luttinger, C. C. Carmack, and J. Lein, *Proc. Soc. Exp. Biol. Med.* **107**, 455 (1961).
40. A. Gourevitch, T. A. Pursiano, and J. Lein, *Antimicrob. Ag. Chemother.* p. 318 (1963).
41. A. Gourevitch, S. Wolfe, and J. Lein, *Antimicrob. Ag. Chemother.* p. 576 (1962).
42. J. M. T. Hamilton-Miller, *Biochem. J.* **87**, 209 (1963).
43. C. K. Hancock, E. A. Meyers, and B. T. Yager, *J. Amer. Chem. Soc.* **83**, 4211 (1961).
44. C. Hansch, *in* "Physico-Chemical Aspects of Drug Action" (E. J. Ariëns, ed.), Vol. 7, p. 141. Pergamon Press, Oxford, 1968.
45. C. Hansch, *Farmaco, Ed. Sci.* **23**, 293 (1968).
45a. C. Hansch, *Accounts Chem. Res.* **2**, 232 (1969).
46. C. Hansch and S. M. Anderson, *J. Org. Chem.* **32**, 2583 (1967).
47. C. Hansch and E. W. Deutsch, *J. Med. Chem.* **8**, 705 (1965).
48. C. Hansch and A. R. Steward, *J. Med. Chem.* **7**, 691 (1964).
49. C. Hansch, A. R. Steward, S. M. Anderson, and D. Bentley, *J. Med. Chem.* **11**, 1 (1967).
50. J. C. Hanson, A. A. W. Long, J. H. C. Nayler, and E. R. Stove, *J. Chem. Soc.* p. 5976 (1965).
51. J. C. Hanson, J. H. C. Nayler, T. Taylor, and P. H. Gore, *J. Chem. Soc.* p. 5984 (1965).

52. G. A. Hardcastle, D. A. Johnson, C. A. Panetta, A. I. Scott, and S. A. Sutherland, *J. Org. Chem.* **31**, 897 (1966).
53. K. R. Henery-Logan and A. M. Limburg, *Tetrahedron Lett.* p. 4915 (1966).
54. J. R. E. Hoover, A. W. Chow, R. J. Stedman, N. M. Hall, H. S. Greenberg, M. M. Dolan, and R. J. Ferlauto, *J. Med. Chem.* **7**, 245 (1964).
54a. J. P. Hou and J. W. Poole, *J. Pharm. Sci.* **58**, 1510 (1969).
55. J. Iwasa, T. Fujita, and C. Hansch, *J. Med. Chem.* **8**, 150 (1965).
56. K. Izaki, M. Matsuhashi, and J. L. Strominger, *J. Biol. Chem.* **243**, 3180 (1968).
57. H. H. Jaffé *Chem. Rev.* **53**, 191 (1953).
58. K. A. Jensen, P. J. Dragstedt, I. Kioer, E. J. Nielsen, and E. Fredericksen, *Acta Pathol. Microbiol. Scand.* **28**, 407 (1951); *Chem. Abstr.* **45**, 9732 (1951).
59. J. R. Johnson, R. B. Woodward, and R. Robinson, *in* "The Chemistry of Penicillin" (H. T. Clarke, J. R. Johnson, and R. Robinson, eds.), p. 440. Princeton Univ. Press, Princeton, New Jersey, 1949.
60. J. E. Kasik and L. Peacham, *Biochem. J.* **107**, 675 (1968).
61. T. Knott, A. Lange, and R. Volkening, *Arzneim.-Forsch.* **15**, 331 (1965).
62. E. T. Knudsen, G. N. Rolinson, and R. Sutherland, *Brit. Med. J.* **3**, 75 (1967).
63. C. M. Kunin, *J. Lab. Clin. Med.* **65**, 416 (1965).
64. C. M. Kunin, *Clin. Pharmacol. Ther.* **7**, 166 (1966).
65. C. M. Kunin, *Antimicrob. Ag. Chemother.* p. 1025 (1966).
66. C. M. Kunin and M. Finland, *J. Clin. Invest.* **38**, 1509 (1959).
67. J. E. Leffler and E. Grunwald, "Rates and Equilibria of Organic Reactions." Wiley, New York, 1963.
68. T. Leigh, *J. Chem. Soc.* p. 3616 (1965).
69. E. J. Lien, C. Hansch, and S. M. Anderson, *J. Med. Chem.* **11**, 430 (1968).
70. B. Lynn, *Antibiot. Chemother.* *(Basel)* **13**, 123 (1965).
71. L. Magni, B. Ortengren, B. Sjöberg, and S. Wahlqvist, *Scand. J. Clin. Lab. Invest.* **20**, 195 (1967).
72. M. J. Mardle, J. H. C. Nayler, D. W. Rustidge, and H. R. J. Waddington, *J. Chem. Soc.,* C p. 237 (1968).
73. H. H. Martin, *Annu. Rev. Biochem.* **35**, Part 2, 457 (1966).
74. V. Meyer and J. J. Sudborough, *Ber. Deut. Chem. Ges.* **27**, 1580 and 3146 (1894).
75. R. G. Micetich and R. Raap, *J. Med. Chem.* **11**, 159 (1968).
76. D. B. Miller, J. H. C. Nayler, and H. R. J. Waddington, *J. Chem. Soc.,* C p. 242 (1968).
77. P. Naumann and B. Kempf, *Arzneim.-Forsch.* **15**, 331 (1965).
78. R. P. Novick, *Biochem. J.* **83**, 229 (1962).
79. E. F. Panarin, M. V. Solovsky, and O. N. Ekzemplyarov, *Antibiotiki* **12**, 643 (1967).
79a. E. F. Panarin and M. V. Solovsky, *Antibiotiki* **15**, 426 (1970).
80. J. T. Park and J. L. Strominger, *Science* **125**, 99 (1957).
81. A. Percival, W. Brumfitt, and J. de Louvois, *J. Gen. Microbiol.* **32**, 77 (1963).
82. Y. G. Perron, W. F. Minor, L. B. Crast, A. Gourevitch, J. Lein, and L. C. Cheney, *J. Med. Pharm. Chem.* **5**, 1016 (1962).
83. K. E. Price, A. Gourevitch, and L. C. Cheney, *Antimicrob. Ag. Chemother.* p. 670 (1967).
84. A. Quilico, *in* "The Chemistry of Heterocyclic Compounds—5 and 6 Membered Compounds with N and O" (R. H. Wiley, ed.), p. 41. Wiley (Interscience), New York, 1962.
85. H. D. C. Rapson and A. E. Bird, *J. Pharm. Pharmacol.* **15**, Suppl., 222T (1963).
86. H. C. Richards, J. R. Housley, and D. F. Spooner, *Nature (London)* **199**, 354 (1963).
87. M. Ridley, *Brit. Med. J.* **3**, 305 (1967).
88. O. P. W. Robinson, *Brit. J. Clin. Pathol.* **18**, 593 (1964).

89. G. N. Rolinson, *in* "Recent Advances in Medical Microbiology" (A. P. Waterson, ed.), p. 254. Churchill, London, 1966.

90. G. N. Rolinson and F. R. Batchelor, *Antimicrob. Ag. Chemother.* p. 654 (1963).

91. G. N. Rolinson and R. Sutherland, *Brit. J. Pharmacol.* **25**, 638 (1965).

92. I. F. Rollo, G. F. Somers, and D. M. Burley, *Brit. Med. J.* **1**, 76 (1962).

93. J. E. Rosenblatt, A. C. Kind, J. L. Brodie, and W. M. M. Kirby, *Arch. Intern. Med.* **121**, 345 (1968).

94. S. B. Rosenmann and G. H. Warren, *Antimicrob. Ag. Chemother.* p. 611 (1962).

94a. S. B. Rosenmann, L. S. Weber, G. Owen, and G. H. Warren, *Antimicrob. Ag. Chemother.* p. 590 (1967).

95. L. D. Sabath, M. Jago, and E. P. Abraham, *Biochem. J.* **96**, 739 (1965).

96. L. S. Schanker, *Advan. Drug Res.* **1**, 71 (1964).

97. W. Scholtan, *Arzneim.-Forsch.* **13**, 347 (1963).

98. W. Scholtan, *Arzneim.-Forsch.* **18**, 505 (1968).

98a. J. C. Sheehan and K. R. Henery-Logan, *J. Amer. Chem. Soc.* **79**, 1262 (1957).

99. J. T. Smith and J. M. T. Hamilton-Miller, *Nature (London)* **197**, 976 (1963).

100. J. L. Strominger, K. Izaki, M. Matsushashi, and D. J. Tipper, *Fed. Proc., Fed. Amer. Soc. Exp. Biol.* **26**, 947 (1967).

101. N. P. Sullivan, A. T. Symmes, H. C. Miller, and H. W. Rhodehamel, *Science* **107**, 169 (1948).

102. R. Sutherland, *J. Gen. Microbiol.* **34**, 85 (1964).

103. R. Sutherland and O. P. W. Robinson, *Brit. Med. J.* **2**, 804 (1967).

104. J. L. Szabo, C. D. Edwards, and W. F. Bruce, *Antibiot. Chemother.* **1**, 499 (1951).

105. R. W. Taft, *in* "Steric Effects in Organic Chemistry" (M. S. Newman, ed.), p. 598. Wiley, New York, 1956.

106. E. H. Thiele and H. J. Robinson, *Appl. Microbiol.* **16**, 228 (1968).

107. J. M. Thorp, *in* "Absorption and Distribution of Drugs" (T. B. Binns, ed.), p. 64. Livingstone, Edinburgh and London, 1964.

108. D. J. Tipper and J. L. Strominger, *Proc. Nat. Acad. Sci. U.S.* **54**, 75 (1965).

109. S. B. Tuano, L. D. Johnson, J. L. Brodie, and W. M. M. Kirby, *N. Engl. Med. J.* **275**, 635 (1966).

110. H. Vanderhaege, G. Parmentier, and E. Evrard, *Nature (London)* **200**, 891 (1963).

111. G. H. Warren, *Chemotherapia* **10**, 339 (1965-1966).

112. I. M. Weiner and G. H. Mudge, *Amer. J. Med.* **36**, 743 (1964).

113. E. Wise and J. Park, *Proc. Nat. Acad. Sci. U.S.* **54**, 75 (1965).

Chapter 9 The Design of Peptide Hormone Analogs

J. Rudinger

I. Introduction

Since du Vigneaud and his co-workers demonstrated in 1953 (*569, 570*) that the synthesis of complex physiologically active peptides is feasible, considerable effort has been devoted to the synthesis of naturally occurring peptides and their structural analogs. With the successive isolation and structural elucidation of further biologically active natural peptides the scope of this work has broadened and with improvements in the methods and techniques of peptide synthesis it has become more productive, sometimes to the point of routine. Well over a thousand peptides have by now been prepared in this context and it becomes relevant to inquire how the problems of drug design are being met in this special field.

A. SPECIAL FEATURES OF PEPTIDES AS DRUGS

Peptides differ from most other drugs in several respects which are, or should be, important for the structural design and biological investigation of structural analogs.

1. Peptides are built up of obvious and stereotyped structural units—the amino acids. This trivial fact understandably dominates the synthetic procedures which, with rare exceptions, use amino acids as the starting materials; but it has also had an almost hypnotic effect on interpretative thinking which tends to consider individual amino acids and their side chains rather than properties of the molecule as a whole, or of topochemical regions (see *220, 434, 439, 489, 492, 515*) involving parts of several, not necessarily adjacent amino acid residues.

2. Their molecules are relatively large—this is obvious when we compare a small peptide hormone such as oxytocin (MW 1008) with a large steroid drug such as dexamethasone (MW 382). Moreover, linear or even cyclic peptides have a great deal of conformational freedom. This is presumably limited by noncovalent interactions but the extent and manner of such conformational stabilization is as yet virtually unknown. It is therefore difficult to define the topochemical regions important for biological activity and to predict the effects of structural changes on the overall topochemistry of the molecule. Results and concepts drawn from the rapidly developing field of structural protein chemistry should be of assistance here.

3. Peptides are metabolically less stable than most classes of drugs because of the ubiquity of peptidases with varied specificity. A knowledge of the distribution and disposition would therefore be exceptionally important in the design of peptide drugs. However, such knowledge is particularly difficult to obtain by conventional methods because of the analytical difficulties in identifying small amounts of peptides or their degradation products in the presence of large amounts of chemically similar endogenous materials (proteins and peptides).

4. The design of potential peptide drugs is almost invariably based on natural prototypes—peptide hormones, toxins, or antibiotics. Only exception-

ally has a screening approach predominated in the search for biologically active peptides.* In this review, only the design of hormone analogs and certain closely related compounds will be considered.

5. The peptide hormones are among the biologically most active compounds known. Not infrequently doses in the picomole (10^{-12} mole) range are active. As a consequence, even analogs less active by two or three orders of magnitude than the prototype are still very potent compounds by pharmacological standards and activities lower by five or six orders of ten can often still be detected.

6. Peptide hormones may have more than one distinct effect even in physiological concentrations. In higher concentrations, they generally act on a wide range of target tissues or organs. Changes in structure may alter the activity profile and thereby change the specificity even to the point where an "unphysiological" effect may predominate.

7. As a result of evolutionary processes the naturally occurring peptide hormones may differ in structure and also in physiological function in different species, classes, and phyla. By evolutionary mechanisms, too, families of structurally related peptides with different activity profiles have come to serve different physiological functions within the same organism. The study of such series or families can provide early information on structure–activity relations and suggest not only further structural variations but also additional biological systems as potential targets.

B. Scope of the Review and Some General Considerations

The structures of the hormonal peptides which have been subjected to variation in synthetic analogs are given in Table I together with their most important biological effects. Included are angiotensin and the kinins, although their physiological function as hormones has not been established; amphibian toxins such as caerulein, phyllokinin, and the insect venom, polistes kinin, because of their obvious relation to the mammalian peptides with which they are grouped; and the toxins eledoisin and physalaemin because their pharmacology, if not their structure is related to that of the kinins and the approach to the design of analogs has been the same as for true peptide hormones. Work on peptide antibiotics will be referred to only occasionally in particular contexts. Secretin, glucagon, and the calcitonin group of hormones have not been included; although they have been successfully synthesized (68, 196, 427, 520, 603) no analogs have been reported within the period covered by this review. Certain partial sequences which do not themselves occur naturally but have been the subject of extensive structural variations are also listed.

---

* As in screening for antibacterial (510–512) or antiviral (368) activity or in the design of "carriers" for potential carcinostatics (40–42, 301, 519).

A few words should be said about the ribonuclease-S system. The enzyme, pancreatic ribonuclease A, can be cleaved with subtilisin to afford an eicosa-peptide (S-peptide) and a residual protein (S-protein) of 104 amino acids. Either fragment alone is inactive but together they form a noncovalent complex (ribonuclease-S) with practically full ribonuclease activity (*418*). It has been appreciated (*213, 351, 429, 443*) that this system constitutes a useful model for peptide hormones and their receptors and analogs of S peptide have, in fact, been designed along much the same lines as analogs of the peptide hormones (*160, 216, 505*). Although this work has been very interesting and instructive it is not directly concerned with the design of drugs and will therefore be referred to only sporadically to illustrate specific points.

The problem of designing analogs of biologically active peptides is coextensive in its experimental aspects with the study of structure–activity relations. The difference is one of emphasis: Whereas in a discussion of structure–activity relationships it is primarily the information gained in such studies which is of interest, a discussion of design will be concerned with the ways in which such information can best be obtained and in turn utilized for the guidance of further synthetic work.

The structure–activity relationships for analogs of the peptide hormones have repeatedly been summarized and discussed in reviews and monographs covering the whole field* (*214, 220, 491, 637, 477, 478*) or dealing with specific hormones [oxytocin and vasopressin (*451, 78, 30, 431,* especially *439; 587, 32, 33,* especially *34* and *444; 643*); the angiotensins (*504, 384, 490*); bradykinin (*473*); the corticotropins (*230, 323, 214, 489, 490, 491, 216, 407*) and melanotropins (*213, 230, 323, 74, 489, 490, 491, 407, 312*); gastrin (*349, 350*); and insulin (*600*)]. A number of symposia have been devoted to the peptide hormones and their synthetic analogs (*99, 454, 145, 431, 147, 18, 340*) or have included important contributions on this topic (*95, 629, 94, 402, 55, 92*).

This chapter is not intended to recapitulate or even summarize the information which is thoroughly and adequately presented in these reviews; rather will an attempt be made to describe some of the approaches used in exploring the field and the actual structure–activity relations will be referred to only to illustrate the results of such approaches. No attempt will be made to treat the subject exhaustively.

Obviously the word design implies a particular purpose and we must ask what purpose the synthesis of analogs is to serve. Generally speaking, one aim is to obtain analogs which have some advantage over the natural hormone in a practical way; and another, to gain knowledge of various aspects of hormone action including physiological, biochemical, and molecular mechanisms of action. These aims are not distinct. Few would deny that results of

---

* In this paragraph references will be listed in chronological order for greater convenience in selecting recent reviews.

practical significance are hardly ever obtained without some contribution from a knowledge of structure–activity relations at a more than purely empirical level, and, on the other hand, significant advances in analytical knowledge can and should be applied to the design of useful compounds. However, the approach of a particular investigator to the problem of analog design will frequently be biased toward one or other of these aims.

As regards the more generally conceived approaches to structure–activity relations, their biological motivation can often be fairly defined by the question "let's see what happens if ..." and in discussing this work in the first part of this chapter we shall therefore emphasize the structural aspect—the way in which particular structural alterations were decided on and achieved. Pure empiricism has been rare; usually, more or less rational or at least systematic approaches have been used although, as in other fields, chance observations have often served as starting points for lines of thought, and design, independent of the original concept.

Practical utility or potential, as a more stringently defined aim, can result from any one of a number of features such as increased potency, increased selectivity (even at the expense of potency), a modified (generally prolonged) time course of action, greater stability, the ability to inhibit the action of the natural hormone, the presence of useful "markers," or even simplified synthesis. We shall discuss some approaches to these goals under separate headings in the second part of this chapter.

Sometimes the biological end effect aimed at and the principles of design followed to achieve it are explicitly stated. More often, however, the motivation of such work is only implicit or even obscure, or the lines of research directed toward such aims developed from incidental observations rather than a priori considerations. Most leading investigators in this field have at some time set out their ideas on the subject in reviews or lectures and the appropriate papers should be consulted for the authentic views of Bernardi (*8, 51*), Bodanszky (*70*), Boissonnas and Berde (*32, 36, 37, 73–76*), Bumpus and Page (*384, 531*), Havinga (*202, 203*), Hofmann (*213, 215, 216, 220, 230*), Li (*323, 407*), Morley (*349–351*), Nicolaides (*366*), Rudinger and Šorm (*275, 434, 439, 440, 443, 445*), Schröder and Lübke (*332, 336, 469*), Schwyzer (*486–490, 492, 504*), Stewart and Woolley (*537, 540–542*), and du Vigneaud (*266, 563*). If, in interpreting the intentions and reasoning of these or other authors, I have read too extensively between the lines of their published work and imputed to them thoughts or motives which were foreign to them, I ask to be forgiven.

C. Nomenclature and Symbolism

The abbreviations for amino acid residues and substituent groups (*254*) and the designation of synthetic modifications of natural peptides (*255*)

TABLE I

STRUCTURES OF SOME PEPTIDE HORMONES AND RELATED PEPTIDES,[a] AND SOME CHARACTERISTIC BIOLOGICAL TEST SYSTEMS

Neurohypophysial Hormones

Oxytocin:

$$\overset{1}{Cys}-\overset{2}{Tyr}-\overset{3}{Ile}-\overset{4}{Gln}-\overset{5}{Asn}-\overset{6}{Cys}-\overset{7}{Pro}-\overset{8}{Leu}-\overset{9}{Gly}-NH_2$$

Arginine vasopressin:

$$Cys-Tyr-Phe-Gln-Asn-Cys-Pro-Arg-Gly-NH_2$$

Lysine vasopressin:

$$Cys-Tyr-Phe-Gln-Asn-Cys-Pro-Lys-Gly-NH_2$$

Vasotocin:

$$Cys-Tyr-Ile-Gln-Asn-Cys-Pro-Arg-Gly-NH_2$$

Oxytocin contracts the uterus *in vitro* and *in situ*, lowers the blood pressure of the fowl, and increases the milk-ejection pressure in lactating mammals. The vasopressins cause antidiuresis and increase the blood pressure of the rat. Vasotocin increases the osmotic flow of water through the toad bladder or frog skin and stimulates the active transport of sodium by the same membranes. Each hormone shows in some degree the activities characteristic of the others (see, e.g., 33). Lysine vasopressin has been found in some *suina*, arginine vasopressin in all other mammals. Mesotocin ([Ile^8]-oxytocin), isotocin ([Ser^4,Ile^8]-oxytocin) and glumitocin ([Ser^4,Gln^8]-oxytocin) have been found in lower vertebrates.

Corticotropin–Melanotropin–Lipotropin Family

α-Melanotropin:

$$\overset{1}{Ac}-\overset{}{Ser}-\overset{2}{Tyr}-\overset{3}{Ser}-\overset{4}{Met}-\overset{5}{Glu}-\overset{6}{His}-\overset{7}{Phe}-\overset{8}{Arg}-\overset{9}{Trp}-\overset{10}{Gly}-\overset{11}{Lys}-\overset{12}{Pro}-\overset{13}{Val}-NH_2$$

β$_p$-Melanotropin: Asp-Ser-Glu-Gly-Pro-Tyr-Lys-Met-Glu-His-Phe-Arg-Trp-Gly-Ser-Pro-Pro-Lys-Asp

"Pentamelatrin":

$$\overset{1}{His}-\overset{2}{Phe}-\overset{3}{Arg}-\overset{4}{Trp}-\overset{5}{Gly}$$

α$_p$-Corticotropin:

$$\overset{1}{Ser}-\overset{2}{Tyr}-\overset{3}{Ser}-\overset{4}{Met}-\overset{5}{Glu}-\overset{6}{His}-\overset{7}{Phe}-\overset{8}{Arg}-\overset{9}{Trp}-\overset{10}{Gly}-\overset{11}{Lys}-\overset{12}{Pro}-\overset{13}{Val}-\overset{14}{Gly}-\overset{15}{Lys}-\overset{16}{Lys}-\overset{17}{Arg}-\overset{18}{Arg}-\overset{19}{Pro}-\overset{20}{Val}-$$
$$\overset{21}{Lys}-\overset{22}{Val}-\overset{23}{Tyr}-\overset{24}{Pro}-\overset{25}{Asp}-\overset{26}{Gly}-\overset{27}{Ala}-\overset{28}{Glu}-\overset{29}{Asp}-\overset{30}{Gln}-\overset{31}{Leu}-\overset{32}{Ala}-\overset{33}{Glu}-\overset{34}{Ala}-\overset{35}{Phe}-\overset{36}{Pro}-\overset{37}{Leu}-\overset{38}{Glu}-\overset{39}{Phe}$$

"Tetracosactide":

$$\overset{21}{Lys}-\overset{22}{Val}-\overset{23}{Tyr}-\overset{24}{Pro}$$

The corticotropins stimulate adrenal synthesis and release of corticosteroids. Their metabolic actions include a hypoglycemic effect and lipolytic action on adipose tissue or fat cells. They have melanotropic activity. The melanotropins cause melanin dispersion in amphibian melanocytes. They have lipolytic and traces of corticotropic activity. The lipotropins (not shown) contain β-melanotropin sequences in larger structures; their most conspicuous action is lipolysis (see, e.g., 312, 407). Porcine corticotropin and β-melanotropin are shown; other mammalian corticotropins differ in sequence positions 25–33.

Angiotensins

	1	2	3	4	5	6	7	8	
Angiotensin$_b$ II:	Asp–Arg–Val–Tyr–Val–His–Pro–Phe
Angiotensin$_e$ II:	Asp–Arg–Val–Tyr–Ile –His–Pro–Phe
Angiotensin$_e$ I:	Asp–Arg–Val–Tyr–Ile –His–Pro–Phe–His–Leu
"Renin substrate":	Asp–Arg–Val–Tyr–Ile –His–Pro–Phe–His–Leu–Leu–Val–Tyr–Ser–...

Angiotensins II contract smooth muscle (uterus, ileum) and constrict blood vessels, causing an increase in blood pressure in rats and other mammals. Other effects (interaction with the adrenergic and cholinergic systems, renal actions) have been studied with synthetic analogs only exceptionally (see, e.g., 384, 388, 504). Subscript b stands for bovine, e for equine.

Kinins

	1	2	3	4	5	6	7	8	9
Bradykinin:		Arg–Pro–Pro–Gly–Phe–Ser–Pro–Phe–Arg
Kallidin:	Lys–Arg–Pro–Pro–Gly–Phe–Ser–Pro–Phe–Arg
Methionyl-lysyl-bradykinin:	Met–Lys–Arg–Pro–Pro–Gly–Phe–Ser–Pro–Phe–Arg
Phyllokinin:		Arg–Pro–Pro–Gly–Phe–Ser–Pro–Phe–Arg–Ile–Tyr–SO_3H
Polistes kinin:	⎕–Glu–Thr–Asn–Lys–Lys–Leu–Arg–Gly–Arg–Pro–Pro–Gly–Phe–Ser–Pro–Phe– Arg

The kinins cause contraction of uterine, some intestinal, and bronchial smooth muscle. They cause vasodilation and therefore have a hypotensive effect in mammals. Capillary permeability is increased (see, e.g., 146, 544).

TABLE I—*continued*

Eledoisin and Physalaemin

Eledoisin:

$$\underset{1}{\text{Glu}}-\underset{2}{\text{Pro}}-\underset{3}{\text{Ser}}-\underset{4}{\text{Lys}}-\underset{5}{\text{Asp}}-\underset{6}{\text{Ala}}-\underset{7}{\text{Phe}}-\underset{8}{\text{Ile}}-\underset{9}{\text{Gly}}-\underset{10}{\text{Leu}}-\underset{11}{\text{Met}}-\text{NH}_2$$

Physalaemin:

$$\underset{1}{\text{Glu}}-\underset{2}{\text{Ala}}-\underset{3}{\text{Asp}}-\underset{4}{\text{Pro}}-\underset{5}{\text{Asn}}-\underset{6}{\text{Lys}}-\underset{7}{\text{Phe}}-\underset{8}{\text{Tyr}}-\underset{9}{\text{Gly}}-\underset{10}{\text{Leu}}-\underset{11}{\text{Met}}-\text{NH}_2$$

"*Hexeledoisin*":

$$\underset{1}{\text{Ala}}-\underset{2}{\text{Phe}}-\underset{3}{\text{Ile}}-\underset{4}{\text{Gly}}-\underset{5}{\text{Leu}}-\underset{6}{\text{Met}}-\text{NH}_2$$

The actions of eledoisin and physalaemin are similar to those of the kinins. They contract smooth muscle preparations and cause strong peripheral vasodilation leading to a decrease in blood pressure (see, e.g., *146, 545a*).

Gastrin–Cholecystokinin-pancreozymin–Caerulein Family

Gastrin I:
(porcine)

$$\underset{1}{\text{Glu}}-\underset{2}{\text{Gly}}-\underset{3}{\text{Pro}}-\underset{4}{\text{Trp}}-\underset{5}{\text{Leu}}-\underset{6}{\text{Glu}}-\underset{7}{\text{Glu}}-\underset{8}{\text{Glu}}-\underset{9}{\text{Glu}}-\underset{10}{\text{Glu}}-\underset{11}{\text{Ala}}-\underset{12}{\underset{\mid}{\text{Tyr}}}-\underset{13}{\text{Gly}}-\underset{14}{\text{Trp}}-\underset{15}{\text{Met}}-\underset{16}{\text{Asp}}-\underset{17}{\text{Phe}}-\text{NH}_2$$
$$\text{SO}_3\text{H}$$

Caerulein:

$$\text{Glu}-\text{Glu}-\text{Asp}-\underset{\mid}{\text{Tyr}}-\text{Thr}-\text{Gly}-\text{Trp}-\text{Met}-\text{Asp}-\text{Phe}-\text{NH}_2$$
$$\text{SO}_3\text{H}$$

Phyllocaerulein:

$$\text{Glu–Glu–Tyr–Thr–Gly–Trp–Met–Asp–Phe–NH}_2$$
$$\text{SO}_3\text{H}$$

Cholecystokinin–pancreozymin:

$$\cdots\text{–Arg–Asp–Tyr–Met–Gly–Trp–Met–Asp–Phe–NH}_2$$
$$\text{SO}_3\text{H}$$

"*Tetragastrin*":

$$\overset{1}{\text{Trp}}\text{–}\overset{2}{\text{Met}}\text{–}\overset{3}{\text{Asp}}\text{–}\overset{4}{\text{Phe}}\text{–NH}_2$$

The gastrins stimulate secretion of acid and pepsin in the stomach and increase gastric tone and motility. Cholecystokinin-pancreozymin characteristically stimulates pancreatic secretion and contracts the gallbladder. Each hormone has to some extent the effects of the other and caerulein has the activities of both as well as a hypotensive action (see, e.g., *8, 556*).

Insulin (bovine):

A 1 2 3 4 5 6 7 8 9 10 11 12 13 14 15 16 17 18 19 20 21 A

Gly–Ile–Val–Glu–Gln–Cys–Cys–Ala–Ser–Val–Cys–Ser–Leu–Tyr–Gln–Leu–Glu–Asn–Tyr–Cys–Asn

Phe–Val–Asn–Gln–His–Leu–Cys–Gly–Ser–His–Leu–Val–Glu–Ala–Leu–Tyr–Leu–Val–Cys–Gly–Glu–Arg–Gly–Phe–Phe–Tyr–Thr–Pro–Lys–Ala

B 1 2 3 4 5 6 7 8 9 10 11 12 13 14 15 16 17 18 19 20 21 22 23 24 25 26 27 28 29 30 B

Of the varied effects exerted by insulin only the hypoglycemic action and the stimulation of lipogenesis and glucose oxidation by adipose tissue and fat cells have been utilized in tests with crude synthetic analogs.

[a] Names in quotation marks are proposed trivial names for synthetic compounds repeatedly used as prototypes in further structural variations.

follow the Tentative Rules of the IUPAC-IUB Commission on Biochemical Nomenclature as far as possible. To obviate the necessity for designating [Val⁵]- and [Ile⁵]-angiotensins by this "analog" convention in the text, they will be distinguished by the suffixes b (for bovine) and e (for equine), respectively, where necessary.

In some cases active fragments of full hormone sequences have been the objects of extensive structural modifications and will frequently be referred to in the text. For the reader's convenience I have taken the liberty of endowing some of these with ad hoc trivial names as shown in Table I.

II. Structural Aspects of Design

A. SOME GENERAL RULES

As will emerge in the course of this chapter, success in the design of peptide hormone analogs is a matter of detailed exploration rather than general rules. However, some such rules, which may by many be regarded as trivial, have been formulated and this seems the appropriate place to deal with them.

It is sometimes explicitly and very often tacitly assumed that the effect of several structural changes made in one molecule on the activity will be additive. For example, if one modification leads to a relative potency of a and a second modification to potency b, then according to this "additivity rule" the combination of both modifications in the same molecule would be expected to afford an analog with activity $a \times b$. This rule has been elaborated in a "vector diagram" (75) and has been invoked in the design of analogs (e.g., 242, 619). Examples of both the validity of this rule and its failures are too numerous to be discussed here and may be extracted by the diligent reader from the material in this chapter and from the appropriate reviews. There is no doubt that consciously or subconsciously many investigators will continue to give it some weight when incorporating known changes into the design of new analogs. Conspicuous failures of the additivity rule may themselves be of great interest as indicating compensatory or potentiating interactions and may be well worth following up.

One particular corollary of the rule is worth restating. If, for any reason (generally convenience of synthesis) structural changes are made in a molecule already modified with appreciable loss of activity, then a further decrease in potency below the limits of detection must be interpreted with some caution. For example, if a change which in the prototype molecule would leave 1% of residual activity—often an appreciable potency still—is made in a simplified structure which itself has only 1% of the original activity, then the additivity rule predicts that the product will have 1/10,000 of the activity of the prototype, an activity which may well be classified as "nil." Examples of such situations are given in Section II,B,1.

With reference to these and similar cases it has been recommended (490) as a general rule of procedure that changes in structure should be made initially one at a time, and that the native hormones or highly active analogs should be used as the basis of structural change. A further extension of this "rule of small changes" proposes that, in order to separate steric from chemically functional effects, structural changes should be made isosteric or "isofunctional" whenever possible (111, 273, 434, 438); illustrations are given in Section II,C,4. These rules do not imply that drastic structural changes should never be made. Especially in the initial stages of synthetic variation such changes, made with minimal synthetic effort, can economically help to map out the lines or limits of more detailed structural exploration. However, the conclusions drawn from the results of profound structural modifications should be treated with the appropriate reservations.

It has also been proposed as a general rule (542) that biological activity is more sensitive to changes at the carboxyl end than at the amino end of the peptide chain. Though this may be true for some peptides and for some changes the validity of this rule is hardly sufficiently general to make it a useful guide in designing analogs.

B. Changes in Peptide Chain Length

1. Shortening at the Amino and Carboxyl Ends

The question: What length of the peptide chain is necessary for activity? generally obtrudes itself in the earliest stages of the investigation of a peptide hormone. Some information on this point may be obtained already in the course of degradative structural studies and the answer may indeed determine whether, or with what effort, synthesis is possible. Without doubt the observation that the fragment of 28 amino acids obtained from natural porcine corticotropin (39 amino acids) by treatment with pepsin was active, as was the fragment with four further amino acids removed from the carboxyl end (26, 518), greatly encouraged peptide chemists to initiate synthetic work. At the present time reports of biological activity for hydrolytic fragments of, e.g., growth hormone (see 315, 326) or parathyroid hormone (401, 408, 552) give promise that the synthesis of active peptides might be a less formidable undertaking than synthesis of the full peptide chains of the natural hormones.

Further evidence on the chain length requirements for activity generally emerges in the course of synthetic work: The fragments obtained are often tested for activity in the standard assays even before the sequence is completed.

In this way, the molecules of corticotropin and the melanotropins have been explored particularly by Hofmann, Li, Schwyzer, and their respective coworkers. Slight residual corticotropin activity was detected in sequences containing 16 (*235, 499*), 13 (*231*) or even 10 amino acids (*361*). Systematic investigations of peptides of intermediate chain lengths [17 (*329, 405*), 18 (*405*), 19 (*327, 405, 500*), 20 (*222*), 23 (*171, 232, 234*), 24 (*287, 495*), 26 (*406*), 28, and 32 (*20, 548, 549*)] have eventually given the picture of dependence of activity on chain length exemplified in Fig. 1 for steroidogenic potency *in vivo* (see

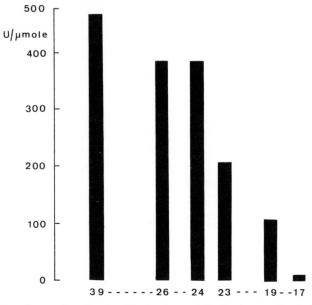

Fig. 1. Dependence of corticosteroid-releasing activity *in vivo* on the chain length of peptides representing amino-terminal sequences of corticotropin. Numbers under columns denote chain length, activities (*361*) are expressed as units per micromole (*407*).

214, 220, 230, 361, 407, 489–491). A similar chain length dependence is observed for the corresponding amides (*20, 361, 405, 407*). Although differences in assay systems or assay procedures, routes of administration, choice of standards, methods for expressing the results (weight or molar basis), purity of the preparations (e.g., water content) and other variables have led to somewhat varying and even controversial results the overall picture which has emerged, regardless of detail, is the same: Peptides including the first 10 to 16 amino acids have minimal activity indicating that all the functionally essential groups are contained within this sequence; with the addition of the arginine residues in positions 17 and 18 the activity rises sharply to become commensurate (in the amides) with that of the full sequence of 39 amino acids in the natural hormones. Whether or not there is a further progressive increase in molar potency with chain length from 19 to 39 appears to be still a matter of dispute and probably depends on the conditions of the assay (*93, 120, 355, 481, 548, 549, 575*).

In early degradative work leucine aminopeptidase was found to inactivate the corticotropins. It was concluded that "one, or both, of the first two amino

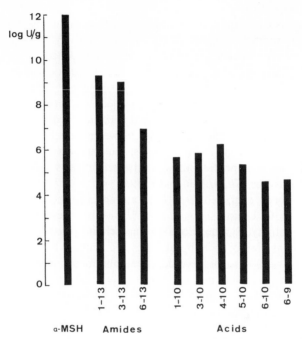

Fig. 2. Melanin-dispersing activity in frog skin *in vitro* of peptides representing shortened sequences of α-melanotropin (α-MSH). The numbers under the columns indicate the sequences, activities are in units per gram on a logarithmic scale. From results summarized in references *361* and *407*.

acids ... appear to be necessary for physiological activity" (*602*). Synthesis of a des-Ser^1 derivative, corticotropin-(2–23)-docosapeptide amide (*173*), showed that activity (in the ascorbic acid depletion test) is decreased by about 35–45 % upon omission of this one amino acid; a further shortening of the chain at the amino end does not appear to have been explored by synthesis.

Similar results are available for the melanophore-expanding (melanotropic) activity of peptides derived from melanotropin or corticotropin sequences (see *164, 213, 214, 220, 312, 407, 489–491*, and Fig. 2). For some time, α-melanotropin-(6–10)-pentapeptide (*221, 228, 330, 496*) ("pentamelatrin") was thought to represent the smallest active fragment. Peptides lacking the tryptophan or histidine residues have generally been found inactive (*226, 230, 312, 614*; but see *361*). Although the activity of pentamelatrin is a millionfold less than that of α-melanotropin, peptides of intermediate chain length [6 (*283, 285, 325*); 7 (*285, 286, 331*); 8 (*225, 226, 229*); 10 (*231, 285*); and 11 (*189*)] as well as the (unacetylated) full tridecapeptide sequence (*189, 231*) have activities increasing with chain length (Fig. 2). The synthetic hormone was available for comparison (*188, 494*).

Only after this work was completed was the tetrapeptide, His–Phe–Arg–Trp, prepared and found to have essentially the same activity as the pentapeptide (*379*). Presumably the subdivision of the chain motivated by synthetic convenience (glycine in a carboxyl-terminal position) had concentrated attention on the penta- rather than the tetrapeptide fragment. Possibly for similar reasons no peptides intermediate in size between sequences 6–10 and 6–13, which differ in activity by a factor of about 500, have been prepared.

For peptides intermediate in length between α-melanotropin and the corticotropin sequence the melanophore-stimulating activity decreases up to the hepta- or octadecapeptide amide and then remains essentially constant on a molar basis (see *220, 312, 361, 407, 491*).

Insulin has been degraded from both amino (*90*) and carboxyl (see *101, 334*) ends of both chains. Even des$^{B23-B30}$-insulin (desoctapeptide-insulin) retains some activity. Synthesis of shortened chains (combined with replacements of several amino acids by alanine; see Section II,C,3) has indicated that B-chain-(4–27)-tetracosapeptide after combination with chain A gives a product with good activity, and some activity is obtained even with the B-chain-(5–27)-tricosapeptide (*598*); the products have not yet been isolated in a pure state so that quantitative comparisons cannot be made.

In the case of eledoisin it was noted in the course of degradative studies (*9a*) that the action of trypsin did not lead to complete inactivation of the natural peptide but no attempts to identify the active fragment are mentioned. Synthetic studies carried out mainly by Bernardi and his co-workers, Lübke and Schröder, and Sandrin and Boissonnas soon revealed that carboxyl-terminal sequences as short as the tetra- and pentapeptide had detectable activity on ileum preparations (*100, 476*) and eledoisin-(6–11)-hexapeptide amide ("hexeledoisin") or higher sequences had considerable potency *in vitro* and *in vivo* (*47, 476, 547*). Systematic variation of the peptide chain length showed that a maximum in potency is, in fact, attained with the nona- or decapeptide which are more active than the natural undecapeptide (or its possible precursors with terminal glutamic acid or glutamine) (*43, 47, 332, 333, 450*). A similar dependence of activity on chain length is observed in series where constant amino acid replacements have been made (e.g., [Asn⁵] or [Val⁸]) (*43, 332, 333*) and probably for the physalaemin sequence (*43,*

49, 460), although in this series the hypotensive effect is apparently highest in the native undecapeptide (*43, 49*).

On the other hand, omission of the carboxyl-terminal methionine already leads to complete loss of activity (*100*).

A still more dramatic shortening of the peptide chain has proved possible in the case of the gastrins. Here again a synthetic intermediate, the carboxyl-terminal gastrin-(14–17)-tetrapeptide amide (*12, 13*) ("tetragastrin") proved to possess the whole range of activities of the natural hormone (*556*) though it has about 10% of the potency in equimolecular amounts. A lengthening of the peptide chain by the protected sequence 9–13 (*354, 556*) increases potency but so does the attachment of certain other acylating moieties (*349, 350, 354*) so that the effect must be regarded as nonspecific. The high potency of so short a fragment has prompted extensive work on analogs particularly by Morley and his colleagues.

In the case of cholecystokinin-pancreozymin, the synthetic octapeptide (*641*) corresponding to the carboxyl-terminal sequence of this tritriaconta-peptide has recently been found to be even more potent in eliciting the typical responses than the native hormone.

The role, if any, of the amino acids additional to those essential for activity, e.g., in the corticotropins, melanotropins, eledoisin, or gastrin has been the subject of speculation. Where they increase potency they may be providing "attachment sites" additional to the functionally essential "active site" (*213, 215, 220*), with effects also on specificity. More generally, the concept of subdivision of sequences into "words" has been elaborated, particular "words" containing the information necessary for activation of the receptor, specific binding to different receptor sites, transport, inactivation, etc. (*492, 493*). Even sequences apparently without further effect on activity such as the "head" of gastrin (*351*) or the carboxyl terminus of the corticotropins may have such functions (see Section III,D,1). It is surprising that more efforts have not been made to explore the specificity of these subsidiary regions by variations of the sequences (see Section II,B,2).

In angiotensin removal of the amino-terminal aspartic acid by Edman degradation led to some loss of activity, further removal of the arginine gave an inactive product (*525*) as did enzymic removal of the carboxyl-terminal phenylalanine (*321*). Synthetic analogs of both bovine (*424, 487, 504*) and equine (*97, 384*) angiotensins II prepared by the groups of Bumpus and Page and of Schwyzer accordingly showed that the des-Asp[1] derivatives retained 25–50% of the biological activity whereas the des-(Asp[1], Arg[2]) analogs had only 1–2% (*97*) or no detectable activity (*487, 504*). Omission of the carboxyl-terminal phenylalanine practically destroyed activity (*424, 487, 504*).

The bradykinin analog shortened by one residue at the amino end, des-Arg[1]-bradykinin (*365, 366*), retains some vasodilator activity but the des-

Arg^9 analog is inactive, as of course is the des-(Arg^1, Arg^9) heptapeptide (*128, 366*).

Removal of the carboxyl-terminal glycine amide residue from oxytocin with chymotrypsin (*23*) or from the vasopressins with trypsin (*568*) causes inactivation. Synthetic analogs shortened at the carboxyl end by three amino acid residues (*414*) or by a single residue (*260*), in each case with retention of a terminal amide group, had very low activity and in some assays (vascular effects) inhibitor properties (see Section III,C,1). Removal of the amino-terminal hemicystine residue in this case is a far-reaching structural change since it leads to disruption of the ring structure. Examination of a continuous series of acyclic peptides representing sequences shortened at the amino end by one to five amino acid residues, with the sulfur of the remaining hemicystine residue (position 6) blocked by a benzyl group, has revealed inhibitor pro-perties in the S-benzyloxytocin-(6–9)-tetrapeptide and -(2–9)-octapeptide amides (*383*) (see Section, III,C,1).

Where relatively small fragments of a sequence have been found to have some activity it is, of course, tempting to use this fragment rather than the full sequence as a starting point for further structural modification. However, it must be kept in mind that if the activity of the fragment itself is already relatively low a further loss of potency due to, e.g., substitution may give a product which no longer has detectable activity at accessible concentrations whereas a similar loss of activity caused by the same modification of an initially more potent, longer sequence may still give analogs of measurable activity (see Section II,A). It is therefore dangerous to draw conclusions about the *absolute* requirement for activity of particular structural features on the basis of such modifications of weakly active sequences (*312, 490*). By way of example, the replacement of tyrosine by phenylalanine in des-(Asp^1, Arg^2)-angiotensin$_e$ II leads to a product considered inactive (*97, 384*) but the analog resulting from the same replacement in the fully active [Asn^1]-angiotensin$_b$ II retains distinct activity (2–10 %) (*423, 487, 504*) and any conclusion about the function-ally essential role of the tyrosine hydroxyl group would therefore be fallacious. The significance of some of the results obtained by structural variations in the minimally active pentamelatrin must be subject to similar reservations (*312*).

2. *Chain Extension*

Lengthening of the peptide chain in hormonal peptides is a variation which occurs in nature, as in the corticotropin–melanotropin–lipotropin family; the kinins; and the gastrin–caerulein–pancreozymin group (see Table I). The natural examples have shown that this structural modification can change potency and specificity as well as metabolic and distribution behavior; to what extent the former changes result from the latter is an interesting question which has hardly been approached experimentally. The known (kinins, angiotensins) or suspected (e.g., corticotropin, the neurohypophysial hormones) occurrence of natural inactive precursors lends added interest to this approach and it is surprising that it has not been pursued more actively. Nor has there been any systematic attempt to investigate to what extent the sequences additional to the common heptapeptide core of the corticotropin–melanotropin–lipotropin family must have specific structures, or to what extent they may be replaced by more generalized sequences. In the gastrin (*349, 350, 354*) and eledoisin–physalaemin (*47, 49, 336, 450, 476, 547*) groups of peptides variations in the inessential sequences (largely elisions rather than replacements) indicate a low degree of specificity.

Additional amino acids have been attached to the amino end of oxytocin (*191, 275, 279, 289, 567*) or lysine vasopressin (*191, 290, 624, 626*) in efforts to change specificity (*191*) or to prolong action (*29, 277, 279, 447*); the details are discussed in Sections III,B,2 and D,5.

Chain extension of bradykinin at the amino end, in derivatives which can be regarded as analogs of the natural kinins kallidin, methionyl-lysyl-bradykinin, and polistes kinin (Table I) changes potency and, as is now known, modifies metabolic behavior (see Section III,D,1). Most analogs of this type are active, sometimes more active than bradykinin (*468, 538*). By contrast, chain extension at the carboxyl end appears to give less active analogs (*537*); however, here again the natural "analog" phyllokinin is highly active.

Extension of the peptide chain of angiotensin II at the carboxyl end by the sequence His–Leu gives the natural precursor, angiotensin I, which is active *in vivo* (see Section III,D,5). The corresponding amide is also active but when the added sequence is Pro–Phe the product is inert (*487, 504*) presumably because it cannot be enzymically converted to the active octapeptide. Acylation at the amino end with poly-(*O*-acetylserine) gives an active derivative (*15*).

3. Elision and Intercalation of Residues

Shortening of the peptide chain by omission (elision) of residues from within the sequence drastically changes the steric relations of the side chains in the regions remaining on either side of the site of elision. Such "frame shifts" often lead to complete or almost complete loss of activity. Frequently, the residual activity is of the same order as would result from complete omission of one of the "frame-shifted" sequences. For instance, in the corticotropins sequence 1–10 appears to be essential for activity and the basic tetrapeptide sequence 15–18 contributed strongly to potency without being essential for activity. Omission of the connecting sequence 11–14 causes practically the same loss of potency (by a factor of about 10^{-4}) as complete omission of the whole carboxyl-terminal segment, 11–18 (*328, 407*).

Analogs of bradykinin with proline residues missing from positions 7 (*81, 82, 367, 501*), 2, and both 7 and 2 (*82, 190*) were prepared by accident rather than design. Together with some others (*82, 190*), they resulted from, eventually successful (*80*), attempts to synthesize bradykinin on the basis of incomplete structural information. Only the des-Pro² derivative had some (1 %) bradykinin-like activity (*82*).

In oxytocin, omission of Pro⁷ or Leu⁸ (as also of the carboxyl-terminal Gly⁹) (*260*) has the same effect on activity as omission of the whole carboxyl-terminal tripeptide sequence Pro–Leu–Gly (*414*).

Elisions within the amino-terminal sequences of eledoisin or gastrin which contribute little to activity have no marked effect (*47, 450, 547*). However, in caerulein the elision of amino acids between the tyrosine sulfate residue and the terminal tetrapeptide amide sequence has a similar effect as omission of either the sulfate group or of the tyrosin sulfate (*7, 8*).

Generally speaking it seems that the result of an elision is roughly equivalent to that of a multiple substitution at one or the other side of the site of elision. It therefore seems that this type of structural change is not very informative.

The same considerations apply to intercalation of amino acid residues within an active sequence which again cause a "frame-shift." The insertion of an extra tyrosine in position 2a of oxytocin has afforded an inhibitor (*193*) (see Section III,C,4) but doubling of the tyrosine in angiotensin$_b$ II (*424, 504*) or for that matter doubling the isoleucine residue in oxytocin itself (*37*) merely caused extensive or complete loss of activity. Intercalation of a glycine residue in *endo*-Gly⁴ᵃ-bradykinin gives a fairly active analog (*369*) but the same change in positions 3a or 4a of tetragastrin, or doubling the phenylalanine residue in this peptide, destroys activity (*350*).

C. MODIFICATION OF SIDE CHAINS

By far the most popular approach to the modification of peptide structure has been by replacement of constituent amino acids with others.

1. *Replacement with Protein-Constituent Amino Acids*

If mutual replacements of protein-constituent ("natural") amino acids are made at random they do not, by definition, fall within the scope of "design." Where such amino acids are used as offering defined structural relations to the residue being replaced (omission of side chains, replacement with glycine or alanine; basic side chains, interchange of arginine and lysine; isomerism, leucine and isoleucine; etc.) they form special cases of the structural approaches discussed below.

Where a substitution is made for the same amino acid in different positions within the same sequence interesting information can emerge regardless of the rationale by which the substituting amino acid is chosen. For example, in angiotensin$_b$ II replacement of Val^3 by leucine does not change the pressor activity, whereas the same substitution for Val^5 decreases potency by 75% (487, 504) and position 5 is also more sensitive when alanine is the replacing amino acid (298, 299). In bradykinin, replacement of arginine by lysine (365, 366, 463) or alanine (464, 469) is more damaging in position 1 than in position

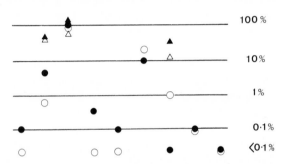

Fig. 3. Replacement of individual amino acid residues in bradykinin with alanine (circles) and of the proline residues with sarcosine (triangles). Contractile action of the analogs on guinea pig ileum (open symbols) and hypotensive effect (filled symbols) in rabbits (alanine substitutions) or guinea pigs (sarcosine substitutions). Activities are expressed as percentages of the activity of bradykinin and displayed on a logarithmic scale. Results from Schröder (469, 473) and Yanaihara et al. (616).

9 and there is a dramatic difference in the sensitivities to change at the three proline positions (464, 616) (Fig. 3).

The choice of replacements will necessarily be limited to protein-constituent amino acids where the variation is based on structural relations of natural peptides forming a family or evolutionary line (Section III,E).

To predict the effect of replacements by natural amino acids Sneath (535) has proposed an approach through numerical taxonomy. Degrees of similarity between the amino acids are calculated by statistical evaluation of numerous properties and four "vectors" corresponding to composite groups of properties are extracted by principal component analysis. The correlation is then analyzed between changes in biological activity and changes in the degree of similarity or in particular vectors. The procedure has been applied to the potency data for 31 peptides of the oxytocin–vasopressin group and to 13 angiotensin derivatives. It is concluded that "... predictions of the biological activity of new peptides ... would probably be better than chance, though not of high accuracy."

This approach is essentially a statistical expression and refinement of what the chemist has by experience come to regard as the degree of resemblance between amino acids and of the rule-of-thumb that major changes in chemical properties are likely to cause greater changes in biological activity. A detailed critique of this interesting treatment is outside the scope of this review. However, it should be noted that it can only be applied to individual groups of compounds when a fair amount of experimental material on structure–activity relations is already available and that it is limited (at least provisionally) to the protein-constituent amino acids though there seems to be no reason in principle why it should not be extended to others provided a sufficient number of properties is determined for each new amino acid. Furthermore, and this appears to be a crucial point, it treats the properties of the amino acids and of the whole molecule in an integrative rather than an analytical manner. For instance, it gives equal weight to all positions in the peptide chain alike although experience shows them to be of unequal significance, and it combines (even in the vector presentation) the steric, physical, and chemically functional properties of side chains instead of attempting to distinguish their separate contributions at any given site. Similarly it subsumes biological activity under a single numerical parameter, ignoring such phenomena as partial agonism or inhibition, duration of the response, etc. For these reasons it seems unlikely that the method in its present general form will contribute much to the design of analogs.

In the following sections amino acid replacements will be considered from the point of view of the structural relations, regardless of the classification into "natural" (protein-constituent) and "unnatural."

2. Substitution or Omission of Terminal or Side Chain Reactive Groups

The reactive (chemically functional) side chain substituents are not unnaturally the first to attract the attention of the organic chemist (72, 73, 76, 236, 238, 563, 571). Although the importance of the nonfunctional side chains has come to be increasingly appreciated (111, 298, 299, 359) the reactive groups including the terminal amino and carboxyl groups still remain favorite targets for structural modification.

The role of such groups can be examined by substitution or by omission. The two procedures are by no means equivalent (see 238, 336, 563) presumably because of the opposite steric effects involved in the two structural changes. Some examples are given in Table II.

a. Substitution of Reactive Groups. In favorable cases chemically functional groups can be selectively substituted even in the native hormones [e.g., insulin

TABLE II

COMPARISON OF EFFECTS ON ACTIVITY OF SUBSTITUTING OR OMITTING
CHEMICALLY REACTIVE GROUPS

Prototype and analogs	Activity[a]		References
Oxytocin	Uterotonic in vitro	Avian depressor	
1-Desamino	160	180	109, 236, 266
N^α-Methyl	0.4	0.01	279, 615
N^α-Acetyl	0.35	Inh.	85
[Phe²]- (2-desoxy-)	12	6	72, 257
[Tyr(Me)²]- (O-methyl-)	1.5 Inh.	Inh.	278, 306, 316
Angiotensin_b II	Pressor		
[Phe⁴]- (4-desoxy-)	10		423, 487, 504
[Tyr(Me)⁴]- (O-methyl-)	0.2		118, 474
Bradykinin	Hypotensive		
[Ala⁶]- (6-desoxy-)	10[b]		464
[Ser(CO·NH₂)⁶]- (O-carbamyl-)	1.3[c]		127, 366
Corticotropin-(1–20)- eicosapeptide amide	Steroidogenic, adrenal ascorbic acid depletion		
[Abu⁴]- (4-de(methylmercapto)-)	20–40		223
[Met(O)⁴]-(?) (oxidized)	Practically none		
[Gln⁵,Lys(For)¹⁰]-α-Melano- tropin	Frog skin darkening in vitro		
[Abu⁴]- (4-de(methylmercapto)-)	2		223
[Met(O)⁴]- (oxidized)	0.1		230

[a] Activities expressed as percentages of the activity of the prototype.
[b] Rabbit.
[c] Guinea pig.

(see 334); corticotropin (581); oxytocin (533, 534)]. Here we shall mainly be concerned with synthetic derivatives.

Analogs of oxytocin (85, 110, 172, 533, 534) and the vasopressins (105, 172, 543) with the terminal α-amino group acylated* have low activity and some-

* Only acyl groups other than aminoacyl or peptidyl are considered here; see Sections II,B,2 and III,D,5.

times (*85*, *543*) inhibitor properties (see Section III,C,1). By contrast, acylation of the terminal amino group of the angiotensins even with bulky substituents (*15*, *123*) gives active compounds. Acetylbradykinin has fair vascular activity (*529*, *540*) with some inhibitor properties on capillary permeability (*537*). In the corticotropin–melanotropin series N^α-acetylation increases the melanotropic but decreases the corticotropic activity of a given sequence (*164*, *189*, *214*, *220*, *318*, *361*, *581*), following in this the natural pattern.

Carboxyl-terminal sequences of those peptides in which the amino-terminal portion is in any case inessential (eledoisin–physalaemin, gastrin) may be made more or less potent by acylation, in dependence on the substituting groups (*336*, *349*, *354*).

Introduction of the formyl group as a relatively stable protecting group for the ε-position of lysine (*224*) has made N^ϵ-formyllysine derivatives readily available, sometimes as synthetic intermediates. N^ϵ-Formyl derivatives of α-melanotropin or partial corticotropin or melanotropin sequences (*214*, *220*, *232*, *233*, *606*, *613*) may have melanotropic potency but their corticotropic activity is greatly decreased or abolished. Larger substituents (tosyl) also reduce melanotropic activity considerably (*226*, *233*).

Side chain formylation in lysine vasopressin reduces activity (*79*) to about the same extent as replacement of lysine by citrulline (*66*). A variety of acyl groups have been introduced into the lysine side chain of eledoisin sequences (*48*, *50*, *336*) in efforts to increase potency or persistence (see Section III,D,4).

It seems likely that introduction of suitable substituents into lysine side chains identified as inessential for activity will increasingly be exploited to attach "markers" (Section III,F), reactive groups (Section III,C,5) and other modifying groups to hormone molecules.

Nitroarginine peptides may also serve as synthetic intermediates. Where they have been examined [bradykinin (*69*, *70*), angiotensin$_b$ II (*202*, *422*, *487*, *504*), a melanotropin sequence (*224*)] they proved less active than the arginine prototypes.

Substitution of histidine has hardly been studied. In an already relatively inactive analogue of angiotensin$_e$ II an *im*-benzyl substituent destroys activity (*271*). Substitution of a shortened ribonuclease S peptide with a carboxymethyl group in position 3 (but not in position 1) of the imidazole ring converts it into a competitive inhibitor (*160*).

Esters, as blocked derivatives of carboxyl end groups, have had little attention. The methyl ester of corticotropin-(1–16)-hexadecapeptide (*499*) has some activity and angiotensin$_b$ II methyl ester is appreciably more active than the corresponding amide, perhaps because the ester is hydrolyzed to the acid in tissues (*487*, *504*). Conversion of free terminal carboxyl groups to amides [angiotensin$_b$ II (*422*, *487*, *504*) and bradykinin (*537*)] or conversely "deblocking" of the terminal carboxamide groups of the natural peptide amides [oxytocin or vasopressin (*133, 139, 140, 342*), carboxyl-terminal fragments of eledoisin (*100, 450*) or gastrin (*182, 350, 354*)] causes profound loss of activity in those cases where the carboxyl or carboxamide group is close to (or part of?) the minimal active region. The vasopressinoic acids can act as inhibitors (*133, 140, 342*) (see Section III,C,1). By contrast, the amides of the corticotropin-(1–17)-, -(1–18)-, -(1–19)-, and -(1–23)-peptides are more active than the free acids (*382, 405, 575*) (see Section III,D,1). Angiotensin$_b$-I-amide is also rather active (*487, 504*) presumably because the amide group is acceptable to the "converting enzyme" (Section III,D,5). Side chain amide–acid interconversions are discussed below (Section II,C,4,c).

Methylation or ethylation of the phenolic hydroxyl group of oxytocin (*277, 278, 316, 630*) or lysine vasopressin (*521, 619*) leads to analogs with inhibitor properties (see Section III,C,1), as does *N,O*-acetylation or carbamoylation of oxytocin (*533, 534*). The same change in angiotensin$_b$ II merely decreases activity (*118, 474*). *O*-Acetylation of serine in α-melanotropin (*164*) and its carbamoylation in bradykinin (*127*) reduces but does not abolish activity.

Oxidation of methionine to the sulfoxide or sulfone can also be regarded as a functional substitution. It greatly depresses or abolishes activity in peptides of the corticotropin and melanotropin (*214, 223*), gastrin (*350, 354*), and eledoisin (*100, 450*) series. In all these cases, omission (Section II,C,3,b) or isosteric replacement (Section II,C,4,d) has given active compounds.

Substitution of chemically reactive groups will no doubt continue to be a favorite structural modification, especially because of its synthetic simplicity. However, it is most informative when it forms part of a more general structural exploration of the reactive sites as described in the following sections.

b. Omission of Reactive Groups. In a particularly systematic study du Vigneaud and his co-workers have eliminated the chemically functional groups of the oxytocin molecule, the phenolic hydroxyl and α-amino group and the three carboxamide groups, one by one and sometimes several at a time (see Table III). Similar though less complete investigations have been made with the vasopressins by the same authors and by Boissonnas, Guttmann, and Huguenin (*77, 177, 245, 247, 249, 300, 546*). The most dramatic result has been the increase in uterotonic, avian depressor, and milk-ejecting activity achieved by omission of the amino group from oxytocin (*109, 236, 266, 571*) and generally, though not invariably, from oxytocin analogs modified at other sites in the molecule (see Table III, and e.g., *163, 566, 590, 592*). In the vasopressin series the most important property of "desamino" analogs is their generally increased antidiuretic and decreased pressor activity, leading to a useful shift in selectivity (see Section III,B,2; Table VII).

Whereas removal of the carboxamide group from the side chain in position 4 of oxytocin (glutamine) has little effect on activity, loss of this group from position 5 (asparagine) and from the carboxyl end of the chain causes a drastic though not complete loss of activity (Table III) together with the appearance of partial agonism or inhibitor properties (*88, 108*).

Removal of the sulfur from oxytocin was carried out in the course of degradative studies (*560*) and destroyed activity (see *28*). Synthesis of the desthiooxytocin—[Ala^1,Ala^6]-oxytocin (*272*)—and the desthiovasopressins (*248*) confirmed that these analogs did, indeed, have minimal activities (*248, 399*). However, this case illustrates the limitations of the conclusions which can be drawn about the biologically functional role of chemically reactive groups

TABLE III

EFFECT OF OMISSION OF CHEMICALLY FUNCTIONAL GROUPS ON SOME
BIOLOGICAL ACTIVITIES OF OXYTOCIN[a]

| Oxytocin analog | Activity (% of oxytocin) | | | References |
	Uterotonic *in vitro* (rat)	Depressor (fowl)	Milk-ejecting (rabbit)	
1-Desamino-	150	190	120	*109, 236, 266*
2-Desoxy-	6	12	15	*72, 257*
4-Decarboxamido-	14	21	55	*565*
5-Decarboxamido-	0.05	0.05	0.25	*192, 565*
9-Decarboxamido-	1.4	<0.004	1	*88*
1-Desamino-2-desoxy-	3.8	13	15	*238*
1-Desamino-4-decarboxamido-	17	38	66	*89*
2-Desoxy-4-decarboxamido-	0.3	0.7	—	*89*
1-Desamino-2-desoxy-4-decarboxamido-	Nil	Negligible	—	*89*

[a] Essentially after du Vigneaud (*563*) and Branda and du Vigneaud (*89*).

from their omission since it has turned out (*273, 438, 485*) that the disulfide group as such is not in fact important for activity provided isosteric relations are maintained (see Section II,C,4,d).

Similar modifications by omission of reactive groups have been made in other peptides. Elimination of the α-amino group increases and prolongs the activity of the angiotensins II (*15, 384, 419, 425, 487*) (see Section III,D,1) but in bradykinin the same change (*269*) decreases potency. In comparison with the [D-Ser^1]-derivatives of some corticotropin analogs the desamino (i.e. [1-β-hydroxypropionic acid]) derivatives are somewhat less active (*130*).

Omission of the terminal carboxamide group from *t*-butyloxycarbonyl-tetragastrin abolishes activity (*182, 350*), omission of the carboxyl group from bradykinin greatly decreases potency (*269*).

The omission of the tyrosine hydroxyl group, that is, replacement of tyrosine by the readily available phenylalanine, has given moderately active analogs of angiotensin$_e$ II (*423, 487, 504*) (see Table II) and of corticotropin-(1–23)-tricosapeptide amide (position 2) (*173*). Substitution of phenylalanine for tyrosine in positions 14 and 19 of the insulin chain A also gives active products after combination with chain B (*239, 593–596, 600*). Replacement of serine by alanine, equivalent to omission of the hydroxyl group, does not greatly change the activity of bradykinin (*464*) and corticotropin-(1–23)-tricosapeptide amide (position 3) (*173*). In all those cases, therefore, the hydroxyl groups are not essential for activity.

Omission of the methylmercapto group of methionine is realized by replacement with α-aminobutyric acid. The [Abu^4]-analog of corticotropin-(1–20)-eicosapeptide amide and of partially blocked α-melanotropin had the same or somewhat lower potencies in all assays as the methionine peptides, showing that the methylmercapto group is not essential for biological function (*223, 227*) (see Table II). In hexeledoisin substitution of α-aminobutyric acid for methionine practically abolishes activity (*100, 450*) and here again the importance of the sulfur is better judged from isosteric replacement (Section II,C,4,d). A similar if less marked difference between omission and isosteric replacement of the methylmercapto groups is found with tetragastrin (*350, 353, 354*).

3. *Omission of Side Chains*

The role of whole side chains, both chemically functional and nonfunctional, has been examined by their omission. Replacement by glycine is equivalent to elimination of the whole side chain, replacement by alanine of all beyond the β-carbon atom. Because the steric properties of glycine are drastically different from those of all other amino acids the use of alanine rather than glycine should give a better approximation to the original conformation of the peptide backbone. In substitution for proline, sarcosine would be expected to maintain the properties of the backbone better than either glycine or alanine; N-methylalanine which should be closer still does not seem to have been examined as a replacement for proline.

Schröder has replaced each amino acid of bradykinin in turn with an alanine residue (*462, 464, 469, 473, 480*). The result is shown in Fig. 3 together with the effect of substituting sarcosine for proline (*616*). The sensitivity of the proline positions to replacement with alanine or with sarcosine follows the same series but the potencies clearly show that at positions 2 and 7 sarcosine is more acceptable than alanine. There is no gross difference between the replacement of Ser^6 or Pro^7 with glycine (*70, 71, 462, 469*) and with alanine (*464, 469*).

In angiotensin$_e$ II Smeby, Bumpus, and their colleagues have placed alanine

TABLE IV

Effect of Omission and Inversion of Side Chains on the Uterotonic and Avian Depressor Activities of Oxytocin[a]

Position	Glycine			Replacement with Alanine			D-Enantiomer		
	Uterotonic	Avian depr.	Ref.	Uterotonic	Avian depr.	Ref.	Uterotonic	Avian depr.	Ref.
Cys[1]	—	—	—	0.0002[b]	—	399	0.4	0.04	237, 279
Tyr[2]	<0.002	<0.002	136	—	—	—	1.5[c]	7.5	137
Ile[3]	<0.002	<0.002	136	—	—	—	—	—	—
Gln[4]	0.62	1.2	136, 165	7.5	14	192	0.02	0.2	138
Asn[5]	—	—	—	<0.007	<0.007	192, 565	0.04	0.08	138
Cys[6]	—	—	—	0.0002[b]	—	399	0.004	nil	338
Pro[7]	15	0.3	52	—	—	—	2.9	<0.001	156
Leu[8]	3.3	1.6	256	30	29	256, 590	4.4	4.4	461

[a] Activities on the rat uterus in vitro in media without magnesium, and on the fowl blood pressure expressed approximately as percentages of the activities of oxytocin.

[b] Simultaneous substitution for Cys[1] and Cys[6].

[c] Inhibitor properties.

in positions 3 (*299*), 4 (*509*), 5 (*298*), 6 (*555*), 7 (*508*), and 8 (*386*). The [Ala³]- is more active than the [Ala⁵]-analog, as in similar substitutions with leucine (*487, 504*). The other analogs have low activity or none; [Ala⁸]-angiotensin$_e$ II has some inhibitor properties (*555*). Replacement of the proline with sarcosine has apparently not been tried.

The results for oxytocin are less complete (Table IV) but it will be noted that in the two cases where both alanine and glycine have been substituted (positions 4 and 8) the alanine analogs are distinctly more active. Replacement of the cystine by two alanines has been discussed (Section II,C,2,b).

In a systematically pursued program Weitzel, Weber, and their co-workers have introduced alanine at 11 positions in chain A and at 9 positions in chain B of sheep insulin (*239, 593–598, 600, 648*). In many cases two or more such replacements were made simultaneously (e.g., *593, 598*). Many of the syntheses were carried out by the solid-phase method without isolation of intermediates, and activities were assessed on the crude mixtures formed from the appropriately modified A and B chains under recombination conditions without isolation of the products. For these reasons only positive results are significant, showing that the changes made do not destroy the activity of the product.* In this way it was established that the side chains of Gln⁵, Val¹⁰, Ser¹², Tyr¹⁴, Gln¹⁵, Asn¹⁸, or Asn²¹ of chain A (*239, 593–596, 600, 648*) and of Asn³, Gln⁴, His⁵, Ser⁹, His¹⁰, Thr²⁷, or Pro²⁸ (*597, 598*) of chain B are not essential for insulin action. When the two hemicystine residues in positions A6 and A11 were replaced by alanine the product had low but definite activity (*595, 600*) and the intrachenar disulfide bond of chain A is therefore not functionally required (see also Section II,C,4,d). In spite of its limitations this approach has obviously yielded valuable information.

4. *Isosteric and Isofunctional Replacements*

a. Some General Considerations. Replacement of one side chain by another in general may have both steric consequences—changing the conformation, or conformational freedom, of the peptide molecule or altering the topography of the molecular surface—and results which may be called chemically functional in the widest sense. In this sense functionality is taken to mean not only reactivity but also charge, hydrogen-bonding capacity, and lipophilic or hydrophilic properties. Unless analogs are designed with this dichotomy in mind it is often difficult or impossible to interpret the biological results of a structural change in molecular terms. Rudinger has suggested (*111, 434, 438*) that to this end substitutions should be made as nearly as possible either isosteric

---

* Lack of activity could signify either that the synthesis had not given the desired peptide sequence, or that the insulin analog was inactive, or that it had not been formed because the structural modification hindered proper linking of the disulfide bridges.

or "isofunctional." It is, of course, recognized that precisely isosteric relations are hardly ever achieved and that "functionality" in this context is a relative term; for example, the relevant functionality of a lysine side chain might in different situations be its charge, the hydrophilic character or hydrogen-bonding capacity of the amino group, or even the lipophilic properties of the four methylene groups. An examination of functionality will therefore often involve a series of graded substitutions. It is obvious that this type of approach will more often than not require the use of specially designed and prepared "unnatural" amino acids and this may be the reason why the principle outlined above has not been more generally followed.

In the succeeding paragraphs the relation between some amino acid side chains will be considered from this point of view and some examples of structural explorations on this basis will be given.

b. Arginine and Lysine. Replacement of arginine by lysine, a change which occurs naturally in porcine vasopressin and the β-melanotropins, has been a popular structural modification also in synthetic analogs, partly perhaps because of the synthetic difficulties caused by arginine. The two amino acids are approximately isofunctional; both side chains will be protonated in the physiological pH range though, of course, arginine is much the stronger base. They are also similar sterically in that both place the positive charge at about the same distance from the peptide chain but the guanidino group is larger than the aminomethylene group replacing it in lysine. For this reason citrulline, isosteric with arginine but uncharged, and ornithine, with the same functional group as lysine but a shorter side chain, should be included for more detailed comparisons (see Fig. 4). Further shortening of the side chain in α,γ-diaminobutyric acid has been examined (*578, 625, 628*) but of the homologs of arginine, only homoarginine has been used in a single instance (*203*). Nitroarginine (see Section II,C,2,a) would seem to be less suitable than citrulline for checking the importance of arginine basicity since the additional substituent greatly increases the size. The use of N^ϵ-trimethyllysine salts (*202*) deserves more attention.

In bradykinin the arginine positions have been explored by Bodanszky, by Nicolaides, and by Schröder and their co-workers. The two arginine residues have been replaced separately by lysine (*365, 366, 463*), ornithine (*365, 366, 480*), and citrulline (*69, 70, 128, 365, 366, 377*); both have been replaced simultaneously with lysines (*463, 469, 602a*), citrullines (*69, 70, 377*), nitroarginines (*69, 70*), and α,γ-diaminobutyric acids (*578*). Unfortunately, the assays varied from case to case so that a complete picture of biological activities is not available. However, lysine is evidently the most acceptable replacement in both positions and ornithine appears preferable to citrulline. Position I is more sensitive to change than position 9 and of the doubly substituted analogs only those with lysine and nitroarginine retain some activity.

Replacement of the arginine in pentamelatrin with ornithine (*67, 69, 113, 330, 609, 610*), lysine (*113, 609, 610*), or citrulline (*67, 69*) has been studied by Bodanszky, by Li, and by Yajima with their co-workers. The results are difficult to evaluate because the arginine peptide itself already has very low activity. There now seems to be agreement that the ornithine analog is inactive in the accessible dose range (*67, 69, 113, 609, 610*) though skin-lightening properties have been reported for this as for the citrulline derivative (*67, 69*). The lysine analog has decreased (*609, 610*) or no detectable (*113*) activity. Substitution of lysine (*113*) or ornithine (*553*) in position 8 of longer corticotropin sequences reduces but does not abolish their melanotropic activity and depresses their corticotropic potency about a hundredfold. On the other hand, replacement of the arginine residues in positions 17 and 18 of active corticotropin sequences by lysine (*124, 130, 194, 421, 583*) or by ornithine (*125, 126, 554, 583*) as carried out by Boissonnas and Guttmann and by Riniker and Rittel and their co-workers has given highly active analogs.

Otsuka et al. (*380, 381*) have prepared analogs in which the terminal tetrapeptide sequence, Lys–Lys–Arg–Arg, of [Gly^1]-corticotropin-(1–18)-octadecapeptide has been replaced by Arg–Arg or by Lys–Arg–Arg–NH$_2$, a change which can be regarded as an elision of lysine or replacement of lysine by arginine in a shortened sequence. The compounds are less active than the normal octadecapeptide or its amide (*382*).

In vasopressin, the substitution of lysine for arginine in position 8 has been carried out by Nature; the effect of shortening the side chain in ornithine (*246*) and α,γ-diaminobutyric acid (*625, 628*) is shown in another context in Table VII (Section II,B,2). The further examination of this position has not been very systematic.* Histidine decreases vasopressin-like activity sharply (*292*), about as much as leucine (*83, 291*) and much more than citrulline (*66*). The low activity of the histidine analog must therefore be ascribed to its unsuitable steric features rather than to decreased basicity (see *439*). This is confirmed by the relatively high pressor activities of [8-alanine]- (*590*) and [8-N^ϵ-formyl-lysine]-vasopressin (*79*). Isosteric replacement of a methylene group in the lysine side chain by sulfur ("thialysine" or S-β-aminoethylcysteine) gives an active compound (*207*) as expected. However, the obvious replacement of lysine by norleucine and by β-hydroxynorleucine which would more precisely define the functions of the side chain has not yet been reported. An [8-p-aminophenylalanine]-vasopressin would also be interesting, as would an [8-δ-(2-imidazolyl)norvaline] analog.

* Recently Zaoral, Kolc, and Šorm (*649*) have completed the series of homologous substitutions in position 8 of vasopressin by the synthesis of the [8-α,β-diaminopropionic acid] derivative. The complete series has also been prepared with the basic amino acids in the D configuration and the effects of chain length and configuration on the antidiuretic and pressor activities have been discussed.

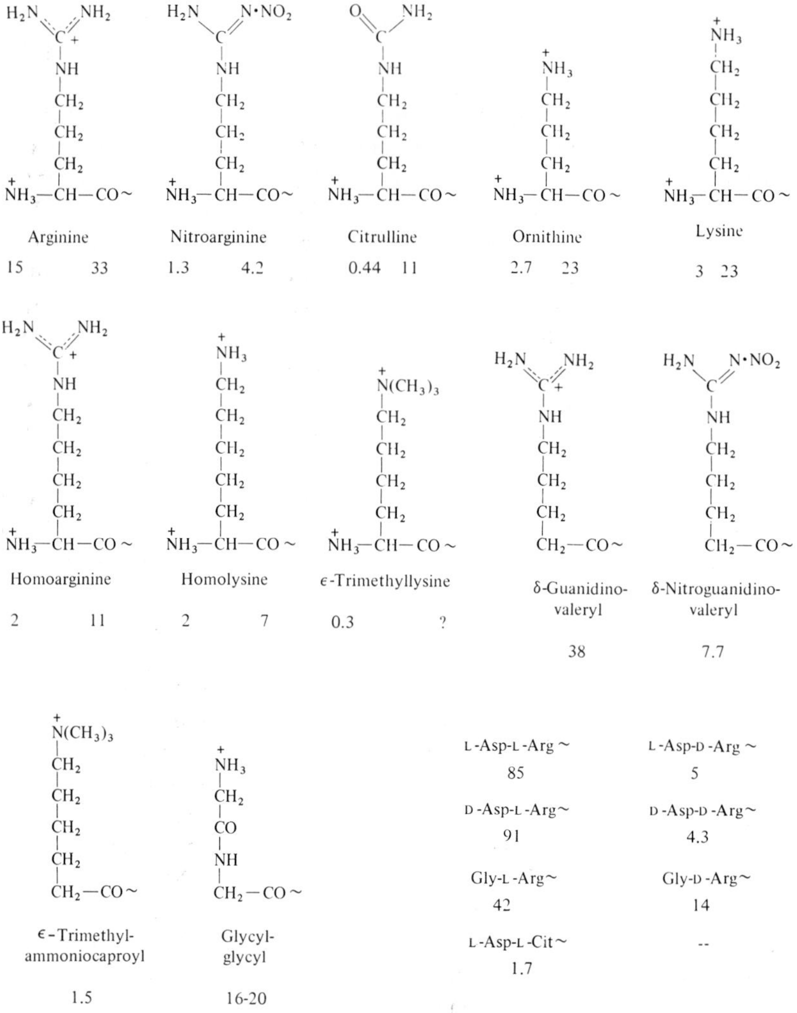

Fig. 4. Variations in position 2 of des-Asp¹-angiotensin_e II (structural formulas) and positions 1 and 2 of angiotensin_e II (abbreviated formulas). Numbers give rat pressor response as a percentage of the response to a standard preparation. Where given, activities on left and right are for the L and D derivative, respectively. Results from Havinga, Schattenkerk *et al.* (202, 203, 456), for the [Gly¹,Gly²] derivative from Jorgensen *et al.* (271).

In the angiotensins II position 2 has been varied by Schröder, by Schwyzer and Riniker and in a particularly thorough study by Havinga, Schattenkerk, and their co-workers. Nitroarginine (422, 487, 504), ornithine (423, 487, 504), and lysine (465) replaced arginine in angiotensin_b II with an effectiveness decreasing in this order. The set was extended by the preparation of the analogs of angiotensin$_e$ II, its des-Asp^1 and [Gly^1] derivatives shown in Fig. 4 (*202, 203, 456*). The series systematically explores the effect of the distance of the functional substituent from the α-carbon atom; of its basicity and dimensions; and of its hydrogen-bonding capacity on the activity, and also the effect of the presence and configuration of a free or aminoacylated α-amino group in this position. The inclusion of quaternary ammonium compounds is particularly noteworthy. It is concluded that for optimal effectiveness the side chain should have both a positive charge (preferably diffuse) and the ability to act as a hydrogen bond donor; that the distance of the group from the α-carbon (at least in the des-Asp^1 series) is not critically important; and that D or desamino residues in this position confer higher potency in the des-Asp^1 series but that the D-isomers have lower potency when they are aminoacylated (*202, 203, 456*) (see Section II,C,4,i). An interesting supplement to the series is provided by [Gly^1, Gly^2]-angiotensin$_e$ II (*271*) whose activity is ascribed to its ability to take up a conformation in which the α-amino group occupies the site of the basic side chain substituent (*271*) (Fig. 4).

Additional analogs designed to test this hypothesis of course immediately come to mind such as those in which glutamine, α-aminoadipic acid δ-amide, the corresponding amidines, and ω-methylated derivatives of arginine or the appropriate desamino compounds occupy this position.

c. Aspartic Acid, Glutamic Acid, and Their Amides. The aminodicarboxylic acids and their ω-amides form a convenient natural set in which the carboxamide and carboxyl groups are nearly isosteric and the length of the side chain varies by one methylene group. The amides have been used to replace the acids in several cases, probably because they are more readily available and synthetically more convenient than the ω-esters (usually benzyl or *t*-butyl) which are the usual starting materials in work with the acids.

In fragments of corticotropin or melanotropin glutamine can replace glutamic acid in position 5 without appreciable loss of activity (*214, 229–231, 233, 283, 285, 458, 606*) but this is not surprising since glycine is also acceptable in this position (*458*). In the angiotensins again position 1 can accommodate not only aspargine (*428, 487, 504*) but a number of other amino acids including glutamine, glutamic or pyroglutamic acid (*118, 470*), as well as glycine (*202, 423, 456, 487, 504*) or isoleucine (*298*).

On the other hand, the aspartyl residue of gastrin and its shorter chain analogs seems to be critical for activity (*350, 351, 354*). Morley, Gregory and their colleagues have made a very detailed examination of the structural requirements in this position (*184, 350*) (see Fig. 5). With the carboxyl group intact the steric situation has been changed either by lengthening (glutamic acid) or by shortening (aminomalonic acid) the side chain; changing its configuration; altering its spacing from the carboxyl terminus by intercalating a methylene group, without (β-aminoglutaric acid) or with (β-aspartyl) simultaneous shortening of the side chain; and by altering its spacing from other functional groups by transferring the carboxymethyl substituent from the α-carbon to the preceding nitrogen (iminodiacetic acid or N-carboxymethyl-glycine). On the other hand, the carboxyl group has been omitted (alanine);

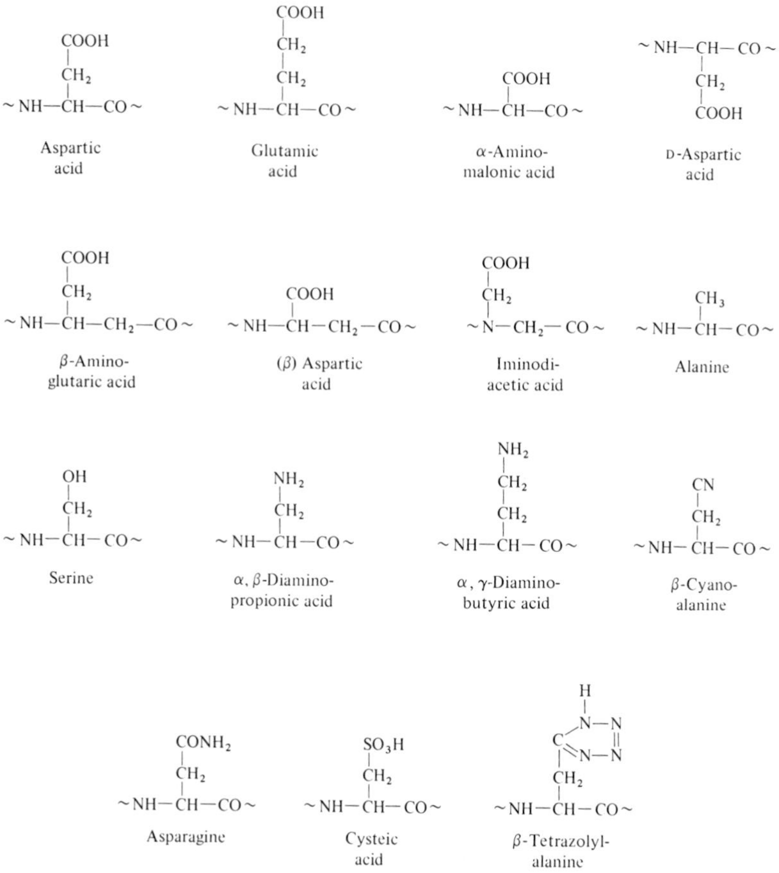

$$
\begin{array}{llll}
& \quad\text{COOH} & & \\
& \quad|\;\;\;\; & & \\
\quad\text{COOH} & \quad\text{CH}_2 & & \sim\text{NH}-\text{CH}-\text{CO}\sim \\
\quad| & \quad| & \quad\text{COOH} & \quad| \\
\quad\text{CH}_2 & \quad\text{CH}_2 & \quad| & \quad\text{CH}_2 \\
\quad| & \quad| & \quad\text{CH} & \quad| \\
\sim\text{NH}-\text{CH}-\text{CO}\sim & \sim\text{NH}-\text{CH}-\text{CO}\sim & \sim\text{NH}-\text{CH}-\text{CO}\sim & \quad\text{COOH} \\
& & & \\
\quad\text{Aspartic} & \quad\text{Glutamic} & \quad\alpha\text{-Amino-} & \quad\text{D-Aspartic} \\
\quad\text{acid} & \quad\text{acid} & \quad\text{malonic acid} & \quad\text{acid}
\end{array}
$$

Fig. 5. Variations in the aspartic acid position of tetragastrin derivatives. From Morley (*350, 351*).

replaced with the hydrophilic hydroxyl, amino, or aminomethylene groups (serine, α,β-diaminopropionic and α,γ-diaminobutyric acids); the polar, neutral cyano group (β-cyanoalanine); the nearly isosteric, hydrophilic, but neutral carboxamide group (asparagine); or the strongly acidic sulfonic acid grouping (cysteic acid). Of all these compounds only the [D-Asp³] and the [βAsp³]-analog showed marginal (less than 1%) activity and it is considered possible (*350*) that this may have been due to contamination with a trace of the L-α-aspartyl isomer. All other analogs were completely inactive. The effectiveness of the rather reactive cyanomethyl and methoxycarbonyl-methyl esters is probably explained by their hydrolysis to the acids (*350*).

A biologically equivalent replacement for the carboxyl group was eventually found in the tetrazolyl grouping, chosen because it has an acid dissociation constant similar to that of the carboxyl group and a similar disposition of at least the nearer heteroatoms (*351*). This work, then, establishes the necessity

TABLE V

SIDE CHAINS IN POSITION 4 OF OXYTOCIN: EFFECT OF CHAIN LENGTH, BRANCHING AND POLAR SUBSTITUENTS ON BIOLOGICAL ACTIVITY

Amino acid in position 4	Activity (% of oxytocin)			References
	Uterotonic *in vitro* (rat)	Depressor (fowl)	Milk-ejection (rabbit)	
Glycine	0.5	1.1	4.1	*136, 165*
Alanine	6.6	13	55	*192*
α-Aminobutyric acid	13	21	58	*565*
Norvaline	11	20	44	*163*
Norleucine	3.7	10	21	*163*
Valine	25.5	25	102	*566*
Isoleucine	6.8	16	45	*241*
Leucine	2.4	8.7	16	*241*
Serine	39	45	57	*192*
Asparagine	20	40	60	*259*
N^ω-Methylasparagine	7.5	23.5	?	*204*
Ornithine	11	32	31	*205*
Glutamic acid	0.1	0.3	2.7	*389*

for a grouping roughly isoelectronic with the carboxyl group and of the same acidity in the precise position in which the one methylene group of the side chain places it. This group may be both critical for function and important for attachment since none of the inactive analogs appear to act as antagonists (*350, 351*).

The glutamine in position 4 of oxytocin is at a site of natural variation (isotocin is [Ser^4, Ile^8]-oxytocin). Omission of the carboxamide group has given an active compound (*565*) and the effect of alkyl chains of various lengths and modes of branching has been examined (*136, 163, 165, 192, 241, 565, 566*) mainly by du Vigneaud and his school, with the results shown in Table V.

Maximal activity was found at 3 carbons and branching (in [Val⁴]-oxytocin) further increased potency. On the other hand, hydrophilic substituents attached to, or replacing, alkyl groups in a linear side chain invariably increase activity (see Ser vs Ala or Abu; Asn vs Ala or Nva; and Orn vs Nva or Nle in Table V). The N^{ω}-methylasparagine isomer of oxytocin in which the amide group is, as it were, shifted down the chain (204) is less active than the asparagine analog (295) in which the side chain is simply shortened. This position could be further probed by placing, e.g., threonine* or allothreonine, the β-methyl-asparagines, or α-amino-β-ureidopropionic acid in this position. An interesting feature is the very low activity of the desamido derivative, [Glu⁴]-oxytocin (389), which is sterically and functionally closest to the prototype. The negative charge which this side chain carries must have a profound influence at some stage of hormone action, perhaps at a transport barrier.

By contrast, the asparagine carboxamide at position 5 is not readily replaced. Its omission in [Ala⁵]-oxytocin (192, 565) or displacement in [Gln⁵]-oxytocin (295) practically abolishes activity, apparently with a loss of both affinity and intrinsic activity (108). The substitutions by valine (588) and ornithine (205) are not very informative; α-aminobutyric and α,β-diaminobutyric acid would approximate the steric properties of asparagine somewhat better and, of course, cysteic acid S-amide would make a very interesting replacement.

d. Methionine and Cystine. The role of the methylmercapto group of methionine has been examined by replacement with α-aminobutyric acid (equivalent to omission; see Section II,C,2,b) or with norleucine or S-ethyl-cysteine (isosteric substitution). While omission of the methylmercapto group in a corticotropin derivative may somewhat reduce activity (223, 227) replacement of methionine with norleucine, together with some other changes, has given analogs more active than the prototype (84, 130, 194). A direct comparison of exactly corresponding derivatives with α-aminobutyric acid and norleucine has not been made so far.

In derivatives of tetragastrin isosteric replacement of methionine by nor-leucine or S-ethylcysteine preserves full activity, whereas replacement by norvaline or α-aminobutyric acid leads to distinctly less active compounds (350, 353). It should be noted that both in corticotropin sequences (170) and in gastrin (25) or benzyloxycarbonyltetragastrin (349, 350, 353) the branched leucine is also acceptable in place of methionine.

In active sequences of eledoisin or physalaemin the methionine position is more selective. Replacement with alanine (476), α-aminobutyric acid, or norvaline (450) reduces activity to less than 5% whereas replacement with

---

* Since completion of this manuscript Manning, Coy, and Sawyer (638) have prepared [4-threonine]-oxytocin and shown it to have greater uteronic and avian depressor potency than oxytocin itself.

norleucine (450) or S-ethylcysteine (48, 460) preserves at least 15% of the potency. Leucine is not acceptable here in place of methionine (100).

The disulfide bridges of the neurohypophysial hormones have been thought to participate functionally in the mechanism of action. A disulfide interchange reaction at the receptors was presumed to initiate the response (see, e.g., 409). One point in favor of this hypothesis was the failure to detect any biological activity in "desthiooxytocin" ([Ala^1,Ala^6]-oxytocin), an analog formally derived by omission of the disulfide group (28, 272) (see Section II,C,2,b). However, this structural alteration not only eliminates disulfide reactivity but also has drastic steric consequences since it converts a cyclic into a much more flexible linear peptide. To separate these effects Rudinger and Jošt designed an analog which was approximately isosteric with an active molecule but had

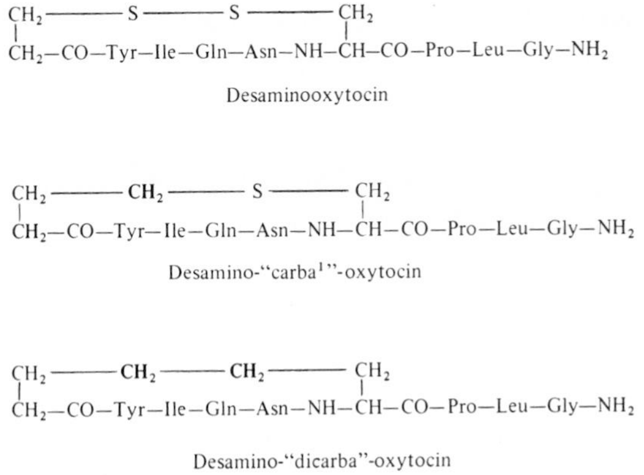

$$CH_2 \underline{\hspace{1cm}} S \underline{\hspace{1cm}} S \underline{\hspace{1cm}} CH_2$$
$$CH_2 - CO - Tyr - Ile - Gln - Asn - NH - CH - CO - Pro - Leu - Gly - NH_2$$

Desaminooxytocin

$$CH_2 \underline{\hspace{1cm}} CH_2 \underline{\hspace{1cm}} S \underline{\hspace{1cm}} CH_2$$
$$CH_2 - CO - Tyr - Ile - Gln - Asn - NH - CH - CO - Pro - Leu - Gly - NH_2$$

Desamino-"carba^1"-oxytocin

$$CH_2 \underline{\hspace{1cm}} CH_2 \underline{\hspace{1cm}} CH_2 \underline{\hspace{1cm}} CH_2$$
$$CH_2 - CO - Tyr - Ile - Gln - Asn - NH - CH - CO - Pro - Leu - Gly - NH_2$$

Desamino-"dicarba"-oxytocin

Fig. 6. Isosters of oxytocin lacking the disulfide bond.

no disulfide grouping, by formally replacing one sulfur atom of the disulfide bridge in desaminooxytocin with a methylene group, i.e., replacing "desamino-cystine" in positions 1,6 of oxytocin with S-γ-carboxypropylcysteine ("des-aminocystathionine") (Fig. 6). The resulting desamino-"carba"-analog had hormonal activity (91, 273, 397, 438, 485) proving that disulfide reactivity is not required to initiate biological responses. Replacement of both sulfur atoms of the bridge by methylene groups in oxytocin (273) and the vasopressins (201, 448) has also given rather potent analogs.

This example illustrates the utility of designs separating steric from functional factors. The "desthio" derivatives of the vasopressins (248) and oxytocin (399) have since been found to have very weak hormonal activities, lower by four to six orders of magnitude than those of the "carba" analogs but the importance of the disulfide group is obviously much better estimated from isosteric replacement.

An insulin A-chain in which the cystine in positions 6,11 was replaced by cystathionine (274, 276) has been combined with chain B to give a product with insulin activity, again showing that the intrachenar disulfide bridge is not required for hormonal activity. The same conclusion has also been reached in this case by replacing the cystine with two alanine residues (see Section II,C,3).

Walter and du Vigneaud have replaced one or both sulfur atoms of oxytocin or desaminooxytocin with selenium to give a series of highly active analogs (584, 589, 591, 592). This isologous replacement preserves both the steric properties and the fundamental reactivity of the prototype.

e. Histidine. Histidine is unique among protein-constituent amino acids because of the special properties of its imidazole group—its pK, ability to act as a proton donor or acceptor, and imide reactivity among others. It has been implicated in the catalytic function of several enzymes and there has

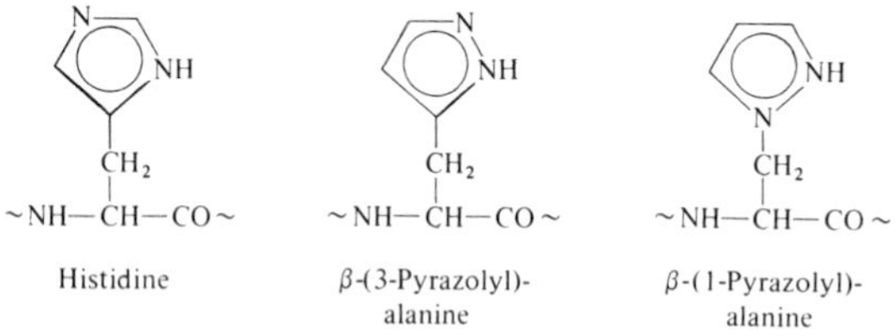

Fig. 7. Pyrazolylalanines as isosters of histidine.

been a tendency to regard it as essential also for the activity of the hormones in which it is found. The apparent reluctance until recently to test this point experimentally is all the more surprising. In angiotensin$_b$ II histidine has been replaced by phenylalanine (466) and lysine (474), presumably because these amino acids approximate, respectively, the steric properties and the basicity of histidine. Both analogs retain low (1 and 0.1%) pressor activity.

Hofmann has introduced β-(3-pyrazolyl)alanine (Fig. 7) as a close isoster of histidine which differs, however, from the prototype in its acid–base properties and the position of one nitrogen atom (218). Incorporation of this amino acid in place of histidine into angiotensin$_b$ II (14, 217) and into [Gln^5]-corticotropin-(1–20)-eicosapeptide amide (219) gave hormone analogs with high pressor and corticotropic–melanotropic activity, respectively, proving that the special acid–base properties are unimportant for the hormonal activity. By contrast, the ribonuclease-S-peptide-(1–12)-dodecapeptides with β-(1-pyrazolyl)alanine and β-(3-pyrazolyl)alanine in place of histidine form inactive complexes with the S-protein, confirming the importance of histidine for ribonuclease action (159, 160, 218).

Hofmann and Bowers (633) have now used the same substitution to show that histidine as such is not essential to the biological activity of the thyreo-tropin-releasing hormone, pyroglutamylhistidylproline amide.

f. Phenylalanine and Tyrosine. The substitution of phenylalanine for tyrosine constitutes omission of a reactive group (Section II,C,2,b). The reverse replacement has been carried out extensively, as in lysine vasopressin (*77*), the antiotensins II (*474, 523*), an eledoisin hexapeptide (*48*) and positions 5 (*469, 480*) and 7 (*459*) of bradykinin. The activity is generally reduced, in some cases (vasopressin, bradykinin position 5) drastically.

However, for a proper understanding of the consequences of phenylalanine–tyrosine replacements it is again necessary to separate steric and functional effects and among the latter to distinguish between the properties of the hydroxyl group as an acidic, a hydrogen-bonding, or a reactive substituent as well as its possible effect on the electron density of the aromatic ring. By a proper choice of suitably substituted derivatives it may often be possible to do this.

Thus [Tyr^8]-angiotensin$_e$ II has a lower direct musculotropic effect but retains most of the hypertonic activity of the parent compound (*387, 555*; but see *474*). Methylation of the tyrosine further reduces the hypertonic potency but *restores* the direct musculotropic activity (*555*). On these grounds it is suggested that the decreased effect on the ileum is due to misalignment of the molecule by hydrogen bonding (*555*).

Morley, Gregory, and their colleagues have designed a series of tetra-gastrin analogues to test the role of the phenylalanine (*181, 349, 350*). Sub-stitution of the aromatic ring in the *p*-position with groups of varying size and character (methyl, methoxyl, nitro, fluoro) does not grossly affect activity and replacement by hexahydrophenylalanine* (*β*-cyclohexylglycine) is also acceptable, showing that the aromatic character of the side-chain is immaterial. However, replacement by tyrosine abolishes activity—a surprising effect for which the special properties of the unsubstituted hydroxyl group must be responsible. Side chains such as that of alanine, leucine, and valine also reduce or destroy activity, indicating that certain requirements of shape and, apparent-ly, lipophilicity must also be met.

Rudinger, Jošt, and Šorm with their colleagues have made a rather thorough study of position 2 in oxytocin (Fig. 8), stimulated by the finding that some of the analogs modified in this position have inhibitor properties. When [Tyr(Me)^2]-oxytocin was found to act as an inhibitor of oxytocin (*29, 277, 278, 316*) the known (*72, 257*) [Phe^2]-oxytocin was reexamined (*278, 443*) to determine whether mere omission of the hydroxyl group would have similar effects. The compound was found to behave as a partial agonist and, under

---

* The cyclohexane ring, while topologically flat, is "thicker" than the benzene ring. In some situations *β*-cyclopentylalanine might give a better steric approximation to phenyl-alanine than *β*-cyclohexylalanine.

suitable conditions, even as an inhibitor of oxytocin (*309, 443, 444*; see also *108*) showing that the hydroxyl group probably participates in, but is not essential for, the function of the hormone–receptor complex. The inhibitor properties were, however, accentuated when *p*-substituents (other than hydroxyl) of increasing size (methyl, ethyl = methoxyl, ethoxyl) were introduced, indicating an additional steric effect. The similarity of the ethyl and

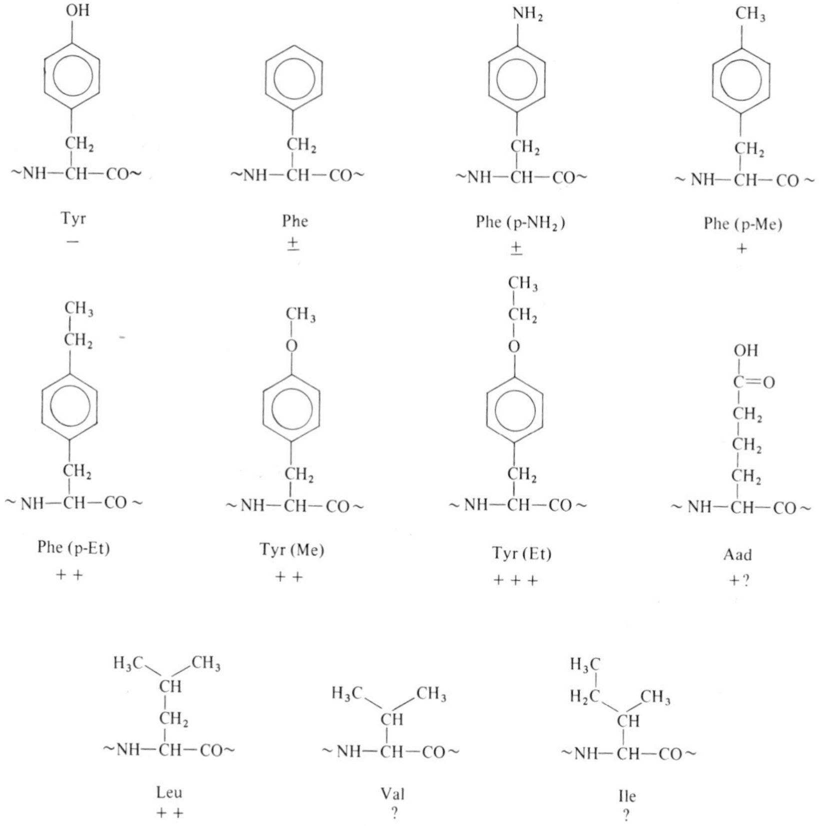

OH
$\sim$NH—CH—CO$\sim$
Tyr
$-$

$\pm$
$\sim$NH—CH—CO$\sim$
Phe
$\pm$

NH$_2$
$\sim$NH—CH—CO$\sim$
Phe (p-NH$_2$)
$\pm$

CH$_3$
$\sim$NH—CH—CO$\sim$
Phe (p-Me)
$+$

CH$_3$ CH$_2$
$\sim$NH—CH—CO$\sim$
Phe (p-Et)
$+ +$

CH$_3$ O
$\sim$NH—CH—CO$\sim$
Tyr (Me)
$+ +$

CH$_3$ CH$_2$ O
$\sim$NH—CH—CO$\sim$
Tyr (Et)
$+ + +$

OH C=O CH$_2$ CH$_2$ CH$_2$
$\sim$NH—CH—CO$\sim$
Aad
$+ ?$

H$_3$C CH$_3$ CH CH$_2$
$\sim$NH—CH—CO$\sim$
Leu
$+ +$

H$_3$C CH$_3$ CH
$\sim$NH—CH—CO$\sim$
Val
?

H$_3$C H$_2$C CH$_3$ CH
$\sim$NH—CH—CO$\sim$
Ile
?

Fig. 8. Variations in position 2 of oxytocin. The plus signs denote tendency to inhibition on an arbitrary scale. Aad is α-aminoadipic acid. For references, see text.

methoxyl derivative show that the lipophilic properties of the substituent are of minor importance and since [2-*p*-aminophenylalanine]-oxytocin (*436*) also acted as a partial agonist the critical property of the hydroxyl group is one which cannot even be imitated by the amino group (*433, 434, 444*).

Replacement of the tyrosine with leucine (*240, 277, 278*), valine (*240*), or isoleucine (*87*) decreased activity (drastically in the leucine and valine analogs) and in the case of [Leu^2]-oxytocin partial agonism was observed (*305, 309, 444*). If the conclusions about the role of the hydroxyl group are correct similar anomalies should also be shown by [Ile^2]- and [Val^2]-oxytocin but suitable experimental conditions may be required to demonstrate them (see Section III,C,2). In an attempt to restore an acidic group to approximately the position of the tyrosine hydroxyl, [2-α-aminoadipic acid]-oxytocin has been prepared (*345*). Preliminary experiments show that this, too, is a partial agonist with very low potency. Perhaps α-aminopimelic acid may more accurately reproduce the dimensions of the tyrosine.

The oxytocic potency of [Ile^2]-oxytocin approximates that of the [Phe^2]-analog, suggesting that the *sec*-butyl group (but not the isobutyl side chain of leucine) is equivalent to benzyl in its contribution to binding and relevant steric properties.

Little systematic variation has been carried out with the tyrosine in angiotensin. It has been replaced by phenylalanine (*423, 487, 504*), *O*-methyltyrosine (*118, 474*), and alanine (*509*) in the full sequence and with phenylalanine, *p*-fluorophenylalanine, and thienylalanine in des-Asp^1, Arg^2-angiotensin$_e$ II (*97, 384*). Of these only [Phe^4]-angiotensin$_b$ II and the corresponding asparagine derivative are reasonably active (*487, 504*). However, since des-Asp^1, Arg^2-angiotensin II itself has greatly reduced activity and its [Phe^4]-derivative was found inactive (*97, 384*) no final conclusions can be drawn about the replacements with thienylalanine and *p*-fluorophenylalanine. In any case one would like to see the series extended by, e.g., *p*-methylphenylalanine and *p*-aminophenylalanine to distinguish between possible roles of the aromatic substituent.

In a modified physalaemin heptapeptide amide replacement of tyrosine by phenylalanine, *O*-methyltyrosine, *m*-tyrosine, and *p*-fluorophenylalanine had little effect on activity (*49*), perhaps not unexpectedly since this is a site of natural variation, occupied by isoleucine in eledoisin.

In bradykinin replacement of the phenylalanine in position 8 by *p*-fluorophenylalanine (*364, 366*), and *O*-methyltyrosine (*540*) increases potency whereas replacement with tyrosine decreases it (*459*). However, since each of these analogs was tested in a different assay system it is difficult to draw any more general conclusions from these results. In position 5 introduction of a *m*-trifluoromethyl substituent into the ring also increases potency (*369*). Again a more systematic exploration of these effects would be welcome.

g. Aliphatic Amino Acids. Replacements of aliphatic amino acids have often been confined to the naturally occurring alanine, valine, leucine, and isoleucine. Comparison of isoleucine with valine and alanine can, indeed, give information about the importance of side chain length and comparison of leucine with valine and isoleucine about the importance of β-branching. Thus, while the natural [Val^5]- and [Ile^5]-angiotensins and their [Asn^1]

derivatives are about equally active Schwyzer has shown that [Asn[1], Leu[5]]-angiotensin$_b$ II has appreciably lower activity (*487, 504*) so that β-branching of the side chain is important. In position 3 leucine can replace valine without loss of activity (*487, 504*) and only shortening of the chain in [Ala[3]]-angiotensin$_e$ II reduces activity by one-third (*299*).

Only rarely have α-aminobutyric acid, norvaline, or norleucine been used to supplement the information obtained with the protein-constituent amino

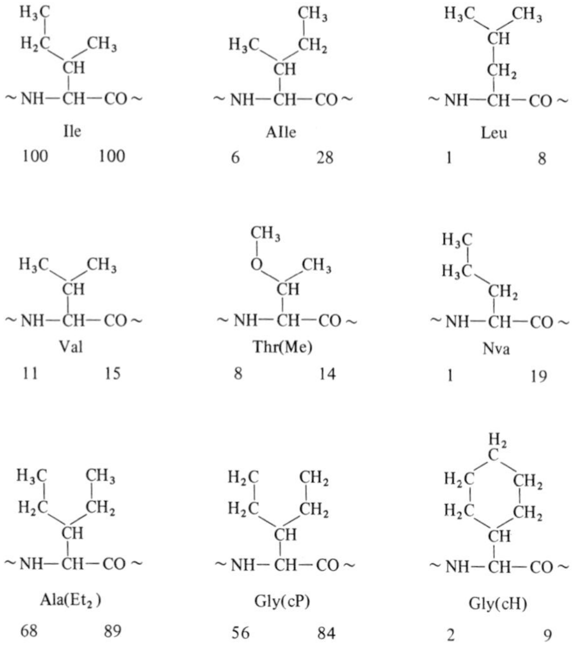

Fig. 9. Variations of the aliphatic side chain in position 3 of oxytocin. The numbers give approximate potencies, as percentages of the activity of oxytocin, in the assay on the rat uterus *in vitro* (medium without magnesium) (left) and the guinea pig intramammary gland pressure (right). Ala(Et$_2$) is β,β-diethylalanine, Gly(cP) cyclopentylglycine, Gly(cH) cyclohexylglycine. From Rudinger *et al.* (*111, 143, 359*).

acids (see, e.g., *163, 256, 359*) and apart from *O*-methylthreonine (see below) more intricate isosters such as β-dimethylaminoalanine for leucine or threonine and allothreonine for valine do not appear to have been used.

As an example of a more systematic variation of an aliphatic side chain we may consider position 3 in oxytocin. Early experiments showed that replacement of isoleucine by valine lowers potency by about an order of ten, replacement by leucine still more (*83, 437*). Further experiments by Rudinger and his colleagues showed that the isomeric norleucine, the stereoisomeric alloisoleucine, and the lower homolog norvaline (see Fig. 9) all were poor replacements for isoleucine (359). Now whereas the low potency of the [Leu³]- and [aIle³]-oxytocins might be ascribed to steric changes induced by the "misplaced" methyl groups the decreased activities of the merely "demethylated" [Val³]- and [Nva³]-analogs suggested that this side chain might be important for lipophilic binding (359). To confirm this interpretation and eliminate the possibility that second-order steric effects due to the smaller side chains might be responsible, a side chain was required which would be isosteric with that of isoleucine but would have a different "functionality" in the sense of decreased lipophilicity. Accordingly, the isoleucine was replaced by O-methylthreonine (111). The activity profile of the analog was similar to that of [Val³]-oxytocin demonstrating that it was the "functionality" and not the steric effect of the missing methylene group which is important. If this conclusion is correct, replacement of the oxygen by the more lipophilic sulfur (in β-methylmercapto-α-aminobutyric acid) should largely restore potency.

The decreased potency of the alloisoleucine as against the valine derivative suggested that the "misplaced" methyl group makes no contribution to activity but rather lowers it. A steric effect was suspected and for confirmation the same methyl group was formally incorporated into oxytocin itself, as the side chain of β,β-diethylalanine. The activity of this analog was, indeed, about half that of oxytocin just as the activity of [aIle³]-oxytocin was about half that of [Val³]-oxytocin (143) proving the existence of a steric effect and, incidentally, providing an example of the "additivity rule" (see Section II,A). Conformational stabilization of the diethylalanine side chain by (formal) crosslinking of the two δ positions, in a cyclopentylglycine side chain, hardly changed the activity profile, suggesting that the conformation of diethylalanine (and presumably of isoleucine) in the active form of the molecule was similar to that of the carbon atoms in cyclopentane (143). By such systematic variations of the lipophilic and steric properties it therefore proved possible to establish the importance of lipophilic binding together with a rather high degree of stereospecificity.

Recently a similar exploration of position 5 in [Asn¹]-angiotensin II has been carried out by Jorgensen and his co-workers (634). The results confirm the importance of β-branching but, beyond that, lipophilicity alone seems to determine the potency without any steric restrictions such as are found in the oxytocin series.

h. Terminal Groups. As replacements of a terminal amino group, a methyl group should be roughly isosteric and a hydroxyl group in addition partly isofunctional. No such replacements have as yet been reported at critical sites. They should prove particularly interesting in oxytocin where omission of the amino group increases potency.

The approximately isosteric and partly isofunctional interchange of terminal

(Section II,C,2,a) and side chain (Section II,C,4,b) carboxyl and carboxamide groups has already been discussed. Bernardi and his colleagues have shown (48) that in hexeledoisin replacement of the carboxamide by a (neutral, electrophilic) nitrile group maintains a much higher activity than its replacement by the more closely isosteric but ionized carboxyl group (100, 450). It would be of interest to incorporate this modification also into gastrin or oxytocin.

The hydrazide and methylamide analogs of *t*-butyloxycarbonyltetragastrin are fully active, the piperidide has decreased activity and the methyl ester or dimethylamide is inactive (182, 350). On the other hand, in the eledoisin series the methyl ester retains some activity (460) whereas the hydrazide (460) and dimethylamide (48) are almost inactive. Evidently the steric and polar factors will be difficult to disentangle in these instances.

i. D-Amino Acids. It is obvious that the side chains of enantiomeric amino acids are fully identical functionally but in a peptide chain replacement of an L- by a D-amino acid residue may lead to profound steric changes. We would expect that such changes at the ends of the peptide chain would least affect the overall topochemistry of the molecule and could be equivalent merely to displacing the terminal carboxyl (carboxamide) or amino groups. The consequences of a similar change within the chain will vary from case to case and are difficult to predict. Nevertheless such changes have proved popular, particularly in the search for enzyme-resistant derivatives (see Section III,D,1) and inhibitors (Section III,C,3), all the more so when this search was rewarded with success in several instances.

In oxytocin replacements by D-amino acids have been made at all positions except 3 (see Table IV). It is interesting to compare the effect of omitting and inverting side chains. The two structural changes in some cases do, but in others do not have parallel effects. In lysine vasopressin replacement of L- by D-proline leaves some antidiuretic but abolishes pressor activity (303); in its effect on pressor activity it resembles other structural changes which "misplace" the terminal carboxamide group. Vasopressin analogs with basic D-amino acids in position 8 (621–623, 625, 627) have proved of great interest because of their high antidiuretic selectivity and potency (see Table VII). Again, metabolic factors may be involved (Sections III,D,1 and 3).

The "all-D" isomers, or enantiomers, of pentamelatrin (200, 608), oxytocin (162), [Asn[1]]-angiotensin$_b$ II (471, 579), bradykinin (540, 541, 577), and tetragastrin (121, 350, 354) have been prepared; all except the first, which is an inhibitor, were inactive. The reversed-sequence all-D ("retro-enantio") analogs are discussed in Section II,D,4.

Nicolaides with his colleagues and Stewart and Woolley between them have replaced all the amino acids in bradykinin (except of course glycine) with the D-enantiomers singly (127, 364, 366, 369, 370, 540) or several at a time (*540*). The [D-Phe^5]-, [D-Ser^6]-, and [D-Phe^8]-bradykinins had fair activity, the others low. The derivative with all three prolines in the D configuration had inhibitor properties (*540*).

In glycyl-hexeledoisin again all the amino acids (except glycine) have been replaced by their enantiomers singly or in pairs (*335, 479*). All except the D-alanine derivative in which the substitution is in any case outside the minimal active region had very low activity.

TABLE VI

MELANOTROPIC ACTIVITY OF DIASTEREOMERS OF
PENTAMELATRIN

Diastereomer					Activity[a]	Reference
His–Phe–Arg–Trp–Gly						
L	L	L	L	—	100[a]	
D	L	L	L	—	Inh.	604, 607
L	D	L	L	—	330–3300	457, 612
L	L	D	L	—	Nil	604, 609
L	L	L	D	—	330	607
D	D	L	L	—	180	612
D	L	D	L	—	10	609
D	L	L	D	—	Inh.	612
D	D	D	L	—	Inh.	611
L	D	D	L	—	70	611
L	D	L	D	—	3300	609
L	D	D	D	—	Inh.	611
D	D	D	D	—	Inh.	200, 608

[a] As percentage of the activity of pentamelatrin which is 3×10^4 U/gm; "Inh." is inhibition or a lightening response. For discussion, see Yajima (*604, 610*).

Eight diastereomeres of tetragastrin have been reported (*121*). The analogs with D-tryptophan or D-methionine were less active than the parent compound, those with D-aspartic acid or D-phenylalanine marginally active perhaps because of contamination with the L-isomers (*350, 354*). Multiple substitutions as far as the results have been reported (*354*) destroy activity.

The results of Schwyzer and Riniker and of Havinga and Schattenkerk for positions 1 and 2 in the angiotensins II provide an interesting study. The [D-Asp^1]- and [β-D-Asp^1]-angiotensins$_b$ II have increased potency and prolonged effects (*419, 425*). Similarly in des-Asp^1-angiotensin$_e$ II the diastereomers with the terminal amino acid (arginine, lysine, citrulline etc.) in the D configuration consistently have the higher potency but when an amino acid (glycine, D- or L-aspartic acid) is added in position 1 the [D-Arg²] derivative is less active than the [L-Arg²] diastereomer (see Fig. 4; Section II,C,4,b). These differences are evidently related to metabolic factors; apparently it is the configuration of the amino-terminal residue in each case which affects the metabolic stability.

Numerous melanotropin and corticotropin fragments with D-amino acids in sequence 6–9 have been prepared (see Table VI). This work was originally prompted by the observation that alkali treatment of these hormones and related peptides prolongs and increases their activity (see Section III,D,1) but some of the compounds, most of which were prepared by Yajima and his co-workers (see *604, 609*), proved of interest as antagonists rather than agonists. On the other hand, substitution of D-amino acids in the *N*-terminal sequence of corticotropin has afforded analogs with high potency and in some cases protracted activity (*84, 284, 421*) (see Section III,D,1).

D. Changes in the Peptide Backbone

It is sometimes assumed that the backbone of peptide linkages only serves as a sort of framework supporting the amino acid side chains whose arrangement is then responsible for the topochemical features related to the binding and activity of peptides. However, recent evidence from X-ray crystallographic work on enzymes has suggested that groups of the peptide backbone may participate in substrate binding (*65*). The possibility that in biologically active peptides, too, the peptide chain might have a functional in addition to its purely steric role makes structural changes in the backbone particularly interesting. Certainly it is the point of attack of proteolytic enzymes and appropriate modifications might be expected to confer metabolic stability (see Section III,D,1).

Modifications of the peptide backbone have involved substitution on the imino nitrogen or α-carbon atoms; intercalation of methylene or imino groups in the backbone (the insertion or omission of whole amino acid residues has been discussed in Section II,B,3); more or less isosteric replacements of atoms or groups within the backbone, including reversal of the direction of amide bonds; and in a broader sense attempts to stabilize particular conformations of the peptide chain.

1. *Methylation*

N-methylation of amide bonds, which is sometimes motivated by the hope of obtaining metabolically stable analogs (*244, 277*), profoundly alters both the stereochemistry and the chemistry (hydrogen-bonding capacity) of the backbone amide group. It is therefore not surprising that the replacement of glycine by sarcosine in oxytocin (104), lysine vasopressin (343), or bradykinin (469) and the replacement of tyrosine or phenylalanine and tryptophan by their N-methyl derivatives in oxytocin (244, 277) and benzyl-oxycarbonyltetragastrin (181, 183, 349, 350) greatly reduces or even abolishes activity. On the other hand, replacement of methionine by N-methylnorleucine in the same tetragastrin derivative gives an active product (350, 353). Replacement of proline by sarcosine (616) can be regarded as a side chain omission (II,C,3) rather than alteration of the backbone. Although optically active $C_{(\alpha)}$-methyl derivatives of some natural amino acids are available they do not seem to have been exploited in analog design. α-Phenylalanine, which is a C-methyl derivative of phenylglycine rather than phenylalanine, is not acceptable in place of phenylalanine in tetragastrin (181, 350) but the phenylglycine analog would be required for comparison to show the effect of C-methylation as such.

Substitutions with $C_{(\alpha)}$-branched amino acids (α-methylalanine, 1-aminocyclopentanecarboxylic acid) are increasingly being used in the study of active conformations (see Section II,D,5).

2. Intercalation of Methylene and Imino Groups

As in the case of amino acid interpolations in the peptide chain (Section II,B,3) the insertion of single methylene and imino groups would be expected to alter the spacing of the side chains and the topochemistry of the molecule appreciably. The structural change is likely to have less effect if it changes the steric relations of, or within, a sequence which is not important for activity, or if it alters the spacing of only one side chain or an endgroup as in substitutions for terminal amino acids of the peptide chain. Generally speaking, this is what is experimentally found.

Single methylene groups can be inserted in the peptide chain by using β-rather than α-amino acids (Fig. 10b,c). Presumably because of the effort required to prepare optically active substituted β-amino acids, particularly those with side chains in the α position (Fig. 10c), β-alanine has been most frequently used in such structural modifications. It has replaced glycine in oxytocin and vasopressin (139, 140) with considerable loss and aspartic acid in tetragastrin (184, 350) with complete loss of activity. The glycine and alanine in terminal penta- and heptapeptide sequences of gastrin (121, 350, 354) and eledoisin (472), respectively, can be replaced by β-alanine with retention of high potency but these changes are in any case in inessential regions of the parent molecules. β-Alanine is also acceptable in place of serine in the amino-terminal position of corticotropin-(1–23)-tricosapeptide amide (170), possibly with some metabolic stabilization (see Section III,D,1,a).

The two "homophenylalanines", L-3-amino-4-phenylbutyric acid (type b in

Fig. 10) and 3-amino-2-benzylpropionic acid (type c) have been substituted for phenylalanine in the carboxyl-terminal position of angiotensin$_e$ II (*387*). The latter replacement reduces pressor activity about thousandfold, the former only about tenfold. The benzyloxycarbonyltetragastrin derivative containing β-aminoglutaric in place of aspartic acid is inactive (*184, 350*).

In β-aspartyl and γ-glutamyl analogs the lengthening of the backbone necessarily involves also shortening of the side chain. In the "permissive" amino-terminal position of angiotensins this change, in fact, affords highly active analogs (*419, 425*) (see Section III,D,1) but in the very critical position

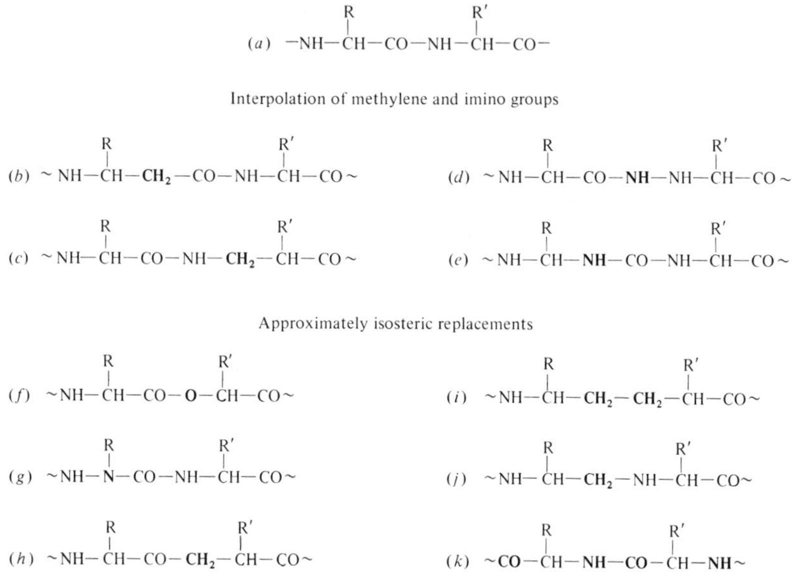

$$(a) \quad -NH-\overset{R}{\underset{|}{CH}}-CO-NH-\overset{R'}{\underset{|}{CH}}-CO-$$

Interpolation of methylene and imino groups

$$(b) \sim NH-\overset{R}{\underset{|}{CH}}-\mathbf{CH_2}-CO-NH-\overset{R'}{\underset{|}{CH}}-CO\sim \qquad (d) \sim NH-\overset{R}{\underset{|}{CH}}-CO-\mathbf{NH-NH}-\overset{R'}{\underset{|}{CH}}-CO\sim$$

$$(c) \sim NH-\overset{R}{\underset{|}{CH}}-CO-NH-\mathbf{CH_2}-\overset{R'}{\underset{|}{CH}}-CO\sim \qquad (e) \sim NH-\overset{R}{\underset{|}{CH}}-\mathbf{NH}-CO-NH-\overset{R'}{\underset{|}{CH}}-CO\sim$$

Approximately isosteric replacements

$$(f) \sim NH-\overset{R}{\underset{|}{CH}}-CO-\mathbf{O}-\overset{R'}{\underset{|}{CH}}-CO\sim \qquad (i) \sim NH-\overset{R}{\underset{|}{CH}}-\mathbf{CH_2-CH_2}-\overset{R'}{\underset{|}{CH}}-CO\sim$$

$$(g) \sim NH-\overset{R}{\underset{|}{\mathbf{N}}}-CO-NH-\overset{R'}{\underset{|}{CH}}-CO\sim \qquad (j) \sim NH-\overset{R}{\underset{|}{CH}}-\mathbf{CH_2-NH}-\overset{R'}{\underset{|}{CH}}-CO\sim$$

$$(h) \sim NH-\overset{R}{\underset{|}{CH}}-CO-\mathbf{CH_2}-\overset{R'}{\underset{|}{CH}}-CO\sim \qquad (k) \sim CO-\overset{R}{\underset{|}{CH}}-NH-CO-\overset{R'}{\underset{|}{CH}}-NH\sim$$

Fig. 10. Modifications of the peptide backbone. Interpolated or substituted groups are shown in boldface type.

3 of tetragastrin the β-aspartyl analog retains only marginal activity and even this may be due to contamination with traces of the α-isomer (*350*).

The [4-isoglutamine] (*416*) and [5-isoasparagine] (*337*) isomers of oxytocin, prepared originally to eliminate these alternative structures for the native hormone, have only minimal potency; the former also has some inhibitor properties (*415*). [βAla^4]-Oxytocin is also practically inactive (*339*) though the [Gly^4] analog retains appreciable activity (*137, 165*) so that it is not the loss of the side chain in this position which is primarily responsible.

In disulfide-bridged peptides such as the neurohypophysial hormones or insulin the cystine side chain may be regarded as part of the "backbone" of

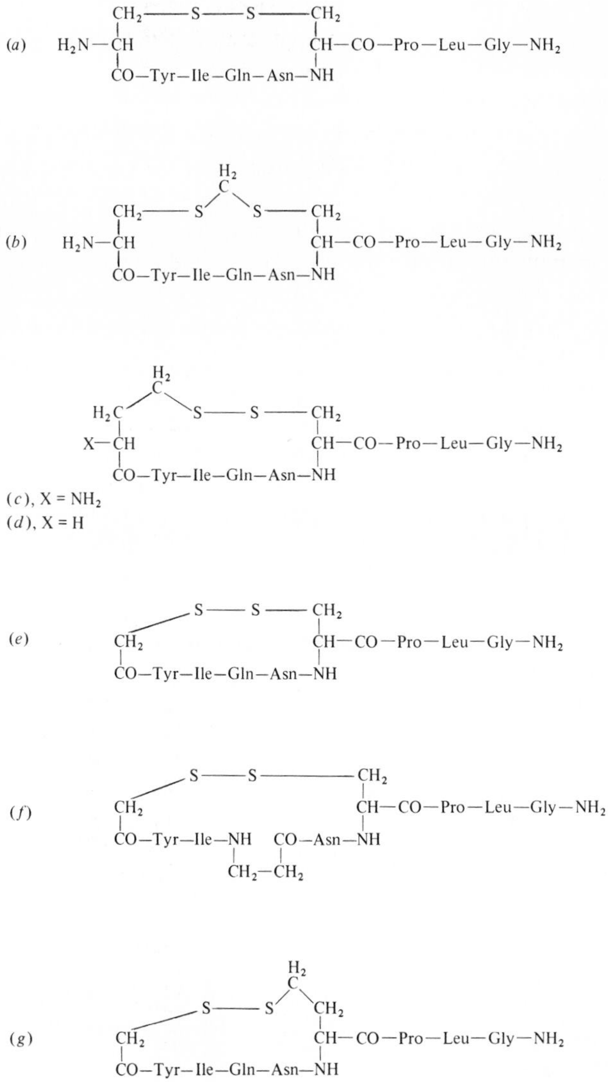

(a)
$$CH_2 \longrightarrow S \longrightarrow S \longrightarrow CH_2$$
$$H_2N \longrightarrow CH \qquad\qquad CH \longrightarrow CO \longrightarrow Pro \longrightarrow Leu \longrightarrow Gly \longrightarrow NH_2$$
$$CO \longrightarrow Tyr \longrightarrow Ile \longrightarrow Gln \longrightarrow Asn \longrightarrow NH$$

(b)
$$\overset{H_2}{C}$$
$$CH_2 \longrightarrow S \qquad S \longrightarrow CH_2$$
$$H_2N \longrightarrow CH \qquad\qquad CH \longrightarrow CO \longrightarrow Pro \longrightarrow Leu \longrightarrow Gly \longrightarrow NH_2$$
$$CO \longrightarrow Tyr \longrightarrow Ile \longrightarrow Gln \longrightarrow Asn \longrightarrow NH$$

$$\overset{H_2}{C}$$
$$H_2C \qquad S \longrightarrow S \longrightarrow CH_2$$
$$X \longrightarrow CH \qquad\qquad CH \longrightarrow CO \longrightarrow Pro \longrightarrow Leu \longrightarrow Gly \longrightarrow NH_2$$
$$CO \longrightarrow Tyr \longrightarrow Ile \longrightarrow Gln \longrightarrow Asn \longrightarrow NH$$

(c), X = NH₂
(d), X = H

(e)
$$S \longrightarrow S \longrightarrow CH_2$$
$$CH_2 \qquad\qquad CH \longrightarrow CO \longrightarrow Pro \longrightarrow Leu \longrightarrow Gly \longrightarrow NH_2$$
$$CO \longrightarrow Tyr \longrightarrow Ile \longrightarrow Gln \longrightarrow Asn \longrightarrow NH$$

(f)
$$S \longrightarrow S \longrightarrow CH_2$$
$$CH_2 \qquad\qquad CH \longrightarrow CO \longrightarrow Pro \longrightarrow Leu \longrightarrow Gly \longrightarrow NH_2$$
$$CO \longrightarrow Tyr \longrightarrow Ile \longrightarrow NH \quad CO \longrightarrow Asn \longrightarrow NH$$
$$CH_2 \longrightarrow CH_2$$

(g)
$$\overset{H_2}{C}$$
$$S \longrightarrow S \qquad CH_2$$
$$CH_2 \qquad\qquad CH \longrightarrow CO \longrightarrow Pro \longrightarrow Leu \longrightarrow Gly \longrightarrow NH_2$$
$$CO \longrightarrow Tyr \longrightarrow Ile \longrightarrow Gln \longrightarrow Asn \longrightarrow NH$$

Fig. 11. Changes in the size of the ring in oxytocin. *a*, Oxytocin; *b*, [1,6-djenkolic acid]-; *c*, [1-hemihomocystine]-; *d*, [1-(3-mercaptobutyric acid)]-; *e*, [1-mercaptoacetic acid]-; *f*, [1-mercaptoacetic acid, 4-β-alanine]-; *g*, [1-mercaptoacetic acid, 6-hemihomocystine]-oxytocin. For references, see text.

the heterodetic (486) ring. In oxytocin (Fig. 11a) insertion of a methylene group into this ring either between the sulfur atoms (485) (Fig. 11b) or by substitution of hemihomocystine for hemicystine in position 1 (263) (Fig. 11c) sharply decreases activity, as does the same change in the desaminoanalog [1-(3-mercaptobutyric acid)]-oxytocin (264) (Fig. 11d). Jarvis, du Vigneaud, and their co-workers in a systematic study of this problem (266) have further shown that omission of a methylene group from the ring, a change which is possible in the desamino series, gives in [1-mercaptoacetic acid]-oxytocin (267) (Fig. 11e) an analog with fair potency. An interesting situation arises when ring expansion at one site is compensated by ring contraction at another. In [1-mercaptoacetic acid, 4-β-alanine]-oxytocin (265) (Fig. 11f) the ring size remains unchanged but the peptide bonds and the side chains of the tyrosine and isoleucine residues in positions 2 and 3 are displaced by one atom of the backbone; the analog apparently has even less activity than [βAla^4]-oxytocin, showing that the effect of the two changes is additive rather than compensating. Even where both the added and the eliminated methylene group are in the bridge portion of the molecule as in [1-mercapto-acetic acid, 6-homohemicystine]-oxytocin (266) (Fig. 11g) there is con-siderable loss of activity though the compound should be approximately isosteric with oxytocin.

The incorporation of α-hydrazino acids into the peptide chain, with the β-nitrogen atom as part of the amide bond (Fig. 10d), is equivalent to inserting an NH group into the chain. Analogs of this type have been derived from oxytocin (375) and [Asn^5]-eledoisin-(4–11)-octapeptide (185, 371). [NH·Gly^2]-Oxytocin* has low activity with inhibitor properties, the [NH·Gly^9] and [NH·Phe^7] derivatives of the eledoisin sequence have fair (20%) and low (1%) activity, respectively.

An imino group can also be intercalated between the α-carbon and carbonyl group to give a urea derivative (Fig. 10e). Such compounds are generally obtained by mischance rather than design, as byproducts in peptide synthesis by the azide procedure, and they should be readily accessible. Apparently the only analogs of this type deliberately made and evaluated, the "homo-α'-aza-tyrosine" derivatives of [Asn^1]- and [βAsp^1]-angiotensin$_b$ II, have relatively high activity (25% as against the parent compounds) (419, 426).

3. Substitution within the Backbone

More subtle changes in the backbone result when groups within the peptide chain are replaced approximately isosterically. The most frequent change of

---

* By a logical extension of the rules of nomenclature (254) the hydrazino acids can be named and symbolized as N-amino derivatives of the corresponding amino acids, i.e., NH·Gly is the hydrazinoacetyl residue.

this type has been replacement of amino acids by hydroxy acids, equivalent to replacing amide by ester linkages (Fig. 10f). Such "depsipeptide" analogs have been studied by Shemyakin, Shchukina, and their co-workers in the angiotensin (507) and bradykinin (411, 513, 514, 517) systems. The effect of substitution varies with the position (Fig. 12). In bradykinin, an ester bond in position 3–4 greatly lowers activity, in position 5–6 leaves it unchanged, and in position 7–8 even increases potency in vivo (411) presumably for metabolic reasons (Section III,D,1,c). Similar differences are shown by the angiotensin analogs. In a tetragastrin derivative substitution of β-phenyllactic acid for

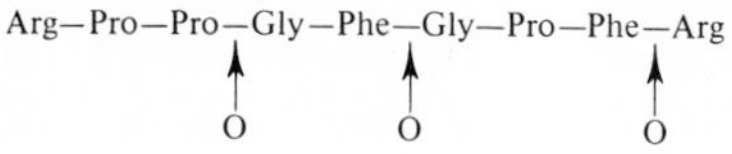

Arg—Pro—Pro—Gly—Phe—Gly—Pro—Phe—Arg

	O	O	O
Hypotensive	0.07	12	400
Uterotonic	0.005	20	50
Capillary permeability	0.07	30	25

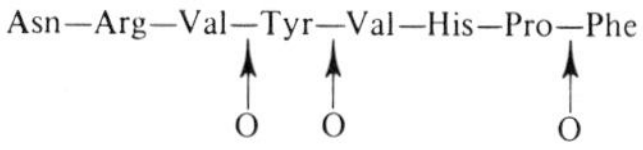

Asn—Arg—Val—Tyr—Val—His—Pro—Phe

	O	O	O
Hypertensive	0.06	3.0	10
Uterotonic	0.05	0.1	0.1

Fig. 12. Activities of depsipeptide analogs of [Gly⁶]-bradykinin and [Asn¹]-angiotensin b II. Effects on rat blood pressure, rat uterus in vitro and capillary permeability in the rabbit skin determined from minimal effective doses and expressed as percentages of the activities of the parent compounds. Location of ester bond indicated by arrows. From Shchukina, Shemyakin et al. (411, 507, 513, 517).

phenylalanine gives a marginally active analog, perhaps because the compound is chemically unstable (350).

Apart from minor differences in geometry and solvation the CO—NH and CO—O groups differ fundamentally in their ability to form hydrogen bonds; loss of activity may indicate that hydrogen bonding is required either to maintain conformation or for interaction with the receptor.

A second possibility which has been explored mainly by Niedrich and his colleagues is the replacement of an α-CH group by a nitrogen atom (Fig. 10g). Such "aza" analogs (168) are approximately isosteric except that the arrangement of the side chain can correspond to that of either an L- or a D-amino acid. Apart from this one would expect the topochemistry of the parent molecule to be largely unchanged (*373*) and active analogs should result. This, indeed, is the case with [9-semicarbazide]-oxytocin (*372*) and [5-α-azaasparagine]-eledoisin-(4–11)-octapeptide (*374*) which are as potent, or more potent, than the parent compounds. The low potency (less than 1 %) recorded for [3-α-azavaline]-angiotensin$_b$ II (*209*) is therefore surprising.

The reverse replacement of the peptide NH group by CH_2 (Fig. 10*h*) is formally attractive but experimentally difficult to achieve. In particular, the preparation of the required intermediates with the correct side chain configuration would be a synthetic task of some complexity and the optical stability of the resulting ketones would be expected to be low. The replacement of the CO—NH by a CH_2—CH_2 sequences (Fig. 10*i*), equivalent to replacing the peptide backbone by a paraffin chain, encounters the first of these obstacles but not the second; it could most readily be realized for glycine-containing sequences. Replacement of glycine amide by ethylene diamine in lysine vasopressin (*620*) is the only example so far of replacing a carbonyl with a methylene group (Fig. 10*j*); the resulting analog has only low potency. The changes shown in Figs. 10*i* and *j* are isosteric only in the sense that they do not alter the number of atoms in the main chain and substitution for the carbonyl only (Fig. 10*j*) in addition turns a neutral (amide) into a basic (amino) nitrogen.

4. *Reversal of Peptide Bonds*

A radical change in the backbone which might yet be expected to produce minor changes in side chain topochemistry is the (formal) reversal of the direction of the peptide bonds (Fig. 10*k*). This can be achieved by construction of a reversed sequence from amino acids of the opposite (enantiomeric) configuration. Such "retro-enantio" isomers most closely resemble the prototypes when the peptides are cyclic (*64, 515*). In noncyclic retro-enantio isomers the positions of the endgroups remain reversed. The design of such analogs could no doubt be improved by omission of the amino endgroup where this is known to be inessential and introduction of a "false" terminal carboxyl or carboxamide group could be achieved by terminating the chain at the amino end by a (suitably substituted) malonic or malonamic acid unit.

Apart from the endgroup problem there remains, of course, some degree of nonequivalence in the attachment of the side chain to the normal and reversed system of peptide bonds—this is extreme in the case of proline (*576*) where the end of the side chain can be regarded as reattached to the backbone—and the possibility that the peptide groups themselves take part in receptor binding and activation.

Ovchinnikov, Shemyakin, and their colleagues have shown that retro-enantio isomers of the cyclodepsipeptide antibiotics and of a simplified gramicidin S structure (with the proline residue replaced by glycine) are biologically active (*515, 516*). However, the reversed-sequence, all-D analogs of [Gly^9]-bradykinin (*540, 576, 577*) and of α-melanotropin-(6–10)-penta-peptide (*114*) have proved inactive (*576, 577*) or almost inactive (*540*) as agonists and ineffective as inhibitors (*114, 540, 576, 577*). In the case of brady-kinin the presence of three proline residues makes it likely that the topology of the two molecules is, in fact, rather different (*576*) and recent work (*269*) has shown, by omission of the endgroups, that these are of considerable importance for activity.

5. Conformational Stabilization

One approach to limiting the uncertainties about the active conformation of peptide molecules is through the introduction of additional crosslinks which would greatly limit the number of conformations accessible to the peptide chain and to the whole molecule. This approach has not been explored extensively, probably because there are no plausible hypotheses indicating which among the many possible conformations should be aimed at; because it is difficult to design bridges which would not, by their additional bulk, introduce new ambiguities; and because such designs would generally be difficult to realize synthetically.

The only ventures in this direction so far have been the conversions of linear into homodetic cyclic peptides: the synthesis of a [Gly^7]-cyclokallidin (*341*) and cyclization of a des-Asp^1,Arg^2-angiotensin hexapeptide (*270*) which itself unfortunately already has low activity. Both products were practically inactive. Cyclization of the peptide chain, though chemically the simplest way of limiting conformational freedom, would not be expected to succeed where the endgroups are known to be essential.

A more subtle form of conformational stabilization has been attempted by attaching a poly-(O-acetylserine) chain to the terminus of angiotensin (*15*). This was based on the hypothesis (*531*) that angiotensin has an α-helical conformation in its interaction with the receptor. The analogue was active (*15*) but no evidence for an effect on the conformation of the angiotensin sequence has been provided. O-Acetylserine in any case is more likely to support the formation of β-structures than of an α-helix.

Recently, substitutions in the peptide backbone or side chains are being used to limit the range of possible backbone conformations by hindering free rotation around the $C_{(\alpha)}$–CO and N–$C_{(\alpha)}$ bonds, and thereby to narrow the possibilities which need be considered for the active conformation of the molecule. Jorgensen and his co-workers (*634*) have introduced β-branched and unbranched aliphatic side chains (see Section II,C,4,g) and also α-methylalanine (α-aminoisobutyric acid), cycloleucine (1-aminocyclopentane-carboxylic acid), and D- or L-proline into position 5 of [Asn^1]-angiotensin II and concluded that a conformational preference of $\phi \sim -120°$ and $\psi \sim +120°$ at $C_{(\alpha)}$ of the amino acid in position 5 correlates well with high pressor potency. Substitutions with α-methylalanine and cycloleucine in this and other positions of angiotensin II have also been reported by others (639, 642).

In the model system of ribonuclease-S, X-ray crystallography has revealed the three-dimensional picture of the active conformation and S-peptide should therefore be a particularly suitable object for studies of this type.

III. Biological Aspects and Practical Aims of Design

A. SIMPLIFIED SYNTHESIS

Structural alterations designed to simplify synthesis become relevant when peptide drugs are to be made on a large scale. In the very first synthetic analogs of a peptide hormone to be designed, oxytocin was modified at position 3 partly because this is a site of variation in the natural hormones (83, 437) but also because the isoleucine in this position was at that time still one of the least accessible amino acids (437). As it turned out replacement of isoleucine by valine or leucine (83, 359, 437) decreased the activity so that the analogs were not attractive for practical use.

In the synthesis of the angiotensins asparagine was originally used in position 1 as a protected form of aspartic acid (428, 504) but since the asparagine-containing intermediates were themselves highly active, [Asn^1]-angiotensin$_b$ II (428) was chosen as the standard derivative for production.

However, it is for the long chain peptide hormones that the problem of simplifying structure—essentially, reducing the chain length—becomes important or even critical. Although the full sequences of bovine (503) and even human (19, 20) corticotropins have been synthesized by now it is hardly thinkable that these could have been produced as synthetic drugs at the time (1961–1963) when the production of highly active shorter fragments (see Section II,B,1), in particular the tetracosactide of Schwyzer and Kappeler (287, 495) and the (1–23)-tricosapeptide amide of Geiger, Sturm, and Siedel (171), became feasible.

The replacement of methionine by norleucine which was incorporated together with other changes in a corticotropin analog (84) eliminates the complications arising from oxidation of the methionine and thereby not only increases stability (84) but also simplifies synthesis. Replacement of the arginine residues in positions 17 and 18 of shortened corticotropin sequences (130, 194, 421) in addition to increasing potency (Section III,B,2) should also simplify synthesis.

The very short sequences required for high gastrin activity (see Section II,B,1) no doubt encouraged production of a gastrin analog for diagnostic use. "Pentagastrin," Boc–βAla–Trp–Met–Asp–Phe–NH$_2$, was chosen from among several highly active analogs for this purpose (*121, 350, 354*).

B. Increased Potency and Selectivity

1. *Increased Potency*

Because many peptide hormones are extremely potent there has been little incentive to a search for more potent analogs. Increased selectivity (see Section III,B,2) or duration of action (Section III,D) has generally been considered more important. However, analogs more active than the natural peptides have been repeatedly encountered. In many cases the increase in potency resulted from structural changes which were designed, or might have been expected, to increase resistance toward inactivating enzymes; desamino-oxytocin (*236, 571*), [βAsp^1]-angiotensin$_b$ II (*420, 425*), a depsipeptide brady-kinin analog (*411*), desamino-[D-Arg^8]-vasopressin (*562, 623*) and corticotropin derivatives with *N*-terminal D-serine (*84, 124, 125, 130, 268, 284, 420*), β-hydr-oxypropionic acid (*130*), and β-alanine (*170*) are cases in point. Often the potency measured in terms of the intensity of the response was increased with-out any apparent change in the duration of the effect or with only a slight increase. The possible pharmacokinetic basis of these findings is discussed in Section III,D,3.

Insulin, which is consumed in enormous amounts, is one hormone in which increased potency would be exceedingly welcome. The discovery that some nonmammalian insulins have a higher potency than those of mammals (see Section III,E) may provide a pointer to the design of more active analogs.

2. *Increased Selectivity*

As has been pointed out (Section 1,A) the peptide hormones generally act on more than one organ or tissue. In some instances the concentrations required differ so greatly that this alone ensures sufficient selectivity. In other situations it is desirable to increase the selectivity still further or, on the other hand, to accentuate an effect which in the natural hormone is less prominent and probably nonphysiological.

Examples of both kinds are provided by the neurohypophysial hormones. Thus vasopressin analogs have been developed which have a higher anti-diuretic : pressor activity ratio than the parent hormones and are improved antidiuretic agents (Table VII). Huguenin, Boissonnas, and their colleagues combined the finding that omission of the phenolic hydroxyl group from arginine vasopressin (but not from lysine vasopressin; see below) decreases the pressor but hardly affects the antidiuretic potency (245) with the observation that omission of the α-amino group from lysine vasopressin (300) and arginine vasopressin (247, 249) increases the antidiuretic but decreases the pressor activity and developed the highly potent and selective antidiuretic

TABLE VII

SELECTIVITY OF SOME VASOPRESSIN ANALOGS: ANTIDIURETIC AND PRESSOR ACTIVITIES IN THE RAT AND THEIR RATIO[a]

Vasopressin analog	Potency (% of [Arg^8]-vasopressin)		
	Antidiuretic (A)	Pressor (P)	Ratio P/A
[Lys^8]-	62	68	1.1
[Phe^2,Lys^8]-	5	14	2.7
[Orn^8]-	22	90	4.1
[Phe^2,Orn^8]-	4	38	9.6
[Ile^3,Orn^8]-	0.62	26	41
[Phe^2,Ile^3,Orn^8]-	0.14	30	220
1-Desamino-[Orn^8]-	50	89	1.8
1-Desamino-[Phe^2,Orn^8]-	3.2	11	3.5
1-Desamino-[Ile^3, Orn^8]-	17	67	3.9
1-Desamino-[Phe^2,Ile^3,Orn^8]-	1	25	25
			A/P
[Arg^8]-	100	100	1
[Phe^2,Arg^8]-	87	30	2.9
1-Desamino-[Arg^8]-	325	92	3.5
1-Desamino-[Phe^2,Arg^8]-	200	7.2	27
[D-Arg^8]-	28	1	28
1-Desamino-[D-Arg^8]-	218[b]	2.8	79

[a] From Huguenin (243) and Zaoral, Kolc, and Šorm (623).
[b] For low dose range (about 10 pg/100 gm).

agent, desamino-[Phe^2,Arg^8]-vasopressin (247, 546). On the other hand, Zaoral and Šorm had noted that substitution by a basic D-amino acid in position 8 sharply decreased the pressor activity but left relatively high antidiuretic potency (621, 622, 625, 627). Further modification by omission of the amino group gave another highly active and selective compound, desamino-[D-Arg^8]-vasopressin (623), which shows some clinical promise (562).

Conversely, the vascular effects of vasopressin which probably play no physiological role were less affected by omission of the phenolic hydroxyl group from lysine vasopressin than was the antidiuretic activity (Table VII) and the resulting [Phe^2,Lys^8]-vasopressin (77) has found application as a selective vasoconstrictor agent (39, 186, 208). A further increase in this ratio, and an absolute increase in pressor activity, could be achieved by placing ornithine in position 8 (242, 246) and isoleucine in position 3 (35, 36, 242). Omission of the amino group, as was to be expected (see above) again accentuates the antidiuretic properties (243).

There are indications that even the vascular effects of the neurohypophysial hormones can be more or less selective for particular types of blood vessels or vascular beds (4, 31, 36); changed selectivity can also result from sustained release of the active peptide from "hormonogen" analogs (116) (see Section III,D,5). The design of analogs with more precisely defined vascular effects will, however, require much more detailed pharmacological analysis than has hitherto been customary. Altura's work on the microcirculation (3) is an excellent example of such an approach.

In the case of oxytocin it was noted that the milk-ejection activity was generally less sensitive to structural changes than the uterotonic or vascular effects (359, 400, 451) and several analogs of oxytocin were considered for practical use as galactogogues: [3-alloisoleucine]-oxytocin (281, 359, 400), [4-glycine]-oxytocin (165) and desamino-[4-α-aminobutyric acid]-oxytocin (86, 564). However, Krejčí and Poláček have shown (398) that the increased ratio of milk-ejection to in vitro uterotonic activity may be an experimental artefact due to the convention of assaying for uterotonic activity in vitro in the absence of magnesium and for the effect on the mammary gland, in vitro or in vivo, in the presence of magnesium. If the activities are assayed under comparable conditions the apparent selectivity largely disappears, at least for the analogues modified in position 3. Nevertheless, an improved ratio of milk-ejection to vascular and antidiuretic activity (all assayed in vivo) remains as an advantage, particularly when the peptide is to be given sublingually or as a spray and the dosage is therefore difficult to control precisely.

[2-O-Methyltyrosine]-oxytocin (277, 278, 316) has an oxytocin-like action on the uterus in situ (306) but inhibits the vascular effects of oxytocin under similar conditions (304, 316). Evidently as a result of this selectivity it stimulates labor in humans without the attendant clinically undesirable increase in blood lactate which appears to be a result of the vasoconstrictor action exerted by oxytocin (but not by the analog) in the uterine and placental circulation (211, 212).

Modification of the terminal glycine amide group is often more damaging to the vascular effects than to other activities. It is therefore not entirely unexpected that mono- or dimethylation of this group in derivatives of desaminooxytocin leaves appreciable uterotonic but abolishes avian depressor activity (550). More detailed pharmacological studies of these and related compounds will be awaited with interest.

Structural modifications designed to improve the selectivity of vasopressin as a corticotropin-releasing factor (191) have been based on the report (455) that a porcine hypophysial peptide with strong corticotropin-releasing activity contained serine and histidine in addition to the component amino acids of lysine vasopressin. Attachment of histidyl-seryl or seryl-histidyl sequences to the amino terminus of oxytocin and lysine vasopressin (191) did, indeed, increase the relative but decreased the absolute corticotropin-releasing activity (131, 166). It was suspected (432) that the increased corticotropin-releasing specificity may be a consequence of the "hormonogen" character of the peptides rather than any relation to a specific natural peptide. Attachment of three glycine residues (290) instead of the histidine and serine was, in fact, found to give the same effect (417).

The diuretic and natriuretic activity of [Leu^4]-oxytocin (107) and [Leu^4,Ile^8]-oxytocin (442, 506) may be an example of a situation in which a "new" activity appears because another more prominent one has been eliminated. The natural neurohypophysial hormones are well known to have natriuretic and diuretic effects (see 33) but these can be demonstrated only under special conditions because they are generally masked in the standard assays by the conspicuous antidiuretic activity. A mere suppression of the antidiuretic effect might therefore be sufficient to give prominence to the interesting natriuretic action. Leucine is the only one in a series of amino acids substituted in this position which is reported to elicit these effects (163) and additional changes in other parts of the molecule will no doubt be made in an effort to accentuate them. Omission of the amino group appears to restore some antidiuretic activity (see 163). This example incidentally emphasizes the need for a thorough pharmacological analysis if novel starting points for design are not to be missed.

Gastrin analogs were early tested for a wide range of effects (354, 556). Although some dissociation of activities was observed it was concluded that there was no marked selectivity in a qualitative sense (354) and the practical incentive was toward the design of an inhibitor rather than an agonist of increased selectivity (351). The discovery of caerulein (11, 45) and phyllocaerulein (6, 46) and their structural and pharmacological relation (6, 8, 153) to both gastrin and pancreozymin-cholecystokinin (356, 357) has reopened this problem (7, 8, 51) since "gastrin-like," "pancreozymin-cholecystokinin-like," and hypotensive activities are here carried by the same molecule. So far it has been found (5, 7, 8) that the O-sulfated tyrosine residue separated by two amino acid residues from the carboxyl-terminal tetrapeptide sequence shared with the two hormones is critical for activity on the gallbladder but not for the "gastrin-like" effects (351, 352, 641). Presumably this situation will stimulate more work directed toward selectively acting peptides.

Among the other classes of peptides there seems to have been little induce-ment toward, and search for, more selectivity. It is symptomatic that most analogs of angiotensin and bradykinin with a few exceptions (*97, 132, 385, 537, 616*) have been tested only on one or two pharmacological preparations (see *477*) and the tests chosen have, moreover, differed from one laboratory to another. Where changes have been observed in the relative activities on blood vessels (measured *in vivo*) and smooth muscle (uterus, intestine) *in vitro* these may have been due to changes in metabolic behavior rather than tissue specifities (see Section III,D,1,c). As in the case of vasopressin analogs it would seem worth while to search for changes in specificity for different segments of the vascular tree, or different vascular beds, by more differentiated assay systems.

The recent finding that structural changes in position 8 of angiotensin can dissociate the direct musculotropic effects from the indirect effects mediated by inhibition of norepinephrine uptake into sympathetic (*387*) or release of acetylcholine from parasympathetic nerve endings (*555*) reveals a new and interesting aspect of specificity for these peptides. Thus [8-alanine]- and [8-(DL-3-amino-3-benzylbutyric acid)]-angiotensin$_e$ II have very little pressor activity yet inhibit cardiac norepinephrine uptake (*387*). Replacement of phenylalanine in angiotensin$_e$ II with tyrosine (but not with O-methyltyrosine) reduces the direct musculotropic effect on the guinea pig ileum more than the acetylcholine-mediated contractile effect, while [Ala^8]-angiotensin$_e$ II acts as an inhibitor (*555*). Although the possible systemic resultants of these specificity changes are not clear the findings again illustrate the way in which detailed pharmacological analysis can give new directions to the design of analogs.

In the corticotropin–melanotropin family the effects of chain length (see Section II,B,1) and acetylation (Section II,C,2,a) which have been defined in the course of systematic studies give such specificity that no additional differ-entiation is required. The corticotropin-releasing activity of peptides with partial melanotropin sequences has been reported (*169, 285, 286*) but no systematic structural studies designed to increase this effect seem to have been made. The metabolic effects (e.g., *318, 319, 404, 551*) and actions on the nervous system (e.g., *155, 310*) also have been studied without, however, being deliberate aims for analog design.

3. *Suppression of Immunoreactivity*

Most peptide and protein hormones are antigenic (able to react with specific antibodies) and, under suitable conditions, immunogenic (able to induce antibody formation). Antigenicity must also be regarded as a form of bio-logical activity which may present serious problems (neutralization of hormonal effects, autoimmune endocrinopathies, allergic reactions) particularly with the larger peptide (or protein) hormones and with peptides which are administered chronically. Although antisera produced against a particular polypeptide by different species or individuals, or even the several antibodies in the antiserum of a single individual, may be directed against different regions of the antigenic molecule certain regions will tend to be more generally antigenic than others. If such antigenic regions do not coincide with the regions required for physiological activity—and on general grounds there is no reason why they should, provided the molecule is sufficiently large—then it should be possible to decrease antigenicity while preserving activity.

It was to be suspected that the species-specific sequences 25–33 of the natural corticotropins would be particularly immunogenic in other species and, indeed, tetracosactide is only weakly immunogenic (*17, 161, 572*) and reacts only very weakly with anticorticotropin antibodies (*154, 161, 253*). Shorter sequences are even less immunoactive (*17, 154, 253*) while some of them still retain good hormonal activity (see Section II,B,1). This is an additional bonus of shortened sequences.

The elimination of antigenicity is likely to be especially important in the case of insulin. Though no insulin analogs have yet been obtained in a sufficiently pure state for a quantitative determination of potency on the one hand and antigenicity on the other, this line of structural design is likely to be intensively pursued in the coming years.

Even so small a peptide as vasopressin can be immunogenic and it has been suspected that the vasopressin resistance of some patients with cephalic diabetes insipidus may result from an immune reaction to the exogenous vasopressins (*430*). In one such patient who was refractory to both arginine and lysine vasopressin the analog, desamino-[D-Arg^8]-vasopressin, produced a good response (*562*). Synthetic peptide hormone analogs, though not specifically designed for the purpose, may therefore be worth trying in place of the normal (isolated or synthetic) hormones where an immune reaction is suspected.

C. ANTAGONISTS

Approaches to the design of antagonists may be based, in general terms, on the receptor theory of drug action.* This predicts that if a hormone analog is still capable of binding to the specific hormone receptor but is modified in

---

* An a priori approach has been based on the nucleic acid triplet code for amino acids: The anticodons corresponding to the polynucleotide code "message" for the active peptide were retranslated into amino acid sequences and the corresponding peptides synthesized (*351*). The procedure, while original, is somewhat analogous to a search for antonyms by spelling words backward and seems about as likely to afford success.

such a way that the peptide–receptor complex is incapable of whatever primary process is required to initiate the response, then such an analog will act as a competitive inhibitor. For the deliberate *ab initio* design of an inhibitor on this basis it would be necessary to know which regions of the hormone molecule are involved in binding only and which are directly or indirectly required for the biochemical functionality of the hormone–receptor complex (it is, of course, possible for a given group to contribute to both). Generally such knowledge itself only emerges from studies of structure–activity relationships and most clearly from observations of partial agonism or antagonism. To break into this vicious circle the design of effective inhibitors generally extrapolates from empirically acquired knowledge or from analogies with other groups of compounds.

1. *Modification of Chemically Reactive Groups*

One plausible assumption which might be made a priori concerns the possible role of chemically reactive groups. If it were to be assumed that the inert (unsubstituted) side chains are largely responsible for binding the hormone to the specific receptors but that reactive side chain substituents are required for the functionality of the resulting complex then the blocking or omission of such reactive groups (see Section II,C,2) would be expected to afford competitive inhibitors. Such reasoning seems to be implicit in several researches in this field.

Early work with analogs of oxytocin and vasopressin and of the melanotropins indicated that, contrary to naively chemical expectation, the chemically reactive side chain substituents are not required for activity (see, e.g., *230, 435, 563,* and Section II,C,2). However, this conclusion had to be to some extent revised when it was found that the oxytocin derivative in which the phenolic hydroxyl group of the tyrosine was blocked by methylation ([Tyr(Me)²]-oxytocin; "methyloxytocin") behaved as a partial agonist or inhibitor (*27, 277, 278, 304–307, 316, 443*) and—what is even more important in principle—that even the analog in which the hydroxyl group was merely omitted, [Phe²]-oxytocin, showed such behavior under suitable conditions (*108, 309, 443, 444*). With these observations as the starting point the familiar pattern of structural modification was then initiated (see Section II,C,4,f) and more universal inhibitors were obtained either by increasing the size of the *p*-substituent replacing the tyrosine hydroxyl group (*117, 433, 444, 630*) or by also substituting the terminal amino group (*61–63, 110*). Additional substitution of the amino group in *N*-carbamoyl-*O*-methyloxytocin gives a highly effective antagonist which, unlike methyloxytocin itself (*306*), inhibits the action of oxytocin on the uterus and mammary gland also *in vivo* (*61–63*). *N,O*-Disubstitution in the dicarbamoyl (*533*) and diacetyl (*534*) derivatives of oxytocin also confers inhibitor properties but their range has not yet been defined.

By analogy with the results for oxytocin the [2-O-methyltyrosine] (521, 574, 619) and [2-O-ethyltyrosine] (619) analogs of lysine vasopressin were synthesized and found to inhibit the actions of both oxytocin and vasopressin (304, 444, 574, 619), the O-ethyl derivative again being the more effective (304, 444). The result of additional N^{α}-substitution has not yet been examined in the vasopressin series.

Presumably by analogy (118) O-methyltyrosine has also been substituted for tyrosine in [Asn¹]-angiotensin$_b$ II (118, 474). The analog had low activity, much lower than that produced by mere omission of the hydroxyl group (487, 504), but apparently no inhibitor properties. Similar reuslts have been obtained with [Tyr(Me)⁴] analogs of other angiotensin II derivatives (631).

Also by analogy, O-methyltyrosine has been substituted for phenylalanine in bradykinin (540). Whatever the validity of the analogy in this case the [Tyr(Me)⁵,Tyr(Me)⁸]-bradykinin and several of its derivatives were indeed found to inhibit the action of bradykinin on the rat uterus though the effect was variable and a bradykinin-like action supervened at higher concentrations. The vascular effects of these analogs have not yet been reported. Similar results were also produced when the phenylalanines were replaced by leucines and in addition serine by threonine (539, 540).

Returning to the molecule of oxytocin we may note that omission of the asparagine carboxamide group not only greatly decreases activity (192, 565) but also changes its character by decreasing the maximal response of the uterus even to saturation doses (108) (partial agonism). It remains to be seen if suitable substitution in this position can restore some of the affinity while maintaining or increasing the functional deficiency. The [Val⁵]- and [Orn⁵]-oxytocins (205, 588) offer no promise in this respect.

It has already been pointed out (444) that changes in the terminal carboxamide group of glycine amide—its omission (88), displacement by chain lengthening (139, 140, 375) (see Section II,D,2), by chain shortening (260) (see Section II,B,1), or by introduction of D-leucine into the penultimate position (461), as also hydrolysis of the amide group (133, 139, 140, 158, 342) (see Section II,C,2,a)—all cause the appearance of antagonism in one or both of the blood pressure assays and in some cases a decrease in the maximal response of the uterus in vitro (108, 139) or inhibition together with uterotonic action (375). To decide whether the inhibitor properties of [NH·Gly⁹]-oxytocin (375) were associated with the hydrazide group or with the chain lengthening the "aza" isoster, [9-semicarbazide]-oxytocin, was prepared (372) which also has a hydrazide grouping but maintains the position of the terminal amide group. The high potency of this analog, together with the inhibitor properties of [βAla⁹]-lysine vasopressin (140) which has no hydrazide grouping but a lengthened chain, confirmed that it is the misalignment of the terminal amide group with which inhibition can be correlated.

Little effort seems to have been made to develop and exploit the properties of this group of inhibitors or potential inhibitors until recently. The finding (*133, 342*) that [Gly·OH^9,Arg^8]-vasopressin ([Arg^8]-vasopressinoic acid) inhibits the vasopressin-induced antidiuresis in the rat (and the activity of kidney medullary adenyl cyclase) is likely to change this situation, because of clinical interest in an "antiantidiuretic" compound.

A beautifully clear-cut case of antagonism has been observed between two of the natural neurohypophysial hormones. Jard and Morel have found that the antidiuretic and natriuretic action of vasotocin on the frog kidney is inhibited by oxytocin. Examination of a series of analogs indicated a functional role in this organ for the basic side chain substituent in position 8 and a critical role in receptor binding for the isoleucine residue in position 3 (*261, 262, 348*). Unfortunately, these findings have no obvious relevance to the mammalian kidney and presumably for this reason have not been followed up by further structural variations.

The diuretic and "anti-vasopressin" effect of [Leu^4]-oxytocin (*107*) and [Leu^4,Ile^8]-oxytocin (*442*) (synthesized in another context; see Section III,E) may be connected with their natriuretic activity (*107, 506*) though [Leu^4,Ile^8]-oxytocin also inhibits the hydroosmotic effect of oxytocin on the toad bladder (*142*).

Any evidence for the involvement of a particular group in the function of a hormone–receptor complex naturally makes that group a particularly challenging target. The great sensitivity of the aspartic acid residue in tetragastrin derivatives to structural change has been interpreted as indicating such a role (*350, 351*). However, since none of the inactive compounds modified in this positions behaved as obvious antagonists this would seem to be a case where the same group also makes an important contribution to binding.

The hypothesis that the disulfide bond of the neurohypophysial hormones was functionally involved in the process initiating responses in the toad bladder and kidney (see, e.g., *409*) was one of the motives for designing "carba" analogs of these hormones (*273, 438*) (see Section II,C,4,d); if the hypothesis had been correct these analogs, being isosteric with oxytocin, should have been bound to the receptors by noncovalent interactions but, lacking the disulfide group, should have been unable to initiate a response: They should have been competitive inhibitors. In point of fact the compounds are highly potent agonists and thereby disprove the hypothesis instead of validating the principle of antagonist design.

However, synthetic analogs of oxytocin with the hemicystine residues replaced by alanines (*272*) (see Section II,C,2,b) or serines (*360*) in addition to showing feeble oxytocin-like activity can act as inhibitors of oxytocin on the rat uterus (399). Independently it was found (383) that the carboxyl-terminal tetrapeptide and octapeptide amide sequences of oxytocin (with S-benzylcysteine in position 6) are oxytocin antagonists; in the latter case inhibition is consistently competitive (pA_2 5.7) though the specificity has not been established in any of these cases.

Such results might have been taken to indicate a functional requirement for the disulfide group if it were not for the fact that isosters lacking the S—S group are potent agonists, as has just above been noted. An interpretation of the inhibitor properties of the acyclic analogs has been proposed in terms of "nonproductive" binding, with functionally important groups (tyrosine?) misaligned on the receptor because of the greater conformational freedom of the acyclic molecules (399). This rationalization does not hold out hopes of designing much more potent inhibitors of this type because the same conformational freedom will also result in weakened binding to the receptor.

[Ala⁸]-Angiotensin$_e$ II has no contractile action on the guinea pig ileum but in high doses inhibits the response to angiotensin given subsequently (555). This effect is discussed in terms of tachyphylaxis rather than inhibition but it is specific and presumably competitive. It will be interesting to explore the structural and pharmacological range of this behavior. Conceivably it may be due to misalignment resulting from elimination of a binding site rather than from a functional (in the chemical or biological sense) role of the phenyl group.

Recently, Marshall and his co-workers (640) have found that [Phe⁴,Tyr⁸]-angiotensin$_b$ II, an analog in which the tyrosine and phenylalanine residues of the native hormone are interchanged, acts as a specific competitive inhibitor of angiotensin in vitro and in vivo.

A survey of these results gives rise to the suspicion that chemically reactive groups may, after all, be involved in the function of the hormone–receptor complexes at least in some cases. In the model system, ribonuclease-S, the imidazole ring of histidine (159, 160, 218) and the amino group of lysine (505) are certainly involved in enzyme action. If, however, more than one such group participates but no single one is essential, the elimination of one of them may decrease efficacy without causing inhibition.

2. Pharmacological Desiderata in the Search for Antagonists

In this connection it is relevant to examine the pharmacological situation, and again work on oxytocin analogs can be instructive.

It has been noted that methyloxytocin can behave as a full agonist, partial agonist, or antagonist according to the test object and experimental conditions (305–307, 316, 443, 444). If a normal assay procedure designed to give quantitative results is used (e.g., a 2 + 2 dose procedure) partial agonism may well be missed if the doses are in the lower range. Rudinger and Krejčí (443) have emphasized that with peptides, as with other drugs, full dose–response curves should be recorded wherever possible if anomalies are to be detected. It was, indeed, obedience to this principle which revealed the partial agonist character in the action on the isolated rat uterus of 9-decarboxamido- and 5-decarb-oxamido-oxytocin (*108*) and oxytocinoic acid (*139*) and also, unexpectedly, of lysine vasopressin and other neurohypophysial hormone analogs with phenylalanine in position 3 (*585, 586*). It has also revealed partial agonism when applied to work with the toad bladder (*141*) and vascular smooth muscle strips (*3*).

Furthermore, those conditions which ensure high sensitivity of the uterine strip and are therefore favored for assay purposes (intensive estrogen pretreatment, relatively high calcium concentrations, addition of magnesium, high temperature) are exactly those under which the anomalous properties are least in evidence. As the conditions are made "worse," with attendant decrease in the sensitivity of the assay, partial agonism and eventually antagonism appear (*306, 307, 444*). With analogs such as [Phe²]-oxytocin conditions have to be made very "bad" (uteri from spayed rats washed free of calcium and restored to a medium low in calcium) before inhibition can be seen (*309, 444*) and this is presumably why its anomalous properties were missed in earlier work. Creation of "bad" assay conditions evidently decreases the efficiency of the stimulus–response coupling, a situation which not only decreases sensitivity but also leads to disappearance (mobilization) of the receptor reserve and thereby reveals decreased intrinsic activity (*309, 636*).

Whatever the mechanism, the experimental observation remains that the favored assay conditions are not necessarily the best for detecting partial agonism or antagonism and that, if antagonists are to be screened for, special conditions should be developed which may well be such that no self-respecting pharmacologist would use them for assay purposes.

By following these two principles, recording full dose–response curves and developing special experimental conditions, wherever this is feasible, structural features leading to partial agonism should be more readily detected and once such features are identified the design of inhibitors can be attempted, as described for the work starting from methyloxytocin in Section II,C,4,f. It may well be that such an approach would also lead to antagonists in those groups of peptides where the search has so far shown little success.

3. *Diastereomers*

In pentamelatrin certain replacements of L- by D-amino acids (originally made in the expectation of protracted effects: see Section III,D,1) afforded analogs which inhibit the melanotropic action of the all-L-pentapeptide. The very systematic work with this sequence is summarized in Table VI and it will be noted that the all-D-pentamelatrin is such an inhibitor. When three further (L) amino acids were added to this core to complete the carboxyl-terminal sequence of α-melanotropin, in [D-His^6,D-Phe^7,D-Arg^8,D-Trp^9, Lys(For)^{11}]-α-melanotropin-(6–13)-octapeptide amide, the product was an antagonist of the corresponding all-L-peptide but further extension by L-amino acids at the amino end reversed the inhibitor properties: [D-His^6,D-Phe^7, D-Arg^8,D-Trp^9]-α-melanotropin had normal melanotropic activity (605).

A similar analog of tetracosatide with the sequence Glu^5–Trp^9 in the D configuration (284) had no adrenal-stimulating or lipotropic activity and did not inhibit the lipotropic activity of tetracosatide (284). However, recently it has been found to inhibit the stimulating effect of tetracosactide on the adenyl cyclase of a fat-cell membrane preparation (56).

In all these cases it is unclear whether the diastereomerism is merely one way of "misplacing" functionally required groups or whether more subtle relations are involved. Analogs in which suspect groups (indole, guanidine) are omitted or preferably replaced isosterically would be useful for comparison.

With or without specific reference to the inhibitor properties of all-D-pentamelatrin the all-D analogs of other active peptides have also been synthesized (see Section II,C,4,i); none was an inhibitor.

Numerous analogs with only one or a few D-amino acids have also been prepared (Section II,C,4,i), in some cases at least in the hope of obtaining antagonists. [D-Tyr^2]-Oxytocin does have some inhibitor (as well as agonist) properties when tested on the isolated rat uterus (137). This is in line with the properties of other analogs modified in position 2 (see Section II,C,4,f and III,C,1) and may not be specifically due to the diastereomeric relation. It was also noted that some (unspecified) D-amino acid analogues of eledoisin have weak antagonist properties (332, 479) but no details have been given. [D-Pro^2, D-Pro^3,D-Pro^7]- and des-Arg^1-[D-Arg^9]-bradykinin have been reported to show inhibitor, as well as agonist, properties when tested on the isolated rat uterus (540). No inhibitors have been detected among the diasteromers of angiotensin or of tetragastrin.

4. Increase in Size of the Molecule

It has been a widely accepted rule in the pharmacology of cholinergic and adrenergic substances that an increase in the size of the molecule will tend to produce antagonists. At first sight the properties of the O-substituted analogs of oxytocin and vasopressin would seem to support a similar rule even for peptides. However, since the desoxy derivative, with the molecule *decreased* in size, also has inhibitor properties under suitable conditions it must be the absence of the hydroxyl group which is the primary source of such properties.

With explicit reference to this rule (540) and to experience in the "strepogenin" field (539) the serine in bradykinin was replaced by threonine; simultaneously one or both phenylalanines were replaced by leucine. Compounds with some inhibitor activity were obtained but as no antagonist properties have been reported for [Thr^6]-bradykinin itself (127, 539) or for analogs in which the size of the side chain in position 6 was increased for instance by carbamoylation of the serine (127) or by its replacement with asparagine (366), phenylalanine, or tosyllysine (540) it seems that the replacement of the phenylalanine residues by leucine is more important for the observed inhibition than the (formal) C-methylation of the serine. It has been noted (Section III,C,1) that other modifications in the phenylalanine positions also cause antagonism (540).

In empirical agreement with the "size rule" a doubly C-methylated oxytocin, [1-penicillamine]-oxytocin, and its desamino derivative are potent inhibitors of the uterotonic effect of oxytocin though no rationale was invoked in the design of these analogs (106, 482). Substitution with only one methyl group (483) or replacement of the other hemicystine (484) did not afford inhibitors.

The endo-Tyr^{2a}-analog of oxytocin was also found to have inhibitor properties (193). In other cases similar doubling of tyrosine or other residues (see Section II,B,3) did not lead to antagonists. It has been suggested (444) that the inhibitor properties of the endo-Tyr^{2a} derivative may be due to displacement of the functional tyrosine hydroxyl group from its proper position. In this sense it may be related to the inhibitors considered under Section III,C,1.

5. Specific Irreversible Inhibitors

Specific irreversible inhibitors of the peptide hormones analogous to the "site-directed irreversible inhibitors" of enzymology or "affinity labels" of immunology, or indeed to some classes of irreversible inhibitors from other fields of pharmacology, would constitute extremely valuable tools for studying the pharmacology and molecular biology of hormone action as well as potential drugs. The design of such inhibitors requires that a suitable chemically reactive group should be attached to the hormone structure in such a way that the ability of the molecule to bind to the specific receptors is not impaired. In the latter respect the problem of design is similar to that encountered in introducing "marker" groups (see Section III,F). What a "suitable" group is in this context cannot be decided a priori since the structure of the receptor is completely unknown and potential targets for the "anchor" group can only be guessed at. As a general requirement common to all such systems the group must be sufficiently stable to survive for a reasonable time in the medium used for the experiment (including the nonspecific components of the target tissue) but sufficiently reactive to become attached in the time during which the molecule is kinetically immobilized on the receptor. In peptide hormones, the "anchor" group must also be compatible with the functional groups already present in the peptide moiety, otherwise it would obviously spend itself by intra- or intermolecular reaction with its carrier peptide.

The pitfalls attaching to the use of such compounds once they have been designed and synthesized—nonspecific binding, "silent" receptors, and others—need not concern us here.

Since [2-*p*-aminophenylalanine]-oxytocin was available from other work (*436*) (see Section II,C,4,f) its diazotisation was attempted; after all, the compound is a substituted aniline. However, at the pH required for experiments with tissues (uterus, frog skin) the diazonium salt decomposed rapidly and no irreversible inhibition was observed.

The introduction of substituents such as chloroacetyl into hexeledoisin (*336*) or 4-chloro-6-dimethylamino-2-triazolyl into a lysyl-tetragastrin (*349, 350*) may have been intended to serve a similar purpose though no experiments have been described. Other possibilities have been discussed with particular reference to gastrin (*351*).

In spite of the slow start it can be predicted that this line of design will be very actively pursued in the near future.

D. Modification of Metabolism and Distribution

The metabolic phases of hormone action have received a good deal of attention as the target for analog design, partly no doubt because of the practical attractions of hormone derivatives with protracted action but presumably also because rather more is known, or surmised, about the molecular aspects of inactivation than about, say, the molecular events at the tissue receptors.

Several approaches have been explored in efforts to obtain protracted action. The most obvious aims to modify the structure of the peptide in such a way as to make the molecule resistant toward the enzymes assumed to be responsible for its inactivation. Alternatively, peptides may be designed which, though they are themselves inert in relation to the receptors, have a "sparing" effect by acting as competitive substrates or as inhibitors of enzymes destroying the active peptides. Again, attempts may be made to slow down excretion of the active peptide or more generally to modify its distribution properties in such a way as to prevent or slow down "dilution" into the organism. Finally, derivatives may be designed from which the active peptide is expected to be released gradually by enzyme action or chemically. Examples of each of these approaches will be given below.

1. Conferring Resistance to Enzymes

Ideally the design of enzyme-resistant analogs should be based on knowledge of the enzymes actually responsible for disposition of the hormone under physiological conditions. In actual practice possible sites of enzymic attack are often designated on general grounds even without experimental evidence—the ends of the chain as being susceptible to aminopeptidases or carboxypeptidases, peptide bonds involving basic or aromatic amino acids as being sensitive to trypsin- or chymotrypsin-like enzymes, etc. Alternatively, a survey may be made of the mode of inactivation by blood plasma or serum and by tissue homogenates and the design of analogs may be based on the findings.

The structural changes made to block inactivation may include substitution (methylation, acylation) or omission of the terminal amino group, and conversion of terminal carboxyl to carboxamide groups; methylation of potentially susceptible peptide bonds or their replacement by ester bonds; and the introduction of D- for L-amino acid residues or of other "unnatural" residues expected to balk the enzymes. From the results achieved so far it seems that the chemical means of conferring enzyme resistance are generally available but that the biochemical and pharmacokinetic knowledge (see Section III,D,3) brought to bear on the problem is often insufficient to achieve the desired effect.

a. Corticotropin and Melanotropin. Although there appears to be no published work on the mode of inactivation of corticotropin *in vivo* it has long been known that treatment of corticotropin or melanotropin preparations with hot dilute alkali prolongs and sometimes intensifies the melanin-dispersing action (e.g., *313*). The corticotropic action (measured by corticosteroid blood levels) of an alkali-treated corticotropin preparation was not increased (*322*). It has been suspected (*403*) and later proved (*176, 320, 391*) that this treatment causes racemization of some of the amino acid residues in the chain, particularly arginine and phenylalanine. Hydrolysis of peptide bonds and conversion of arginine to ornithine also occur (*176, 391*). The prolonged action was thought to result from increased resistance to inactivating enzymes. These observations prompted the synthesis of melanotropin analogs containing ornithine (*330*) or citrulline (as a possible alternative degradation product of arginine) (*69*) and preparation of a number of pentamelatrin analogs in which phenylalanine (*330, 457, 612*), arginine (*604, 609*), histidine and tryptophan (*607*), or several of these amino acids (*200, 604, 608, 609, 611, 612*) (see Table VI) were replaced by the D-enantiomers. Some of these compounds proved interesting as inhibitors (Section III,C,3) but only one, [D-Phe^2,Orn^3]-pentamelatrin, had prolonged action (*330*). It has recently been suggested that other effects than mere enzyme resistance may be involved (*312, 407*).

Human serum has been shown to inactivate the corticotropin-(1–26)-, -(1–19)-, and -(1–18)-peptides, at rates increasing in this order, under conditions which leave the activity of native corticotropin unchanged (*130, 252*). Corticotropin-(1–18)-octadecapeptide amide is inactivated more slowly than the free acid (*252*). These observations may explain the increased potency of the heptadeca-, octadeca-, nonadeca-, and tricosapeptide amides (*382, 405, 575*) as against the acids, and the shorter duration of the response to tetracosactide (*314, 582*) and other abbreviated sequences (*548, 549*) as against corticotropin (see *252*). An alternative explanation of the higher potency of the amides has been given in terms of the net charge in this region of the molecule (*405, 407*).

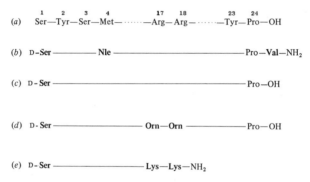

Fig. 13. Tetracosactide (*a*) and four corticotropin derivatives with prolonged action. For references, see text.

Although there seems to be no biochemical evidence that aminopeptidases are important for the disposition of corticotropin, derivatives with D-serine in the amino-terminal position, designed to be resistant to aminopeptidases (*84, 284*), have under some conditions shown prolonged action (as measured by corticosteroid levels *in vivo*) as well as high potency. In the [D-Ser^1,Nle^4,Val-NH$_2$^{25}]-corticotropin-(1–25)-pentacosapeptide (Fig. 13*b*) of Boissonnas, Guttmann, and Pless (*84*) both the amino and the carboxyl terminus are made enzyme-resistant and oxidative inactivation is precluded by replacement of methionine with norleucine. This derivative has high potency (*129*) and in humans the duration of the response is longer than that of tetracosactide (*134*) and equivalent to that of β-corticotropin (*167, 280*). The prolonged time course is more evident after intravenous than after intramuscular or subcutaneous injection (*167, 268*) and this has been ascribed to the presence of additional inactivating enzymes in muscle tissue (*167*). On the other hand, the [D-Ser^1]- and [D-Ser^1,Orn^{17},Orn^{18}]-corticotropin-(1–24)-tetracosapeptides as well as [D-Ser^1,Lys^{17},Lys^{18}]-corticotropin-(1–18)-octadecapeptide amide

(Fig. 13c–e), derivatives prepared by Riniker, Rittel, Kappeler, and their co-workers (284, 421), have prolonged effects as compared with tetracosactide when given to rats subcutaneously in higher doses as well as intravenously (124–126). The last two peptides also have prolonged effects when injected intramuscularly in humans (583). Increased potency is also shown by [D-Ala^1]- (384), [βAla^1]-, and desamino derivatives (130) of active corticotropin sequences but no studies on the duration of the response to these analogs have been reported so far.

TABLE VIII

INTENSITY AND DURATION OF PRESSOR RESPONSES TO ANALOGS OF ANGIOTENSIN$_b$ II MODIFIED IN POSITION 1 AND STABILITY OF THE PEPTIDES IN RAT SERUM AND KIDNEY EXTRACTS[a]

	Pressor response[b]		Half-life[c]	
Derivative	Intensity	Duration	Serum	Kidney extract
Angiotensin$_b$ II	100	100	100	100
[L-βAsp^1]-	150–200	200–300	430	260
[D-αAsp^1]-	150–200	200–300	500	340
[D-βAsp^1]-	150–200	200–300	500	200
1-Desamino-	50	200–300	330	280

[a] From Riniker (419). All parameters are expressed as percentages of those for angiotensin$_b$ II.

[b] Nephrectomized rats; intensity of response to equal doses and duration of response to equipressor doses.

[c] Relative time for 50% inactivation; serum from nephrectomized rats.

It must be admitted that none of the peptides discussed in the preceding paragraph when injected as aqueous solutions will reach the duration of action shown by depot preparations of β-corticotropin or tetracosactide (e.g., 167, 280). Thus zinc phosphate depot preparations may raise the plasma corticoid levels for 24–32 hr (e.g., 53, 250, 376, 410).

b. Angiotensin. The most conspicuous mode of degradation of the angiotensins in rat blood serum or human plasma is by aminopeptidase action (98, 296, 358, 412). Accordingly, analogs resistant to aminopeptidases (296, 412) such as those with a D-α-aspartyl, L- or D-β-aspartyl, or "desaminoaspartyl" (succinyl) group in the amino-terminal position (420, 425) do show protracted hypertensive action in the nephrectomized rat (96) (Table VIII) and in humans (251). No prolonged effect was found when the β-aspartyl isomer or the

N-phenylthiocarbamyl derivative (378) [which is also inactivated more slowly than angiotensin by blood or plasma (135)] were tested in dogs (135, 251). However, the β-aspartyl analog raised the blood pressure when injected subcutaneously in dogs, whereas angiotensin II in a corresponding dose did not (251).

For a number of other analogs which were found to be (296) or a priori should be resistant to aminopeptidases—the compounds with terminal γ-glutamyl, pyroglutamyl, or D-asparaginyl residues (118, 470) or with the terminal amino group carrying p-nitrobenzoyl, p-aminobenzoyl (123) or poly-(O-acetylserine) (15) substituents—the duration of action has not been reported (15, 470) or found normal (118).

The prolongation of the response to the β-aspartyl analog (1.5–2-fold) is much less than would be expected from the differences in overall inactivation rates by plasma (Table VIII) including the contribution of an endopeptidase (135, 412) which is also present. It has been pointed out (e.g., 98, 135, 210, 528) that the bloodstream is unlikely to be the chief site of physiological inactivation. Clearance studies have shown that angiotensin is largely (65–80%) removed from the blood by a single passage through the hepatic (54, 60, 178, 210, 317, 344), renal (22, 60, 210, 317), and limb (22, 60, 178, 210) circulations. In liver homogenates a chymotrypsin-like endopeptidase (135, 412) and a specific carboxypeptidase (618) are found. However, the ester and amide of [Asn^1]-angiotensin$_b$ II and des-Asp^1-[D-Phe^8]-angiotensin$_b$ II (487, 504) which should be resistant to carboxypeptidases, and [Asn^1,D-Tyr^4]-angiotensin$_b$ II (489) which should not be attacked by chymotrypsin-like enzymes, have low or very low but qualitatively apparently normal activities. Such attempts to block possible additional loci of inactivation therefore do not appear promising.

The occurrence of angiotensin tachyphylaxis in certain vascular preparations has been linked with the absence of inactivating enzymes from these tissues. Suitable plasma fractions can reverse the tachyphylaxis induced in cat aortic strips by [Asn^1]-angiotensin but not that induced by [βAsp^1]-angiotensin II (297). In normal and nephrectomized rats the pressor response to angiotensin II showed tachyphylaxis but the response to [Asn^1]-angiotensin$_b$ II did not (449). These observations suggest the interesting possibility that tachyphylaxis might more generally be varied by changing the metabolic susceptibility of analogs.

c. *Kinins.* Bradykinin is inactivated in blood plasma by a carboxypeptidase [carboxypeptidase N (148, 149, 142)] and also by a second enzyme, an endopeptidase cleaving the Pro^7-Phe^8 bond (617). Of the analogs potentially resistant to the carboxypeptidase [D-Arg^9]-bradykinin (370, 540) and also decarboxybradykinin (269) have very low vasodilator activity. No protracted effect has been noted and the half-life of the [D-Arg^9] derivative in the circulation is the same as that of bradykinin (370). The depsipeptide analog [7-

glycine, 8-β-phenyllactic acid]-bradykinin has a prolonged effect which has been ascribed to its slower inactivation (by 20–35%) in plasma (411). Although it has been suggested (411) that the presence of the ester bond may reduce the susceptibility of the neighboring terminal amide bond to carboxypeptidase N it seems as likely that it is the resistance of the ester bond itself to the (at that time undefined) endopeptidase which is reponsible for the effect.

Bradykinin amide (537), bradykinyl-glycine, and bradykinyl-arginine (537, 542) do not appear to have been tested in vivo. However, the natural peptide phyllokinin, bradykinyl-isoleucyl-tyrosine-O-sulfate (9, 10, 44), did show distinctly protracted vasodepressor action (9, 10). This effect is reduced, or disappears, when the sulfate ester grouping is absent and the potency also greatly decreases (9). It will be interesting to determine whether the sulfate grouping affects the distribution pattern of the peptide or its susceptibility to enzymes. The implications for the design of analogs are obvious.

Several enzymes inactivating bradykinin have been identified in kidney homogenates (149–151) but recently it has been found that the lung is the organ mainly responsible for the disposition of bradykinin in vivo, some 80% of the peptide being extracted by a single passage through the lungs (57, 58, 157, 561). In the lungs bradykinin is destroyed by hydrolysis of the Arg^1–Pro^2 bond and also at a second site, possibly the Ser^6–Pro^7 bond (446).

It will be of interest to reexamine some of the numerous known bradykinin analogs from this point of view. Kallidin and several of its derivatives are less active than bradykinin when tested on smooth muscle in vitro but more active as vasodilators in vivo (468); for lysyl-lysyl-kallidin the ratio of potencies (referred to bradykinin) on rabbit blood pressure and the guinea pig ileum is as high as 40–50 (468). It may well be that the high in vivo activities owe more to differences in disposition in the organism than to differences in the tissue receptors (e.g., ileum vs vascular smooth muscle; no activities on vascular smooth muscle in vitro have been reported for these compounds). A natural bradykinin analog, polistes kinin, is 10 times more active than bradykinin when injected into the jugular vein but 6 times less active by the intraaortic route (538) and in this case it has been shown experimentally that the peptide is not removed by the lung (538). Nevertheless neither kallidin (545) nor the extended-chain kallidin derivatives (144, 467, 468) show protracted effects on blood pressure.

Acetylbradykinin (537, 542) and desaminobradykinin (269) are relatively active in vitro (20–50% of bradykinin potency) but do not appear to have been tested in vivo. The phenylalanines in positions 5 and 8 have been replaced with leucine with the expressed aim of conferring resistance to chymotrypsin-like enzymes (539, 540) but no results for the action of these compounds in vivo have been recorded.

d. Oxytocin and Vasopressin. The primate pregnancy serum "oxytocinase" inactivating both oxytocin and vasopressin was identified as an aminopeptidase (*524, 558, 559*). In liver cell sap inactivation was found to proceed by reduction of the disulphide bond followed by aminopeptidase degradation (see *447*). Reduction of the disulfide bond also appears to be the first step during inactivation by the uterus (*16*).

In the hope of preventing aminopeptidase attack oxytocin analogs were prepared in which the amino-terminal hemicystine was methylated or replaced by hemi-D-cystine (*277, 279*; see also *237, 615*) or in which the susceptible Cys–Tyr peptide bond was methylated (*244, 277*). All these compounds proved to have very low activity. The highly active desaminooxytocin prepared in a different context (*236, 571*) would also be expected to be resistant and was, in fact, found to be stable on incubation with leucine aminopeptidase (*180*) or human pregnancy serum (*179*). However, none of these analogs, whether of high or low potency, initially showed a prolonged effect in any of the standard pharmacological assay systems (*29, 109*; but see *108*). The final possibility that it is reduction of the disulfide bond which determines the rate at which the response decays was eliminated when the time course of the antidiuretic response to the nondisulfide "carba" analogs (see Section II,C,4,d) and to oxytocin was found to be identical (*397*).

These unexpected results prompted some of the pharmacokinetic considerations and the further experiments on disposition set out in Section III,C,3.

Introduction of D-amino acids into position 8 of vasopressin (*621–623, 625, 627*) might be expected to stabilize the resulting analogs toward trypsin-like enzymes. Some of them have shown very high antidiuretic potencies (Table VII, Section III,B,2) but it is not quite clear if, in doses which evoke a submaximal response in terms of intensity, they have a prolonged effect (*562*).

2. Inhibition of Inactivating or Activating Enzymes

The design of peptides with a "sparing" action on the active hormones is attractive in principle because relatively simple peptides might suffice, the specificity requirements of the enzymes are likely to be less strict than those of the receptors, and there might even be a possibility of developing irreversible ("site-directed") inhibitors of the enzyme. On the other side the uncertainty about the physiologically important inactivating enzymes makes the choice of a target arbitrary and the pharmacokinetic situation would probably be very complex.

Certain *S*-benzylated fragments of oxytocin as well as the *S*-benzyl and desthio derivatives of the full sequence were found to be good competitive inhibitors of the pregnancy serum and tissue "oxytocinases" *in vitro* (e.g., *28*). However, no potentiation or prolongation of the response to oxytocin has been noted *in vivo*.

In the case of angiotensin and the kinins the activation as well as the inactivation mechanism can be a target for the design of active peptide derivatives. Compounds which behave as competitive substrates or as reversible or irreversible inhibitors of the activating enzymes ought to be useful pharmacological tools and, should the pathophysiological role of these systems be established, starting points for the development of drugs.

Surprisingly little work has been done in this direction. Angiotensin II is produced in two stages, the protein precursors (angiotensinogens) being cleaved by renin or renin-like enzymes to give the decapeptide angiotensin I from which the octapeptide angiotensin II is produced by a "converting enzyme" (for reviews, see *384, 388, 504, 528*). The physiological site of conversion is the lung (*21, 59, 362, 561*) though some conversion also takes place elsewhere in the organism (*59, 536*; but see *362, 561*). An octapeptide ester containing the sequence around the renin-susceptible Leu–Leu bond, which is itself a relatively poor renin substrate, in low concentrations inhibits the renin-induced formation of angiotensin I from a tetradecapeptide precursor or from purified angiotensinogens in aqueous solution but not in serum (*529*). The tetrapeptide methyl or ethyl esters with the sequences Leu–Leu–Val–Tyr and Leu–Leu–Val–Phe inhibit angiotensin formation in serum but high concentrations (about 5 mM) are required (*302*); it is not stated if the peptides are themselves hydrolyzed by renin. Some other peptides which can serve as renin substrates without releasing angiotensin (*413, 528*) do not appear to have been tested as inhibitors of angiotensin formation (competitive substrates) in this system.

Analogs of angiotensin I which have weak or no pressor activity are evidently not attacked by the converting enzyme and could conceivably act as inhibitors of this enzyme. Several such analogs are known (*187, 504, 525*) but the only one which has apparently tested for this effect, [D-Phe[8]]-angiotensin I, does not inhibit the converting enzyme (*187*). It is not recorded if hippuryl-histidyl-leucine, a substrate for converting enzyme (*119*), inhibits the conversion of angiotensin I to angiotensin II.

Bradykinin, kallidin, or methionyl-lysyl-bradykinin are similarly released from precursors, the kininogens, by a family of enzymes, the kallikreins (see *146, 197, 392, 544, 557, 580, 601*). Activation of the kininogens appears to involve cleavage of an Arg–Ser bond. No attempts to design peptides as inhibitors of this activation have been reported.

3. Some Pharmacokinetic Considerations

In many of the instances discussed in Section III,D,1 the examination of the analogs for protracted effects has evidently been rather perfunctory. In some cases no results for the time course of a suitable response are reported even where the analogs were explicitly designed to be enzyme-resistant. In

most of the work the results were judged only by visual inspection of time–
effect curves and in many such experiments, as published graphs show, the
doses of the analog and reference compounds were not matched to give the
same maximal intensity of the response; the curves differ in their maxima
and are difficult to compare. In other experiments doses evoking supramaximal
(in terms of intensity) responses were used so that a difference in duration may
merely be a reflection of the excess dose.

Pliška (393) has discussed the measurement and expression of time-course
differences for responses *in vivo* with particular reference to the neurohypophysial hormones and their analogs. The persistence of the response is expressed
by a "formal elimination constant" which is the exponential constant for
the decrease in the concentration of the peptide as calculated from the decay
of the response, or as the "index of persistence" which is the ratio of
decay of the response, or as the "index of persistence" which is the ratio of
this coefficient for a standard to that for the analog. Various methods for
determining these parameters are described including one which is based on
the comparison of dose–response curves using the *total* (time-integrated)
effect as a measure of the response (conventionally in measurement of blood
pressure changes it is the maximal pressure difference, or intensity of the effect
which is taken as the response). The most exact and reproducible results were
obtained (395) by direct analysis of the decay curves after a steady state
response had been achieved by infusion of the peptide. Similar procedures
could no doubt be applied more generally.

Such inadequacies apart it emerges as a striking conclusion of the work
summarized in Section III,D,1 that analogs designed to be resistant to inactivating enzymes have only rarely shown the anticipated protracted effects, and
even then only to a moderate degree. Several causes may be responsible for
this failure. Often the molecular site of inactivation has only been surmised
rather than experimentally established—in the case of corticotropin admittedly
with some practical success. In other cases enzymes detected in the serum or
in tissue homogenates have been assumed to be responsible for the physiological inactivation although, as has repeatedly been shown or argued (e.g.,
22, 135, 210, 396, 445, 528, 561), this assumption is by no means valid. Several
alternative pathways for disposition may often be available. Finally, the
suspicion (445) that it may be pharmacokinetically naive to expect enzyme
resistance automatically to result in protracted action has proved justified.
Pliška has shown (394) by mathematical analysis of a three-compartment
pharmacokinetic model that in certain situations only changes in inactivation
within the receptor compartment will affect the time course of the response,
whereas changes in other compartments may cause only an increase in the
intensity of the response without appreciable change in the time course. (The
receptor compartment is defined as that distribution space from which the
drug can reach the receptors without passing a transport barrier.) The pre-
valence of such situations would explain not only the failure to achieve

prolonged effects even where enzyme resistance has demonstrably been achieved but also the increased potency repeatedly found together with, or instead of, protracted action for such enzyme-resistant analogs (e.g., [βAsp^1]-angiotensin$_b$ II, lysyl-lysyl-kallidin, the [D-Ser^1]-corticotropin derivatives and perhaps desamino-[D-Arg^8]-vasopressin; see Section III,D,1). In this connection it is interesting to note that homogenates of aorta inactivate the desamino-, [βAsp^1]-, and [Arg^1]-analogs more slowly than angiotensin II (98) and it may be this property of a target tissue, rather than the aminopeptidase activity of plasma, which is responsible for the prolonged effects (251, 412) of such analogs.

These considerations show the importance of more relevant biochemical and pharmacokinetic information. Recent techniques for determining clearance by individual organs or vascular regions, used to such good effect by Biron and by Vane and their co-workers for the study of angiotensin and bradykinin (57–60, 157, 362, 536, 561) (see Section III,D,1) should provide such information at the level of the organism. The elegant oil-immersion technique for isolated tissues developed by Kalsner and Nickerson (282) can in turn give information about disposition in some target tissues and this, as has been noted, is particularly important for the design of long-acting analogs. The technique has already been used (308) to confirm that the prolonged effects of desamino-[Tyr(Me)^2]-oxytocin on the uterus and mammary gland in vivo (62, 288) are associated with a decreased rate of inactivation by oil-immersed tissue. It is to be hoped that these, and other, methods will be more extensively used to provide the information necessary for the truly rational design of analogs with modified metabolic properties.

4. Modifying Distribution

Very little work has been done with the expressed aim of modifying the distribution properties of biologically active peptides. This is hardly surprising since the basis for the design of such analogs, a knowledge of the distribution behavior of peptides in general, and of particular hormones, is almost completely lacking.

Attempts to change the distribution properties by incorporating lipophilic residues in the carboxyl-terminal heptapeptide fragment of physalaemin (e.g., asparagine replaced by glutamic acid γ-t-butylamide, lysine by phenylalanine, methionine by S-butylcysteine), by doubling the size of the molecule through joining two units with bridges attached to the α- or ϵ-amino groups of the lysine or to the sulfur in a cysteine or homocysteine side chain, or by attaching active heptapeptides to soluble polymeric carriers all failed to give derivatives with prolonged hypotensive action (460). On the other hand, derivatives of the carboxyl-terminal heptapeptide sequence of eledoisin with lipophilic acyl groups (butyryl, valeryl) bound to the N^ϵ-amino group of lysine (*48*) elicited hypotensive responses of reduced initial intensity and increased duration when injected in a suitable solvent (diacetin) (*50*). Since the effect was dependent both on the structure of the peptide and on the solvent used for intramuscular injection it seems likely that it is the primary resorption process which is modified. No protracted effects were found with a similar series of acyl derivatives (*336*) which were presumably injected intravenously.

5. *Hormonogens*

Angiotensin and the kinins are formed *in vivo* by activation of naturally occurring hormonogens. Most of the synthetic analogs with lengthened peptide chains prepared so far have contained sequences corresponding to those identified in the protein precursors.

A tetradecapeptide isolated from partial enzymic digests of angiotensinogens (*526*) has been synthesized in this form (*530*) or with asparagine replacing the amino-terminal aspartic acid (*346*). Although these peptides are converted to angiotensin I by renin (*346, 347, 526, 530*) it has been concluded from the activity of the peptide *in vitro*, the rapid onset of the pressor response, and the slope of the dose–response relation that the pressor effect of the [Asn^1]-tetradecapeptide is due to the compound itself rather than to angiotensin released from it *in vivo*. The somewhat longer duration of the response is explained by the greater stability of the tetradecapaptide toward plasma and not by its conversion to angiotensin (*346*).

By contrast, angiotensin I which is the primary product of renin action has little or no activity except under conditions where conversion to angiotensin II is feasible (*206, 384, 527, 528*). Here again, however, the time course of the response is closely similar to that for angiotensin II (*527*) presumably because of the kinetics of the system (*528*).

Only few variations have been made in the structure of angiotensin I. The carboxyl-terminal leucine has been removed enzymically (*525*), the histidyl–leucyl sequence has been replaced by doubling the prolyl-phenylalanyl sequence of angiotensin II (*487*) and the L-phenylalanine has been replaced by the D-isomer (*187*). All the products have low pressor activity, indicating that they are not attacked by converting enzyme. The terminal amide of angiotensin I has hypertensive action (*487*) though it has yet to be shown if this is due to conversion into angiotensin II. The tetradecapeptide "renin substrate" is not attacked by the converting enzyme (*526*).

For a better understanding of the activating system and, possibly, the achievement of modified metabolic behavior it would certainly be of interest to prepare a wider range of angiotensin derivatives extended at the carboxyl end of the peptide chain.

Isolated (*198, 199*) or synthetic (*475*) fragments of bradykininogen with the bradykinin sequence amino-terminal have very low activities *in vivo* unless they are preincubated with activating enzymes. This contrasts with the relatively high, and prolonged, activity of the natural analog phyllokinin (*9*) which, however, is thought to be active of itself and not by release of bradykinin. Nor is there any indication that synthetic analogs extended at the carboxyl end by arginine, glycine (*537, 540, 542*) or isoleucyl-tyrosine (*44*) act as hormonogens.

Rudinger, Rychlík, and Šorm and their co-workers have designed synthetic hormonogens of oxytocin and lysine vasopressin by attaching additional amino acids and short peptide chains to the terminal amino group (*277, 279, 289*). Similar modifications were made independently as a way of blocking the amino group (*567*) and in efforts to change specificity (*191*) (see Section III,B,2).

Compounds such as glycyl-, leucyl-, prolyl-, or leucyl-glycyl-glycyl-oxytocin (*279, 289, 567*) did, in fact, show the properties expected of hormonogens. They had consistently higher potencies *in vivo* than *in vitro* (*29, 447*) and their effects *in vivo* generally developed more slowly than the responses to oxytocin or vasopressin and always decayed more slowly (*29, 447, 567*). The magnitude and time course of the response, which could be followed particularly well in the assay for antidiuretic activity, depended on the nature of the added amino acid or peptide sequence (*29, 447*). Thus leucyl-oxytocin had a rather high potency and relatively short action and prolyl- or glycyl-glycyl-oxytocin had low potency but very long-lasting effects (Table IX). Similar relations were found in a series of N^α-aminoacyl and N^α-peptidyl derivatives of lysine vasopressin (*290, 624, 626*). Such a structural dependence would be expected from an activation process (*29, 447*): Rapid activation gives a high level of hormone but quickly exhausts the hormonogen, slow activation builds up only low hormone levels from the same concentration of hormonogen but the release is sustained for a longer time. Aminopeptidases seem to be chiefly (*29, 447*) but not exclusively (*290*) responsible for activation. To give more direct proof of the enzymic nature of the activation two analogs were designed (*279, 289*) which should be resistant to the common aminopeptidases but similar to the hormonogens in all other respects. One of these, sarcosyl-oxytocin, showed the expected low activity *in vitro* and *in vivo* with a normal (i.e., oxytocin-like) time course of action. The other, D-leucyl-oxytocin, had still lower potency but caused a protracted response which, however, is ascribed (*29*) to contamination with traces of the L-leucyl isomer.

In some experiments especially with the less active analogs a biphasic avian depressor, rat pressor, or antidiuretic response was recorded with an early time course similar to that for oxytocin or vasopressin passing into one typical for the hormonogens (*29, 447*). This is thought to result from superposition of the response to the hormonogen itself, in its quality as a structural analog of the hormone, and the response of the hormone liberated from the hormonogen (445). This behavior can be mathematically modelled in the three-compartment pharmacokinetic system (394) mentioned in Section III,D,3 (Fig. 14).

An unexpected feature was the inhibition of the response to oxytocin and vasopressin observed after active or subthreshold doses of some hormonogens, especially in the avian depressor and milk-ejection assays. It was found that infusion of oxytocin at low rates can mimic this effect (as well as the response to the hormonogen) so that this phenomenon gives additional support to the characterisation of the analogs as hormonogens (29, 445).

TABLE IX

Some Properties of Aminoacyl and Peptidyl Derivatives of Oxytocin
(Synthetic Hormonogens)

N^α-Substituent	Uterotonic action[a]			Antidiuretic action[a]	
	in vitro A	in vivo B	Ratio B/A	Potency	Index of persistence[b]
Leu-	5	18	3.5	9	2.9
Phe-	0.6	10	17	6.8	2.6
Gly-	0.07	0.8	11	4.4	3.2
Pro-	0.13	1.5	11	0.17	4.3
Gly–Gly-	0.16	1.5	9	0.8	4.0
Leu–Gly–Gly-	0.05	4	80	0.13	5.0
Sar-	0.46	0.34	0.8	0.83	1.0

[a] Approximate potencies as percentages of the activity of oxytocin. Results from Beránková-Ksandrová et al. (29).
[b] For definition, see Pliška (393) and Section III,D,3.

In rats with hereditary diabetes insipidus (Brattleboro strain) which provide a good pathophysiological model for the clinical condition the antidiuretic effect of glycyl-glycyl-glycyl-vasopressin also persisted a good deal longer than that of lysine vasopressin after injection of aqueous solutions of both peptides. However, as in the case of the long-acting corticotropins (Section III,D,1,a) depot forms of vasopressin gave a longer response still (311). On the other hand, the sustained release of vasopressin from the hormonogen has vascular effects beneficial in haemorrhagic shock (115, 116) so that this line of design may after all lead to practically useful results.

It has been pointed out (534) that "hormonogen" properties can also be obtained by introducing substituents removed at a convenient rate by a nonenzymic reaction (e.g., hydrolysis) under conditions *in vivo*. Carbamoyl substituents on the phenolic hydroxyl groups of tyrosine have been discussed in this context but no results have yet been reported.

From considerations similar to those set out in Section III,D,3 it is evident

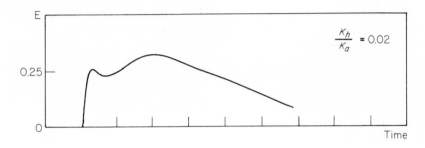

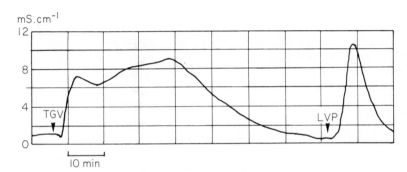

Fig. 14. Time course of the antidiuretic response to N^α-glycyl-glycyl-glycyl-[8-lysine]-vasopressin compared with the computed time course for a three-compartment model. *Bottom*: Tracing of record of urine conductivity from a hydrated, ethanol-anesthetized rat following injection of N^α-glycyl-glycyl-glycyl-[8-lysine]-vasopressin (TGV; 20 ng) and of lysine vasopressin (LVP; 0.2 ng); ordinate: specific conductivity of urine in millisiemens/cm; abscissa: time. *Top*: Computed time course of the response to a hormonogen with some inherent activity; ordinate: effect in machine units; abscissa: machine time; K_h and K_a are the assumed dissociation constants of the peptide–receptor complexes for the hormonogen and hormone, respectively; for other parameters of the model system, see Pliška (*394*). From the results of Pliška (*394*).

that sustained-release effects will only be observed when certain pharmacokinetic conditions as to compartmentation of the hormonogen and hormone, rates of activation and inactivation, elimination of both peptides, etc. are met. It is probably for this reason that some of the angiotensin and bradykinin derivatives apparently meeting the structural criteria for hormonogens have failed to show the expected biological behavior.

E. EVOLUTIONARY ASPECTS

Two main lines of thought concerning the design of analogs may originate from evolutionary considerations. The first attempts to anticipate presumed but as yet undiscovered members of an evolutionary line of hormones and so to serve the comparative endocrinologist by supplying him with chemical and biological information about the "missing link." The other approach aims more generally at exploiting the information on structure–activity relationships emerging from a comparison within natural families of hormones.

An early example of the first kind is provided by the synthesis of the "hybrid" neurohypophysial hormone analogs in which, on the basis of the vasopressin structure, the isoleucine in position 3 of oxytocin was replaced by phenyl-alanine (83, 291) or the leucine in position 8 by arginine (293). These efforts were rewarded when the latter compound, [Arg^8]-oxytocin or "vasotocin," was identified as the endogenous hormone of lower vertebrates (294, 390, 452). [Ile^8]-Oxytocin, prepared originally as a straightforward structural analog (38, 258) was later predicted as a link ("mesotocin") between oxytocin and the fish hormone isotocin ([Ser^4,Ile^8]oxytocin) (1) and duly found in amphibians (2).

Deliberate attempts have lately been made, from considerations of the mechanism of protein evolution, to predict the structure of other as yet undiscovered evolutionary intermediates (174, 175, 441, 442, 573) and the predicted structures, [Pro^4]- (453), [Pro^4,Ile^8]- (442, 453), [Pro^4,Gln^8]- (453), [Gln^8]- (24), and [Leu^4,Ile^8]-oxytocin (442), have been synthesized.

More often, comparative endocrinology has been the source rather than the beneficiary of analog design. Thus the chain length requirements for corticotropic and melanotropic activity are already to some extent indicated by the properties of the natural members of this hormone family and the discovery of the lipotropins (324) extends the knowledge of the structural dependence of lipotropic action already obtained from the other natural hormones and synthetic analogs (e.g., 318, 319, 404, 551).

Presumably, if the structures and properties of caerulein (11, 45) or phyllo-caerulein (6, 46) had by historical accident been known before those of gastrin (12, 13) this would of itself have directed synthetic effort toward the carboxyl end of the gastrin molecule. In the event comparison of the natural peptides gastrin, caerulin, and cholecystokinin-pancreozymin in their actions on the gallbladder (5) indicated the importance of the tyrosine-O-sulphate residue for the cholecystokinin type of activity in parallel with the results for synthetic caerulein analogs (7, 9, 351, 352).

A comparison of the structures of natural insulins (122, 334, 532) and calcitonins (see 363) reveals many "inessential" structural features. An obvious further step would be the design and synthesis of a "generalized" molecule which incorporates at each variable site that amino acid which is most readily accessible or synthetically least troublesome. Also, the hormones of some lower species are more active than those of mammals [chicken (295, 532) or turkey (599) insulin, salmon calcitonin (195, 363)] and we may anticipate attempts to incorporate structural features of such nonmammalian hormones into more typical mammalian sequences.

There is a third, as yet unexploited possibility for relating comparative endocrinology and the design of analogs. It would require us to deduce potential pharmacological effects of a particular family of peptide hormones in man or mammals generally from their physiological role in lower orders. By setting up suitable pharmacological tests it should then be possible to search for and develop such effects in synthetic hormone analogs. The bottleneck of this approach is often our ignorance of nonmammalian endocrinology. The still obscure function of the neurohypophysial hormones in lower vertebrates is a case in point.

F. INTRODUCTION OF MARKERS, CONJUGATION

It has been realized for some time that a knowledge of the conformation of peptide molecules is fundamental to an understanding of their topochemistry, the true "structure" in relation to biological action. Recent improvements in physicochemical methods of conformational analysis have made this problem experimentally accessible. However, some of the experimental complexities involved can be greatly simplified if the molecule of interest is modified by inclusion of suitable "markers," "labels," "probes," or "reporter groups" and the design of such molecules is likely to be of growing importance.

For the determination of full three-dimensional structures by X-ray crystallography heavy-atom labels are still desirable. It may be that this consideration in part motivated the synthesis of oxytocin isologs with the heavier selenium replacing sulfur (584, 589, 591, 592); in any case the analogs are being exploited to this end (112). The replacement of phenylalanine by p-bromophenylalanine in [Asn^1]-angiotensin$_b$ II (487, 504) was certainly made with similar possibilities in mind. Unfortunately, no amount of design can overcome the reluctance of many biologically active peptides to yield the crystals required for X-ray analysis.

Analogs with suitably modified (generally simplified) structure, although not specifically designed for this purpose, are proving useful in analyzing the information obtained, e.g., by optical rotatory dispersion and circular dichroism (646) or by proton magnetic resonance spectroscopy (645, 647). More deliberate efforts in this direction will presumably be made in the near future.

As nuclear magnetic resonance markers phthaloyl groups (*497*) have been introduced into gramicidin S (*498*). Improvements in proton magnetic resonance spectroscopy make such markers less important but it may be predicted that fluorine-containing derivatives will find such use because of the small size and favorable magnetic resonance properties of the fluorine atom. Trifluoroacetyl substituents have been considered in this context (*522*) but direct substitution of hydrogens or hydroxyl groups in amino acid side chains by fluorine should give a better approximation to isosteric conditions and a wider choice of locations.

Schwyzer has pointed out that suitably placed charge-transfer donors and acceptors should be useful as conformational probes. In tryptophan-containing peptides the indole side chain itself can act as a donor. Preliminary model studies have been carried out (*102, 103*) and application to biologically active peptides may soon be expected.

Measurements of fluorescence and fluorescence polarization can give valuable information about the environment of fluorescent groups and its changes by intermolecular interactions (e.g., binding to macromolecules). The tyrosine and tryptophan residues in peptides provide built-in fluorescent probes but molecules containing markers with superior fluorescence properties may also be designed. Following this line of thought Schwyzer has recently described the preparation and use of a tetracosactide derivative carrying a dansyl (1-dimethylaminonaphthalene-5-sulfonyl) substituent in the side chain of the lysine in position 21 (*502, 644*).

The efficient design of analogs carrying markers or probes generally presupposes some knowledge of structure–activity relations. A structural change which would simultaneously alter the biologically important properties of the molecule would be self-defeating. Biological activity of the modified molecule provides the best evidence that the information obtained by physicochemical investigations is really relevant.

Cuatrecasas (*632*) has attached a macromolecular "marker" (Sepharose) to insulin through the amino groups in position B1 and in the lysine side chain in order to prevent entry of the hormone into the cell. The high insulinlike activity of the conjugate proves that the primary site of insulin action is at the cell membrane.

Derivatives in which peptides are attached to carrier macromolecules to improve immunogenicity need not retain hormonal activity. Most frequently, structurally more or less undefined products of this kind are prepared by condensation reactions but occasionally attachment through links precisely located on the peptide molecule is preferred. For attachment by the diazo coupling reaction *p*-aminobenzoyl or *p*-aminophenylacetyl groups have been introduced into oxytocin, lysine vasopressin (*172*), and angiotensin (*123*).

Where it is anticipated that several different markers, carriers, or reactive groups (see also Section III,C,5) may be attached in turn to the same molecule it should prove economical to build into the peptide a common "bridge" element terminating with a specifically reacting attachment site to which the various markers or other moieties can be linked.

IV. Conclusions

It will probably depend on the prejudices of each reader whether he, or she, will conclude after reading this chapter that efforts to design analogs of the peptide hormones have in some degree been successful. In the author's opinion—influenced no doubt by his own prejudices—two lessons emerge from this survey for future work, one addressed to the chemist and one to the pharmacologist. The chemist should be less reluctant in his molecular architecture to abandon the facile use of ready-made bricks, the protein-constituent amino acids, and to undertake sometimes quite intricate syntheses to meet the designs which will best answer a given purpose. The pharmacologist, on the other hand, should be more ready to adapt his attitudes and techniques to the special problem of investigating the manifold properties and potential of synthetic hormone analogs, as distinct from (or in addition to) carrying out standard assays to determine potencies of routinely produced structural variants. If these lessons are learned the design of peptide hormone analogs should become not only a more interesting but also a more fruitful activity.

ACKNOWLEDGMENTS

During the writing of this review the author enjoyed the support of the Swiss National Foundation for Scientific Research (Grant No. 4883) and the hospitality of Professor R. Schwyzer's laboratory.

REFERENCES

1. R. Acher, J. Chauvet, M. T. Chauvet, and D. Crépy, *Biochim. Biophys. Acta* **58**, 624 (1962).
2. R. Acher, J. Chauvet, M. T. Chauvet, and D. Crépy, *Biochim. Biophys. Acta* **90**, 613 (1964).
3. B. M. Altura, *Amer. J. Physiol.* **219**, 222 (1970).
4. B. M. Altura and S. G. Hershey, *Angiology* **18**, 428 (1967).

5. M. S. Amer, *Endocrinology* **84**, 1277 (1969).
6. A. Anastasi, *Experientia* **25**, 8 (1969).
7. A. Anastasi, L. Bernardi, G. Bertaccini, B. Bosisio, R. de Castiglione, V. Erspamer, O. Goffredo, and M. Impicciatore, *Experientia* **24**, 771 (1968).
8. A. Anastasi, L. Bernardi, G. Bosisio, R. de Castiglione, O. Goffredo, G. Bertaccini, V. Erspamer, and M. Impicciatore, *in* "Peptides 1968; Proc. 9th Eur. Peptide Symp." (E. Bricas, ed.), p. 247. North-Holland Publ., Amsterdam, 1968.
9. A. Anastasi, G. Bertaccini, and V. Erspamer, *Brit. J. Pharmacol.* **27**, 479 (1966).
9a. A. Anastasi and V. Erspamer, *Arch. Biochem. Biophys.* **101**, 58 (1963).
10. A. Anastasi, V. Erspamer, G. Bertaccini, and J. M. Cei, *in* "Hypotensive Peptides" (E. G. Erdös, N. Back, and F. Sicuteri, eds.), p. 76. Springer, Berlin, 1966.
11. A. Anastasi, V. Erspamer, and R. Endean, *Experientia* **23**, 699 (1967).
12. J. C. Anderson, M. A. Barton, P. M. Hardy, G. W. Kenner, J. K. MacLeod, J. Preston, and R. C. Sheppard, *in* "Proc. 7th Eur. Peptide Symp., 1964" (V. Bruckner and K. Medzihradszky, eds.); *Acta Chim. Acad. Sci. Hung.* **44**, Spec. Issue p. 178 (1965).
13. J. C. Anderson, M. A. Barton, R. A. Gregory, P. M. Hardy, G. W. Kenner, J. K. MacLeod, J. Preston, R. C. Sheppard, and J. S. Morley, *Nature (London)* **204**, 933 (1964).
14. R. Andreatta and K. Hofmann, *J. Amer. Chem. Soc.* **90**, 7334 (1968).
15. K. Arakawa, R. R. Smeby, and F. M. Bumpus, *J. Amer. Chem. Soc.* **84**, 1424 (1962).
16. L. Audrain and H. Clauser, *Biochim. Biophys. Acta* **30**, 191 (1958).
17. E. A. Axelrod, A. C. Trakatellis, and K. Hofmann, *Nature (London)* **197**, 146 (1963).
18. N. Back, L. Martini, and R. Paoletti, eds., "Pharmacology of Hormonal Polypeptides and Proteins." Plenum Press, New York, 1968.
19. S. Bajusz, K. Medzihradszky, Z. Paulay, and Zs. Lang, *Acta Chim. Acad. Sci. Hung.* **52**, 335 (1967).
20. S. Bajusz, Z. Paulay, Zs. Lang, K. Medzihradszky, L. Kisfaludy, and M. Löw, *in* "Peptides; Proc. 8th Eur. Peptide Symp., 1966" (H. C. Beyerman, A. von de Linde, and W. Maassen van den Brink, eds.), p. 237. North-Holland Publ., Amsterdam, 1967.
21. Y. S. Bakhle, *Nature (London)* **220**, 919 (1968).
22. Y. S. Bakhle, A. M. Reynard, and J. R. Vane, *Nature (London)* **222**, 956 (1969).
23. T. Barth, V. Pliška, and I. Rychlík, *Collect. Czech. Chem. Commun.* **32**, 1058 (1967).
24. J. W. M. Baxter, T. C. Wuu, M. Manning, and W. H. Sawyer, *Experientia* **25**, 1127 (1969).
25. J. Beacham, P. H. Bentley, G. W. Kenner, J. J. Mendive, and R. C. Sheppard, *in* "Peptides; Proc. 8th Eur. Peptide Symp., 1966" (H. C. Beyerman, A. van de Linde, and W. Maassen van den Brink, eds.), p. 235. North-Holland Publ., Amsterdam, 1967.
26. P. H. Bell, K. S. Howard, R. G. Shepherd, B. M. Finn, and J. H. Meisenhelder, *J. Amer. Chem. Soc.* **78**, 5059 (1956).
27. Z. Beránková, I. Rychlík, K. Jošt, J. Rudinger, and F. Šorm, *Collect. Czech. Chem. Commun.* **26**, 2673 (1961).
28. Z. Beránková and F. Šorm, *Collect. Czech. Chem. Commun.* **26**, 2557 (1961).
29. Z. Beránková-Ksandrová, G. W. Bisset, K. Jošt, I. Krejčí, V. Pliška, J. Rudinger, I. Rychlík, and F. Šorm, *Brit. J. Pharmacol.* **26**, 615 (1966).
30. B. Berde, "Pharmacologie des hormones neurohypophysaires et de leurs analogues synthétiques." Masson, Paris, 1963.
31. B. Berde, *in* "Advances in Oxytocin Research," p. 11. Pergamon Press, Oxford, 1965.
32. B. Berde, *in* "Pharmacology of Hormonal Polypeptides and Proteins" (N. Back, L. Martini, and R. Paoletti, eds.), p. 53. Plenum Press, New York, 1968.
33. B. Berde, ed., "Handbuch der experimentellen Pharmakologie," Vol. 23. Springer, Berlin, 1968.

34. B. Berde and R. A. Boissonnas, *in* "Handbuch der experimentellen Pharmakologie" (B. Berde, ed.), p. 802. Springer, Berlin, 1968.
35. B. Berde, R. A. Boissonnas, R. L. Huguenin, and E. Stürmer, *Experientia* **20**, 42 (1964).
36. B. Berde and A. Cerletti, *Klin. Wochenschr.* **42**, 1159 (1964).
37. B. Berde, A. Cerletti, and H. Konzett, *in* "Oxytocin" (R. Caldeyro-Barcia and H. Heller, eds.), p. 247. Pergamon Press, Oxford, 1961.
38. B. Berde and H. Konzett, *Med. Exp.* **2**, 317 (1960).
39. B. Berde, H. Weidmann, and A. Cerletti, *Helv. Physiol. Pharmacol. Acta* **19**, 285 (1961).
40. F. Bergel, J. M. Johnson, and R. Wade, *J. Chem. Soc.* p. 3802 (1962).
41. F. Bergel, J. M. Johnson, and R. Wade, *in* "Peptides; Proc. 6th Eur. Peptide Symp., 1963" (L. Zervas, ed.), p. 241. Pergamon Press, Oxford, 1966.
42. F. Bergel and J. A. Stock, *J. Chem. Soc.* p. 3658 (1960).
43. L. Bernardi, *in* "Hypotensive Peptides" (E. G. Erdös, N. Back, and F. Sicuteri, eds.), p. 86. Springer, Berlin, 1966.
44. L. Bernardi, G. Bosisio, R. de Castiglione, and O. Goffredo, *Experientia* **22**, 425 (1966).
45. L. Bernardi, G. Bosisio, R. de Castiglione, and O. Goffredo, *Experientia* **23**, 700 (1967).
46. L. Bernardi, G. Bosisio, R. de Castiglione, and O. Goffredo, *Experientia* **25**, 7 (1969).
47. L. Bernardi, G. Bosisio, F. Chillemi, G. de Caro, R. de Castiglione, V. Erspamer, A. Glaesser, and O. Goffredo, *Experientia* **20**, 306 (1964).
48. L. Bernardi, G. Bosisio, F. Chillemi, G. de Caro, R. de Castiglione, V. Erspamer, A. Glaesser, and O. Goffredo, *Experientia* **21**, 695 (1965).
49. L. Bernardi, G. Bosisio, F. Chillemi, G. de Caro, R. de Castiglione, V. Erspamer, and O. Goffredo, *Experientia* **22**, 29 (1966).
50. L. Bernardi, R. de Castiglione, G. B. Fregnan, and A. H. Glaesser, *J. Pharm. Pharmacol.* **19**, 95 (1967).
51. L. Bernardi, R. de Castiglione, O. Goffredo, and G. Bosisio, *Farmaco, Ed. Sci.* **24**, 639 (1969).
52. Zh. D. Bespalova, V. F. Martynov, and M. I. Titov, *Zh. Obshch. Khim.* **38**, 1684 (1968).
53. G. M. Besser, P. W. P. Butler, and F. S. Plumpton, *Brit. Med. J.* **4**, 391 (1967).
54. C. A. Beuzeville and H. D. Lauson, *Fed. Proc., Fed. Amer. Soc. Exp. Biol.* **24**, 525 (1965).
55. H. C. Beyerman, A. van de Linde, and W. Maassen van den Brink, eds., "Peptides; Proc. 8th Eur. Peptide Symp., 1966." North-Holland Publ., Amsterdam, 1967.
56. L. Birnbaumer and M. Rodbell, *J. Biol. Chem.* **244**, 3477 (1969).
57. P. Biron, *Clin. Res.* **16**, 112 (1968).
58. P. Biron and R. Charbonneau, *Rev. Can. Biol.* **27**, 75 (1968).
59. P. Biron and C. G. Huggins, *Life Sc.* **7**, Part 1, 965 (1968).
60. P. Biron, P. Meyer, and J. C. Pannissett, *Can. J. Physiol. Pharmacol.* **46**, 175 (1968).
61. G. W. Bisset and B. J. Clark, *Nature (London)* **218**, 197 (1968).
62. G. W. Bisset, B. J. Clark, I. Krejčí, I. Poláček, and J. Rudinger, *Brit. J. Pharmacol.* **40**, 342 (1970).
63. G. W. Bisset and D. G. Smyth, unpublished data; see Smyth (*534*, footnote on p. 1592).
64. K. Bláha, I. Frič, and J. Rudinger, *Collect. Czech. Chem. Commun.* **34**, 3497 (1969).
65. C. C. F. Blake, L. N. Johnson, G. A. Mair, A. C. T. North, C. D. Phillips, and V. R. Sarma, *Proc. Roy. Soc. Ser. B* **167**, 378 (1967).
66. M. Bodanszky and C. A. Birkhimer, *J. Amer. Soc.* **84**, 4943 (1962).
67. M. Bodanszky, M. A. Ondetti, C. A. Birkhimer, and P. L. Thomas, *J. Amer. Chem. Soc.* **86**, 4452 (1964).
68. M. Bodanszky, M. A. Ondetti, S. D. Levine, V. L. Narayanan, M. von Saltza, J. T. Sheehan, N. J. Williams, and E. F. Sabo, *in* "Peptides; Proc. 8th Eur. Peptide Symp., 1966" (H. C. Beyerman, A. van de Linde, and W. Maassen van den Brink, eds.), p. 242. North-Holland Publ., Amsterdam, 1967.

69. M. Bodanszky, M. A. Ondetti, B. Rubin, J. J. Piala, J. Fried, J. T. Sheehan, and C. A. Birkhimer, *Nature* (*London*) **194**, 485 (1962).
70. M. Bodanszky, M. A. Ondetti, J. T. Sheehan, and S. Lande, *Ann. N.Y. Acad. Sci.* **104**, 24 (1963).
71. M. Bodanszky, J. T. Sheehan, M. A. Ondetti, and S. Lande, *J. Amer. Chem. Soc.* **85** 991 (1963).
72. M. Bodanszky and V. du Vigneaud, *J. Amer. Chem. Soc.* **81**, 1258 (1959).
73. R. A. Boissonnas, in "Polypeptides which Affect Smooth Muscle and Blood Vessels" (M. Schachter, ed.), p. 7. Pergamon Press, Oxford, 1960.
74. R. A. Boissonnas, *Symp. Deut. Ges. Endokrinol.*, *8th* p. 197 (1962).
75. R. A. Boissonnas, *Proc. 1st Int. Pharmacol. Meet.*, *1961* p. 232 (1963).
76. R. A. Boissonnas, *Ann. Endocrinol.* **26**, Suppl. 5bis, 635 (1965).
77. R. A. Boissonnas and S. Guttmann, *Helv. Chim. Acta* **43**, 190 (1960).
78. R. A. Boissonnas, S. Guttmann, B. Berde, and H. Konzett, *Experientia* **17**, 377 (1961).
79. R. A. Boissonnas, S. Guttmann, R. L. Huguenin, P.-A. Jaquenoud, and E. Sandrin, *Helv. Chim. Acta* **46**, 2347 (1963).
80. R. A. Boissonnas, S. Guttmann, and P.-A. Jaquenoud, *Helv. Chim. Acta* **43**, 1349 (1960).
81. R. A. Boissonnas, S. Guttmann, and P.-A. Jaquenoud, *Helv. Chim. Acta* **43**, 1481 (1960).
82. R. A. Boissonnas, S. Guttmann, P.-A. Jaquenoud, H. Konzett, and E. Stürmer, *Experientia* **16**, 326 (1960).
83. R. A. Boissonnas, S. Guttmann, P.-A. Jaquenoud, and J.-P. Waller, *Helv. Chim. Acta* **39**, 1421 (1956).
84. R. A. Boissonnas, S. Guttmann, and J. Pless, *Experientia* **22**, 526 (1966).
85. R. A. Boissonnas, J.-F. Pechére, and S. Guttmann, unpublished results; see Boissonnas *et al.* (*78*).
86. L. A. Branda, S. Drabarek, and V. du Vigneaud, *J. Biol. Chem.* **241**, 2572 (1966).
87. L. A. Branda, V. J. Hruby, and V. du Vigneaud, *Mol. Pharmacol.* **3**, 248 (1967).
88. L. A. Branda and V. du Vigneaud, *J. Med. Chem.* **9**, 169 (1966).
89. L. A. Branda and V. du Vigneaud *J. Biol. Chem.* **241**, 4051 (1966).
90. D. Brandenburg and H. A. Ooms, in "Protein and Polypeptide Hormones" (M. Margoulies, ed.), p. 482. Excerpta Med. Found., Amsterdam, 1968; D. Brandenburg, *Hoppe-Seyler's Z. Physiol. Chem.* **350**, 741 (1969).
91. T. Braun, K. Jošt, and J. Rudinger, *Experientia* **24**, 1060 (1968).
92. E. Bricas, ed., "Peptides 1968; Proc. 9th Eur. Peptide Symp." North-Holland Publ., Amsterdam, 1968.
93. P. J. Brombacher, H. J. Buytendijk, and F. Maesen, *Z. Klin. Chem. Klin. Biochem.* **7**, 291 (1969).
94. V. Bruckner and K. Medzihradszky, eds., "Proc. 7th Eur. Peptide Symp., 1964"; *Acta Chim. Acad. Sci. Hung.* **44**, Spec. Issue (1965).
95. K. J. Brunings and P. Lindgren, eds., *Proc. 1st Int. Pharmacol. Meet.*, *1961*, Vol. 7, p. 232. Pergamon Press, Oxford, 1963.
96. H. Brunner and D. Regoli, *Experientia* **18**, 504 (1962).
97. F. M. Bumpus, P. A. Khairallah, K. Arakawa, I. H. Page, and R. R. Smeby, *Biochim. Biophys. Acta* **46**, 38 (1961).
98. F. M. Bumpus, R. R. Smeby, I. H. Page, and P. A. Khairallah, *Can. Med. Assoc. J.* **90**, 190 (1964).
99. R. Caldeyro-Barcia and H. Heller, eds., "Oxytocin." Pergamon Press, Oxford, 1961.
100. B. Camerino, G. de Caro, R. A. Boissonnas, E. Sandrin, and E. Stürmer, *Experientia* **19**, 339 (1963).
101. F. H. Carpenter, *Amer. J. Med.* **40**, 750 (1966).

102. J.-P. Carrión, D. A. Deranleau, B. Donzel, K. Esko, P. Moser, and R. Schwyzer, *Helv. Chim. Acta* **51**, 459 (1968).
103. J.-P. Carrión, B. Donzel, D. Deranleau, K. Esko, P. Moser, and R. Schwyzer, *in* "Peptides; Proc. 8th Eur. Peptide Symp., 1966" (H. C. Beyerman, A. van de Linde, and W. Maassen van den Brink, eds.), p. 177. North-Holland Publ., Amsterdam, 1967.
104. W. D. Cash, L. McC. Mahaffey, A. S. Buck, D. E. Nettleton, C. Romas, and V. du Vigneaud, *J. Med. Pharm. Chem.* **5**, 413 (1962).
105. W. D. Cash and B. L. Smith, *J. Biol. Chem.* **238**, 994 (1963).
106. W. Y. Chan, R. Fear, and V. du Vigneaud, *Endocrinology* **81**, 1267 (1967).
107. W. Y. Chan, V. J. Hruby, G. Flouret, and V. du Vigneaud, *Science* **161**, 280 (1968).
108. W. Y. Chan and N. Kelley, *J. Pharmacol. Exp. Ther.* **156**, 150 (1967).
109. W. Y. Chan and V. du Vigneaud, *Endocrinology* **71**, 977 (1962).
110. A. Chimiak, K. Eisler, K. Jošt, and J. Rudinger, *Collect. Czech. Chem. Commun.* **33**, 2918 (1968).
111. A. Chimiak and J. Rudinger, *Collect. Czech. Chem. Commun.* **30**, 2592 (1965).
112. C. C. Chiu, I. L. Schwartz, and R. Walter, *Science* **163**, 925 (1969).
113. D. Chung and C. H. Li, *J. Amer. Chem. Soc.* **89**, 4208 (1967).
114. D. Chung and C. H. Li, *Biochim. Biophys. Acta* **136**, 570 (1967).
115. J. H. Cort, J. Hammer, M. Ulrych, Z. Píša, T. Douša, and J. Rudinger, *Lancet* **2**, 840 (1964).
116. J. H. Cort, M. F. Jeanjean, and A. E. Thomson, *Amer. J. Physiol.* **214**, 455 (1968).
117. J. H. Cort, J. Rudinger, B. Lichardus, and I. Hagemann, *Amer. J. Physiol.* **210**, 162 (1966).
118. M. A. Cresswell, R. W. Hanson, and H. D. Law, *J. Chem. Soc., C* p. 2669 (1967).
119. D. W. Cushman and H. S. Cheung, *Fed. Proc., Fed. Amer. Soc. Exp. Biol.* **28**, 3019 (1969).
120. T. S. Danowski, K. Hofmann, F. A. Weigand, and J. H. Sunder, *J. Clin. Endocrinol. Metab.* **28**, 1120 (1968).
121. J. M. Davey, A. H. Laird, and J. S. Morley, *J. Chem. Soc., C* p. 555 (1966).
122. M. O. Dayhoff, "Atlas of Protein Sequence and Structure 1969." *Natl. Biomed. Res. Found.*, Silver Springs, Maryland, 1969.
123. S. D. Deodhar, *J. Exp. Med.* **111**, 419 (1960).
124. P. A. Desaulles, R. Riniker, and W. Rittel, *in* "Protein and Polypeptide Hormones" (M. Margoulies, ed.), p. 489. Excerpta Med. Found., Amsterdam, 1968.
125. P. A. Desaulles and W. Rittel, *Mem. Soc. Endocrinol.* **17**, 125 (1968).
126. P. A. Desaulles and W. Rittel, *Proc. Roy. Soc. Med.* **60**, 906 (1967).
127. H. A. DeWald, M. K. Craft, and E. D. Nicolaides, *J. Med. Chem.* **6**, 741 (1963).
128. H. A. DeWald and E. D. Nicolaides, *J. Med. Chem.* **7**, 50 (1964).
129. W. Doepfner, *Experientia* **22**, 527 (1966).
130. W. Doepfner, *Proc. 3rd Int. Congr. Endocrinol., 1968.* Excerpta Med. Found., p. 407. Amsterdam, 1969.
131. W. Doepfner, R. Stürmer, and B. Berde, *Endocrinology* **72**, 897 (1963).
132. V. H. Donaldson and O. D. Ratnoff, *Proc. Soc. Exp. Biol. Med.* **125**, 145 (1967).
133. T. Douša, O. Hechter, R. Walter, and I. L. Schwartz, *Science* **167**, 1134 (1970).
134. W. W. Downie, K. Whaley, M. A. Wright, M. A. Bell, and A. K. Taylor, *Brit. Med. J.* **4**, 487 (1968).
135. A. E. Doyle, W. J. Louis, and E. C. Osborn, *Aust. J. Expt. Biol. Med. Sci.* **45**, 41 (1967).
136. S. Drabarek, *J. Amer. Chem. Soc.* **86**, 4477 (1964).
137. S. Drabarek and V. du Vigneaud, *J. Amer. Chem. Soc.* **87**, 3974 (1965).

138. A. S. Dutta, N. Anand, and K. Kar, *J. Med. Chem.* **9**, 497 (1966).
139. A. S. Dutta, N. Anand, and K. Kar, *Indian J. Chem.* **4**, 488 (1966).
140. A. S. Dutta, N. Anand, and R. C. Srimal, *Indian J. Chem.* **7**, 3 (1969).
141. P. Eggena, I. L. Schwartz, and R. Walter, *J. Gen. Physiol.* **52**, 465 (1968).
142. P. Eggena, I. L. Schwartz, and R. Walter, *J. Gen. Physiol.* **56**, 250 (1970).
143. K. Eisler, J. Rudinger, and F. Šorm, *Collect. Czech. Chem. Commun.* **31**, 4563 (1966).
144. D. F. Elliott and G. P. Lewis, *Biochem. J.* **95**, 437 (1965).
145. E. G. Erdös, ed., *Ann. N.Y. Acad. Sci.* **104**, Art. 1 (1963).
146. E. G. Erdös, *Advan. Pharmacol.* **4**, 1 (1966).
147. E. G. Erdös, N. Back, and F. Sicuteri, eds., "Hypotensive Peptides." Springer, Berlin, 1966.
148. E. G. Erdös and E. M. Sloane, *Biochem. Pharmacol.* **11**, 585 (1962).
149. E. G. Erdös and H. Y. T. Yang, *Int. Symp. Vasoactive Polypeptides: Bradykinin and Related Kinins, Riberão Prêto, 1966* (M. Rocha e Silva and A. Rothschild, eds.), p. 239. Soc. Bras. Farm. Ter. Exp., São Paulo, Brazil, 1967.
150. E. G. Erdös and H. Y. T. Yang, in "Hypotensive Peptides" (E. G. Erdös, N. Back, and F. Sicuteri, eds.), p. 235. Springer, Berlin, 1966.
151. E. G. Erdös and H. Y. T. Yang, *Life Sci.* **6**, 569 (1967).
152. E. G. Erdös, H. Y. T. Yang, L. L. Tague, and N. Manning, *Biochem. Pharmacol.* **16**, 1287 (1967).
153. V. Erspamer, G. Bertaccini, G. de Caro, R. Endean, and M. Impicciatore, *Experientia* **23**, 702 (1967).
154. J.-P. Felber and M. L. Aubert, in "Protein and Polypeptide Hormones" (M. Margoulies, ed.), p. 373. Excerpta Med. Found., Amsterdam, 1968.
155. W. Ferrari, G. L. Gessa, and L. Vargiu, *Ann. N.Y. Acad. Sci.* **104**, 330 (1963).
156. J. J. Ferraro and V. du Vigneaud, *J. Amer. Chem. Soc.* **88**, 3847 (1966).
157. S. H. Ferreira and J. R. Vane, *Brit. J. Pharmacol.* **30**, 417 (1967).
158. B. M. Ferrier and V. du Vigneaud, *J. Med. Chem.* **9**, 55 (1966).
159. F. M. Finn and K. Hofmann, *J. Amer. Chem. Soc.* **89**, 5298 (1967).
160. F. M. Finn, J. P. Visser, and K. Hofmann, in "Peptides 1968; Proc. 9th Eur. Peptide Symp." (E. Bricas, ed.), p. 330. North-Holland Publ., Amsterdam, 1968.
161. N. Fleischer, J. R. Givens, K. Abe, W. E. Nicholson, and G. W. Liddle, *Endocrinology* **78**, 1067 (1966).
162. G. Flouret and V. du Vigneaud, *J. Amer. Chem. Soc.* **87**, 3775 (1965).
163. G. Flouret and V. du Vigneaud, *J. Med. Chem.* **12**, 1035 (1969).
164. E. Flückiger, *Pharmakologie* **245**, 168 (1963).
165. A. P. Fosker and H. D. Law, *J. Chem. Soc.* p. 4922 (1965).
166. F. Fraschini, G. Mangili, L. Martini, and M. Motta, in "Oxytocin, Vasopressin and Their Structural Analogues; Proc. 2nd Int. Pharmacol. Meeting, 1963" (J. Rudinger, ed.), Vol. 10, p. 75. Pergamon Press, Oxford, 1964.
167. M. Friedman, *Experientia* **25**, 416 (1969).
168. J. Gante, *Fortschr. Chem. Forsch.* **6**, 358 (1966).
169. M. P. de Garilhe, C. Gros, J. Porath, and E. B. Lindner, *Experientia* **16**, 414 (1960).
170. R. Geiger, H.-G. Schröder, and W. Siedel, *Justus Liebigs Ann. Chem.* **726**, 177 (1969).
171. R. Geiger, K. Sturm, and W. Siedel, *Chem. Ber.* **97**, 1207 (1964).
172. R. Geiger, K. Sturm, and W. Siedel, *Chem. Ber.* **101**, 1223 (1968).
173. R. Geiger, K. Sturm, G. Vogel, and W. Siedel, *Z. Naturforsch. B* **19**, 858 (1964).
174. I. I. Geschwind, *Amer. Zool.* **7**, 89 (1967).
175. I. I. Geschwind, *Colloq. Int. Cent. Nat. Rech. Sci.* No. 177, 386 (1969).
176. I. I. Geschwind and C. H. Li, *Arch. Biochem. Biophys.* **106**, 200 (1964).

177. D. Gillesen and V. du Vigneaud, *J. Biol. Chem.* **242**, 4806 (1967).
178. J. A. Goffinet and P. J. Mulrow, *Clin. Res.* **11**, 408 (1965).
179. J. Golubow, W. Y. Chan, and V. du Vigneaud, *Proc. Soc. Exp. Biol. Med.* **113**, 113 (1963).
180. J. Golubow and V. du Vigneaud, *Proc. Soc. Exp. Biol. Med.* **112**, 218 (1963).
181. H. Gregory, D. S. Jones, and J. S. Morley, *J. Chem. Soc., C* p. 531 (1968).
182. H. Gregory, A. H. Laird, J. S. Morley, and J. M. Smith, *J. Chem. Soc.* p. 522 (1968).
183. H. Gregory and J. S. Morley, *J. Chem. Soc., C* p. 910 (1968).
184. H. Gregory, J. S. Morley, J. M. Smith, and M. J. Smithers, *J. Chem. Soc., C* p. 715 (1968).
185. R. Grupe and H. Niedrich, *Chem. Ber.* **100**, 3288 (1967).
186. U. Guhl, *Schweiz. Med. Wochenschr.* **91**, 798 (1961).
187. S. Guttmann, *Helv. Chim. Acta* **44**, 721 (1961).
188. S. Guttmann and R. A. Boissonnas, *Helv. Chim. Acta* **42**, 1257 (1959).
189. S. Guttmann and R. A. Boissonnas, *Experientia* **17**, 265 (1961).
190. S. Guttmann and R. A. Boissonnas, *Helv. Chim. Acta* **44**, 1713 (1961).
191. S. Guttmann and R. A. Boissonnas, *Helv. Chim. Acta* **45**, 2517 (1962).
192. S. Guttmann and R. A. Boissonnas, *Helv. Chim. Acta* **46**, 1626 (1963).
193. S. Guttmann, P.-A. Jaquenoud, R. A. Boissonnas, H. Konzett, and B. Berde, *Naturwissenschaften* **44**, 632 (1957).
194. S. Guttmann, J. Pless, and R. A. Boissonnas, *in* "Proc. 7th Eur. Peptide Symp., 1964" (V. Bruckner and K. Medzihradszky, eds.); *Acta Chim. Acad. Sci. Hung.* **44**, Spec. Issue p. 141 (1965).
195. S. Guttmann, J. Pless, R. L. Huguenin, E. Sandrin, H. Bossert, and K. Zehnder, *Helv. Chim. Acta* **52**, 1789 (1969).
196. S. Guttmann, J. Pless, E. Sandrin, P.-A. Jaquenoud, H. Bossert, and H. Willems, *Helv. Chim. Acta* **51**, 1155 (1968).
197. E. Habermann, *in* "Hypotensive Peptides" (E. G. Erdös, N. Back, and F. Sicuteri, eds.), p. 116. Springer, Berlin, 1966.
198. E. Habermann, *Naunyn-Schmiedebergs Arch. Pharmakol. Exp. Pathol.* **251**, 187 (1965).
199. E. Habermann, *Naunyn-Schmiedebergs Arch. Pharmakol. Exp. Pathol.* **253**, 474 (1966).
200. K. Hano, M. Koida, K. Kubo, and H. Yajima, *Biochem. Biophys. Acta* **90**, 201 (1964).
201. S. Hase, T. Morikawa, and S. Sakakibara, *Experientia* **25**, 1239 (1969).
202. E. Havinga and C. Schattenkerk, *Tetrahedron* Suppl. **8**, 313 (1966).
203. E. Havinga, C. Schattenkerk, G. H. Visser, and K. E. T. Kerling, *Rec. Trav. Chim. Pays-Bas* **83**, 672 (1964).
204. R. T. Havran, I. L. Schwartz, and R. Walter, *Mol. Pharmacol.* **5**, 83 (1969).
205. R. T. Havran, I. L. Schwartz, and R. Walter, *J. Amer. Chem. Soc.* **91**, 1836 (1969).
206. O. M. Helmer, *Amer. J. Physiol.* **188**, 571 (1957).
207. P. Herman and M. Zaoral, *Collect. Czech. Chem. Commun.* **30**, 2817 (1965).
208. S. G. Hershey and B. M. Altura, *Schweiz. Med. Wochenschr.* **96**, 1467 (1966).
209. H.-J. Hess, W. T. Moreland, and G. T. Laubach, *J. Amer. Chem. Soc.* **85**, 4040 (1963).
210. R. L. Hodge, K. K. F. Ng, and J. R. Vane, *Nature (London)* **215**, 138 (1967).
211. J. Hodr, Z. K. Štembera, S. Kazda, V. Brotánek, and J. Rudinger, *Abh. Deut. Akad. Wiss. Berlin, Kl. Med.* p. 359 (1966).
212. J. Hodr, Z. K. Štembera, V. Brotánek, J. Rudinger, and J. Vondráček, *in* "Intrauterine Dangers to the Foetus," p. 445. Excerpta Med. Found., Amsterdam, 1967.
213. K. Hofmann, *Brookhaven Symp. Biol.* **13**, 184 (1960).
214. K. Hofmann, *Annu. Rev. Biochem.* **31**, 213 (1962).
215. K. Hofmann, *Harvey Lect.* **59**, 89 (1963).

216. K. Hofmann, *Metab., Clin. Exp.* **13**, 1275 (1964).
217. K. Hofmann, R. Andreatta, J. P. Buckley, W. E. Hagemann, and A. P. Shapiro, *J. Amer. Chem. Soc.* **90**, 1654 (1968).
218. K. Hofmann and H. Bohn, *J. Amer. Chem. Soc.* **88**, 5914 (1966).
219. K. Hofmann, H. Bohn, and R. Andreatta, *J. Amer. Chem. Soc.* **89**, 7126 (1967).
220. K. Hofmann and P. G. Katsoyannis, *in* "The Proteins" (H. Neurath, ed.), 2nd ed., Vol. 1, p. 53. Academic Press, New York, 1963.
221. K. Hofmann and S. Lande, *J. Amer. Chem. Soc.* **83**, 2286 (1961).
222. K. Hofmann, T. Liu, H. Yajima, N. Yanaihara, C. Yanaihara, and J. L. Humes, *J. Amer. Chem. Soc.* **84**, 1054 (1962).
223. K. Hofmann, J. Rosenthaler, R. D. Wells, and H. Yajima, *J. Amer. Chem. Soc.* **86**, 4991 (1964).
224. K. Hofmann, E. Stutz, G. Spühler, H. Yajima, and E. T. Schwartz, *J. Amer. Chem. Soc.* **82**, 3727 (1960).
225. K. Hofmann, T. A. Thompson, and E. T. Schwartz, *J. Amer. Chem. Soc.* **79**, 6087 (1957).
226. K. Hofmann, T. A. Thompson, M. E. Woolner, G. Spühler, H. Yajima, J. D. Cipera, and E. T. Schwartz, *J. Amer. Chem. Soc.* **82**, 3721 (1960).
227. K. Hofmann, R. D. Wells, H. Yajima, and J. Rosenthaler, *J. Amer. Chem. Soc.* **85**, 1546 (1963).
228. K. Hofmann, M. E. Woolner, G. Spühler, and E. T. Schwartz, *J. Amer. Chem. Soc.* **80**, 1486 (1958).
229. K. Hofmann, M. E. Woolner, H. Yajima, G. Spühler, T. A. Thompson, and E. T. Schwartz, *J. Amer. Chem. Soc.* **80**, 6458 (1958).
230. K. Hofmann and H. Yajima, *Recent Progr. Horm. Res.* **18**, 41 (1962).
231. K. Hofmann and H. Yajima, *J. Amer. Chem. Soc.* **83**, 2289 (1961).
232. K. Hofmann, H. Yajima, T.-Y. Liu, and N. Yanaihara, *J. Amer. Chem. Soc.* **84**, 4475 (1962).
233. K. Hofmann, H. Yajima, and E. T. Schwartz, *J. Amer. Chem. Soc.* **82**, 3732 (1960).
234. K. Hofmann, H. Yajima, N. Yanaihara, T.-Y. Liu, and S. Lande, *J. Amer. Chem. Soc.* **83**, 487 (1961).
235. K. Hofmann, N. Yanaihara, S. Lande, and H. Yajima, *J. Amer. Chem. Soc.* **84**, 4470 (1962).
236. D. B. Hope, V. V. S. Murti, and V. du Vigneaud, *J. Biol. Chem.* **237**, 1563 (1962).
237. D. B. Hope, V. V. S. Murti, and V. du Vigneaud, *J. Amer. Chem. Soc.* **85**, 3686 (1963).
238. D. B. Hope and V. du Vigneaud, *J. Biol. Chem.* **237**, 3146 (1962).
239. S. Hörnle, U. Weber, and G. Weitzel, *Hoppe-Seyler's Z. Physiol. Chem.* **349**, 1428 (1968).
240. V. J. Hruby and V. du Vigneaud, *J. Med. Chem.* **12**, 731 (1969).
241. V. J. Hruby, G. Flouret, and V. du Vigneaud, *J. Biol. Chem.* **244**, 3890 (1970).
242. R. L. Huguenin, *Helv. Chim. Acta* **47**, 1934 (1964).
243. R. L. Huguenin, *Helv. Chim. Acta* **49**, 711 (1966).
244. R. L. Huguenin and R. A. Boissonnas, *Helv. Chim. Acta* **44**, 213 (1961).
245. R. L. Huguenin and R. A. Boissonnas, *Helv. Chim. Acta* **45**, 1629 (1962).
246. R. L. Huguenin and R. A. Boissonnas, *Helv. Chim. Acta* **46**, 1669 (1963).
247. R. L. Huguenin and R. A. Boissonnas, *Helv. Chim. Acta* **49**, 695 (1966).
248. R. L. Huguenin and S. Guttmann, *Helv. Chim. Acta* **48**, 1885 (1965).
249. R. L. Huguenin, E. Stürmer, R. A. Boissonnas, and B. Berde, *Experientia* **21**, 68 (1965).
250. A. Hunger, *J. Mond. Pharm.* **11**, 313 (1968).

251. P. Imhof, H. Brunner, J. Quitt, B. Steinmann, and A. Jacono, *Schweiz. Med. Wochenchr.* **94**, 1199 (1964).
252. H. Imura, M. Hitoshi, M. Shigeru, M. Tadashi, and F. Masaichi, *Endocrinology* **80**, 599 (1967).
253. H. Imura, L. L. Sparks, G. M. Grodsky, and P. H. Forsham, *Clin. Endocrinol.* **25**, 1361 (1965).
254. IUPAC-IUB Commission on Biochemical Nomenclature, *Biochemistry* **5**, 2485 (1966).
255. IUPAC-IUB Commission on Biochemical Nomenclature, *Biochemistry* **6**, 362 (1967).
256. P.-A. Jaquenoud, *Helv. Chim. Acta* **48**, 1899 (1965).
257. P.-A. Jaquenoud and R. A. Boissonnas, *Helv. Chim. Acta* **42**, 788 (1959).
258. P.-A. Jaquenoud and R. A. Boissonnas, *Helv. Chim. Acta* **44**, 113 (1961).
259. P.-A. Jaquenoud and R. A. Boissonnas, *Helv. Chim. Acta* **45**, 1601 (1962).
260. P.-A. Jaquenoud and R. A. Boissonnas, *Helv. Chim. Acta* **45**, 1462 (1962).
261. S. Jard, *J. Physiol. (Paris)* **58**, Suppl. 15 (1966).
262. S. Jard and F. Morel, *Amer. J. Physiol.* **204**, 222 (1963).
263. D. Jarvis, M. Bodanszky, and V. du Vigneaud, *J. Amer. Chem. Soc.* **83**, 4780 (1961).
264. D. Jarvis, B. M. Ferrier, and V. du Vigneaud, *J. Biol. Chem.* **240**, 3553 (1965).
265. D. Jarvis, M. Manning, and V. du Vigneaud, *Biochemistry* **6**, 1223 (1967).
266. D. Jarvis and V. du Vigneaud, *Science* **143**, 545 (1964).
267. D. Jarvis and V. du Vigneaud, *J. Biol. Chem.* **242**, 1768 (1967).
268. M. Jenny, A. F. Muller, and R. S. Mach, *Experientia* **22**, 528 (1966).
269. W. D. Johnson, H. D. Law, and R. O. Studer, *Experientia* **25**, 573 (1969).
270. E. C. Jorgensen and W. Patton, *J. Med. Chem.* **12**, 935 (1969).
271. E. C. Jorgensen, G. C. Windridge, W. Patton, and T. C. Lee, *J. Med. Chem.* **12**, 733 (1969).
272. K. Jošt, V. G. Debabov, H. Nesvadba, and J. Rudinger, *Collect. Czech. Chem. Commun.* **29**, 419 (1964).
273. K. Jošt and J. Rudinger, *Collect. Czech. Chem. Commun.* **32**, 1229 (1967).
274. K. Jošt and J. Rudinger, *Collect. Czech. Chem. Commun.* **33**, 109 (1968).
275. K. Jošt and J. Rudinger, *Colloq. Int. Cent. Nat. Rech. Sci.* No. 177, 13 (1969).
276. K. Jošt, J. Rudinger, H. Klostermeyer, and H. Zahn, *Z. Naturforsch. B* **23**, 1059 (1968).
277. K. Jošt, J. Rudinger, and F. Šorm, *Collect. Czech. Chem. Commun.* **26**, 2496 (1961).
278. K. Jošt, J. Rudinger, and F. Šorm, *Collect. Czech. Chem. Commun.* **28**, 1706 (1963).
279. K. Jošt, J. Rudinger, and F. Šorm, *Collect. Czech. Chem. Commun.* **28**, 2021 (1963).
280. W. Jubiz, C. D. West, and F. H. Tyler, *J. Clin. Endocrinol. Metab.* **28**, 1377 (1968).
281. C. Jungmannová, V. Brotánek, S. Kazda, and J. Rudinger, in "Oxytocin and its Analogues" (R. Klimek and W. Król, eds.), p. 106. Polish Endorcinol. Soc., Kraków, 1964.
282. S. Kalsner and M. Nickerson, *Can. J. Physiol. Pharmacol* **46**, 719 (1968).
283. H. Kappeler, *Helv. Chim. Acta* **44**, 476 (1961).
284. H. Kappeler, B. Riniker, W. Rittel, P. Desaulles, R. Maier, B. Schär, and M. Staehelin, in "Peptides; Proc. 8th Eur. Peptide Symp., 1966" (H. C. Beyerman, A. van de Linde, and W. Maassen van den Brink, eds.), p. 214. North-Holland Publ., Amsterdam, 1967.
285. H. Kappeler and R. Schwyzer, *Experientia* **16**, 415 (1960).
286. H. Kappeler and R. Schwyzer, *Helv. Chim. Acta* **43**, 1453 (1960).
287. H. Kappeler and R. Schwyzer, *Helv. Chim. Acta* **44**, 1136 (1961).
288. E. Kasafírek, K. Eisler, and J. Rudinger, *Collect. Czech. Chem. Commun.* **34**, 2848 (1969).
289. E. Kasafírek, K. Jošt, J. Rudinger, and F. Šorm, *Collect. Czech. Chem. Commun.* **30**, 2600 (1965).

290. E. Kasafírek, V. Rábek, J. Rudinger, and F. Šorm, *Collect. Czech. Chem. Commun.* **31**, 4581 (1966).
291. P. G. Katsoyannis, *J. Amer. Chem. Soc.* **79**, 109 (1957).
292. P. G. Katsoyannis and V. du Vigneaud, *Arch. Biochem. Biophys.* **78**, 555 (1958).
293. P. G. Katsoyannis and V. du Vigneaud, *J. Biol. Chem.* **233**, 1352 (1958).
294. P. G. Katsoyannis and V. du Vigneaud, *Nature (London)* **184**, 1465 (1959).
295. W. Kemmler and K. Rager, *Hoppe-Seyler's Z. Physiol. Chem.* **349**, 515 (1968).
296. P. A. Khairallah, F. M. Bumpus, I. H. Page, and R. R. Smeby, *Science* **140**, 672 (1963).
297. P. A. Khairallah, I. H. Page, F. M. Bumpus, and K. Türker, *Circ. Res.* **19**, 247 (1966).
298. M. C. Khosla, N. C. Chaturvedi, R. R. Smeby, and F. M. Bumpus, *Biochemistry* **7**, 3417 (1968).
299. M. C. Khosla, R. R. Smeby, and F. M. Bumpus, *Biochemistry* **6**, 754 (1967).
300. R. D. Kimbrough, W. D. Cash, L. A. Branda, W. Y. Chan, and V. du Vigneaud, *J. Biol. Chem.* **238**, 1411 (1963).
301. I. L. Knunyants, K. I. Karpavichyus, and O. V. Kil'disheva, *Izv. Akad. Nauk SSSR, Otd. Khim. Nauk.* p. 1024 (1962).
302. T. Kokubu, E. Ueda, S. Fujimoto, K. Hiwada, A. Kato, H. Akutsu, and Y. Yamamura, *Nature (London)* **217**, 456 (1968).
303. J. Kolc, M. Zaoral, and F. Šorm, *Collect. Czech. Chem. Commun.* **32**, 2667 (1967).
304. I. Krejčí, B. Kupková, and I. Vávra, *Brit. J. Pharmacol.* **30**, 497 (1967).
305. Krejčí, I. Poláček, B. Kupková, and J. Rudinger, *in* "Oxytocin, Vasopressin and Their Structural Analogues; Proc. 2nd Int. Pharmacol. Meeting, 1963" (J. Rudinger, ed.), Vol. 10, p. 117. Pergamon Press, Oxford, 1964.
306. I. Krejčí, I. Poláček, and J. Rudinger, *Brit. J. Pharmacol.* **30**, 506 (1967).
307. I. Krejčí, I. Poláček, and J. Rudinger, *Mem. Soc. Endocrinol.* **14**, 171 (1966).
308. I. Krejčí, I. Poláček, and J. Rudinger, *Abstr. 4th Int. Congr. Pharmacol., 1969* p. 208 (1969).
309. I. Krejčí, I. Poláček, and J. Rudinger, unpublished results.
310. W. A. Krivoy, M. Lane, and D. C. Kroeger, *Ann. N.Y. Acad. Sci.* **104**, 312 (1963).
311. J. Kynčl, V. Jelínek, and J. Rudinger, *Acta Endocrinol.* **60**, 369 (1969).
312. S. Lande and A. B. Lerner, *Pharmacol. Rev.* **19**, 1 (1967).
313. F. W. Landgerbe and G. M. Mitchell, *Quart. J. Exp. Physiol.* **39**, 11 (1954).
314. J. Landon, V. H. T. James, R. J. Cryer, W. Wynn, and L. A. W. Frankland, *J. Clin. Endocrinol. Metab.* **24**, 1206 (1964).
315. Z. Laron, *Proc. 2nd Int. Congr. Endocrinol., 1964.* Int. Congr. Ser. No. 83, p. 1195. Excerpta Med. Found., Amsterdam, 1965.
316. H. D. Law and V. du Vigneaud, *J. Amer. Chem. Soc.* **82**, 4579 (1960).
317. W. P. Leary and J. G. Ledingham, *Nature (London)* **222**, 959 (1969).
318. H. E. Lebovitz and F. L. Engel, *Endocrinology* **73**, 573 (1963).
319. H. E. Lebovitz, S. Genuth, and K. Pooler, *Endocrinology* **79**, 635 (1966).
320. T. H. Lee and V. Buettner-Janusch, *J. Biol. Chem.* **238**, 2012 (1963).
321. K. E. Lentz, L. T. Skeggs, K. R. Woods, J. R. Kahn, and N. P. Shumway, *J. Exp. Med.* **104**, 183 (1956).
322. A. B. Lerner, S. Lande, and S. Kulovich, *Proc. 2nd Int. Congr. Endocrinol., 1964* Int. Congr. Ser. No. 83, p. 392. Excerpta Med. Found., Amsterdam, 1965.
323. C.-H. Li, *Recent Progr. Horm. Res.* **18**, 1 (1962).
324. C.-H. Li, L. Barnafi, M. Chretien, and D. Chung, *Nature (London)* **208**, 1093 (1965).
325. C.-H. Li, B. Gorup, D. Chung, and J. Ramachandran, *J. Org. Chem.* **28**, 178 (1963).
326. C.-H. Li and W.-K. Liu, *Experientia* **20**, 169 (1964).
327. C.-H. Li, J. Meienhofer, E. Schnabel, D. Chung, T.-B. Lo, and J. Ramachandran, *J. Amer. Chem. Soc.* **82**, 5760 (1960); **83**, 4449 (1961).

328. C.-H. Li, J. Ramachandran, and D. Chung, *J. Amer. Chem. Soc.* **85**, 1895 (1963); **86**, 2711 (1964).
329. C.-H. Li, J. Ramachandran, D. Chung, and B. Gorup, *J. Amer. Chem. Soc.* **84**, 2460 (1962); **86**, 2703 (1964).
330. C.-H. Li, E. Schnabel, and D. Chung, *J. Amer. Chem. Soc.* **82**, 2062 (1960).
331. C.-H. Li, E. Schnabel, D. Chung, and T.-B. Lo, *Nature (London)* **189**, 143 (1961).
332. K. Lübke, R. Hempel, and E. Schröder, *in* "Proc. 7th Eur. Peptide Symp., 1964" (V. Bruckner and K. Medzihradszky, eds.): *Acta Chim. Acad. Sci. Hung.* **44**, Spec. Issue p. 131 (1965).
333. K. Lübke, R. Hempel, and E. Schröder, *Experientia* **21**, 84 (1965).
334. K. Lübke and H. Klostermeyer, *Advan. Enzymol.* **33**, 445 (1970).
335. K. Lübke and E. Schröder, *Justus Liebigs Ann. Chem.* **684**, 252 (1965).
336. K. Lübke, G. Zöllner, and E. Schröder, *in* "Hypotensive Peptides" (E. G. Erdös, N. Back, and F. Sicuteri, eds.), p. 45. Springer, Berlin, 1966.
337. W. B. Lutz, C. Ressler, E. E. Nettleton, and V. du Vigneaud, *J. Amer. Chem. Soc.* **81**, 167 (1959).
338. M. Manning and V. du Vigneaud, *J. Amer. Chem. Soc.* **87**, 3978 (1965).
339. M. Manning and V. du Vigneaud, *Biochemistry* **4**, 1884 (1965).
340. M. Margoulies, ed., "Protein and Polypeptide Hormones." Excerpta Med. Found., Amsterdam, 1968.
341. J. Meinhofer, *Justus Liebigs Ann. Chem.* **691**, 218 (1966).
342. J. Meienhofer, A. Trzeciak, T. Douša, O. Hechter, R. T. Havran, I. L. Schwartz, and R. Walter, *in* "Peptides 1969; Proc. 10th Eur. Peptide Symp." (E. Scoffone, ed.), p. 157. North-Holland Publ., Amsterdam, 1971.
343. J. Meienhofer and V. du Vigneaud, *J. Amer. Chem. Soc.* **83**, 142 (1961).
344. A. L. Methot, P. Meyer, P. Biron, M. F. Lorain, G. Lagure, and P. Millier, *Nature (London)* **203**, 531 (1964).
345. O. L. Mndzhoyan, K. Jošt, and J. Rudinger, unpublished results; see Rudinger and Jošt (*439*).
346. D. Montague, B. Riniker, H. Brunner, and F. Gross, *Amer. J. Physiol.* **210**, 591 (1966).
347. D. Montague, B. Riniker, and F. Gross, *Amer. J. Physiol.* **210**, 595 (1966).
348. F. Morel and S. Jard, *Amer. J. Physiol.* **204**, 227 (1963).
349. J. S. Morley, *in* "Peptides; Proc. 8th Eur. Peptide Symp., 1966" (H. C. Beyerman, A. van de Linde, and W. Maassen van den Brink, eds.), p. 226. North-Holland Publ., Amsterdam, 1967.
350. J. S. Morley, *Proc. Roy. Soc.*, *Ser B.* **170**, 97 (1968).
351. J. S. Morley, *Fed. Proc.*, *Fed. Amer. Soc. Exp. Biol.* **27**, 1314 (1968).
352. J. S. Morley, *Proc. 3rd Symp. Pancreatic Club, 1968* (in press).
353. J. S. Morley and J. M. Smith, *J. Chem. Soc., C* p. 726 (1968).
354. J. S. Morley, H. J. Tracy, and R. A. Gregory, *Nature (London)* **207**, 1356 (1965).
355. J. L. Mulder, *in* "Protein and Polypeptide Hormones" (M. Margoulies, ed.), p. 786. Excerpta Med. Found., Amsterdam, 1968.
356. V. Mutt and J. E. Jorpes, *Biochem. Biophys. Res. Commun.* **26**, 392 (1967).
357. V. Mutt and J. E. Jorpes, *Eur. J. Biochem.* **6**, 156 (1968).
358. I. Nagatsu, L. Gillespie, J. E. Folk, and G. G. Glenner, *Biochem. Pharmacol.* **14**, 721 (1965).
359. H. Nesvadba, J. Honzl, and J. Rudinger, *Collect. Czech. Chem. Commun.* **28**, 1691 (1963).
360. H. Nesvadba, K. Jošt, J. Rudinger, and F. Šorm, *Collect. Czech. Chem. Commun.* **33**, 3790 (1968).

361. R. L. Ney, E. Ogata, N. Shimizu, W. E. Nicholson, and G. W. Liddle, *Proc. 2nd Int. Congr. Endocrinol.*, *1964* Int. Congr. Ser. No. 83, p. 1184. Excerpta Med. Found., Amsterdam, 1965.

362. K. K. F. Ng and J. R. Vane, *Nature (London)* **218**, 144 (1968).

363. H. D. Niall, H. T. Keutmann, D. H. Copp, and J. T. Potts, *Proc. Nat. Acad. Sci. U.S.* **64**, 770 (1969).

364. E. D. Nicolaides, M. V. Craft, and H. A. DeWald, *J. Med. Chem.* **6**, 524 (1963).

365. E. D. Nicolaides, H. A. DeWald, and M. V. Craft, *J. Med. Chem.* **6**, 739 (1963).

366. E. D. Nicolaides, H. A. DeWald, and M. V. Craft, *Ann. N.Y. Acad. Sci.* **104**, 15 (1963).

367. E. D. Nicolaides, H. A. DeWald, P. G. Shorley, and H. O. J. Collier, *Nature (London)* **187**, 773 (1960).

368. E. D. Nicolaides, H. A. DeWald, R. Westland, M. Lipnik, and J. Posler, *J. Med. Chem.* **11**, 74 (1968).

369. E. D. Nicolaides and M. Lipnik, *J. Med. Chem.* **9**, 958 (1966).

370. E. D. Nicolaides, D. A. McCarthy, and D. E. Potter, *Biochemistry* **4**, 190 (1965).

371. H. Niedrich, *Chem. Ber.* **100**, 3273 (1967).

372. H. Niedrich, *in* "Peptides 1968; Proc. 9th Eur. Peptide Symp." (E. Bricas, ed.), p. 267. North-Holland Publ., Amsterdam, 1968.

373. H. Niedrich, *Chem. Ber.* **102**, 1557 (1969).

374. H. Niedrich, C. Berseck, and P. Oehme, *in* "Peptides 1969; Proc. 10th Eur. Peptide Symp." (E. Scoffone, ed.), p. 370. North-Holland Publ., Amsterdam, 1971.

375. H. Niedrich, B. Wiegershausen, and E. Göres, *in* "Oxytocin, Vasopressin and Their Structural Analogues; Proc. 2nd Int. Pharmacol, Meeting, 1963" (J. Rudinger, ed.), Vol. 10, p. 173. Pergamon Press, Oxford, 1964.

376. G. W. Oertel and D. Wenzel, *Arzneim.-Forsch.* **16**, 1107 (1966).

377. M. A. Ondetti, *J. Med. Chem.* **6**, 10 (1963).

378. E. C. Osborn, W. J. Louis, and A. E. Doyle, *Aust. J. Exp. Biol.* **44**, 475 (1966).

379. H. Otsuka and K. Inouye, *Bull. Chem. Soc. Jap.* **37**, 289 (1964).

380. H. Otsuka, K. Inouye, M. Kanayama, and F. Shinozaki, *Bull. Chem. Soc. Jap.* **38**, 1563 (1965).

381. H. Otsuka, K. Inouye, M. Kanayama, and F. Shinozaki, *Bull. Chem. Soc. Jap.* **38**, 679 (1965).

382. H. Otsuka, K. Inouye, F. Shinozaki, and K. Makoto, *J. Biochem. (Tokyo)* **58**, 512 (1965).

383. N. I. A. Overweg, I. L. Schwartz, B. M. Dubois, and R. Walter, *J. Pharmacol. Exp. Ther.* **161**, 342 (1968).

384. I. H. Page and F. M. Bumpus, *Physiol. Rev.* **41**, 331 (1961).

385. T. B. Paiva and A. C. M. Paiva, *Brit. J. Pharmacol.* **15**, 4 (1960).

386. W. K. Park, R. R. Smeby, and F. M. Bumpus, *Biochemistry* **6**, 3458 (1967).

387. M. J. Peach, F. M. Bumpus, and P. A. Khairallah, *J. Pharmacol. Exp. Ther.* **167**, 291 (1969).

388. W. S. Peart, *Pharmacol. Rev.* **17**, 143 (1965).

389. I. Photaki and V. du Vigneaud, *J. Amer. Chem. Soc.* **87**, 908 (1965).

390. B. T. Pickering and H. Heller, *Nature (London)* **184**, 1463 (1959).

391. B. T. Pickering and C. H. Li, *Arch. Biochem. Biophys.* **104**, 119 (1964).

392. J. V. Pierce, *Fed. Proc., Fed. Amer. Soc. Exp. Biol.* **27**, 52 (1968).

393. V. Pliška, *Arzneim.-Forsch.* **16**, 886 (1966).

394. V. Pliška, *Farmaco, Ed. Sci.* **23**, 623 (1968).

395. V. Pliška, *Eur. J. Pharmacol.* **5**, 253 (1969).

396. V. Pliška, T. Barth, and I. Rychlík, *Experientia* **23**, 196 (1967).

397. V. Pliška, J. Rudinger, T. Douša, and J. H. Cort, *Amer. J. Physiol.* **215**, 916 (1968).
398. I. Poláček and I. Krejčí, *Eur. J. Pharmacol.* **7**, 85 (1969).
399. I. Poláček, I. Krejčí, H. Nesvadba, and J. Rudinger, *Eur. J. Pharmacol.* **9**, 239 (1970).
400. I. Poláček, I. Krejčí, and J. Rudinger, *J. Endocrinol.* **38**, 13 (1967).
401. J. T. Potts, G. D. Aurbach, and L. M. Sherwood, *Recent Progr. Horm. Res.* **22**, 101 (1966).
402. *Proc. 2nd Int. Congr. Endocrinol., 1964* Int. Congr. Ser. No. 83. Excerpta Med. Found., Amsterdam, 1965.
403. M. S. Raben, *J. Clin. Endocrinol. Metab.* **15**, 842 (1955).
404. M. S. Raben, R. Landolt, F. A. Smith, K. Hofmann, and H. Yajima, *Nature (London)* **189**, 681 (1961).
405. J. Ramachandran, D. Chung, and C. H. Li, *J. Amer. Chem. Soc.* **87**, 2696 (1965).
406. J. Ramachandran and C. H. Li, *J. Amer. Chem. Soc.* **87**, 2691 (1965).
407. J. Ramachandran and C. H. Li, *Advan. Enzymol.* **29**, 391 (1967).
408. H. Rasmussen, *J. Biol. Chem.* **235**, 3442 (1960).
409. H. Rasmussen, I. L. Schwartz, R. Young, and J. Marc-Aurele, *J. Gen. Physiol.* **46**, 1171 (1963).
410. J.-G. Rausch-Strooman and R. Petry, *Deut. Med. Wochenschr.* **93**, 1938 (1958).
411. G. A. Ravdel, M. P. Filatova, L. A. Shchukina, T. S. Paskhina, M. S. Surovikina, S. S. Trapeznikova, and T. P. Egorova, *J. Med. Chem.* **10**, 242 (1967).
412. D. Regoli, B. Riniker, and H. Brunner, *Biochem. Pharmacol.* **12**, 637 (1963).
413. A. Reinharz and M. Roth, *Eur. J. Biochem.* **7**, 334 (1969).
414. C. Ressler, *Proc. Soc. Exp. Biol. Med.* **92**, 725 (1956).
415. C. Ressler and J. R. Rachele, *Proc. Soc. Exp. Biol. Med.* **98**, 170 (1958).
416. C. Ressler and V. du Vigneaud, *J. Amer. Chem. Soc.* **79**, 4511 (1957).
417. K. Řežábek, *Česko. Fysiol.* **15**, 399 (1966).
418. F. M. Richards and P. J. Vithayathil, *Brookhaven Symp. Biol.* **13**, 115 (1960).
419. B. Riniker, *Metab., Clin. Exp.* **13**, 1247 (1964).
420. B. Riniker, H. Brunner, and R. Schwyzer, *Angew. Chem.* **74**, 469 (1962).
421. B. Riniker and W. Rittel, *Helv. Chim. Acta* **53**, 513 (1970).
422. B. Riniker and R. Schwyzer, *Helv. Chim. Acta* **44**, 674 (1961).
423. B. Riniker and R. Schwyzer, *Helv. Chim. Acta* **44**, 677 (1961).
424. B. Riniker and R. Schwyzer, *Helv. Chim. Acta* **44**, 685 (1961).
425. B. Riniker and R. Schwyzer, *Helv. Chim. Acta* **47**, 2357 (1964).
426. B. Riniker and R. Schwyzer, *Helv. Chim. Acta* **47**, 2375 (1964).
427. W. Rittel, M. Brugger, B. Kamber, B. Riniker, and P. Sieber, *Helv. Chim. Acta* **51**, 924 (1968).
428. W. Rittel, B. Iselin, H. Kappeler, B. Riniker, and R. Schwyzer, *Helv. Chim. Acta* **40**, 614 (1957); *Angew. Chem.* **69**, 179 (1957).
429. R. Rocchi, F. Marchiori, and E. Scoffone, *Gazz. Chim. Ital.* **93**, 823 (1963).
430. J. Roth, S. M. Glick, L. A. Klein, and M. J. Petersen, *J. Clin. Endocrinol. Metab.* **26**, 671 (1966).
431. J. Rudinger, ed., "Oxytocin, Vasopressin and Their Structural Analogues; Proc. 2nd Int. Pharmacol. Meeting, 1963" Vol. 10. Pergamon Press, Oxford, 1964.
432. J. Rudinger, *in* "Oxytocin, Vasopressin and Their Structural Analogues; Proc. 2nd Int. Pharmacol. Meeting, 1963" (J. Rudinger, ed.), Vol. 10, p. 81. Pergamon Press, Oxford, 1964.
433. J. Rudinger, *Proc. 2nd Int. Congr. Endocrinol., 1964* Int. Congr. Ser. No. 83, p. 1202. Excerpta Med. Found., Amsterdam, 1965.

434. J. Rudinger, *Proc. Roy. Soc., Ser. B* **170**, 17 (1968).
435. J. Rudinger, *Proc. 3rd Int. Congr. Endocrinol., 1968* Int. Congr. Ser. No. 157, p. 419. Excerpta Med. Found., Amsterdam, 1969.
436. J. Rudinger, unpublished results.
437. J. Rudinger, J. Honzl, and M. Zaoral, *Collect. Czech. Chem. Commun.* **21**, 770 (1956).
438. J. Rudinger and K. Jošt, *Experientia* **20**, 570 (1964).
439. J. Rudinger and K. Jošt, *in* "Oxytocin, Vasopressin and Their Structural Analogues; Proc. 2nd Int. Pharmacol. Meeting, 1963" (J. Rudinger, ed.), Vol. 10, p. 3. Pergamon Press, Oxford, 1964.
440. J. Rudinger, K. Jošt, and F. Šorm, *in* "Peptides; Proc. 6th Eur. Peptide Symp., 1963" (L. Zervas, ed.), p. 221. Pergamon Press, Oxford, 1966.
441. J. Rudinger, O. V. Kesarev, and K. Poduška, *Abstr. Commun., 5th FEBS Meet., 1968* Abstr. No. 989 (1968).
442. J. Rudinger, O. V. Kesarev, K. Poduška, B. T. Pickering, R. E. J. Dyball, D. R. Ferguson, and W. R. Ward, *Experientia* **25**, 680 (1969).
443. J. Rudinger and I. Krejčí, *Experientia* **18**, 585 (1962).
444. J. Rudinger and I. Krejčí, *in* "Handbuch der experimentellen Pharmakologie" (B. Berde, ed.), p. 748. Springer, Berlin, 1968.
445. J. Rudinger, V. Pliška, I. Rychlík, and F. Šorm, *in* "Pharmacology of Hormonal Polypeptides and Proteins" (N. Back, L. Martini, and R. Paoletti, eds.), p. 66. Plenum Press, New York, 1968.
446. J. W. Ryan, J. Roblero, and J. M. Stewart, *Biochem. J.* **110**, 795 (1968).
447. I. Rychlík, *in* "Oxytocin, Vasopressin and Their Structural Analogues; Proc. 2nd Int. Pharmacol. Meeting, 1963" (J. Rudinger, ed.), Vol. 10, p. 153. Pergamon Press, Oxford, 1964.
448. S. Sakakibara and S. Hase, *Bull. Chem. Soc. Jap.* **41**, 2816 (1968).
449. M. P. Sambhi and J. D. Barrett, *Circ. Res.* **21**, 327 (1967).
450. E. Sandrin and R. A. Boissonnas, *Helv. Chim. Acta* **47**, 1294 (1964).
451. W. H. Sawyer, *Pharmacol. Rev.* **13**, 225 (1961).
452. W. H. Sawyer, R. A. Munsick, and H. B. van Dyke, *Nature (London)* **184**, 1464 (1959).
453. W. H. Sawyer, T. C. Wuu, J. W. M. Baxter, and M. Manning, *Endocrinology* **85**, 385 (1969).
454. M. Schachter, ed., "Polypeptides which Affect Smooth Muscle and Blood Vessels." Pergamon Press, Oxford, 1960.
455. A. V. Schally, M. Saffran, and B. Zimmermann, *Biochem. J.* **70**, 97 (1958).
456. C. Schattenkerk and E. Havinga, *Rec. Trav. Chim. Pays-Bas* **84**, 653 (1965).
457. E. Schnabel and C. H. Li, *J. Amer. Chem. Soc.* **82**, 4576 (1960).
458. E. Schnabel and C. H. Li, *J. Biol. Chem.* **235**, 2010 (1960).
459. E. Schnabel and J. Meienhofer, unpublished results; see Schröder and Lübke (*477*, p. 122).
460. E. Schnabel and A. Oberdorf, *in* "Protein and Polypeptide Hormones" (M. Margoulies, ed.), p. 224. Excerpta Med. Found., Amsterdam, 1968.
461. C. H. Schneider and V. du Vigneaud, *J. Amer. Chem. Soc.* **84**, 3005 (1962).
462. E. Schröder, *Justus Liebigs Ann. Chem.* **673**, 186 (1964).
463. E. Schröder, *Justus Liebigs Ann. Chem.* **673**, 220 (1964).
464. E. Schröder, *Justus Liebigs Ann. Chem.* **679**, 207 (1964).
465. E. Schröder, *Justus Liebigs Ann. Chem.* **680**, 132 (1964).
466. E. Schröder, *Justus Liebigs Ann. Chem.* **680**, 142 (1964).
467. E. Schröder, *Experientia* **20**, 39 (1964).
468. E. Schröder, *Experientia* **21**, 271 (1965).

469. E. Schröder, in "Peptides 1963; Proc. 6th Eur. Peptide Symp." (L. Zervas, ed.), p. 253. Pergamon Press, Oxford, 1966.

470. E. Schröder, Justus Liebigs Ann. Chem. 691, 232 (1966).

471. E. Schröder, Justus Liebigs Ann. Chem. 692, 241 (1966).

472. E. Schröder, unpublished data; see Schröder and Lübke (477, p. 146).

473. E. Schröder and R. Hempel, Experientia 20, 529 (1964).

474. E. Schröder and R. Hempel, Justus Liebigs Ann. Chem. 684, 243 (1965).

475. E. Schröder and M. Lehmann, Experientia 25, 1126 (1969).

476. E. Schröder and K. Lübke, Experientia 20, 19 (1964).

477. E. Schröder and K. Lübke, "The Peptides," Vol. 2. Academic Press, New York, 1966.

478. E. Schröder and K. Lübke, Fortschr. Chem. Org. Naturst. 26, 48 (1968).

479. E. Schröder, K. Lübke, and R. Hempel, Experientia 21, 70 (1965).

480. E. Schröder, H.-S. Petras, and E. Klieger, Justus Liebigs Ann. Chem. 679, 221 (1964).

481. W. Schuler, B. Schär, and P. Desaulles, Schweiz. Med. Wochenschr. 93, 1027 (1963).

482. H. Schulz and V. du Vigneaud, J. Med. Chem. 9, 647 (1966).

483. H. Schulz and V. du Vigneaud, J. Amer. Chem. Soc. 88, 5015 (1966).

484. H. Schulz and V. du Vigneaud, J. Med. Chem. 10, 1037 (1967).

485. I. L. Schwartz, H. Rasmussen, and J. Rudinger, Proc. Nat. Acad. Sci. U.S. 52, 1044 (1964).

486. R. Schwyzer, Chimia 12, 53 (1958).

487. R. Schwyzer, Helv. Chim. Acta 44, 667 (1961).

488. R. Schwyzer, Proc. 1st Int. Pharmacol. Meet., 1961 Vol. 7, p. 203 (1963).

489. R. Schwyzer, Pure Appl. Chem. 6, 265 (1963).

490. R. Schwyzer, Ergeb. Physiol., Biol. Chem. Exp. Pharmakol. 53, 1 (1963).

491. R. Schwyzer, Annu. Rev. Biochem. 33, 259 (1964).

492. R. Schwyzer, in "Protein and Polypeptide Hormones" (M. Margoulies, ed.), p. 201. Excerpta Med. Found., Amsterdam, 1968.

493. R. Schwyzer, J. Mond. Pharm. 3, 254 (1968).

494. R. Schwyzer, A. Costopanagiotis, and P. Sieber, Chimia 16, 295 (1962); Helv. Chim. Acta 46, 870 (1963).

495. R. Schwyzer and H. Kappeler, Helv. Chim. Acta 46, 1550 (1963).

496. R. Schwyzer and C. H. Li, Nature (London) 182, 1669 (1958).

497. R. Schwyzer and U. Ludescher, Biochemistry 7, 2514 (1968).

498. R. Schwyzer and U. Ludescher, Biochemistry 7, 2519 (1968).

499. R. Schwyzer, W. Rittel, and A. Costopanagiotis, Helv. Chim. Acta 45, 2473 (1962).

500. R. Schwyzer, W. Rittel, H. Kappeler, and B. Iselin, Angew. Chem. 72, 915 (1960).

501. R. Schwyzer, W. Rittel, P. Sieber, H. Kappeler, and H. Zuber, Helv. Chim. Acta 43, 1130 (1960).

502. R. Schwyzer and P. Schiller, Helv. Chim. Acta 54, 897 (1971).

503. R. Schwyzer and P. Sieber, Helv. Chim. Acta 49, 134 (1966); Nature (London) 199, 172 (1963).

504. R. Schwyzer and H. Turrian, Vitam. Horm. (New York) 18, 327 (1960).

505. E. Scoffone, F. Marchiori, L. Moroder, R. Rocchi, and A. Scatturin, in "Peptides 1968; Proc. 9th Eur. Peptide Symp." (E. Bricas, ed.), p. 325. North-Holland Publ., Amsterdam, 1968.

506. E. Sedláková, B. Lichardus, and J. H. Cort, Science 164, 580 (1969).

507. E. P. Semkin, A. P. Smirnova, and L. A. Shchukina, Zh. Obshch. Khim. 38, 2358 (1968).

508. J. H. Seu, R. R. Smeby, and F. M. Bumpus, J. Amer. Chem. Soc. 84, 3883 (1962).

509. J. H. Seu, R. R. Smeby, and F. M. Bumpus, J. Amer. Chem. Soc. 84, 4948 (1962).

510. S. Shankman, V. Gold, and S. Higa, Tex. Rep. Biol. Med. 19, 358 (1961).

511. S. Shankman, S. Higa, H. A. Florsheim, Y. Schvo, and V. Gold, *Arch. Biochem. Biophys.* **86**, 204 (1960).
512. S. Shankman, S. Higa, S. Makineni, and W. Noll, *J. Med. Chem.* **6**, 746 (1963).
513. L. A. Shchukina, G. A. Ravdel', and M. P. Filatova, *Khim. Prir. Soedin.* **2**, 265 (1966).
514. L. A. Shchukina, G. A. Ravdel, M. P. Filatova, and A. L. Zhuze, *in* "Proc. 7th Eur. Peptide Symp., 1964" (V. Bruckner and K. Medzihradszky, eds.); *Acta Chim. Acad. Sci. Hung.* **44**, Spec. Issue p. 205 (1965).
515. M. M. Shemyakin, Yu. A. Ovchinnikov, and V. T. Ivanov, *Angew. Chem.* **81**, 523 (1969).
516. M. M. Shemyakin, Yu. A. Ovchinnikov, V. T. Ivanov, and I. D. Ryabova, *Experientia* **23**, 326 (1967).
517. M. M. Shemyakin, L. A. Shchukina, E. I. Vinogradova, G. A. Ravdel, and Yu. A. Ovchinnikov, *Experientia* **22**, 535 (1966).
518. R. G. Shepherd, S. D. Willson, K. S. Howard, P. H. Bell, D. S. Davies, S. B. Davis, E. A. Eigner, and N. E. Shakespeare, *J. Amer. Chem. Soc.* **78**, 5067 (1956).
519. E. N. Shkodinskaya, O. S. Vasina, A. Ya. Berlin, Z. P. Sof'ina, and L. F. Larionov, *Zh. Obshch. Khim.* **32**, 324 (1962).
520. P. Sieber, M. Brugger, B. Kamber, B. Riniker, and W. Rittel, *Helv. Chim. Acta* **51**, 2057 (1968).
521. W. Siedel, K. Sturm, and R. Geiger, *Chem. Ber.* **96**, 1436 (1963).
522. R. E. Sievers, E. Bayer, and P. Hunziker, *Nature (London)* **223**, 180 (1969).
523. K. M. Sivanandaiah, R. R. Smeby, and F. M. Bumpus, *Biochemistry* **5**, 1224 (1966).
524. I. Sjöholm, *FEBS Lett.* **4**, 135 (1969).
525. L. T. Skeggs and J. R. Kahn, *Circulation* **17**, 658 (1958).
526. L. T. Skeggs, J. R. Kahn, K. E. Lentz, and N. P. Shumway, *J. Exp. Med.* **106**, 439 (1957).
527. L. T. Skeggs, J. R. Kahn, and N. P. Shumway, *J. Exp. Med.* **103**, 295 (1956).
528. L. T. Skeggs, K. E. Lentz, A. B. Gould, H. Hochstrasser, and J. R. Kahn, *Fed. Proc., Fed. Amer. Soc. Exp. Biol.* **26**, 42 (1967).
529. L. T. Skeggs, K. E. Lentz, H. Hochstrasser, and J. R. Kahn, *Can. Med. Ass. J.* **90**, 185 (1964).
530. L. T. Skeggs, K. E. Lentz, J. R. Kahn, and N. P. Shumway, *J. Exp. Med.* **108**, 283 (1958).
531. R. R. Smeby, K. Arakawa, F. M. Bumpus, and M. M. Marsh, *Biochim. Biophys. Acta* **58**, 550 (1962).
532. L. F. Smith, *Amer. J. Med.* **40**, 662 (1966).
533. D. G. Smyth, *J. Biol. Chem.* **242**, 1579 (1967).
534. D. G. Smyth, *J. Biol. Chem.* **242**, 1592 (1967).
535. P. H. A. Sneath, *J. Theor. Biol.* **12**, 157 (1966).
536. P. Stanley and P. Biron, *Experientia* **25**, 46 (1969).
537. J. M. Stewart, *Fed. Proc. Fed. Amer. Soc. Exp. Biol.* **27**, 63 (1968).
538. J. M. Stewart, *Fed. Proc., Fed. Amer. Soc. Exp. Biol.* **27**, 534 (1968).
539. J. M. Stewart and D. W. Woolley, *Biochemistry* **3**, 700 (1964).
540. J. M. Stewart and D. W. Woolley, *in* "Hypotensive Peptides" (E. G. Erdös, N. Back, and F. Sicuteri, eds.), p. 23. Springer, Berlin, 1966.
541. J. M. Stewart and D. W. Woolley, *Nature (London)* **206**, 619 (1965).
542. J. M. Stewart and D. W. Woolley, *Nature (London)* **207**, 1160 (1965).
543. R. O. Studer and W. D. Cash, *J. Biol. Chem.* **238**, 2 (1963).
544. E. Stürmer, *Schweiz. Med. Wochenschr.* **96**, 1667 (1966).
545. E. Stürmer and B. Berde, *J. Pharmacol. Exp. Ther.* **139**, 38 (1963).
545a. E. Stürmer and A. Fanchamps, *Deut. Med. Wochenschr.* **90**, 1012 (1965).
546. E. Stürmer, R. L. Huguenin, R. A. Boissonnas, and B. Berde, *Experientia* **21**, 583 (1965).

547. E. Stürmer, E. Sandrin, and R. A. Boissonnas, *Experientia* **20**, 303 (1964).
548. L. Szporny, G. T. Hajos, Sz. Szeberényi, and G. Fekete, *in* "Pharmacology of Hormonal Polypeptides and Proteins" (N. Back, L. Martini, and R. Paoletti, eds.), p. 195. Plenum Press, New York, 1968.
549. L. Szporny, G. T. Hajos, Sz. Szeberényi, and G. Fekete, *in* "Protein and Polypeptide Hormones" (M. Margoulies, ed.), p. 492. Excerpta Med. Found., Amsterdam, 1968.
550. H. Takashima, W. Fraefel, and V. du Vigneaud, *J. Amer. Chem. Soc.* **91**, 6182 (1969).
551. A. Tanaka, B. T. Pickering, and C. H. Li, *Arch. Biochem. Biophys.* **99**, 294 (1962).
552. C. M. Tashjian, L. Levine, and P. L. Munson, *Endocrinology* **76**, 979 (1965).
553. G. I. Tesser and W. Rittel, *Rec. Trav. Chim. Pays-Bas* **88**, 553 (1969).
554. G. I. Tesser and R. Schwyzer, *Helv. Chim. Acta* **49**, 1013 (1966).
555. A. Toth, F. M. Bumpus, and P. A. Khairallah, personal communication; see Khairallah *et al.* (*635*).
556. H. J. Tracy and R. A. Gregory, *Nature* (*London*) **204**, 935 (1964).
557. I. Trautschold, H. Fritz, and E. Werle, *in* "Hypotensive Peptides" (E. G. Erdös, N. Buck, and F. Sicuteri, eds.), p. 221. Springer, Berlin, 1966.
558. H. Tuppy, *in* "Oxytocin, Vasopressin and Their Analogues; Proc. 2nd Int. Pharmacol. Meeting, 1963" (J. Rudinger, ed.), Vol. 10, p. 67. Pergamon Press, Oxford, 1964.
559. H. Tuppy and H. Nesvadba, *Monatsh. Chem.* **88**, 977 (1957).
560. R. A. Turner, J. G. Pierce, and V. du Vigneaud, *J. Biol. Chem.* **193**, 359 (1951).
561. J. R. Vane, *Brit. J. Pharmacol.* **35**, 209 (1969).
562. I. Vávra, A. Machová, V. Holeček, J. H. Cort, M. Zaoral, and F. Šorm, *Lancet* **1**, 948 (1968).
563. V. du Vigneaud, *Proc. Robert A. Welch Found. Conf. Chem. Res.* **8**, 133 (1964).
564. V. du Vigneaud, *Bull. N.Y. Acad. Med.* [2] **41**, 802 (1965).
565. V. du Vigneaud, G. S. Denning, S. Drabarek, and W. Y. Chan, *J. Biol. Chem.* **238**, PC1560 (1963); **239**, 477 (1964).
566. V. du Vigneaud, G. Flouret, and R. Walter, *J. Biol. Chem.* **241**, 2093 (1966).
567. V. du Vigneaud, P. S. Fitt, M. Bodanszky, and M. O'Connell, *Proc. Soc. Exp. Biol. Med.* **104**, 653 (1960).
568. V. du Vigneaud, H. C. Lawler, and E. A. Popenoe, *J. Amer. Chem. Soc.* **75**, 4880 (1953).
569. V. du Vigneaud, C. Ressler, J. M. Swan, C. W. Roberts, P. G. Katsoyannis, and S. Gordon, *J. Amer. Chem. Soc.* **75**, 4879 (1953).
570. V. du Vigneaud, C. Ressler, J. M. Swan, C. W. Roberts, and P. G. Katsoyannis, *J. Amer. Chem. Soc.* **76**, 3115 (1954).
571. V. du Vigneaud, G. Winestock, V. V. S. Murti, D. B. Hope, and R. D. Kimbrough, *J. Biol. Chem.* **235**, PC64 (1960).
572. A. S. Villanueva, J. H. Ashcroft, and J. P. Felber, *Acta Endocrinol.* (*Copenhagen*) **51**, 88 (1966).
573. J. F. G. Vliegenthart and D. H. G. Versteeg, *J. Endocrinol.* **38**, 3 (1967).
574. G. Vogel and J. Hergott, *Arzneim.-Forsch.* **13**, 415 (1963).
575. H. G. Vogel, *Arzneim.-Forsch.* **19**, 20 (1969).
576. K. Vogler and P. Lanz, *in* "Hypotensive Peptides" (E. G. Erdös, N. Back, and F. Sicuteri, eds.), p. 14. Springer, Berlin, 1966.
577. K. Vogler, P. Lanz, W. Lergier, and W. Haefely, *Helv. Chim. Acta* **49**, 390 (1966).
578. K. Vogler, R. O. Studer, and W. Lergier, *Helv. Chim. Acta* **44**, 1495 (1961).
579. K. Vogler, R. O. Studer, W. Lergier, and P. Lanz, *Helv. Chim. Acta* **48**, 1407 (1965).
580. W. Vogt, *in* "Hypotensive Peptides" (E. G. Erdös, N. Back, and F. Sicuteri, eds.), p. 185. Springer, Berlin, 1966.
581. J. P. Waller and H. B. F. Dixon, *Biochem. J.* **75**, 320 (1960).

582. A. Walser and F. Koller, *Experientia* **19**, 320 (1963).

583. A. Walser and T. Müller, *in* "Protein and Polypeptide Hormones" (M. Margoulies, ed.), p. 487. Excerpta Med. Found., Amsterdam, 1968.

584. R. Walter and W. Y. Chan, *J. Amer. Chem. Soc.* **89**, 3892 (1967).

585. R. Walter, B. M. Dubois, P. Eggena, and I. L. Schwartz, *Experientia* **25**, 33 (1969).

586. R. Walter, B. M. Dubois, and I. L. Schwartz, *Endocrinology* **83**, 979 (1968).

587. R. Walter, J. Rudinger, and I. L. Schwartz, *Amer. J. Med.* **42**, 653 (1967).

588. R. Walter and I. L. Schwartz, *J. Biol. Chem.* **241**, 5500 (1966),

589. R. Walter and R. Schwartz, *in* "Pharmacology of Hormonal Polypeptides and Proteins" (N. Buck, L. Martini, and R. Paoletti, eds.), p. 101. Plenum Press, New York, 1968.

590. R. Walter and V. du Vigneaud, *Biochemistry* **5**, 3720 (1966).

591. R. Walter and V. du Vigneaud, *J. Amer. Chem. Soc.* **87**, 4192 (1965).

592. R. Walter and V. du Vigneaud, *J. Amer. Chem. Soc.* **88**, 1331 (1966).

593. U. Weber, K.-H. Herzog, H. Grossmann, S. Hörnle, and G. Weitzel, *Hoppe-Seyler's Z. Physiol. Chem.* **350**, 1425 (1969).

594. U. Weber, S. Hörnle, G. Griesser, K.-H. Herzog, and G. Weitzel, *Hoppe-Seyler's Z. Physiol. Chem.* **348**, 1715 (1967).

595. U. Weber, S. Hörnle, P. Köhler, G. Nagelschneider, K. Eisele, and G. Weitzel, *Hoppe-Seyler's Z. Physiol. Chem.* **349**, 512 (1968).

596. U. Weber, F. Schneider, P. Köhler, and G. Weitzel, *Hoppe-Seyler's Z. Physiol. Chem.* **348**, 947 (1967).

597. U. Weber and G. Weitzel, *Hoppe-Seyler's Z. Physiol. Chem.* **349**, 1431 (1968).

598. G. Weitzel, K. Eisele, H. Zollner, and U. Weber, *Hoppe-Seyler's Z. Physiol. Chem.* **350**, 1480 (1969).

599. G. Weitzel, W. Oertel, K. Rager, and W. Kemmler, *Hoppe-Seyler's Z. Physiol. Chem.* **350**, 57 (1969).

600. G. Weitzel, U. Weber, S. Hörnle, and F. Schneider, *in* "Peptides 1968; Proc. 9th Eur. Peptide Symp." (E. Bricas, ed.), p. 222. North-Holland Publ., Amsterdam, 1968.

601. E. Werle, *J. Mond. Pharm.* **3**, 291 (1968).

602. W. F. White, *J. Amer. Chem. Soc.* **77**, 4691 (1955).

602a. E. Wünsch, H.-G. Heidrich, and W. Grassman, *Chem. Ber.* **97**, 1818 (1964).

603. E. Wünsch, G. Wendelberger, E. Jaeger, and R. Scharf, *in* "Peptides 1968; Proc. 9th Eur. Peptide Symp." (E. Bricas, ed.), p. 229. North-Holland Publ., Amsterdam, 1968.

604. H. Yajima, *Gunma Symp. Endocrinol.* **5**, 73 (1968).

605. H. Yajima and K. Kawasaki, *Chem. Pharm. Bull.* **16**, 1387 (1968).

606. H. Yajima, K. Kawasaki, Y. Okada, H. Minami, K. Kubo, and I. Yamashita, *Chem. Pharm. Bull.* **16**, 919 (1968).

607. H. Yajima and K. Kubo, *Biochim. Biophys. Acta* **97**, 596 (1965); *Chem. Pharm. Bull.* **13**, 759 (1965).

608. H. Yajima and K. Kubo, *J. Amer. Chem. Soc.* **87**, 2039 (1965).

609. H. Yajima, K. Kubo, and Y. Kinomura, *Chem. Pharm. Bull.* **15**, 504 (1967).

610. H. Yajima, K. Kubo, Y. Kinomura, and S. Lande, *Biochim. Biophys. Acta* **127**, 545 (1966).

611. H. Yajima, K. Kubo, and Y. Okada, *Chem. Pharm. Bull.* **13**, 1326 (1965).

612. H. Yajima, K. Kubo, T. Oshima, K. Hano, and M. Koida, *Chem. Pharm. Bull.* **14**, 775 (1966).

613. H. Yajima, Y. Okada, Y. Kinomura, and E. Seto, *Chem. Pharm. Bull.* **15**, 270 (1967).

614. H. Yajima, Y. Okada, T. Oshima, and S. Lande, *Chem. Pharm. Bull.* **14**, 707 (1966).

615. D. Yamashiro, H. L. Aanning, L. A. Branda, W. D. Cash, V. V. S. Murti, and V. du Vigneaud, *J. Amer. Chem. Soc.* **90**, 4141 (1968).

616. N. Yanaihara, M. Sekiya, K. Takagi, H. Kato, M. Ichimura, and T. Nagao, *Chem. Pharm. Bull.* **15**, 110 (1966).
617. H. Y. T. Yang and E. G. Erdös, *Nature (London)* **215**, 1402 (1967).
618. H. Y. T. Yang, E. G. Erdös, and T. S. Chiang, *Nature (London)* **218**, 1224 (1968).
619. M. Zaoral, E. Kasafírek, J. Rudinger, and F. Šorm, *Collect. Czech. Chem. Commun.* **30**, 1869 (1965).
620. M. Zaoral, J. Kolc, F. Korenczki, V. P. Černěckij, and F. Šorm, *Collect. Czech. Chem. Commun.* **32**, 843 (1967).
621. M. Zaoral, J. Kolc, and F. Šorm, *Collect. Czech. Chem. Commun.* **31**, 382 (1966).
622. M. Zaoral, J. Kolc, and F. Šorm, *Collect. Czech. Chem. Commun.* **32**, 1242 (1967).
623. M. Zaoral, J. Kolc, and F. Šorm, *Collect. Czech. Chem. Commun.* **32**, 1250 (1967).
624. M. Zaoral, V. Pliška, K. Řežábek, and F. Šorm, *Collect. Czech. Chem. Commun.* **28**, 747 (1963).
625. M. Zaoral and F. Šorm, *Collect. Czech. Chem. Commun.* **30**, 611 (1965).
626. M. Zaoral and F. Šorm, *Collect. Czech. Chem. Commun.* **30**, 2812 (1965).
627. M. Zaoral and F. Šorm, *Collect. Czech. Chem. Commun.* **31**, 310 (1966).
628. M. Zaoral and F. Šorm, *Collect. Czech. Chem. Commun.* **31**, 90 (1966).
629. L. Zervas, ed., "Peptides; Proc. 6th Eur. Peptide Symp., 1963". Pergamon Press, Oxford, 1966.
630. A. L. Zhuze, K. Jošt, E. Kasafírek, and J. Rudinger, *Collect. Czech. Chem. Commun.* **29**, 2648 (1964).
631. N. C. Chaturvedi, W. K. Park, R. R. Smeby, and F. M. Bumpus, *J. Med. Chem.* **13**, 177 (1970).
632. P. Cuatrecasas, *Proc. Nat. Acad. Sci. U.S.* **63**, 450 (1969).
633. K. Hofmann and C. Y. Bowers, *J. Med. Chem.* **13**, 1099 (1970).
634. E. C. Jorgensen, S. R. Rapaka, and T. C. Lee, *J. Med. Chem.* (1971) (in press).
635. P. M. Khairallah, A. Toth, and F. M. Bumpus, *J. Med. Chem.* **13**, 181 (1970).
636. I. Krejčí, V. Pliška, and J. Rudinger, *Brit. J. Pharmacol.* **39**, 217P (1970).
637. H. D. Law, *Progr. Medicin. Chem.* **4**, 125 (1965).
638. M. Manning, E. Coy, and W. H. Sawyer, *Biochemistry* **9**, 3925 (1970).
639. G. R. Marshall and E. Flanigan, *Proc. 2nd Amer. Peptide Symp., 1970* (in press).
640. G. R. Marshall, W. Vine, and P. Needleman, *Proc. Nat. Acad. Sci. U.S.* **67**, 1624 (1970).
641. M. A. Ondetti, J. Pluščec, J. T. Sheehan, and N. Williams, *J. Amer. Chem. Soc.* **92**, 195 (1970).
642. W. K. Park, J. Asselin, and L. Berlinguet, *Proc. 2nd Amer. Peptide Symp., 1970* (in press).
643. B. T. Pickering, *in* "Int. Encyclopedia Pharmacol. Therapeut." (H. Heller and B. T. Pickering, eds.), Section 41, Vol. 1, p. 81. Pergamon Press, Oxford, 1970.
644. P. W. Schiller and R. Schwyzer, *Chimia (Switzerland)* **24**, 458 (1970); *Helv. Chim. Acta* (1971) (in press).
645. D. W. Urry, M. Ohnishi, and R. Walter, *Proc. Nat. Acad. Sci. U.S.* **66**, 111 (1970).
646. R. Walter, W. Gordon, I. L. Schwartz, F. Quadrifoglio, and D. W. Urry, *in* "Peptides 1968; Proc. 9th Eur. Peptide Symp." (E. Bricas, ed.), p. 51, North-Holland Publ., Amsterdam, 1968.
647. R. Walter, L. F. Johnson, and D. W. Urry, unpublished results; see Urry *et al.* (*645*).
647. G. Weitzel, U. Weber, K. Eisele, H. Zollner, and J. Martin, *Hoppe-Seyler's Z. Physiol. Chem.* **351**, 263 (1970).
649. M. Zaoral, J. Kolc, and F. Šorm, *Collect. Czech. Chem. Commun.* **35**, 1716 (1970).

Chapter 10   Recent Advances in the Design of Diuretics

George deStevens

I. Introduction

The principal types of diuretics are classified as follows:

1. Osmotic and acidotic.
2. Nitrogen heterocycles (mono- and bicyclic).
3. Organomercurials.
4. Sulfonamides and disulfonamides.
5. Thiazides and hydrothiazides.
6. Aldosterone antagonists and inhibitors of aldosterone secretion.
7. α,β-Unsaturated ketone derivatives.

All of these have been previously considered in depth (*1*) and it shall be the purpose of this chapter to discuss only those groups of compounds which have been developed since 1963. In addition, some speculations will be made with regard to essential groups associated with structure–activity relationships. The areas of osmotic and acidotic diuretics and organomercurials and aldosterone antagonists will not be considered since nothing new has been developed along these lines. The same applies for thiazides and hydrothiazides although these drugs represent the major advance in diuretic therapy to date. The structure–activity relationships of the thiazides and hydrothiazides have been documented in several chapters (*2*), reviews (*3*) and a monograph (*1*).

II. Mono- and Bicyclic Nitrogen Heterocycles

A. PTERIDINES

The group of compounds related to triamterene, although previously

Triamterene

described, offers an interesting prototype which has led to several active diuretics within its class and also some interesting deviations thereof. Within the pteridine group the nature of the substituents not only has a marked effect on the milligram potency of the compound but indeed affects qualitatively the water excretion and the electrolyte pattern. The latter action is worthy of note in this class since one of the characteristics of triamterene and congeners is the marginal effect on potassium excretion.

For example, Wiebelhaus and co-workers (*4*) have shown that in rats the 2-anilino derivative of triamterene is not diuretic but instead elicits a saluretic effect with potassium loss. This alleged minor change in structure alters almost diametrically the properties associated with triamterene (i.e., mild diuresis, good saluresis, and no kaluresis). Other examples of some major modifications of the triamterene molecule are shown in Table I. Although several hundred of these substances have been documented in the patent literature, the few examples cited herein serve to illustrate some key changes which have led to significant qualitative effects.

Within this group Wy-5256 deserves attention (*5*). After Wiebelhaus had

TABLE I

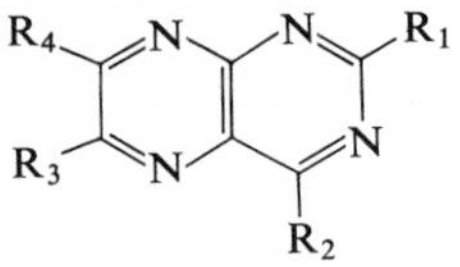

$$R_4 \text{—} N \text{—} N \text{—} R_1$$
$$R_3 \text{—} N \text{—} N$$
$$R_2$$

R_1	R_2	R_3	R_4	H_2O [a]	Na^+ [a]	K^+ [a]
NH_2	NH_2	C_6H_5	NH_2	+	++	−
NHC_6H_5	NH_2	C_6H_5	NH_2	0	++	+
NH_2	NH_2	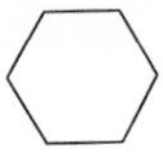 (cyclohexyl)	NH_2	+	++	−
NH_2	NH_2	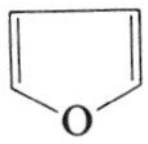 (furanyl)	NH_2	+	++	−
NH_2	NH_2	CH_3	CH_3	+	++	−
C_6H_5	NH_2	$CONH_2$	NH_2	+	++	0
C_6H_5 (Wy-5256)	NH_2	$CONH(CH_2)OCH_3$	$NH(CH_2)_2OCH_3$	++	++	−
C_6H_5	NH_2	$CONH(CH_2)_2$—N(morpholino)O 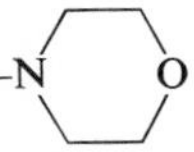	NH_2	++	++	+

[a] (+) Mild effect; (++) good effect; (−) retention of K^+.

noted that replacement of the 2-amino group by a phenyl group and the 6-amino group by the carboxamide group led to no marked change in diuretic properties of triamterene, Santilli (5) and co-workers at Wyeth elaborated extensively on this point. Following the synthesis of a large variety of triamterene-like compounds, it was established that Wy-5256 showed the most interesting effects. This substance in rats and dogs has exhibited the same

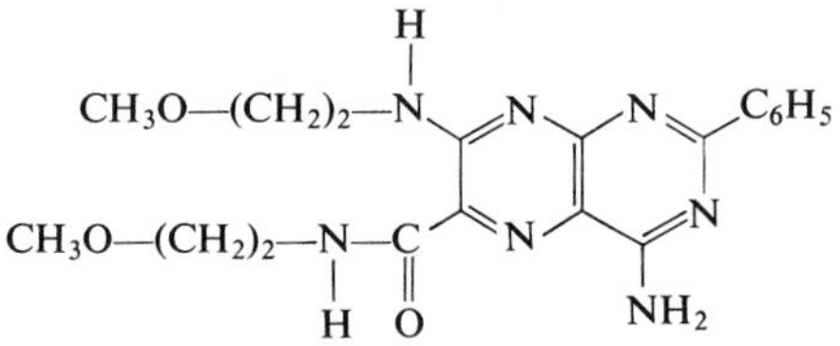

$$CH_3O\text{—}(CH_2)_2\text{—}\overset{H}{N}\text{—}N\text{—}N\text{—}C_6H_5$$
$$CH_3O\text{—}(CH_2)_2\text{—}N\text{—}\overset{}{\underset{H\ O}{C}}\text{—}N$$
$$NH_2$$

Wy-5256

order of diuretic effects as hydrochlorothiazide. However, in contrast to hydrochlorothiazide, it produces a marked increase in total renal blood flow similar to furosemide and ethacrynic acid. The clinical properties of Wy-5256 have not been reported to date.

B. PYRIMIDINES

The pteridine molecule can be considered to be made up of a pyrimidine moeity fused to a pyrazine ring system. Recently, Hofmann *et al.* (*6–8*) at Searle have reported on azidopyrimidines of which SC-16102 seems to show the most important diuretic effects. This substance which bears definite

SC-16102

structural similarities to triamterene and Wy-5256 elicits a pattern of electrolyte excretion qualitatively similar to hydrochlorothiazide in the intact rat. However, it is twice as potent as hydrochlorothiazide. It is also a nonspecific antagonist of vasopressin.

C. PYRAZINES

However, the most significant contribution to come out of the analysis of the pteridine molecule is the development by Cragoe and co-workers (*9–15*) of Merck, Sharp and Dohme Laboratories of the *N*-amidinopyrazinecarb- oxamides. Their work is documented in a series of seven papers describing the structure–activity relationships of over 300 compounds. A summary of the structure–activity relationship is shown and correlated in Scheme 1 and Table II.

The *N*-amidino-3-substituted pyrazinecarboxamides (**IV**) that were pre- pared in this study were assayed for their ability to inhibit the decrease in the urinary ratio of Na/K produced by deoxycorticosterone acetate (DOCA) using the adrenalectomized rat according to the method described previously. The compounds were routinely administered subcutaneously but similar results were obtained when intraperitoneal or oral routes were used. The activity scores are presented in Table II.

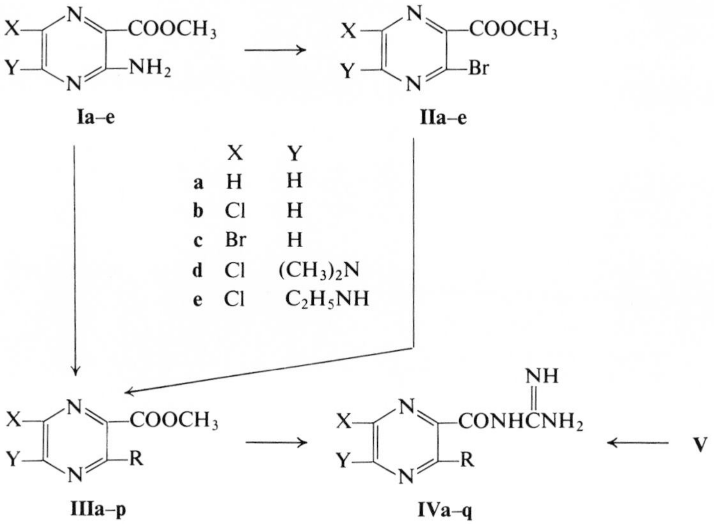

	X	Y	R
a	H	H	HS
b	Cl	H	$(CH_3)_2NCH_2CH_2NH$
c	Cl	H	HS
d	Cl	H	CH_3O
e	Cl	$(CH_3)_2N$	HO
f	Br	H	$C_5H_{10}N$
g	Br	H	$(CH_3)_2N$
h	Br	H	CH_3NH
i	Br	H	CH_3S
j	Br	H	HO
k	Cl	H	*p*-$ClC_6H_4CH_2NH$
l	Cl	H	*p*-$CH_3OC_6H_4CH_2NH$
m	Cl	C_2H_5NH	$CH_2{=}CHCH_2NH$
n	Cl	C_2H_5NH	$CH_3OCH_2CH_2NH$
o	Cl	$(CH_3)_2N$	C_2H_5NH
p	Cl	$(CH_3)_2N$	$HOCH_2CH_2NH$
q	Cl	H	HO (via **V**)

Scheme 1

Using this assay as the criterion of evaluation it can be seen that substitution of the 3-amino nitrogen of *N*-amidino-3-amino-6-bromopyrazinecarboxamide (**VI**) (score equal to +2; this was the initial compound showing activity) results in reduction of activity. Furthermore, the larger groups have a greater effect than the smaller ones; thus, **IVf** is less active than **IVg** and **h**. Similarly,

TABLE II

BIOLOGICAL RESULTS

IV	Rat DOCA-inhib[8] score [a]	Normal rat score [b]
a	±	±1
b	+1	0
c	±	0
d	0	±
e	0	+1
f	±	0
g	+1	0
h	+2	+1
i	±	±
j	0	+3
k	±	0
l	±	0
m	+4	+1
n	+1	+1
o	+3	+2
p	±	+2
q	±	+3

[a] The DOCA-inhibition score[1] is the dose producing reversal of the DOCA Na/K effect: $+4 = <10 \mu g/\text{rat}$, $+3 = 10–50$, $+2 = 51–100$, $+1 = 101–800$, $± = 800$, $0 =$ no activity at $800 \mu g$. Compounds which scored 0 were tested only at a maximum dose of $800 \mu g/\text{rat}$; thus, the possibility exists that activity would be observed at higher doses.

[b] Activity[10] based on increase of urinary electrolyte and volume over control values referred to standards: $+3 =$ activity of hydrochlorothiazide, $+2 =$ chlorothiazide, $0 =$ controls. Compounds with activities between chlorothiazide and controls are scored $+1$ or $±$.

a considerable reduction in activity is observed upon substitution of the 3-amino group of N-amidino-3-amino-6-chloropyrazinecarboxamide (V) (score equal to +3) with relatively large groups (IVb, k, and l). On the other hand, the preparation of N-amidino-3,5-diamino-6-chloropyrazinecarboxamide showed excellent diuretic effects with a score of +4 (see MK-870). Substitution of the 3-amino nitrogen of the more potent 5-amino series, i.e., N-amidino-3-amino-5-ethylamino- (or dimethylamino-) 6-chloropyrazinecarboxamide (VII and VIII) with groups such as allyl or ethyl (IVm and o) produced compounds with potencies equal to or greater than their parents. Substituents bearing hydroxy or alkoxy groups were detrimental to activity (IVp and n).

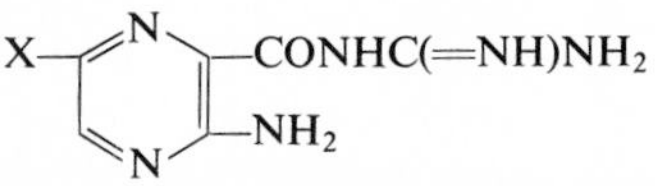

V, X = Cl
VI, X = Br

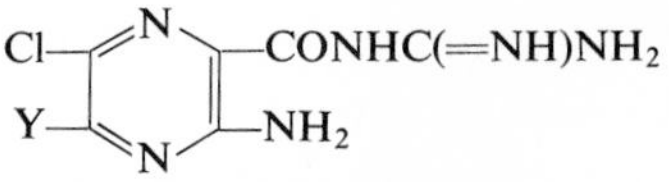

VII, Y = C$_2$H$_5$NH
VIII, Y = (CH$_3$)$_2$N

Replacement of the amino group of **V** by SH (**IVc**) or the amino group of **VI** by SCH$_3$ (**IVi**) produced a marked reduction in activity. Similar decreases in activity were seen when the amino group of **VI**, **V**, or **VIII** was replaced by OH (**IVj, q,** and **e**) or OCH$_3$ (**IVd**).

The compounds recorded in Table II also were tested in normal rats using the intraperitoneal route of administration. The assay and the scoring system have been described previously. The relative activities obtained in this test generally paralleled those observed in the DOCA-inhibition assay. The exceptions were the 3-hydroxy compounds (**IVe, j,** and **q**) which were markedly more active (comparable to their amino analogs **V, VI,** and **VII**) and **IVm** which was considerably less active in the normal rat assay than in the DOCA-inhibition assay.

Finally, Cragoe and co-workers (*14*) reported that substance **IX** is equally

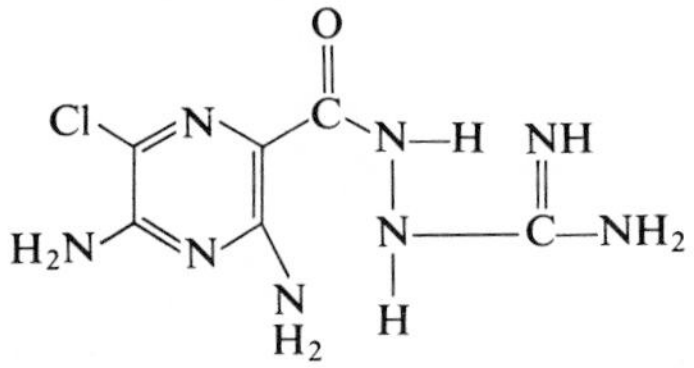

IX

as active as MK-870. However, the cyclization of the guanylhydrazine group of **IX** to form the triazole derivative (**X**) yielded a less potent compound.

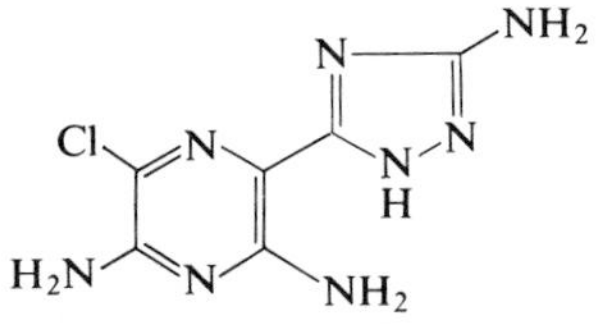

X

The extensive work of the Merck group in the development of the pyrazine diuretics illustrates essentially the necessity of the 3-amino group in pyrazine *N*-amidinocarboxamide for diuretic activity. Having established the basic qualitative character of the diuretic action (that is, diuresis with potassium retention), then further substitutions on the pyrazine ring, such as the 5-amino group, have led to quantitative improvements.

The compound selected for clinical trials was amiloride (MK-870). This substance in experimental animals showed qualitatively an action similar to triamterene. The drug moderately increases sodium elimination, accompanied by bicarbonate and to a lesser extent chloride, and decreases potassium excretion; water diuresis is not pronounced. Amiloride is excreted unchanged by rat, dog, and man. It increases the potential difference and the short circuit current of the isolated ventral skin of the frog and reverses the effects of vasopressin in this preparation (*16*). In this and other pharmacological respects, it resembles triamterene.

MK-870 (Amiloride)

The electrolyte excretion pattern has been essentially confirmed in clinical situations. The natriuretic and antikaliuretic effects of a single oral dose of 20 mg persist for approximately 20 hr (*17*). Amiloride is especially useful in combination with other diuretics in patients with refractory edema or cirrhosis with ascites, and in hypokalemic conditions resulting from the administration of these drugs. Although apparently not itself possessing the hyperglycemic and hyperuricemic characteristics of the thiazides, amiloride does not prevent increases in fasting blood sugar and uric acid concentration induced by hydro-chlorothiazide (*18*). Marked increases in aldosterone secretion with lesser rises in plasma renin have been observed following amiloride administration, presumably the result of potassium retention and renin activation consequent to natriuresis (*19*).

III. Sulfonamides and Disulfonamides

A. 5-Sulfamoylanthranilic Acids

Undoubtedly one of the most clinically successful drugs used within the past three years has been furosemide. Ample evidence has accrued demonstrating that furosemide is several times more active than chlorothiazide and hydrochlorothiazide, following both oral and parenteral administration in both animals and in man, in causing maximum saluretic and diuretic effects. Moreover, the effect is dose-dependent with the plateau or ceiling effects

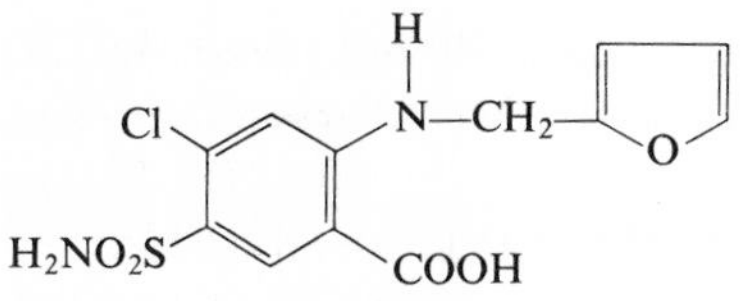

Furosemide

being reached at much higher doses than the thiazides. Due to the tremendous sodium excretion, the potassium ratio appears to be quite acceptable. However, in absolute terms furosemide shows marked potassium excretion. The site of action of this drug is in the proximal and distal tubules as well as in the ascending loop of Henle.

Interestingly enough the structure–activity relationship is rather specific. For example, substitution of the 2-furyl group with thenyl or benzyl leads only to a small diminution in diuretic activity in experimental animals (20). However, substitution of the furyl group with other heterocyclic systems, e.g., pyridyl, oxazolyl, isoxazolyl, thiazolyl, and tetrahydrofuryl, has led to relatively inactive substances (21). Saturation of the furane moiety has also brought about sharp reduction in diuretic activity. Finally, the 4-trifluoromethyl derivative (XI) which was prepared in the CIBA Laboratories according to the method in Scheme 2 was found to be less active than furosemide in experimental animals (22). This result was most surprising since, in general, in the

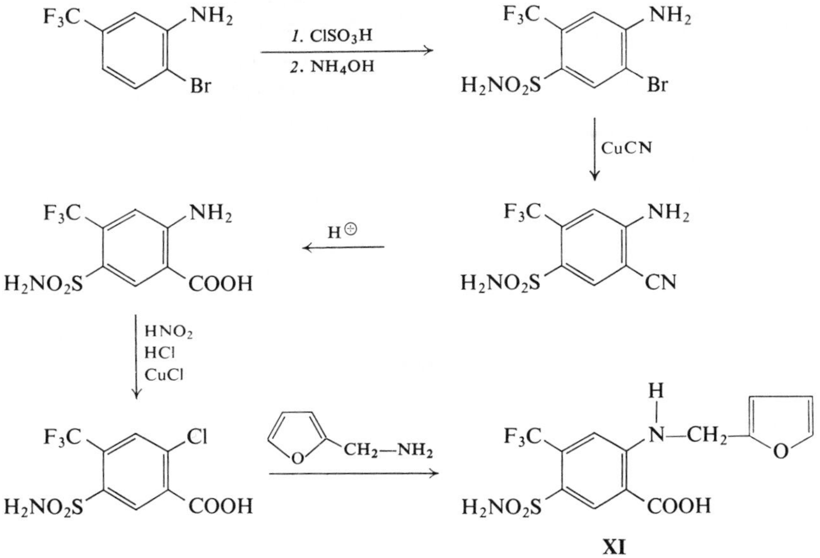

Scheme 2

thiazide series the diuretic and saluretic activities of the 6-chloro- and 6-trifluoromethyl derivatives paralleled one another. The same general relationship applied for the disulfonamide diuretics (*1*).

Recently, Felix and co-workers (*23*) reported their work on the synthesis and diuretic properties of a variety of *N*-alkylaminocarbonyl and *N*-pyrrolylcarbonylanthranilic derivatives. The following two substances were found to have diuretic properties comparable to hydrochlorothiazide.

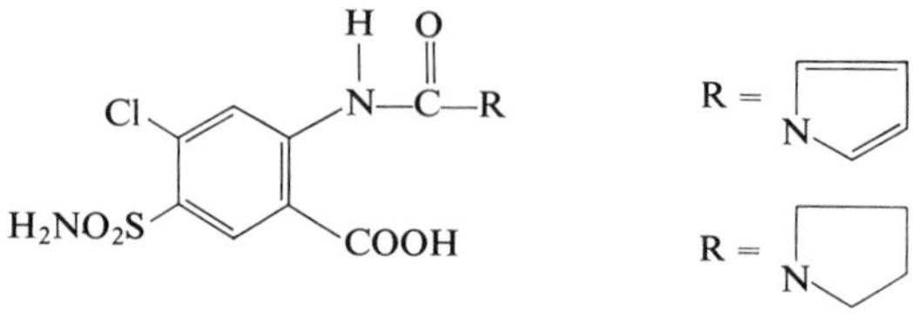

Also note is made of the following substance (**XIV**) which was reported to have a strong action on sodium chloride but little or no effect on potassium (*24*). No clinical reports have been forthcoming.

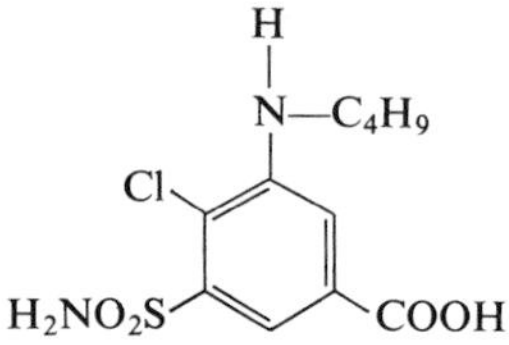

XIV

B. DISULFONAMIDES

Brief comment is herein made to mefruside which is reported to be a potent

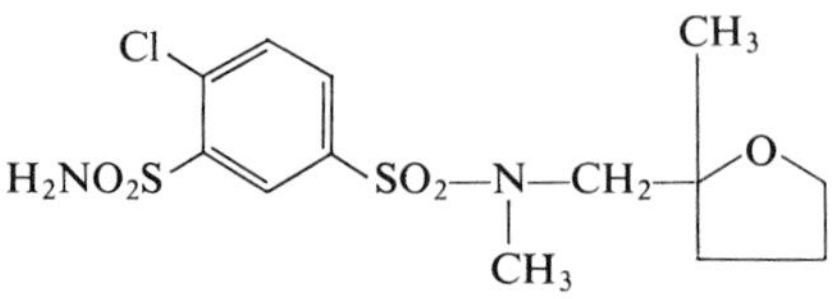

Mefruside

diuretic in animals and in man. The activity of this substance appears to approximate furosemide. It is metabolized to the lactone derivative which is also active. Interestingly, the (−) enantiomers of mefruside and its lactone are severalfold more potent than the (+) antipodes (*25, 26*).

Thus, some of the basic postulates established previously of structural requirements for benzene sulfonamides showing diuretic properties have changed. However, it is clear that the juxtaposition of a chlorine and sulfamyl group on an aromatic ring (benzene or hetero) still holds!

IV. α,β-Unsaturated Ketone Derivatives

ACYLPHENOXYACETIC ACIDS

Compounds of this type containing an α,β-unsaturated acyl group were designed to react with functionally important sulfhydryl groups in a manner similar to that believed to occur with mercurial diuretics (27). Biological data have now appeared indicating that such a reaction indeed does occur *in vivo* as well as *in vitro*. Ethacrynic acid is excreted, in part, in the dog as

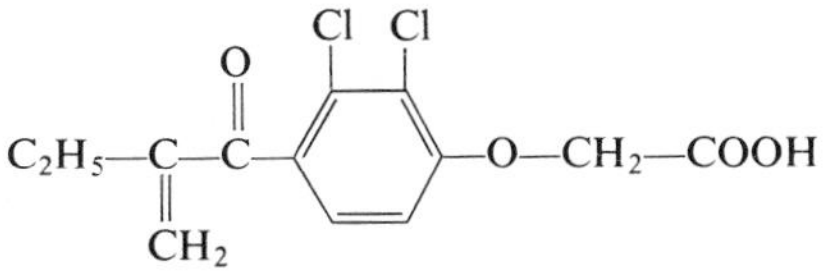

Ethacrynic acid

the cysteine adduct (28); mercurials are known to be excreted as the cysteine conjugates (29). The ethacrynic acid–cysteine adduct was shown to be an active diuretic in man (30). In the dog, ethacrynic acid caused a decrease in protein-bound sulfhydryl groups in kidney cells as do the mercurials. It had no such effect in the rat, a species in which it is not diuretic (31, 32). The uptake of ^{203}Hg-chlormerodrin by slices of renal cortex of the dog and the rat was reduced by ethacrynic acid (33).

Using 13 compounds of this class ranging from highly active to inactive in the dog diuretic assay, little correlation was found between diuretic activity and reactivity toward sulfhydryl (cysteine) in an *in vitro* model system. Better correlation was found with the ability to inhibit *in vitro* Na^+-K^+-(membrane)-ATPase from guinea pig kidney. However, the enzyme derived from the kidney of the dog and the rat was inhibited *in vitro* to approximately the same extent by ethacrynic acid (34). Also, ATPase from the kidneys of rats that had received ethacrynic acid showed substantial inhibition without resulting in diuresis (35).

Substitution on the aromatic nucleus or on the unsaturated acyl group markedly influences diuretic activity as measured in the dog. Compounds without nuclear substituents showed only weak activity. Substitution in the 2-position increased activity modestly while substitution in the 3-position or in the 2,3-positions, especially by chlorine or methyl, gave highly active compounds. Additional substitution in the 5 and/or 6 positions resulted in low activity. However, the 1,4-naphthalene analog was quite active. Substitution on the methylene of the unsaturated acyl group reduced activity; the mono-methyl compounds showed reduced activity and the dimethyl compounds had only low activity. Saturation of the double bond of the acyl group yielded compounds with marginal activity.

Detailed documentation of the pharmacology of ethacrynic acid and some of its congeners has appeared. In dogs, they caused a prompt and profound water diuresis and the excretion of nearly equivalent amounts of sodium and chloride when administered either parenterally or orally. There was some increase in potassium excretion, especially following intravenous administration. They have a steeper dose–response curve and a substantially greater maximal saluretic effect than the thiazides, and at least as great an effect as the organomercurials. Results with combinations indicate a mechanism of action for ethacrynic acid different from that of the thiazides, acetazolamide, and the mercurials. The ascending loop of Henle is a major site of action in the nephron (28, 35). Numerous reports on ethacrynic acid support its clinical efficacy.

Chemical modifications of ethacrynic acid have proved disappointing. First, Topliss and Konzelman (36) prepared two cyclic analogs of ethacrynic acid which showed only marginal diuretic activity.

XV   XVI

A benzofuran analog was also reported to be diuretic but further data has not been presented (37).

XVII

V. Miscellaneous Group

The compounds described within this section represent completely new types of structures which have shown diuretic effects in animals. Little, if anything, is known how these substances act and some have even been shown

to be inactive in humans. However, they are presented in this report to stimulate further work and thinking toward the development of new diuretics.

From the CIBA Laboratories Su-14074 prepared by Walker (*38, 39*) and
Su-15049 prepared by Robison (*40*) were found to cause good diuretic and

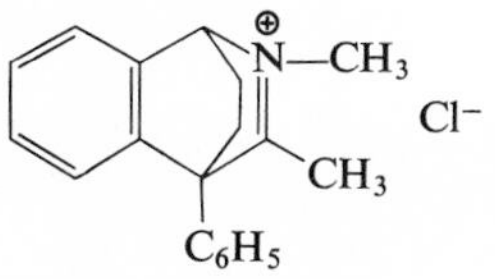

Su-14074

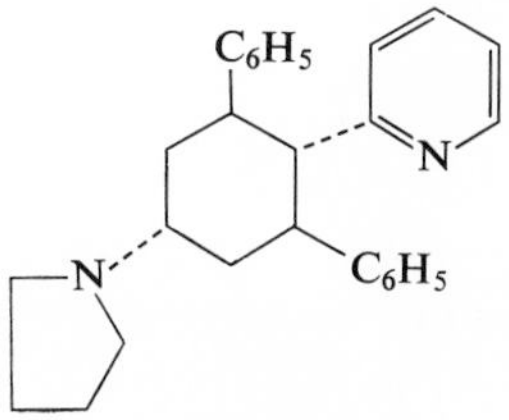

Su-15049

saluretic effects without any effect on potassium excretion when administered
orally to rats and dogs. When tested in humans, these compounds showed
only a mild diuretic effect, but the minimal effect on potassium could be
demonstrated.

Smith and Grostic (*41*) from Upjohn Laboratories reported on the orally
active diuretic agent derivative of anthranilic acid (**XVIII**).

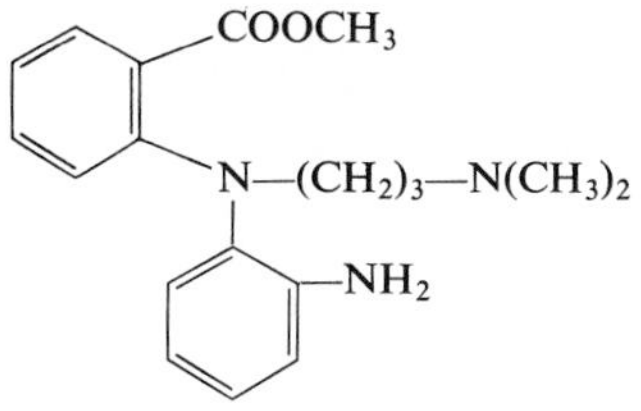

XVIII

Although a definite clinical report on this drug is as yet unavailable, it is
intriguing to note that the major metabolites present in human urine are as
follows:

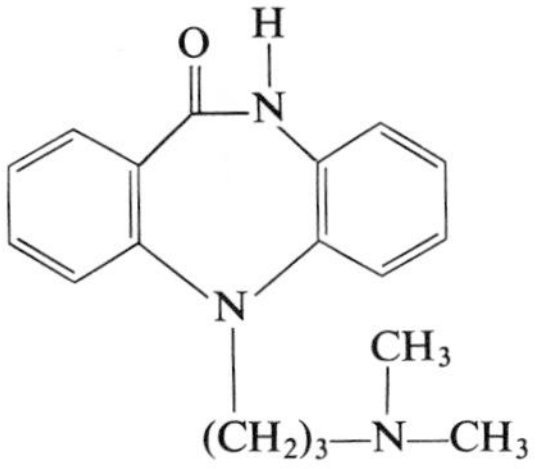

XIX

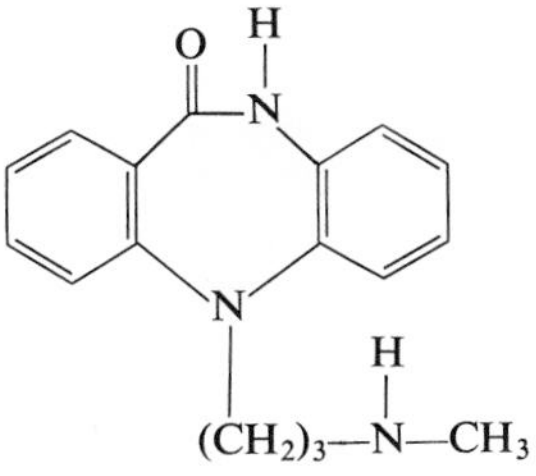

XX

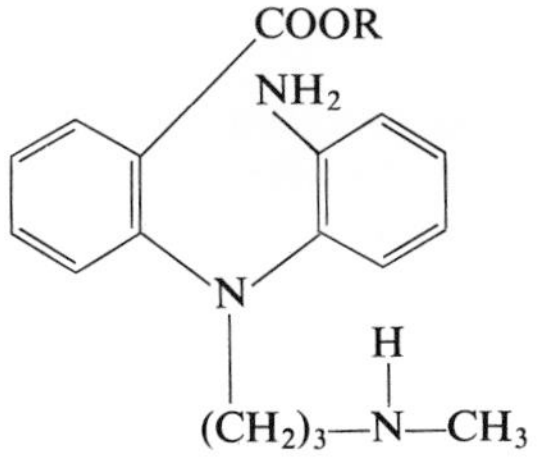

R = CH₃   XXI
R = H   XXII

A heterocyclic compound bearing some semblance to the anthranilic acid derivatives was recently reported by Cummings *et al.* (*42, 43*) from Lederle Laboratories. This substance was not as active in dogs as the thiazides, but

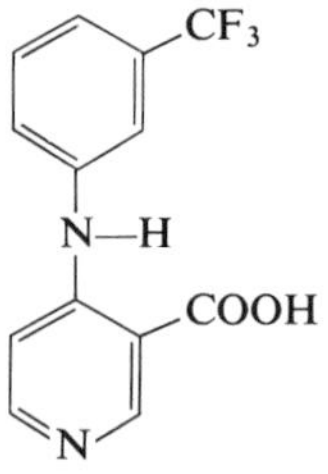

XXIII

at higher doses produced a greater ceiling response similar to that of furosemide and ethacrynic acid. It seems to act in the proximal tubule and the ascending limb of the loop of Henle. However, it lacks an effect in the distal tubule at a site affected by the thiazides and furosemide.

Finally, BS-7161D (pytamine) and BS-7664 reported within the past year are claimed to be very potent compounds (*44*). For example, pytamine administered to rats at 16 mg/kg orally as compared to controls had a 410% increase in water, 455% increase in sodium, and 190% increase in potassium.

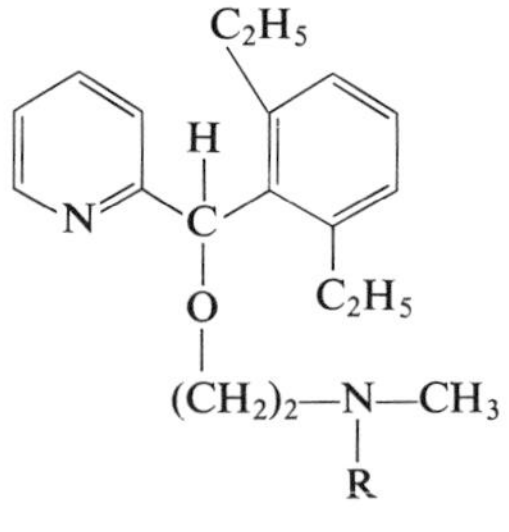

R = H   BS-7664D

R = CH$_3$ BS-7161D Pytamine

REFERENCES

1. G. deStevens, "Diuretics." Academic Press, New York, 1963.
2. G. deStevens, *Encycl. Chem. Tech.* **7**, 248–271 (1965).
3. K. H. Beyer and J. E. Baer, *Pharmacol. Rev.* **13**, 517 (1961).
4. V. D. Wiebelhaus, J. Weinstock, A. R. Maass, F. T. Brennan, G. Sosnowski, and T. Larsen, *J. Pharmacol. Exp. Ther.* **149**, 397 (1965).
5. T. S. Osdene, A. A. Santilli, L. E. McArdle, and M. E. Rosenthale, *J. Med. Chem.* **9**, 697 (1966); **10**, 165 (1967).
6. L. M. Hofmann, *Arch. Int. Pharmacodyn. Ther.* **169**, 189 (1967).
7. L. M. Hofmann, H. A. Wagner, and R. S. Jacobs, *Arch. Int. Pharmacodyn. Ther.* **165**, 476 (1967).

8. L. M. Hofmann, *Proc. Soc. Exp. Biol. Med.* **124**, 1103 (1967).
9. J. B. Bicking, J. M. Mason, O. W. Woltersdorf, Jr., J. H. Jones, S. F. Kwong, C. M. Robb, and E. J. Cragoe, Jr., *J. Med. Chem.* **8**, 638 (1965).
10. E. J. Cragoe, Jr., O. W. Woltersdorf, Jr., J. B. Bicking, S. F. Kwong, and J. H. Jones, *J. Med. Chem.* **10**, 66 (1967).
11. J. B. Bicking, C. M. Robb, S. F. Kwong, and E. J. Cragoe, Jr., *J. Med. Chem.* **10**, 598 (1967).
12. J. H. Jones, J. B. Bicking, and E. J. Cragoe, Jr., *J. Med. Chem.* **10**, 899 (1967).
13. J. H. Jones and E. J. Cragoe, Jr., *J. Med. Chem.* **11**, 322 (1968).
14. K. L. Shepard, J. W. Mason, O. W. Woltersdorf, Jr., J. H. Jones, and E. J. Cragoe, Jr., *J. Med. Chem.* **12**, 280 (1969).
15. J. H. Jones, W. J. Holtz, and E. J. Cragoe, Jr., *J. Med. Chem.* **12**, 285 (1969).
16. J. Eigler, J. Kelter, and E. Renner, *Klin. Wochenschr.* **45**, 737 (1967).
17. F. P. Brunner, *Schweiz. Med. Wochenschr.* **97**, 1542 (1967).
18. D. E. Hutcheon, *Pharmacologist* **9**, 196 (1967).
19. M. B. Bull and J. H. Laragh, *Circulation* **37**, 45 (1968).
20. K. Sturm, W. Siedel and R. Weyer, U.S. Pat. 3,058,882 (1962).
21. L. H. Werner and G. deStevens, unpublished results from the CIBA Laboratories, Summit, New Jersey.
22. L. H. Werner and G. deStevens, Belgian Pat. 689,824 (1967).
23. A. M. Felix, L. B. Czyzewski, D. P. Winter, and R.I. Fryer, *J. Med. Chem.* **12**, 384 (1969).
24. Lovens Kemiske Fab., Belgian Pat. 716,125 (1969).
25. K. Meng and G. Kroneberg, *Arzneim.-Forsch.* **17**, 659 (1967).
26. H. Horstmann, H. Wollweber, and K. Meng, *Arzneim.-Forsch.* **17**, 653 (1967).
27. E. M. Schultz, E. J. Cragoe, Jr., J. B. Bicking, W. A. Bolhofer, and J. M. Sprague, *J. Med. Chem.* **5**, 660 (1962).
28. K. H. Beyer, J. E. Baer, J. K. Michaelson, and H. F. Russo, *J. Pharmacol. Exp. Ther.* **147**, 1 (1965).
29. I. M. Weiner and O. H. Muller, *J. Pharmacol. Exp. Ther.* **113**, 241 (1955).
30. Y. H. Kong, G. V. Irons, Jr., W. M. Ginn, Jr., G. E. Garrison, and E. S. Orgain, *Circulation* **32**, Suppl. II, 128 (1965).
31. R. M. Komorn and E. J. Cafruny, *Science* **143**, 133 (1964).
32. R. M. Komorn and E. J. Cafruny, *J. Pharmacol. Exp. Ther.* **148**, 367 (1965).
33. R. Z. Gussin and E. J. Cafruny, *J. Pharmacol. Exp. Ther.* **149**, 1 (1965).
34. D. E. Duggan and R. M. Noll, *Arch. Biochem. Biophys.* **109**, 388 (1965).
35. J. B. Hook and H. F. Williamson, *Proc. Soc. Exp. Biol. Med.* **120**, 358 (1965).
36. J. G. Topliss and L. M. Konzelman, *J. Pharm. Sci.* **57**, 737 (1968).
37. Geigy, Neth. Pat. 68-10314 (1967).
38. G. N. Walker, French Pat. M-4132 (1966).
39. W. E. Barrett and R. A. Rutledge, *Fed. Proc., Fed. Amer. Soc. Exp. Biol.* **26**, 356 (1967).
40. M. M. Robison, A. A. Renzi, and W. E. Barrett, *Experientia* **23**, 513 (1967).
41. D. L. Smith and M. F. Grostic, *J. Med. Chem.* **10**, 375 (1967).
42. J. R. Cummings, M. A. Ronsberg, E. H. Stokey, and R. Z. Gussin, *Pharmacologist* **10**, 162 (1968).
43. R. Z. Gussin, E. H. Stokey, M. A. Ronsberg, and J. R. Cummings, *Pharmacologist* **10**, 163 (1968).
44. H. Herstel, G. van Hell, D. Mulder, and W. T. Nauta, *Arzneim.-Forsch.* **18**, 827 (1968).

Chapter 11   Design of Biologically Active Steroids

*G. A. Overbeek, J. van der Vies, and
J. de Visser*

I. Introduction

In trying to find new steroidal drugs two starting points may be chosen, which at first sight may seem largely unrelated: (1) structural analogy and (2) physiology and pathology. In terms of methods approach (1) involves chemical exploration with its biological counterpart "screening"; approach (2) involves the biological study of physiological mechanisms and the causes of disease or (in the case of parasitic diseases) the metabolism and requirements of the parasite. A link may develop between these two approaches as soon as it becomes possible to translate the mechanisms of a disorder in chemical or physical terms. So far this is only rarely the case. Even outside the steroid field the only really established examples are the genetically determined enzyme defects. Although in many instances abnormal biochemical reactions leading to the occurrence of "unphysiological" amounts of certain substances, or altered enzymic activity have been detected, it is by no means proven that these should be considered as the primary cause of that particular disease. Nevertheless, these findings may be promising enough to be used as leads for the synthesis of new compounds and as such they become typical examples of approach (2). Another more common link is a methodological one. Quite often methods originally designed for the study of mechanisms of action can be adapted for use as screening methods. In such instances it will usually be necessary to simplify the procedure considerably. Unfortunately the most common link of all is that leads originating from either approach cannot be substantiated by further studies. Examples of both approaches will be presented in this chapter, but for the purpose of elucidating the differences the following two may be mentioned.

Approach (1): By modifying the chemical structure of the natural hormone progesterone its effect on the uterus could be augmented, decreased, prolonged, and even altered in character. Oral activity could be attained.

Approach (2): The bone has a protein part (the matrix) and an inorganic part (calcium salt depot). A steroid would be selected which, on account of its protein anabolic properties, may be expected to promote development of the matrix and, by virtue of its estrogenic activity, to promote calcium deposition.

The activities of the synthetic chemists on one hand and of the pharmacologists and biochemists on the other will be discussed in the following sections.

II. Chemical Exploration and Pharmacological Screening

The chemist starts by synthesizing a particular structure, because he is fascinated either by its chemical singularity or struck by its similarity to known active compounds. This similarity may not be obvious from the ordinary two-dimensional structural formula but only becomes evident if one considers spatial structure, distances between active groups, electron distribution, etc. However, with due reverence to the knowledge and creativity of the chemist, the pharmacologist will have designed a "screening program," a list of methods for the study of as many different activities as he is interested in and feels able to explore. He will usually give priority to the study of the activity expected by the chemist but he will also look for quite different properties that may well be present.*

* Obviously substances obtained purely accidentally, such as intermediates or as side products of a synthesis, can also be studied according to the same pharmacological screening program.

Since the screening program is such an essential part of drug design according to approach (1) and different interpretations of the word "screening" are quite common, it seems necessary to give our definition of pharmacological screening and to elaborate on the underlying principles. Pharmacological screening can be defined as a procedure of systematic testing of substances in a number of widely differing pharmacological tests with the aim of discovering their pharmacological properties. This means that *one* substance can be screened according to a more or less extensive pharmacological program, but when *one or more* substances are studied in *only one test*, this is not considered pharmacological screening. (One could call this "chemical screening," but it is better to avoid the word screening and use the expression "testing.") When screening results in the discovery of an activity, this usually does not mean more than that the active compound probably is one representative of a group of substances having this activity. Hence the finding yields a *lead*, that may be explored, rather than a particular compound that can be developed into a new drug. In order to increase the chances of detecting unknown pharmacological properties tests must be chosen, indicating unrelated activities. In order to be able to screen a reasonable number of substances, tests must be rapid and simple. If possible, one test should allow the detection of more than one activity.

Screening tests do not aim at quantitative measurements, only at the qualitative observation of effects. They are carried out using only one route of administration, one dose, one period of treatment, and one species of animals. These and other experimental conditions are always the same and fixed so that the chances of detection are optimal (e.g., parenteral rather than oral administration and a high but usually subtoxic dose).

It is obvious that in order to screen a reasonable number of compounds one must accept many limitations, and hence also the risk of *not* finding an important activity. In trying too rigidly to avoid this, screening becomes a highly impractical procedure. The same requirement as to the diversity of test methods relates to the choice of compounds to be tested in a screening program: they should not be closely related structurally. Of course, closely related substances may differ considerably with regard to their pharmacological properties, but this is another risk which has to be accepted in order to make screening possible. Testing of *related* compounds starts when exploring the leads found by successful screening, but this second phase of the research procedure is no longer screening. It seems better to screen relatively few substances according to an extensive pharmacological program, rather than to do the opposite. This offers the best chance of finding activities.

In order to maintain the value of a screening program it must be regularly reviewed. Each time one considers which of the screening tests are still up to date and if the activities that can be detected are still of interest. New tests

TABLE I

A HORMONE SCREENING PROGRAM

Name of test	Activities found	Required amount of substance (mg)
Hormone screening test (rats)	Estrogenic Androgenic Glucocorticoid Adrenocorticotropic Gonadotropic Thyrotropic Antithyroidal	~100
Clauberg test sc and oral (rabbits)	Progestational	~20
Litter test (rats)	Inhibition of estrus Inhibition of ovulation Inhibition of egg development Inhibition of nidation Abortifacient Other antifertility effects	~120
Antifertilization test (rabbits)	Inhibition of sperm transport (cervical hostility) Inhibition of sperm capacitation Inhibition of cleavage of fertilized ovum Accelerated transport of eggs	~100
Biochemical screening test (rats)	Blood sugar depressant Blood sugar rising Plasma cholesterol depressant Plasma calcium depressant Lipid-mobilizing Mineralocorticoid Antialdosterone Diuretic Antidiuretic Adrenocorticotropic Glucocorticoid Adverse effects on liver and kidney	~270

should be added when desirable. Table I gives an example of a screening program for hormonal activities as it is used by N.V. Organon, Oss.

The two tests called "hormone screening test" and "biochemical screening test" are good examples of ideal screening tests since, with a number of limitations, i.e., only one animal species, one dose, one mode, and one duration of administration, they provide information on many activities and are relatively simple to carry out. Only the hormone screening test will be described here.

HORMONAL EFFECTS IN IMMATURE MALE AND FEMALE RATS (HORMONE SCREENING TEST)

Purpose: Substances are subjected to the hormone screening test in order to obtain preliminary data on hormonal activities. In general, estrogenic, androgenic, anabolic, gonad inhibitory, or corticoidal effects can be detected.

Test animal: Immature rats, 22–24 days of age and 45–55 gm body weight, are randomly distributed in three groups of 5 males and 5 females.

Standards: Estradiol, testosterone, and hydrocortisone have been tested once and are active at a lower dose than 1 mg daily subcutaneously; new substances are therefore tested in a dose of 1 mg.

Vehicle: Where possible, steroids are dissolved in arachis oil with or without 10% benzyl alcohol. Insoluble steroids are suspended in suspension fluid.

Water-soluble steroidal and nonsteroidal substances are dissolved in physiological NaCl solution.

Water-insoluble nonsteroidal substances are dissolved in arachis oil with or without benzyl alcohol or prepared as suspensions in an appropriate fluid.

Experimental design:

Material administered	Total dose (mg) (net wt)	No. of animals	
		Male	Female
Vehicle		5	5
Substance 1	7	5	5
Substance 2	7	5	5

Quantities required: At least 100 mg of each substance must be available.

Procedure: *a.* After an acclimatization period of 2 days the rats are given daily subcutaneous injections for 7 days. The control group is given the solvent and each of the remaining group is given a daily dose of 1 mg of an unknown substance. The animals are weighed just before the first treatment and 7 days later at the time of autopsy.

b. During the treatment period, the following effects can be observed:

1. Opening of the vagina; if so, vaginal smears are prepared.
2. Local skin reactions at the site of injection.
3. Toxic effects.
4. Behavioral effects.

c. Autopsy: The animals are killed under deep ether anesthesia. Immediately after dissection and removal of adherent tissues the following organs are weighed accurately (error <1%) on a torsion balance: thyroids, thymus, adrenals, spleen, kidneys, testes, ventral prostate, seminal vesicles, levator ani muscle, ovaries, and uterus. Macroscopical observation of the above-mentioned organs and of heart, lungs, liver, stomach, and intestines is necessary. If abnormalities are observed it is necessary to decide whether the organs concerned should also be studied histologically. If deposits of the injected substance are present at the site of injection this fact must be reported.

End points: The average weight of the organs in each treated group is calculated in order to assess whether a decrease or an increase has occurred as compared with the average values of the organs in the control group. By means of the schedule shown in Table II, analysis of the experimental data is facilitated.

TABLE II

CHARACTERISTIC HORMONAL EFFECTS[a]

Organ	Estrogenic (female)	Androgenic (male)	Anabolic	Gonad inhibitory	Corticoidal
Adrenals	>	<			<, <<
Kidneys		>			
Thymus	<	<			<, <<
Spleen	<				
Testes	<	<, =		<	=, >
Seminal vesicles	>	>, >>		<	
Ventral prostate	=	>, >>		<	
Levator ani muscle	<, =, >	>	>		<
Ovaries	<, =	<, =		<, =	
Uterus	>, >>		>		
Vaginal opening	+	+			
Vaginal cornification	+				
Weight gain	<		>		<, <<

[a] *Key:* >, increase in weight; <, decrease in weight; =, no change; +, present.

Innumerable steroids have been synthesized in laboratories all over the world and have been studied for their hormonal activities. Long lists have been published and still longer lists are available in the files of the pharmaceutical industry. However, notwithstanding this vast material it is still only in a very limited way possible to predict the hormonal properties of a newly synthesized steroid. It is easy enough to prepare a list of the main structural characteristics which suggest a certain hormonal activity (Fig. 1). Further substitution in

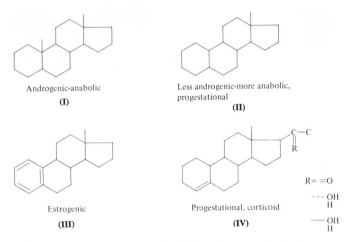

Androgenic-anabolic

(I)

Less androgenic-more anabolic, progestational

(II)

Estrogenic

(III)

Progestational, corticoid

(IV)

$$R= =O$$
$$--- OH \quad H$$
$$— OH \quad H$$

Fig. 1. Structures suggesting the indicated hormonal activities.

these structures reveals a few other rules which are only slightly less primitive. 17α-Alkyl, alkenyl, or alkynyl substitution in **I**, **II**, or **III** induces oral activity. However, it may also abolish all activity (17α-ethylestradiol), or at the same time introduce another property [17α-ethynyl often induces estrogenic activity as in 17α-ethynyl-Δ^4-estren-17β-ol (*13*), or 17α-ethynyl-17β-hydroxy-Δ^4-estren-3-one (*10*) and the corresponding Δ^5 and $\Delta^{5(10)}$ compounds]. A 2-methyl group abolishes the activity in the 11-ketocorticoids. In this case the explanation is that in order to become active the 11-keto group of the compound has to be reduced in the body to 11β-hydroxy. This reduction no longer occurs in the presence of a 2-methyl group (*15*).

The introduction of a 9α-fluoroatom in the corticoids strongly augments the antiinflammatory but also the sodium-retaining properties, but the latter effect can be counteracted by a 16α-methyl or hydroxy group. A further example demonstrates an unexpected finding, i.e., the different effect of the introduction of an α-methyl group at C-6 or C-7 in the already mentioned 17α-ethynyl-Δ^4-estren-17β-ol. 17α-Ethynyl-Δ^4-estren-17β-ol is a *progestational* steroid with additionally a weak estrogenic activity. This could be expected since many 19-nor-Δ^4-C-18 steroids, in particular those with an α-alkyl, alkenyl, or alkynyl group at C-17, are progestational, whereas the 17α-ethynyl group usually introduces some estrogenic activity. Unexpectedly, the estrogenic activity is very strongly augmented by the introduction of a 7α-methyl group, whereas a 6α-methyl group completely abolishes this activity (*12*).

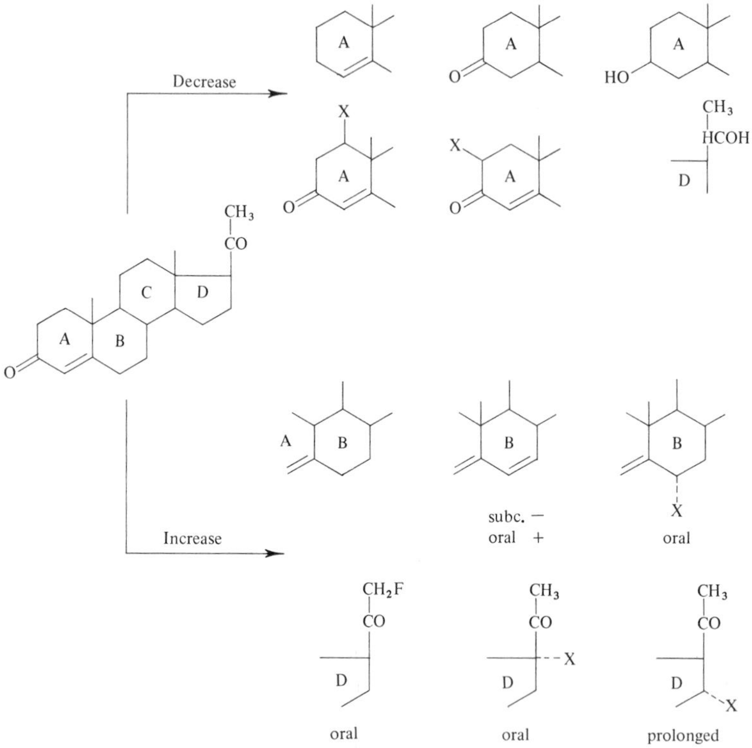

Fig. 2. Effect of structural changes in the progesterone molecule on progestational activity.

Consequently the results of the tests for progestational activity are also strongly affected, thus changing the whole pattern of activity, notwithstanding the minor character of the chemical change.

Another example of the unpredictable changes in activity as the result of chemical changes was already mentioned in the introduction. Figure 2 demonstrates the result of these modifications of the progesterone molecule.

An example of a partly chemical, partly physical approach is provided by studies of van der Vies (*17*) on the absorption and hydrolysis of esters from nandrolone and other long-acting steroids. Either the rate of absorption or, in the case of esterified steroids, the rate of hydrolysis was shown to affect not only the duration of action but also the pattern of activity. Hence by designing simple *in vitro* methods for the determination of these rates it became possible to predict biological effects. Esters of nandrolone are known to have anabolic and androgenic activity as can be demonstrated from their effects on the levator ani muscle and the seminal vesicles or ventral prostate in castrated rats. When nandrolone is esterified with organic acids with increasing chain length the duration of action increases and the androgenic

TABLE III

CORRELATION OF THE DISAPPEARANCE RATES FROM THE GASTROCNEMIUS MUSCLE OF THE RAT (*in Vivo*) AND FROM A PAPER STRIP (ELUTION *in Vitro*) FOR STEROIDS WITH DIFFERENT DURATION OF ACTION

Compound	$T_{1/2}$			
	in vitro	Rank	*in vivo*	Rank
Nandrolone	2	1	0.6	1
Nandrolone phenylproprionate	12	4	25	4
Nandrolone decanoate	33	6	130	6
Nandrolone laurate	75	7	243	7
Progesterone	2.4	2	5.2	2
16α-Ethylprogesterone	5	3	18	3
16α-Ethylprogesterone in castor oil/benzyl benzoate/benzyl alcohol	17	5	28	5

activity becomes less, whereas the anabolic activity remains largely intact (*14*). It was found later (*18*) that these changes could be correlated with the half-life times determined from the disappearance rate from an intramuscular depot and with the rate of elution by plasma from an oil depot on a paper strip. This correlation could even be shown to exist for other (progestational) steroids with different duration of action. These correlations are shown by comparing Fig. 3 for the effect and the duration of action on the levator ani muscle, Fig. 4 for the androgenic activity and Table III for the absorption and elution rates. Since the rates of hydrolysis by plasma are many times higher than the rates of absorption of the nandrolone esters the former is of no importance for the effect *in vivo*; as soon as some ester disappears from the oily depot it is hydrolyzed immediately. This situation does not always exist

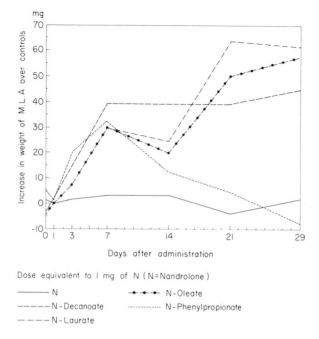

Fig. 3. Myotropic activity and duration of action of various nandrolone esters.

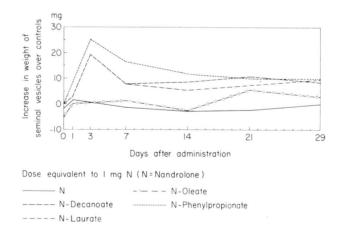

Fig. 4. Androgenic activity and duration of action of various nandrolone esters.

and in the case of the duration of progestational activity of esters of 16α-isopropylnandrolone the effects were found to correlate better with the rates of hydrolysis than with the rates of absorption (Table IV); in this instance, the rates of hydrolysis are relatively much lower. That hydrolysis of the esters of nandrolone is essential for activity was shown by the poor effect of the 3-desoxo analog of nandrolone phenylpropionate. This ester could be shown to be very poorly hydrolyzed by the esterases, which probably explains why

TABLE IV

CORRELATION OF PROGESTATIONAL ACTIVITY AND RATE OF HYDROLYSIS IN PLASMA (*in Vitro*) AND ABSENCE OF CORRELATION OF PROGESTATIONAL ACTIVITY AND ELUTION RATE (*in Vitro*)

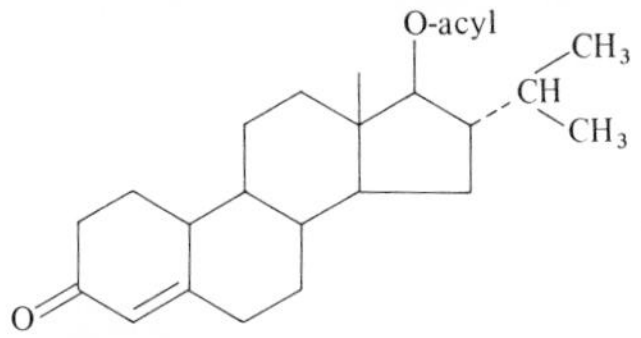

	Elution *in vitro*		Hydrolysis in plasma in 16 hr		Prolonged progestational activity in deciduoma test 1 × 0.25 mg
	$T_{1/2}$ (hr)	Rank	%	Rank	Rank
Ester:					
Acetate	9	1	40	5	6
Trimethyl acetate	11	2	5	1	2
Propionate	13	3	38	4	4
Caproate	18	4	54	6	7
Decanoate	108	7	7	3	2
Palmitate	49	6	6	2	2
Phenylpropionate	22	5	76	7	5

$r = 0.86\ P < 0.05$

it is so much less active than the related nandrolone phenylpropionate (Table V). Hence this retrospective study has furnished methods allowing prospective studies in the future. It has also made it possible, be it in a very limited way, to predict changes in pharmacological properties from the chemical structure of steroids. On the other hand, it has taught again that relatively minor changes like the introduction of a 16α-isopropyl group leads to the prevalance of other factors determining the activity.

Outside the hormone field effects may be more easily predictable. By using the steroid as a peg for attaching various groups known to be associated with certain activities of nonsteroids, the same activities can sometimes be induced

TABLE V

SLOW RATE OF HYDROLYSIS CORRESPONDS WITH POOR ACTIVITY OF 3-DEOXONANDROLONE
PHENYLPROPIONATE IN THE LEVATOR ANI ASSAY

Structure of steroid	Activity in M.L.A. test	Elution in vitro $T_{1/2}$ (hr)	Hydrolysis in plasma, (16 hr) (%)
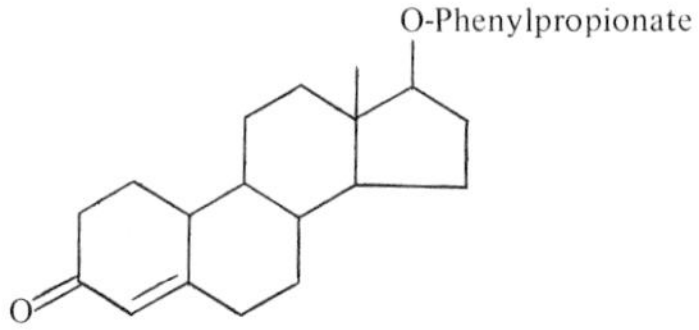 O-Phenylpropionate (structure)	0.25 mg Active	9	99
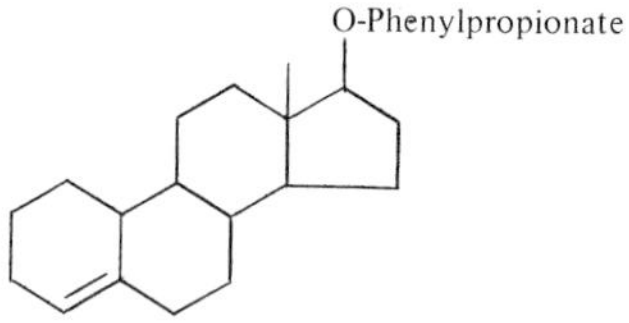 O-Phenylpropionate (structure)	4 mg Inactive	63	11

in steroids. In some instances, the resulting compounds have been shown to have advantages over existing drugs. One of the successful examples of this approach is pancuronium bromide (2β,16β-dipiperidino-5α-androstane-3α,17β-diol diacetate dimethobromide; Fig. 5) a neuromuscular-blocking agent. The compound prepared by Hewett and Savage (7) is a quaternary ammonium base. The nonsteroidal contribution was suggested by choline which was incorporated in the steroid. The compound has about five times the activity of tubocurarine in humans and animals and lacks the histamine-releasing effect of tubocurarine (3, 6). This is another example of what could be expected (neuromuscular-blocking activity) and what was unexpected (the high activity and lack of histamine release). Analogs of pancuronium bromide have been synthesized (5). They have widely different potencies and duration of action. It is interesting that the 3α-monoacetate (dacuronium bromide),

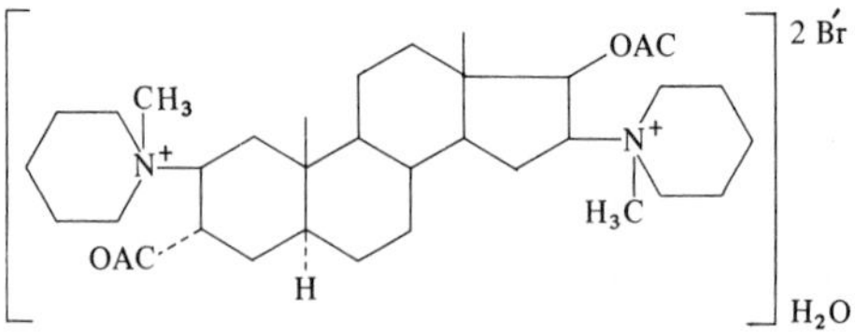

Fig. 5. Chemical structure of pancuronium bromide, a neuromuscular blocker.

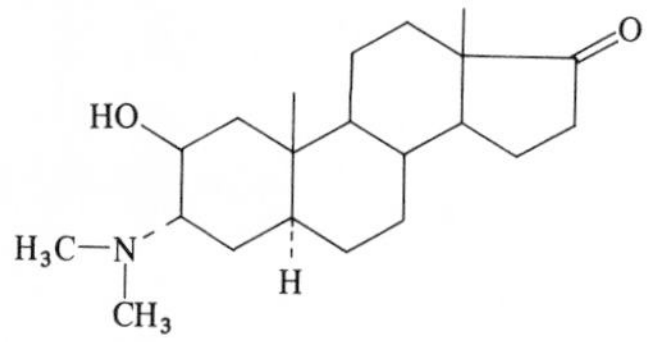

Fig. 6. Chemical structure of 3α-dimethylamino-2β-hydroxy-5α-androstan-17-one, a local anesthetic.

which was found to be only slightly less active in the cat turned out to be considerably less potent in man.

Another example of introduction of groups derived from nonsteroidal drugs was studied by the same group of investigators (1, 8). They found that the introduction of groups typical for local anesthetic compounds could endow steroids with the same activity. In particular, 3α-dimethylamino-2β-hydroxy-5α-androstan-17-one (Fig. 6) was found to be more potent in surface and intracutaneous anesthesia but longer acting in conduction anesthesia with slower onset of action than lidocain.

III. The Biological Study of the Cause of Disease

Whereas in the studies described above the synthetic chemists undertook both the initial thinking and the first part of the practical work, with approach (2) the initiative lies with the biologists and sometimes the biochemists. They have to discover the mechanisms underlying physiological processes and the pathogenesis of a disease in order to find new leads for the design of new drugs. A first example of this kind (although fertility obviously cannot be considered as a "disease") is the search for various types of contraceptives. The study of the physiology of reproduction has taught us that there are many links in the chain of events which might be influenced in the male or the female. The knowledge that gonadotropins are required for ovulation has led to the search for substances inhibiting the production or release of these pituitary hormones. The fact that natural estrogens and progestatives are physiological inhibitors of this type, led Pincus to the use of combinations of synthetic steroids with similar activities for contraceptive purposes. However, since estrogens and progestatives are involved in several other stages of the reproductive process these combinations may have other sites of action as well. These may well be more attractive in view of the obvious desire to interfere as little as possible with physiological processes. Substances not affecting the hypothalamic, pituitary, and ovarian function and acting more peripherally would be preferable, provided a similar degree of protection against pregnancy could be obtained. In trying to achieve this goal it is encouraging to realize how many events have to take place in the fertilized egg in the Fallopian tube and in the uterus, and in particular how delicately these should fit in a very precise time schedule to allow implantation in the endometrium. Another favorable circumstance is the different sensitivity to such hormones as estrogens and progestagens of various organs which should not be influenced. We have no complete knowledge on the sensitivity of all organs involved in the human. It would be extremely useful to perform a systematic study of this kind, although it is realized that what holds for one substance with a particular hormonal activity does not necessarily apply (at least quantitatively) to another one, although qualitatively it may have the same effect. The disturbance of hormonal balance as described for estrogens and progestagens could also be achieved with antiestrogenic and antiprogestational compounds.

At present extensive studies are being performed at physiological levels which may well be past the hormonal stage. These include the requirements for implantation, both with respect to the blastocyst and to the endometrium (11) even at the molecular level. At first sight the general character of these changes as induced in the activity of enzymes occurring all through the body and in the production or action of another unspecific stimulator, e.g., cyclic AMP, appear to offer little hope for obtaining the very specific effect desired for the purpose. Still these studies may turn out to offer practical perspectives. The special local situation as caused by the presence of a "foreign body" like a fertilized egg or a blastocyst may make it possible that only one specifically sensitized site will react to a drug. Also a drug may cause such minor general changes that they do not result in a pharmacological effect, whereas at the activated spot an effect is obtained. The local character of the processes strongly suggests local therapy for which either very low doses of steroids or other drugs could be expected to be effective without causing reactions elsewhere in the body. Not only the fate of the egg can be influenced either before or after fertilization, the sperm cell can also be chosen as the target. In many animal species, probably including man, the sperm, when leaving the male, is infertile and is rendered fertile by a process occurring in the female. This process, called capacitation, can be reversed by substances present in the seminal fluid (decapacitation). The significance of this mechanism is unknown. It may mean a protection of the sperm allowing it to survive during its journey from the testicle to the egg. It seems highly probable that either in the male or in the female the processes of decapacitation and capacitation are influenced by steroid hormones. The further study of the biochemical and of the regulatory processes; including those of other aspects of sperm transport may well lead to new approaches in the contraceptive field, either by treating the male or the female.

Another example of this type, more or less outside the field of endocrinology concerns the search for antiatherosclerotic drugs. In this disease the vessel wall is affected locally, which suggests that even when the vessels are more generally diseased, intimal lesions occurring at weak or very exposed spots may start the development of atheromata. Estrogens can improve the potency of the intima or promote the repair of the initial lesions (1, 2), probably by an effect on the mucopolysaccharides in the vessel wall (16). They also lower the level of the blood lipids, another probable factor in atherosclerosis. Both these actions could be dissociated from the classical "hormonal" estrogenic properties. Why so far the results of clinical studies with these steroids have been rather disappointing is another matter (9). Even the best designed drug may ultimately fail to fulfill expectations. This obviously should not prevent us from following leads that show promise, wherever and however they may have originated.

In rereading this contribution to a volume devoted to drug design the authors feel that the differences between the two approaches are reflected in a typical way by their own presentation. With the first approach the lead is something tangible, it is an existing compound, and every subsequent step in the study is performed with well-defined substances. These may be active or inactive and the study may fail to provide a new drug, but at least the facts are there, which is easy to describe.

With the second approach one starts with a philosophy on largely unexplained events, which are impossible to describe factually as long as the underlying physiological and pathogenic problems are not solved.

This does not mean a preference for one or the other approach. Both may fail and even require as much time for the development of a drug. It is the character of the investigator and his available facilities that will determine which approach he will use.

REFERENCES

1. I. L. Bonta and C. J. de Vos, *Acta Endocrinol.* (*Copenhagen*) **49**, 403 (1965).
2. I. L. Bonta, C. J. de Vos, and A. Delver, *Acta Endocrinol.* (*Copenhagen*) **48**, 137 (1965).
3. I. L. Bonta, E. M. Goorissen, and F. H. Derkx, *Eur. J. Pharmacol.* **4**, 83 and 303 (1968).
4. W. R. Buckett, C. L. Hewett, F. A. Marwick, and D. S. Savage, *Chim. Ther.* **2**, 164 (1967).
5. W. R. Buckett, C. L. Hewett, and D. S. Savage, *Chim. Ther.* **2**, 186 (1967).
6. W. R. Buckett, C. E. B. Marjoribanks, F. A. Marwick, and M. B. Morton, *Brit. J. Pharmacol.* **32**, 671 (1968).
7. C. L. Hewett and D. S. Savage, Belg. Pat. 676,708 (1966).
8. C. L. Hewett and D. S. Savage, *J. Chem. Soc., C* p. 1134 (1968).
9. D. Kritchevsky, *Ann. N.Y. Acad. Sci.* **149**, 1058 (1968).
10. D. A. McGinty and C. Djerassi, *Ann. N.Y. Acad. Sci.* **71**, 500 (1958).

11. A. McLaren, *Nature (London)* **122**, 739 (1969).
12. G. A. Overbeek and J. de Visser, *Acta Endocrinol.* (*Copenhagen*) Suppl. 90, 179 (1964).
13. G. A. Overbeek, Z. Madjerek, and J. de Visser, *Acta Endocrinol.* **41**, 351 (1962).
14. G. A. Overbeek, J. van der Vies, and J. de Visser, "Protein Metabolism." Springer, Berlin, 1962.
15. L. H. Sarett, A. A. Patchett, and S. L. Steelman, *Fortschr.-Arzneimittelforsch.* **5**, 11 (1953).
16. M. Schiff and H. P. Burn, *Arch. Otolaryngol.* **73**, 63 (1961).
17. J. van der Vies, *Acta Endocrinol.* (*Copenhagen*) **49**, 271 (1965).
18. J. van der Vies, *Acta Endocrinol.* (*Copenhagen*) **64**, 656 (1970).

Chapter 12 Rational Elements in the Development of Superior Neuromuscular Blocking Agents

M. Martin-Smith

I. Introduction

In this chapter the term "neuromuscular blocking agent" is used in the now generally accepted sense (*80*) as meaning any drug which abolishes the response of striated muscle to nerve impulses via a primary action about the junction between the somatic motor nerve terminals and the muscle end-plate, whether this action be immediately prejunctional or immediately postjunctional. It therefore excludes drugs predominantly affecting either the axonal conduction of nerve impulses or the contractile mechanism of the muscle, as well as drugs inhibiting transmission between autonomic nerves and cardiac muscle or between autonomic nerves and smooth muscle. The term "curariform drug," on the other hand, is used here in a narrower sense than is employed by some workers, to embrace only those neuromuscular blocking agents which, like (+)-tubocurarine, appear to act predominantly postjunctionally to induce a block of the antidepolarizing type, readily reversed by anticholinesterases. In most instances neuromuscular blocking agents exert their effects in such a way that once paralysis has set in there is no activation of the contractile mechanism of the muscle fibers and so the muscle remains in a state of flaccidity. Accordingly a criterion often employed for the classification of a compound as a neuromuscular blocking agent is that at the height of the paralysis, the muscle will respond normally to direct electrical stimulation. However, in the case of certain muscles of various species, particularly the chicken, blockade of neuromuscular transmission by certain compounds producing a flaccid paralysis in other species is accompanied by a sustained contracture of the muscle which makes normal response to direct electrical stimulation impossible, so this criterion is subject to appropriate reservations.

For the purposes of this chapter the term "cholinergic site" is restricted to its classic meaning of sites involving acetylcholine only, where no subsequent role is played by noradrenaline. "Nicotinic" sites are taken as embracing the neuromuscular junction and autonomic ganglia, and "muscarinic" sites are taken as meaning neuroeffector units innervated by autonomic cholinergic nerves.

In the face of the failure of present-day understanding of drug action to provide accurate prediction of the exact overall biological activity to be found in a given compound (cf. *443*), the neuromuscular blocking agents afford an especially informative group with which to illustrate how intelligent retrospective rationalization of accumulated information may nevertheless still provide a reasonable basis for increasing the chances of successful intentional preparation of new drugs possessing a specified type of activity. Indeed, notwithstanding the prolonged period of clinical use in some countries for the original prototype, (+)-tubocurarine, which might be misconstrued as indicating that no superior agents could be evolved, and despite complications introduced by differences in response in different species as well as in different muscles of the same species, a number of favorable factors conspire to make the neuromuscular blocking agents one of the more suitable groups with which to illustrate the steady development of a rational basis for drug design. These may be listed as follows:

1. Despite a certain lack of direct experimental verification, there exists a highly plausible overall interpretation of normal events at the neuromuscular junction, fully compatible with the specialized microanatomy of the region, and finding strong circumstantial support from studies in a wide range of related fields. Thus there would seem to be good grounds upon which to base logical new approaches to the disruption of the normal functioning of the neuromuscular junction.

2. The different types of pharmacological response elicited by the different types of neuromuscular blocking agent already known, as firmly established on an empirical basis, can be satisfactorily accommodated in terms of different mechanisms of interference with normal events at the neuromuscular junction, thus reinforcing and elaborating the considerations given under 1 above.

3. Both the clinical properties essential in an ideal neuromuscular blocking agent and the undesirable side effects most likely to accompany them are well defined. Thus there exists a clear conception of the particular biological properties being sought in any new compound under consideration for synthesis as a potential neuromuscular blocking agent, while well-established pharmacological tests are immediately available for its rapid preliminary assessment.

4. The neuromuscular blocking agents viewed as a whole represent one of the more favorable instances in which there is discernible a reasonable degree of valid correlation between specific molecular features and the type of

biological activity displayed. Although the optimal requirements of chemical structure to produce neuromuscular blockade differ considerably from one test preparation to another, thus serving to restrict generalizations to those of a broad nature only, within this context key leads are apparent as to the type of molecule most likely to possess the specific properties sought in a superior neuromuscular blocking agent.

It is not the purpose of this chapter to provide an exhaustive catalog of all compounds which have been prepared from rational considerations of one type or another as prospective neuromuscular blocking agents; nor is it intended to attempt a comprehensive account of the vast accumulation of knowledge gleaned from a wide range of scientific disciplines which serves to provide the rational basis underlying the design of these compounds. Rather, the intention is to highlight rational threads discernible amidst the mass of empirical data within the limitations imposed by the shortcomings in the present state of knowledge. This will be attempted by first briefly summarizing what is considered by the author to be the more pertinent background information and then by indicating ways in which these rational elements may be applied, both with reference to selected examples representative of the different types of neuromuscular blocking agents already known and with respect to other potentially rewarding lines of future exploitation. It is hoped that this type of approach may also serve to indicate various general principles capable of application in other areas of drug research.

II. Grosser Morphological Features Influencing the Response to Neuromuscular Blocking Agents

As already implied, marked species differences in the response to certain neuromuscular blocking agents are frequently encountered. In some instances these appear to involve differences in the mechanism of action of the drug in the different species, but in other instances the different responses elicited can be attributed in large measure to differences in the grosser morphology of the muscles concerned and in their methods of innervation (*145, 147, 155, 156, 374, 586*). Thus in order to gain an understanding of how neuromuscular blocking agents, while acting by what would appear to be essentially the same mechanism, may nevertheless elicit different types of response in different species and even with respect to different muscles in the same species, it is necessary to consider the different types of striated muscle found within the animal kingdom.

Although the groups overlap by way of fibers having intermediate properties, fundamentally two extreme types of striated muscle fiber may be distinguished according to the structure of their sarcoplasmic reticulum (*383–385*). One type, described as having a *Felderstruktur*, is histologically characterized by irregularly shaped areas of sarcoplasm containing relatively small numbers of large and poorly defined myofibrils. The other type, described as having a *Fibrellenstruktur*, possesses uniformly distributed myofibrils. Muscle fibers with a *Felderstruktur* receive different innervations in different species. In amphibians and birds, for example, the innervation is by small diameter myelinated motoneurones of the γ-group but the muscle fibers having a *Felderstruktur*, which occur in admixture with fibers having a *Fibrellenstruktur* in the diaphragms of the rat and rabbit, are innervated by the ultimate branches of α-motoneurones. On the other hand, the innervation of muscle fibers exhibiting a *Fibrellenstruktur* would seem to be restricted solely to the branches of large diameter α-motoneurones. A further marked distinction between the two types of muscle fiber is found in the manner in which the innervation is received. In the case of muscle fibers with a *Felderstruktur* each muscle fiber receives along its length many small nerve endings emanating from each of a number of different nerves and the junctions have the appearance of a dense series of small grapelike (*en grappe*) (*153, 154, 267, 268, 270, 283, 568*) bodies set out along the muscle fiber surface. Thus muscle fibers with a *Felderstruktur* are also termed multiply innervated fibers. In contrast, in the case of muscle fibers with a *Fibrellenstruktur* each fiber is innervated either by a single nerve ending or, alternatively, by a strictly limited number of nerve endings (*332, 347*). However, such multiple innervation in *Fibrellenstruktur* fibers is always sparse and the distance between adjacent neuromuscular junctions, which possess discrete (*en plaque*) endplates (*267, 268, 270, 306*), is much greater than is found with *Felderstruktur* fibers. Muscle fibers with a *Fibrellenstruktur* are also referred to as focally innervated fibers. By and large multiply innervated fibers tend to produce a slow graded contraction while focally innervated fibers tend to produce a rapid all-or-none twitch response but there are exceptions within each group. Moreover, each group contains fibers exhibiting a wide range of speed characteristics (*104a*).

Although muscles composed exclusively of multiply innervated fibers may occur in the invertebrates, as, for example, with the big muscles of the lobster claw, within the vertebrata many muscles are composed of a mixture of multiply innervated and focally innervated fibers in various arrangements, with the proportion of the two types varying greatly from muscle to muscle and from species to species (*167, 270, 386, 396*). It is these differences in the proportions of fibers of the two types which underlie some of the differences in response to neuromuscular blocking agents of the depolarizing type by different species and by different muscles in the same species, and which also help to determine the order in which the different muscles become paralyzed. With the notable exception of the four rectus and the two oblique extraocular muscles (*18, 262, 307, 308, 398*), the internal ear muscle (*167*), and the striated muscle in the esophagus (*167*) which contain many densely multiply innervated fibers, mammalian striated muscles are composed predominantly of focally innervated fibers, although multiply innervated fibers also occur in appreciable numbers in the muscle spindles (*82–84, 331*). On the other hand, in amphibians and birds a number of muscles, such as the anterior latissimus dorsi of the chicken, are composed almost entirely of multiply innervated fibers, while others, such as the gastrocnemius muscle of the chicken (*267*), contain approximately equal numbers of focally innervated and multiply innervated fibers and this is the underlying reason why depolarizing neuromuscular blocking agents give rise to a spastic paralysis in the chicken but a flaccid paralysis in mammals, the mechanism of which is discussed more fully later in this chapter.

In general it is considered (*70*) that the cat resembles man most closely in its sensitivity to neuromuscular blocking drugs, but there are a number of instances where this is not so.

III. The Anatomy and Physiology of the Neuromuscular Junction

A. MICROANATOMY

Since detailed knowledge of the intimate microanatomical structure of the neuromuscular junction is mandatory to the complete understanding of its normal functioning, and since knowledge of normal events at the neuromuscular junction in turn is essential to the complete understanding of their disruption, the logical point of departure for any discussion of the rational design of neuromuscular blocking agents must be the consideration of the intimate structural features of this region. Moreover, this approach has other justification in that, while the microanatomy of the neuromuscular junction can be taken as unequivocally established, current concepts of the precise molecular interactions occurring there fall almost entirely within the realms of argument by analogy and intelligent speculation. Thus, initial consideration of morphology permits logical development of theme from the known toward the unknown.

The detailed microanatomy of a typical *en plaque* neuromuscular junction as revealed by a combination of light microscopy and electron microscopy has been fully discussed on a number of occasions (*152, 154, 156, 167, 191, 310, 586, 638*) so it is not necessary to give more than a bare outline here. The essential features can be represented in diagrammatic form as depicted in Fig. 1.

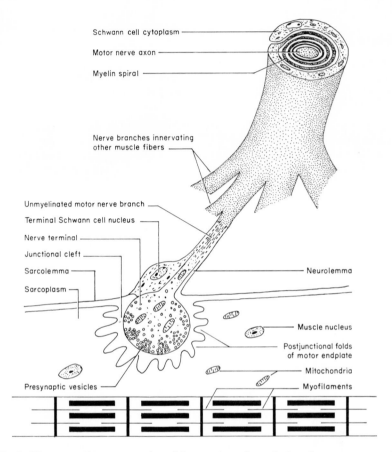

Schwann cell cytoplasm

Motor nerve axon

Myelin spiral

Nerve branches innervating
other muscle fibers

Unmyelinated motor nerve branch

Terminal Schwann cell nucleus

Nerve terminal

Junctional cleft

Sarcolemma

Sarcoplasm

Neurolemma

Muscle nucleus

Postjunctional folds
of motor endplate

Mitochondria

Presynaptic vesicles

Myofilaments

Fig. 1. Diagrammatic representation of the structure of a typical *en plaque* neuromuscular junction.

As the motor nerve axon approaches the bundle of focally innervated muscle fibers which it innervates, it undergoes extensive ramification and the high degree of myelination provided by the encircling Schwann cells disappears. Each ultimate branch of the motor nerve axon then proceeds to a muscle fiber with the one motor nerve innervating something of the order of one hundred or so fibers. At the point of innervation the ultimate ramification of the nerve fiber penetrates the outer membrane or sarcolemma of the muscle fiber while the terminal Schwann cell fuses with the sarcolemma so that continuity is achieved between the Schwann cell membrane or neurolemma and the sarcolemma, thus giving encapsulation of the actual neuromuscular junction. The nerve fiber itself terminates in a bulb-shaped extension fitting into an accommodating indentation of the muscle fiber surface in which the membrane bounding the protoplasm of the muscle fiber is thrown into a number of tubular folds and it is this specialized convoluted region of the muscle fiber membrane in close juxtaposition to the nerve terminal which constitutes the muscle endplate. There is no protoplasmic continuity between the nerve terminal and the muscle fiber, and the well-defined space of ~500–1000 Å in width between them is termed the junctional cleft.

In addition to the clearly discernible mitochondria, the protoplasm of the nerve terminal contains a large number of well-defined small globular bodies of about 500 Å diameter, known as vesicles. The profusion of these vesicles in the nerve terminal close to the junctional cleft, together with other considerations to be discussed presently, gives strong indication that the vesicles have a specialized role essential to the functioning of the neuromuscular junction.

B. PHYSIOLOGY

As already indicated, although the microanatomical features of the neuromuscular junction are firmly established, current interpretation of the intimate events occurring there is by no means unequivocally established. However, there is a substantial body of circumstantial evidence upon which this interpretation is based and it would seem likely that the essential core of present belief is very near the truth.

It is now generally accepted (360), despite opposition from some workers (461), that transmission of the wave of excitation from the nerve to the motor endplate takes place by chemical means since the following facts must be accommodated.

1. The highly specialized microanatomical features of the neuromuscular junction with the lack of any direct protoplasmic continuity between the nerve terminal and the muscle fiber as revealed by electron microscopy (9, 191, 477, 522, 523) would seem anomalous in the extreme if the muscle were simply receiving a direct continuation of the electrical impulse traveling down the nerve.

2. The amount of electrical current involved in the transmission of an impulse along a motor nerve fiber is in itself too small to elicit a direct excitation of the mass of muscle it innervates (360) as can be experimentally demonstrated by placing the cut end of an active nerve fiber in contact with a whole muscle. Thus any explanation of the translation of a nerve impulse into muscular contraction must accommodate a means of amplification of the current conducted by the nerve.

3. Transmission at the neuromuscular junction occurs in one direction only (*359*). A straightforward electrical mechanism would imply the possibility of simple experimental reversal of the direction of transmission which is not the case.

4. There is a time delay in transmission across the neuromuscular junction.

5. Fatigue occurs more readily at the neuromuscular junction than in the nerve or in the muscle (*357, 358, 461*).

6. The selective action shown by the neuromuscular blocking agents at the neuromuscular junction would not be readily explicable in terms of interference with electrical phenomena considered a common property of all conducting membranes.

Available evidence (e.g., *93, 97, 169, 179, 180, 201, 203, 205, 391–393, 482*), including the classic demonstration by Dale, Feldberg, and Vogt (*169*) of the presence in the perfusion fluid from the physostigmine-treated mammalian neuromuscular junction following stimulation of the motor nerve of a substance showing pharmacological properties quantitatively identical to those of a standard solution of acetylcholine (**I**) together with proof (*93*) that this

$$CH_3\overset{\displaystyle CH_3}{\underset{\displaystyle CH_3}{\diagdown}}\overset{+}{N}-CH_2-CH_2-OCOCH_3$$

I

substance is not released as a result of the muscular contraction, makes it amply apparent that the role of chemical transmitter or neurohormone responsible for transferring the excitation across the junctional cleft is best assigned to acetylcholine, although at the same time there is some evidence that this compound may not necessarily be the sole or even the major chemical mediator at all neuromuscular junctions in all species (*429*). There has also been some challenge (*553*) to the accepted view that acetylcholine necessarily acts postjunctionally as required by the classic theory of neurotransmitters. Certainly a prejunctional component to its action, the significance of which is not fully understood, is well established (*31, 144, 329, 446, 509, 514, 515, 517, 518, 553*).

Support for the identity of the neurohormone of the neuromuscular junction as acetylcholine in most species is also afforded by the high and specific sensitivity of this region to acetylcholine (*97, 391, 392*) and by the high concentration there of acetylcholinesterase, the enzyme specifically catalyzing the hydrolytic destruction of acetylcholine (*154, 157*).

There is a considerable body of evidence pointing to the conclusion, which has not gone unchallenged (*303*), that the function of the vesicles present in such profusion in the motor nerve terminals is to act as storage depots of acetylcholine, although as yet it has not proved feasible to achieve physical isolation of these bodies in intact condition and uncontaminated with other components from the neuromuscular junction so as to permit direct chemical analysis in analogous fashion to the successful work (*110, 111, 193, 451, 620, 621*) with the presynaptic vesicles occurring in the primary neurones of the interneuronal synapses of brain tissue. Thus, following earlier fallacious conclusions that mitochondrial binding was responsible for the lack of free diffusion shown by the acetylcholine of nervous tissue (*56, 87, 90*), application of sophisticated centrifugation techniques to guinea pig brain and subsequent analysis of the various fractions (*451, 620, 621*) clearly revealed that the highest concentrations of the neurohormone were associated with the presynaptic vesicles, while analogous studies with rat brain (*110, 111, 193*) revealed the vesicles to contain high concentrations not only of acetylcholine, but also of gangliosides, phospholipids, and cholesterol. In the cases of both the guinea pig and the rat the presynaptic vesicles appeared to have been isolated unchanged as far as could be revealed by electron microscopy. Unfortunately, however, these demonstrations of the storage of acetylcholine by the presynaptic vesicles of brain tissue do not afford unequivocal evidence that the vesicles have a role in transsynaptic transmission. In the first place the evidence (*162, 456*) that acetylcholine does, in fact, have a transmitter function in the brain is somewhat meager and in the second place complications arise from the apparent existence (*202*) of both excitatory and inhibitory transmitters at the interneuronal synapses in the central nervous system. Nevertheless, the obvious morphological similarities between the interneuronal synapse and the neuromuscular junction provide strong circumstantial evidence that there is essentially similar physiological function within the two types of unit. Thus the neurotransmitter role of acetylcholine at the neuromuscular junction is generally considered to point to its having an identical function at interneuronal synapses, while the demonstration of the storage of acetylcholine by the presynaptic vesicles in the brain is considered as legitimate evidence for an analogous role for the vesicles at the neuromuscular junction. It is probably also legitimate to admit as evidence of acetylcholine storage by the vesicles of the somatic motor nerve terminals the demonstrations (*190, 192, 478*) that stimulation of autonomic cholinergic nerves by means of supramaximal pulses leads to a distinct reduction in the number of vesicles in the terminals of these nerves. Again, electron microscopic studies employing the rat diaphragm (*353a,b*) on the effects of the drug HC-3, which selectively depresses the uptake of choline by the nerve terminals, have shown that this compound reduces the number but not the shape or volume of the vesicles in unstimulated preparations. With stimulated preparations it reduces vesicle numbers still further, as well as inducing a fall in vesicle volume, but still leaves the vesicle shape unchanged.

Further evidence that the vesicles in the motor nerve terminals are the storage sites of acetylcholine (*179, 180*) is provided by the observation that when the neuromuscular junction is at rest there is a continual intermittent production of miniature endplate potentials attributable to a continual release of quantal units of chemical mediator, insufficient in themselves to trigger a contractile response in the muscle (*97, 228*), on the grounds that random rupture of individual vesicles would afford a completely rational explanation of this phenomenon. On the other hand, expulsion of acetyl-choline simultaneously from a number of vesicles in response to a nerve impulse would adequately explain the production of a sufficient quantity of the neurohormone to ensure a response by the muscle (*85, 412, 413*). Calculation of the number of molecules of acetylcholine which would fill the volume of a single vesicle based on the assumption that the acetylcholine molecules will occupy the same volume as they do in the crystalline state (*118*) when taken in conjunction with the experimentally determined minimal amount of acetylcholine required to trigger the response of a single muscle fiber (*380*) suggest that something of the order of ten vesicles are involved in the synchronous process.

The exact way in which this simultaneous release of a number of quantal units of acetylcholine is achieved is still largely unestablished, although it is presumably a complex process and must depend upon the physical properties of certain components of the surface of the vesicle. Calcium ions are known to play an essential part (*186, 222, 325, 350, 437*) and it would seem that at least two (*326*) and possibly as many as four (*196b, 505a*) different calcium ion complexes are involved. In the light of the known ability of calcium ions to enter nerves during impulse propagation (*317*) it is possible that calcium ions pass from complex to complex within the terminal membranes during the propagation of the action potential into the nerve terminals (*328, 361*) to play a role in the release of acetylcholine from the vesicles (*184, 256, 326, 426*).

A plausible hypothesis as to the mechanism involved in the synchronous release of multiple quanta of acetylcholine from the presynaptic vesicles into the synaptic clefts of the interneuronal synapses of brain tissue assigns a key role to gangliosides (*111, 112*). These compounds, which are complex glycolipids having molecular constitutions of the type shown in **II** (*397, 402*), are postulated to act by virtue of their ability to exist as monomers or small molecular aggregates in nonpolar solvents on the one hand, but to exist as micellar aggregates having molecular weights of the order of 2 to 3×10^5 in aqueous media (*5, 58, 234, 258, 324, 372, 527, 588*) on the other, with there being an extremely fast rate of dissociation and association on transfer between aqueous and lipid phases. On the assumption that the presynaptic vesicle is made up of a protein matrix filled out with lipid material consisting mainly of cholesterol, phospholipids, and gangliosides (cf. *196a*), it is reasonable to conclude that when the primary neurone is at rest the gangliosides

II

will be in contact with the aqueous cytoplasm and so exist in the form of mixed micelles or lamellar sheets with the phospholipids and cholesterol. Possession of a net negative charge by the vesicles (5) serves to ensure electrostatic repulsion away from the polarized presynaptic membrane with its negatively charged inner surface (42) in the absence of a nerve impulse. However, on arrival of the nerve action potential the reversal of polarization suffered by the presynaptic membrane together with accompanying removal of hydration barriers (32) would be expected to produce physical contact between an appreciable number of vesicles and the lipid material of the membrane (330), causing the gangliosides to dissociate from the aggregated form. The polar acetylcholine molecules, believed to be bound to phosphatidylcholine and cholesterol within the mixed micellar structure (111), would then find themselves in an unfavorable lipid environment and so be forced through the presynaptic membrane into the synaptic cleft. With repolarization of the presynaptic membrane the vesicles, minus the disgorged acetylcholine, would be repelled from the membrane, and the gangliosides, coming into contact with the aqueous cytoplasm within the primary neurone, would once more assume a micellar form. The completion of the cycle would then involve the storage of a fresh supply of acetylcholine within the vesicle, whether this be taken up already formed or in the form of choline prior to subsequent acetylation.

Direct transfer of this hypothesis to events at the neuromuscular junction is handicapped by lack of full knowledge of the chemical entities occurring there but as the general principles involved are not necessarily dependent upon gangliosides and phosphatidylcholine per se (249) it is conceivable that an analogous type of process is in operation.

The role of calcium ions in the release of the acetylcholine from the vesicles is perhaps indicated by investigations (502a) as to the effects of inorganic ions on the distribution of gangliosides in lipid–aqueous biphasic systems. Where calcium ions are present in the lipid phase at concentrations between 5 and 160 mM, the gangliosides partition into the aqueous phase, but when the concentration of calcium ions in the lipid phase falls below 5 mM or rises above 160 mM, the gangliosides enter the lipid phase, while the presence of both protein and calcium ions causes the gangliosides to localize at the lipid–aqueous interface. Sodium, potassium, and magnesium ions do not show analogous effects on the ganglioside distribution. Thus, as has been suggested by Simpson (544a), it seems likely that, after moving through the nerve terminal membrane to the interior, the calcium ions acting in conjunction with the protein of the vesicle serve to orientate the vesicle at the cytoplasm–membrane interface.

Once in the junctional cleft, the liberated acetylcholine is considered to diffuse across the cleft and act on the muscle endplate, but that the process is by no means a simple one is suggested by the existence of the prejunctional component (31, 144, 329, 446, 509, 514, 515, 517, 518, 553) to the actions of the neurohormone, and it may even be that a prejunctional action of the acetylcholine initially liberated in response to a nerve impulse is necessary to achieve liberation of the bulk of the acetylcholine required to act at the muscle endplate (373).

It is assumed that the first step in the reaction of acetylcholine with the sensitive surface of the muscle endplate is the formation of a reversible complex with a specific membrane component which is referred to as the cholinergic receptor and which is generally considered to involve a protein or a phospholipid–protein complex (616). In the case of focally innervated fibers this interaction then triggers the following sequence of events which provides the means of amplification of the current flowing in the nerve impulse.

1. The potential difference between the inside and the outside of the resting endplate membrane, dependent upon its selective permeability to potassium ions with their higher intracellular than extracellular concentrations (42, 360) and to chloride ions (86) with their higher extracellular than intracellular

concentrations, is reduced through the induction of an increased indiscriminate permeability to a variety of small anions and cations (*180, 314, 357–359, 470, 566, 567*). This produces the concurrent generation of a graded, nonpropagating, potential difference between the outer surface of the endplate and the rest of the muscle membrane and it is this potential difference which constitutes the endplate potential (*203–206, 273*).

2. At a critical threshold value the endplate potential induces local circuit currents of high density to flow in the adjacent areas of the muscle fiber membrane (*470*), serving to increase its permeability to sodium ions.

3. Sodium ions pass through the muscle fiber membrane from the exterior along their concentration gradient to reverse the resting potential of the membrane giving rise to a self-propagating "all or nothing" action potential (*314, 340, 470*) which traverses the membrane outward in both directions from the point of innervation toward the tendons and triggers the contractile mechanism to bring about contraction.

4. During the refractory period associated with the propagation of the muscle action potential ($\sim$2 msec), the acetylcholine is hydrolytically destroyed by the enzyme acetylcholinesterase (*15, 438, 463, 554*), the concentration of which would seem to be greatest immediately postjunctionally (*29, 30, 158, 262, 374, 375, 522*), thus permitting repolarization of the muscle endplate (*16, 224, 362, 580, 581*). The remainder of the muscle fiber membrane becomes repolarized due to an efflux of potassium ions down their concentration gradient (*315*) and extrusion of sodium ions via an increased activity of the "sodium pump" mechanism (*150, 176, 194, 316, 366, 555*).

5. As the muscle fiber action potential traverses the membrane there is a rapid release of calcium ions from internal stores within the muscle and these ions pass into the immediate environment of the two contractile proteins actin and myosin, where they produce interaction between these proteins giving rise to shortening and development of tension in the muscle fiber. The speed of shortening is believed to depend upon the adenosinetriphosphatase activity of the particular muscle. When the action potential has passed away from a given section of the muscle fiber, the calcium ions are removed from the environment of the actin and the myosin and are once more sequestered in the store, which is probably located in the interior of the sarcoplasmic reticulum. With the lowering of the calcium ion concentration in their environment the contractile proteins become inactivated and the muscle returns to rest. Fuller details of the excitation–contraction coupling process are given in two recent reviews (*283a, 456a*).

In this way a single nerve impulse gives rise to a single muscle action potential and so there results a single contraction of the muscle fiber of brief duration.

The full chemical identities of the substances responsible for the ion fluxes in the membrane of the muscle fiber are unknown but it is believed that anionic heads of phospholipids play an important role as do conformational changes induced in the membrane proteins during passage of an action potential (536).* The fact that calcium ions act as a stabilizing element in electrical excitation of membranes (244), while there is a competitive interaction between local anesthetics and calcium ions in artificial phospholipid systems as well as in nerve membrane (54, 55, 229, 545), strongly supports the theory that calcium ions associated with the anionic groups of phospholipids perform a "gating" function controlling the fluxes of sodium and potassium ions during the action potential in nerve (272), and hence also in muscle, although whether the calcium ion fluxes initiate the conformational changes in the protein (cf. 249) or occur as a result of them is not established. Recent studies (550) on the pH sensitivity of action potential generation in single muscle fibers indicate that the membrane units associated with the ion fluxes have a $pK_a \approx 5$, which would not be inconsistent (54, 260, 526) with their being the phosphoric group of phosphatidylethanolamine (**III**) or the phosphoric or carboxylic group of phosphatidylserine (**IV**). Further support for the conclusion that it is phosphoryl groups which are actually involved has been provided by the fact that divalent uranyl ions, known to have an ability to complex with phosphate, abolish action potential generation (550) as does treatment (583) of muscle fibers with phospholipase C from *Clostridium welchii*—an enzyme which specifically hydrolyzes the phosphate ester linkage of lecithin (**V**).

It would seem that all conducting membranes are sensitive to acetylcholine, as evidenced, for example, by its effects on nerves, especially mammalian nonmyelinated (C) nerve fibers, where, despite argument to the contrary (e.g., 461), the response would appear to be without physiological significance (520, 521). However, the degree of sensitivity of different membranes to this agent varies considerably. In the case of vertebrate striated muscle, the character of the response to acetylcholine (or to substances with a similar action) is dependent upon the area of each muscle fiber membrane that is highly sensitive to its action. With a fresh preparation of most focally innervated muscles it is only the endplates of the fibers which are sensitive to reasonable concentrations of acetylcholine (97, 157, 228, 393, 453) (although massive doses will affect the rest of the muscle fiber membrane) and application of exogenous acetylcholine in small doses to the endplates from a micropipet by iontophoresis (179, 381, 382, 469, 562) will reproduce the same response in the muscle as occurs under natural physiological activation (182). On the other hand, microinjection of the neurohormone into the interior of the

---

* Further evidence supporting the important role of conformational changes in macromolecules of the muscle membrane during the action potential has recently been obtained (123a) from studies of changes in turbidity, birefringence and fluorescence in suitably treated muscle preparations.

$$CH_2\text{---}O\text{---}\underset{\underset{O}{\|}}{C}\text{---}R$$

$$CH\text{---}O\text{---}\underset{\underset{O}{\|}}{C}\text{---}R'$$

$$CH_2\text{---}O\text{---}\underset{\underset{O}{|}}{\overset{\overset{O}{\uparrow}}{P}}\text{---}OCH_2CH_2NH_2$$

III

$$CH_2\text{---}O\text{---}\underset{\underset{O}{\|}}{C}\text{---}R$$

$$CH\text{---}O\text{---}\underset{\underset{O}{|}}{\overset{\overset{O}{\uparrow}}{P}}\text{---}OCH_2\text{---}CH\text{---}NH_2, \quad C{=}O, \quad O$$

$$CH_2\text{---}O\text{---}\underset{\underset{O}{\|}}{C}\text{---}R'$$

IV

$$CH_2\text{---}O\text{---}\underset{\underset{O}{\|}}{C}\text{---}R$$

$$CH\text{---}O\text{---}\underset{\underset{O}{\|}}{C}\text{---}R'$$

$$CH_2\text{---}O\text{---}\underset{\underset{O}{|}}{\overset{\overset{O}{\uparrow}}{P}}\text{---}OCH_2CH_2\overset{+}{N}{\underset{\diagdown CH_3}{\overset{\diagup CH_3}{\text{---}CH_3}}}$$

V

muscle fiber behind the endplate is without effect (*179–181*). These experiments thus provide compelling evidence that the acetylcholine-sensitive areas are confined to the outer surface of the endplate.

When endogenous acetylcholine is protected against inactivation by prior administration of an anticholinesterase drug, a single nerve impulse will cause the repetitive firing of focally innervated fibers which is manifested as fasciculations in the muscle mass accompanied by a potentiation of the maximal twitch tension. Moreover, since the fasciculations involve synchronous contractions of the muscle fibers within a motor unit, rather than asynchronous fibrillations of individual cells, and since the repetitive muscle action potentials are accompanied by repetitive action potentials in the nerve terminals (*232, 446*), it is clear that some sort of action, direct or indirect, on the nerve terminals is involved with integration via axon reflexes providing the observed synchronization. Accumulated evidence (e.g., *52, 518, 551, 619*) rules out the earlier suggestions (*205, 419*) that the generation of the nerve terminal action potentials results from an ephaptic back-excitation by the action currents generated in the muscle, especially since it is now known (*516, 553*) that the individual spikes of the action potentials in the nerve terminals immediately precede each muscle action potential spike. It would now seem generally agreed that the repetitive muscle action potentials arise directly in response to the repetitive firing of the nerve, but there is some controversy as to whether the anticholinesterase drugs themselves exert a direct action on the nerve terminals. Against evidence (*514, 516, 552*) which has been advanced in support of a direct action on the nerve terminals by the anticholinesterase drugs, all of which appear to induce repetitive firing of focally innervated fibers in response to a single nerve impulse (*31, 52, 509, 515, 517, 594, 617–619*) unless they also possess a postjunctional blocking action (*51*), must be set the possibility that the repetitive nerve action potentials are arising from a depolarizing action of transmitter acetylcholine on the unmyelinated nerve terminal membranes (*329*) in the absence of functional acetylcholinesterase, especially during the enhanced period of excitability corresponding to the negative after-potential.

When the muscle endplate of a focally innervated fiber is exposed to high concentrations of acetylcholine (*19, 639*) in the presence of an anticholinesterase drug so as to prevent its inactivation, whether it be exogenous acetylcholine, or endogenous acetylcholine caused to build up through repeated stimulation of the motor nerve, the large and prolonged endplate potential leads to initial stimulation which is then followed by a block of conduction in the adjacent muscle fiber membrane (*109*). This depolarization block, as it is termed, is characterized by a failure (after an initial brief series of contractions) of the fiber to undergo further contractions since the disappearance of excitability in the muscle fiber membrane immediately surrounding the endplate prevents propagation of an action potential away from the endplate. As manifested at the gross level the end result is a flaccid muscular paralysis.

In the case of multiply innervated muscle fibers a somewhat different situation pertains. Here a high proportion of the surface of the fibers is sensitive to acetylcholine as a result of the multiple innervation and two types of response to nerve impulses are seen. In the first type (which is the sole response given by the multiply innervated fibers of the frog), in place of the propagated all-or-none action potentials characteristic of focally innervated fibers, the muscle fiber membrane responds to the release of acetylcholine at numerous points on its surface by the development of a number of relatively long-lasting localized graded depolarizations (*394, 395*). These may owe their duration, at least in part, to the much lower concentration of acetylcholinesterase occurring in the subneural apparatus of these fibers than occurs with focally innervated fibers (*155, 167*). The localized graded depolarizations affect the contractile mechanism in their immediate vicinity only, but since the junctional regions are densely scattered over a wide area, the nonpropagated depolarizations can activate the contractile mechanism over most of its length. Each localized graded depolarization is analogous (cf. *107, 395*) to the endplate potential in a focally innervated fiber and successive nerve impulses result in the development of a slow graded tension in the fiber instead of repetitive firing as is the case with a focally innervated fiber. The second type of response is seen in the multiply innervated fibers of the fowl and pigeon, which, in addition to their ability to respond in the same way as the multiply innervated fibers of the frog, are also capable of propagated electrical activity (18, 268, 269) similar to that of focally innervated fibers, thus exhibiting characteristics intermediate between the two extreme types.

At one time is was considered (95) that, under normal conditions, the nerve terminals of multiply innervated fibers in contrast to those of focally innervated fibers (487) did not release an excess of acetylcholine—thus providing a safety margin and at the same time making possible the development of the slow graded tension in the fiber in response to successive nerve impulses—but recent work (228a) has revealed that the junctions in multiply innervated chicken muscles are less sensitive to acetylcholine than those in focally innervated muscles. Where high concentrations of acetylcholine are permitted to build up, as in the presence of an anticholinesterase drug, the whole membrane of the fiber becomes progressively further depolarized and keeps the contractile mechanism in a state of continued activation, thus leaving the muscle fiber in a prolonged state of contraction via the excitation–contraction coupling mechanism. These phenomena of graded tension and prolonged contraction thus stand in complete contrast to the situation pertaining with focally innervated fibers. The prolonged contraction produced in the absence of propagating action potentials is termed a contracture and is seen as a rigid paralysis of the muscle mass.

A somewhat similar situation is encountered with chronically denervated focally innervated muscle (17, 266) or with focally innervated muscle exposed to the prolonged action of the local anesthetic marcaine (549). Here, as a result of changes as yet incompletely understood (580) but which appear to involve the absence of acetylcholinesterase (17) as well as changes (274, 583) in the structure of lecithin (V) the main phospholipid of the muscle membrane, increased sensitivity gradually spreads outward from the endplate until in the case of mammalian muscle the entire muscle fiber surface becomes equally as sensitive as the endplate to exogenous acetylcholine. On close arterial injection acetylcholine will induce a quick initial contraction accompanied by a burst of propagated action potentials, followed, if the dose is large enough, by a slow contracture during which all propagated electrical activity ceases and localized potentials bring about progressive depolarization of the whole membrane.

Interestingly, fetal muscle fibers are sensitive to acetylcholine over their entire length but with continued development the chemosensitive zone recedes from the tendon ends until it becomes confined to the adult area at the junctional regions a few weeks after birth (196, 266). The acetylcholine-sensitive area of a chronically denervated muscle fiber also recedes from the tendon ends to the site of the neuromuscular junction when the motor nerve fiber is allowed to reinnervate the former endplate (454) or made to innervate formerly endplate-free parts of the membrane (455). These phenomena make it apparent that intact nerve endings in some way exert a control limiting the chemosensitive area of the muscle fiber membrane, but the manner in which this is achieved is not known, although acetylcholine itself is most probably involved. A further interesting phenomenon is that with denervated muscle, after a time, there is resumption of spontaneous activity at the endplate owing to the Schwann cell taking over production of acetylcholine (47).

C. THE ACETYLCHOLINE RECEPTOR

As already indicated, it is the usual convention to consider acetylcholine as interacting with a component of the postsynaptic membrane, termed the receptor, in order to facilitate description of the initiation of the postsynaptic events involved in the translation of motor nerve impulses into muscular contraction; and since abolition of the response of the receptor to acetylcholine is clearly one way of achieving neuromuscular blockade, a full understanding of the nature and functioning of the receptor becomes fundamental to any rational approach to the intentional design of new neuromuscular blocking agents. However, when due consideration is given to detailed correlation of physiological function with chemical structure at the molecular level, it becomes evident that it is meaningless to consider the actual site of interaction with acetylcholine as a discrete entity in isolation from the other molecular units responsible for passing on the postsynaptic impetus (37), even if the binding site of the neurohormone were to prove to be made up solely from atomic groupings confined within a single macromolecule rather than from functional groupings on different individual molecules suitably disposed in three-dimensional juxtaposition. Furthermore, it is not inconceivable that acetylcholine, in common with other exogenous drug molecules introduced at the postsynaptic membrane, is capable of being bound to a number of sites, only one of which necessarily evokes a train of events manifesting itself as an ultimate physiological or pharmacological response, since ability to complex with appropriate simpler molecules is a fundamental property of macromolecules. Thus, instead of being simply a case of interaction between two molecular species, the problem of drug receptor interaction becomes one of *molecular ecology* in which any primary effects exerted at specific points within the system can be considered only in the context of their influence on all units of a heterogeneous molecular population, presumably composed of an assembly of several macromolecules [which probably include lecithin and at least one protein (*220, 616*)], ordered water molecules (*37*), and inorganic ions. This molecular assembly will obviously be held in a somewhat loose combination in which spatial relationships are crucial and would not be expected to be capable of chemical isolation as a whole. Nor can it be expected that any macromolecule which did in fact contain the full elements of the acetylcholine binding site would necessarily retain a tertiary structure having any close resemblance to the three-dimensional geometry pertaining *in situ* once it was removed from its natural environment. Accordingly it would seem obvious that any attempts to isolate the acetylcholine receptor as a meaningful chemical entity have a very high probability of being abortive, as indeed has proved to be the case with work on the electric organ of the eel *Electrophorus electricus* (*130–134, 212–219, 298–300, 589*), which is considered to have close physiological similarities to mammalian muscle endplates (*4, 129, 231*), and on sciatic nerve tissue (*250, 473*), although work with human skeletal muscle (*280, 281, 467, 468*) has resulted in the isolation of a ribonucleoprotein having some of the properties to be expected of the acetylcholine binding site. It is also apparent (*481*) that a key factor will be the overall rate at which interactions and recovery occur throughout the receptor system *in toto*, although again this cannot be considered in isolation (cf. *12*), especially in the absence of any clear identification of which particular step from among the multiple steps, which are doubtlessly involved between chemoreception and manifestation of response, in fact constitutes the rate-limiting stage.

When exogenous drug molecules, such as those of certain neuromuscular blocking agents, are present at the muscle endplate the pharmacological effects observed are frequently said to result from a competition between the drug molecules and acetylcholine for the cholinergic receptors. This is perhaps an unfortunate expression since it has been misconstrued by some authors as meaning that there is necessarily a competition for the actual acetylcholine binding sites. What is really implied is that the exogenous molecules compete with acetylcholine *for exertion of the predominant influence on the receptor system as a whole*. Although this *may* involve direct competition with acetylcholine for the acetylcholine binding sites, it would seem probable that many of the exogenous drug molecules which produce an effect detectable pharmacologically, in fact, influence the system from areas involving other binding sites. Attempts to take this situation into account have been made as described in Volume I of this treatise using the concept of interaction with "other receptors" (the so-called noncompetitive inhibiting drugs). However, as this distinction can only be made on the basis of dose–response curves, which may not be sensitive enough indicators—especially as their form is so general, complying with the Law of Mass Action, the Langmuir isotherm, and the Michaelis–Menten equation—this approach may not uncover finer differences in basic modes of action.

The very chemical constitutions of macromolecules such as proteins and phospholipids, with their combinations of hydrophilic and lipophilic moieties and reactive functional groups, will provide innumerable potential binding sites for exogenous molecules, and those actually called into play in any given instance may not even be on the same macromolecules as could be involved in the constitution of the acetylcholine binding site. Furthermore, it is conceivable that some exogenous drug molecules could find binding sites such that the receptor system remained uninfluenced with the result that there would be no detectable pharmacological effect. The particular sites which in fact become binding sites can be presumed to vary from drug to drug [as is indeed evidenced by experimentally demonstrable differences in the binding of various radiolabeled neuromuscular blocking agents in the mouse diaphragm (612)], and the selection in any given instance can be expected to depend primarily upon a high thermodynamic favorability of complex formation with the specific drug molecule in question. Obviously the potential binding site offering the most favorable electrostatic, van der Waals, London, and hydrophobic interactions in terms of the chemical topography of a given drug molecule will be the unit most likely to be involved as the binding site for that drug, but there is a strong possibility that several receptor units could be involved either simultaneously or sequentially. Certainly this would not be inconsistent with studies (484) on the "muscarinic" receptors in guinea pig intestinal smooth muscle where analysis of the experimental data by an analog computer has revealed that these receptors are best represented in terms of a multicompartment model (cf. 183), nor would it be inconsistent with the time-dependent changes in the nature of the pharmacological effect (16, 109, 160, 313, 349, 575, 640) and in the nature of their binding in the mouse diaphragm (161, 570, 612) shown by depolarizing neuromuscular blocking agents. The probability of multiple binding sites being involved also casts doubt on the validity of calculations as to the number of individual receptor units in the endplate (607–609, 611). Again, rate phenomena must be taken into consideration (481, 483). Also there is the possibility that more than one molecule of acetylcholine is simultaneously involved (cf. 34a).

The way in which interaction at one point in the receptor system influences the rest of the system, whether it be acetylcholine or an exogenous drug molecule which is implicated, undoubtedly involves the intercession of reversible conformational perturbations (35) or allosteric transitions (136, 356, 457) induced throughout the tertiary structures of the macromolecules, resulting in crucial alterations in the spatial distribution of ionic groups (220, 616) and accompanying redistribution of water molecules. In this way it is possible that the ion fluxes responsible for the depolarization of the endplate (180, 314,

357–359, 470, 566, 567) could be initiated at areas relatively remote from the acetylcholine binding sites rather than at areas in their immediate vicinity.

From the foregoing it is apparent that it is quite impossible to gain full appreciation of structure–action relationships at the cholinergic receptor in molecular terms in the absence of a full knowledge of the precise constitution of the receptor system as a whole (*575*) and, further, that comparisons of the molecular structures of the various drugs acting there, even where these drugs appear to produce identical pharmacological responses, run the grave risk of being grossly misleading since they are based on completely inadequate information. Similarly the different mathematical models which may be used to differentiate various types of dose–response phenomena do little more than underline the real existence of different types of drug–receptor interactions. In themselves they afford no specific indication of the actual molecular processes involved, and it is probable that a number of fundamentally different molecular processes could in fact give similar if not identical dose–response data.

Some fragmentary knowledge of component units of the receptor system is available. As in the case of the membrane groups responsible for the conduction of the muscle action potential, it seems that the negatively charged groups of phospholipids are essential components of the receptor system (*127, 471, 583*) and emphasis on the possible role which these groups or other negatively charged groups have to play is implicit in a simplified pictorial representation of the acetylcholine receptor as a pore in the endplate membrane having a negatively charged rim (*606*), which has certain merits in rationalizing the different types of interference with normal physiological events shown by different groups of neuromuscular blocking agents. That the phosphoryl groups of phosphatidylethanolamine or phosphatidylserine could be involved is, perhaps, indicated by the nature of the pH dependence of the sensitivity of single chronically denervated muscle fibers to acetylcholine (*550*), but lack of knowledge of the exact relationship in biochemical terms between the motor endplate of normal muscle and the membrane of chronically denervated muscle, with its acquired sensitivity to acetylcholine and associated biochemical changes (*274*), prevents unequivocal transfer of this knowledge to the normal endplate. That there are differences between the normal endplate and the membrane of chronically denervated muscle is indicated by the fact that drugs such as (+)-tubocurarine (*81, 424, 434*) and gallamine (*102*), which are devoid of detectable depolarizing activity at the normal endplate region, may initially produce depolarization and a biphasic contraction–contracture response in denervated muscle, since the membrane of denervated muscle unlike the normal endplate exhibits both chemosensitivity and electrical excitability.

It has also been demonstrated that high frequency nerve stimulation, or the application of acetylcholine after inhibition of acetylcholinesterase, produces a disorientation of the regular arrangement of protein particles accompanied by a rearrangement of lipids in the muscle endplate (*167*).

In the light of the necessary similarities between the acetylcholine binding sites initiating postjunctional events and those on acetylcholinesterase, dictated by the fact that both entities have to complex with the same molecular species, attention has recently been focused on the possibility that the dual functions of hydrolysis and postsynaptic activation are, in fact, performed by the same protein (*35, 220, 221, 355, 525, 635, 636, 642, 643*), thus affording ready explanation of the rapidity with which the hydrolysis of the neurohormone is achieved after initiation of postsynaptic events.

Actually a number of variants of this idea have been proposed, but an attractive theme running through several of the proposals (e.g., *220, 221, 564, 616*) is that when the endplate is at rest the choline moieties of lecithin molecules, or other similar units incorporated in the structure of the postsynaptic membrane, are complexed to acetylcholinesterase, and that when acetylcholine molecules cross the junctional cleft they successfully compete with these membrane units for the prerogative of complexing with the enzyme molecules, thus dissociating them from the membrane and simultaneously setting in train events leading to the hydrolysis of the acetylcholine molecules. Certainly the efficacy of lecithinases in liberating acetylcholinesterase from structural material (*401*) would support this hypothesis. Such a process, in which acetylcholine can be regarded as acting as an antimetabolite of the membrane groups, could involve a simple direct displacement of the latter with the acetylcholine molecules then bonding to some or all of the self-same enzyme groups previously involved in the bonding of the membrane groups, as has been suggested by at least two groups of workers (*220, 221, 564*), but this is not necessarily so. Displacement of the membrane groups from the enzyme could equally well occur by a process, such as that portrayed in Fig. 2, in which no enzyme grouping involved in the binding of the enzyme to the membrane is also involved in the bonding of acetylcholine to the enzyme. Moreover, displacement of the membrane from the enzyme can be expected to produce a reorientation of the tertiary structure of the acetylcholinesterase molecule (*627*) and this could occur in such a way as to bring previously remote peptide units into close juxtaposition for the constitution of a multicomponent functional hydrolytic site for the acetylcholine molecule, which can thus be considered to create the conditions necessary for its own destruction in accord with the tenets of the "induced fit" theory (*376–378*). It is to be emphasized, however, that Fig. 2 represents only one of a large number of possibilities, especially since one molecule of acetylcholinesterase appears to possess a large number of hydrolytic sites (*452*), and it is not intended in any way as a literal portrayal of the events which actually take place. It is presented solely in order to focus attention on one general type of process which may reasonably be expected to occur.

Such a model as Fig. 2 could conceivably accommodate evidence which at

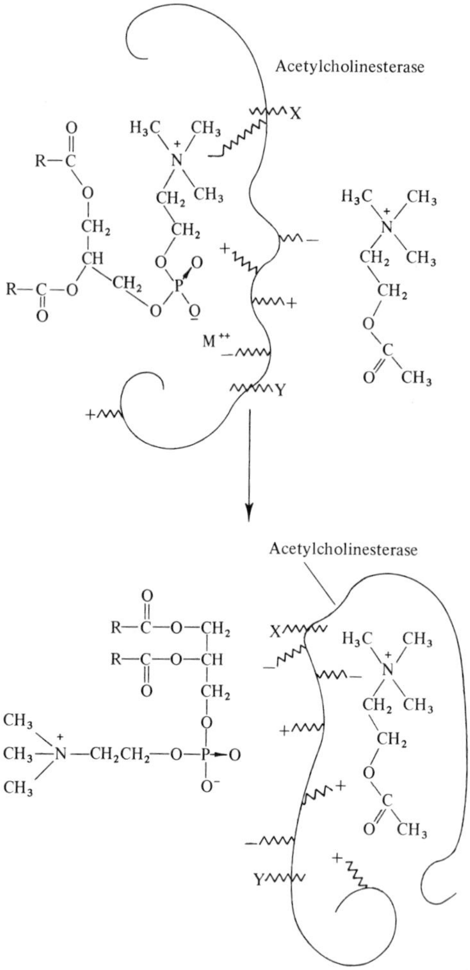

Fig. 2. Schematic representation of displacement of membrane component from acetyl-cholinesterase by acetylcholine via a process in which acetylcholine complexes to sites on the acetylcholinesterase molecule not previously engaged in binding to the membrane component. The constitution of the multicomponent hydrolytic site of the acetylcholinesterase molecule, involving peptide units, which could be far removed from one another in the peptide sequence, is considered to occur via a conformational perturbation as shown. X and Y represent potential cleavage points of the acetylcholinesterase molecule by proteo-lytic enzymes. These are considered to occur in positions such that retention of structural identity by the portion of the acetylcholinesterase molecule lying between them still permits functional activation of postjunctional events through displacement of the membrane component by acetylcholine, but detachment of the portions of the enzyme lying outside these points prevents constitution of the active hydrolytic site.

first sight might seem to militate against acetylcholinesterase being an integral part of the cholinergic receptor. Thus the high cholinolytic potency of atropine but its low affinity for purified acetylcholinesterase (600a) and the blockade of the receptor system by thiol reagents (134a, 221a) but their lack of effect on the isolated enzyme (356a) as well as the opposing relative orders of potencies with respect to receptor activation and acetylcholinesterase inhibition shown by a number of compounds (31a) could be adequately explained by assuming that these compounds attack at sites involving either the membrane unit alone or both the membrane unit and the enzyme molecule. Such attack would not be possible with the free enzyme. Again it is conceivable that displacement of the membrane from the enzyme by acetylcholine can still occur even where the enzyme unit has been modified. Thus the lack of inhibition of postsynaptic events by eserine and the organophosphorus compounds (281a) could have its origin in the enzyme, inactivated as far as its ability to constitute its active hydrolytic site is concerned through prior reaction with these agents, still suffering membrane displacement by acetylcholine.

That allosteric interactions and conformational changes such as those implicated above occur with preparations of acetylcholinesterase completely isolated from any membrane material [a situation where the enzyme may have physicochemical properties considerably different from those it exhibits in situ (37, 546)] is well supported experimentally. Thus it has been demonstrated by spectropolarographic methods (371b) that highly purified acetylcholinesterase from Electrophorus electricus undergoes changes in conformation when interacting with various substrates and inhibitors, while the fact that some neuromuscular blocking agents accelerate the inactivation of acetylcholinesterase by agents esterifying the key serine hydroxyl group of the active site whereas others retard this inactivation finds ready rationalization in terms of the involvement of different conformational changes (37b, 371a). Involvement of different binding sites on acetylcholinesterase with different drug molecules is illustrated by the facts that binding of (+)-tubocurarine to horse plasma cholinesterase is independent of whether or not the enzyme is inhibited by physostigmine or heat (644), that certain neuromuscular blocking agents when well bound to acetylcholinesterase act only as partially competitive inhibitors of acetylcholine hydrolysis even at high concentrations (136a), and that gallamine can accelerate decarbamylation of carbamylated acetylcholinesterase without inhibiting substrate hydrolysis, thus not being bound at the active site of the free enzyme (371a).

Finally, the conformational changes leading to the constitution of the multicomponent functional hydrolytic site in acetylcholinesterase only on interaction with acetylcholine in accord with the "induced fit" theory as outlined in Fig. 2 has close analogy with the situation shown to pertain with carboxypeptidase A (509a).

Similarly, Fig. 2 can be used to offer an explanation for the experimentally observed abolition of acetylcholinesterase activity at innervated endplates in the rat without accompanying alteration in the response of the muscle to acetylcholine (6) when the endplates are exposed to various proteolytic enzymes, if the cleavages of the acetylcholinesterase are confined to peptide linkages outside points X and Y. If this should be the case, there could well be sufficient polypeptide residue left bound to the membrane to be capable of displacement by acetylcholine and so permit initiation of normal post-junctional excitation, but elements of the acetylcholinesterase structure essential to the hydrolytic function are no longer present. Again, the different subcellular locations apparently adopted by radiolabeled neuromuscular blocking agents and by radiolabeled anticholinesterase drugs in the mouse diaphragm, as revealed by autoradiographic studies (606, 607, 612), could result from the two types of drug binding to different parts of the acetylcholin-esterase molecule, with each type inducing markedly different changes in the tertiary structure of the enzyme.

Although neither the full amino acid sequence nor the numerical positions in the linear polypeptide chain of the amino acid residues contributing to the "active site" or "active sites" of acetylcholinesterase [both of which may be subject to species variation (53, cf. 71)] are as yet established, evidence in support of a multicomponent functional hydrolytic site such as that just discussed has been advanced by Krupka (387–389) who also suggests possible conformational changes occurring in the enzyme during the course of the hydrolysis of acetylcholine. In the case of acetylcholinesterase from bovine erythrocytes, Krupka has postulated that at least five individual amino acid residues are implicated in constituting the active hydrolytic site. Of the five functional groups involved, the primary nucleophile, which initiates the hydrolysis through attack on the carbonyl group of the acetylcholine molecule with transfer of the acetyl group to the enzyme (628), would seem, as is the case with a number of esterases (378), to be the hydroxyl group of a serine unit as evidenced by stoichiometric studies employing ^{32}P-labeled diisopropyl-phosphofluoridate which inactivates the enzyme through selective phosphoryl-ation of this group (146, 533). Degradation of the phosphorylated enzyme from the electric eel revealed that the serine residue occurs within the unit Glu–Ser–Ala (533) but there is evidence that the sequence Glu–Ser–Gly–Ala is present in the acetylcholinesterase from bovine erythrocytes (185). Of the remaining four functional groups contributing to the hydrolysis of acetyl-choline, two would appear to be nitrogen atoms—one in each of the imidazole rings of two different histidine residues (387, 388). These basic groups, which have pK 5.5 and 6.3, apparently function, respectively, in aiding the transfer of the acetyl moiety from acetylcholine to the serine hydroxyl group of the enzyme and in the subsequent deacetylation of the acetylated enzyme (629, 630). An acidic group of pK 9.2 (possibly the phenolic group of a tyrosine residue) would appear to provide the proton for the newly generated hydroxyl group in the liberated choline and it is this group together with the imidazole ring nitrogen atom of pK 5.5 which constitute the classic "esteratic site" of acetylcholinesterase (464). The classic "anionic site" responsible for binding the cationic head of the acetylcholine molecule would appear to be a carboxylic anion in the side chain of an aspartic acid or glutamic acid residue. This anion is apparently situated within 5 Å of the imidazole ring nitrogen atom of pK 6.3 and on protonation of the latter suffers neutralization with the result that a newly generated choline molecule is repelled from the enzyme.

It is also possible that in the resting state acetylcholinesterase is actually acetylated on the serine residue rather than having a free serine hydroxyl group (35) and that displacement of the acetyl function to generate the free hydroxyl group capable of initiating the hydrolysis of acetylcholine forms one of the links in the chain of events conferring upon the acetylcholinesterase molecule the dual functions of initiator of postsynaptic events and hydrolytic inactivator of acetylcholine. If this is indeed the case, a function can, perhaps, be assigned to the continual discharge of quantal units of acetylcholine insufficient to activate the muscle endplate in the absence of a nerve impulse as manifested by the production of miniature endplate potentials (97, 228) in that such activity may be necessary to ensure continued acetylation of the acetylcholinesterase (35).

Until further knowledge of the intimate constitution of acetylcholinesterase becomes available, however, the exact processes involved in the hydrolysis of acetylcholine must remain a matter of conjecture, although some appreciation of the considerations which need to be taken into account can be gained from current knowledge of other enzymes. Thus the fact that more than one protein chain is necessary to make up the active form of certain enzymes (295) serves to underline the need to consider the possibility that more than one peptide chain is necessary for the functioning of acetylcholinesterase which is known to deaggregate in solutions of high ionic strength and to reaggregate to a single macromolecule in solutions of low ionic strength (275, 379), while the positions in the peptide sequence in bovine trypsin of the amino acid residues bearing the functional groups actually involved in the hydrolysis of the substrate (474) draws attention to the possibility of analogous distant sequential positions of the units comprising the active site in acetylcholinesterase. In bovine trypsin the active groups responsible for the hydrolytic cleavage of the substrate are the hydroxyl group of a serine residue occurring at position 177 of the peptide chain and the nitrogen atoms of imidazole rings in histidine residues occurring at positions 23 and 40 of the chain—functional groups which are, in fact, identical with three of the five postulated active functional groups of acetylcholinesterase from bovine erthrocytes. Consideration of the structure of bovine trypsin (474) also sheds light on one method by which some of the functional groups constituting the active sites in other enzymes may be held in the correct spatial juxtaposition, despite their being a considerable distance apart in the amino acid sequence, through the utilization of disulfide bridges between half-cystine residues. Thus in bovine trypsin half-cystine residues at positions 25 and 41 form a disulfide bridge in the immediate vicinity of the histidine residues at positions 23 and 40 while a further disulfide bridge between positions 173 and 183 occurs near the serine residue occupying position 177 in the polypeptide chain.

At the same time as the events leading up to the eventual hydrolysis of acetylcholine are occurring within the acetylcholinesterase–acetylcholine complex, other events, set in train by the release of the membrane from the acetylcholinesterase, can be expected to be occurring within the structure of the postsynaptic membrane. These events, which conceivably take place through the intercession of other conformational perturbations and accompanying redistribution of water molecules, can be expected to produce changes in the membrane permeability with the result that the ion fluxes responsible for the depolarization of the endplate are put into operation. Since the depolarization of the endplate is a graded response it would follow that the degree of depolarization is directly proportional to the number of individual membrane units displaced from acetylcholinesterase until the critical level of depolarization is achieved, but undoubtedly a safety factor is incorporated so that effective depolarization will result while a high proportion of acetylcholinesterase molecules remain bound to the membrane (cf. *607*). Such a situation would afford a basis for the concept of "spare receptors" (*475, 558*) but complications arise when this concept is applied to the action of exogenous molecules on account of the probability of the involvement of multiple binding sites and of binding sites not coincident with the acetylcholine binding sites.

Once the hydrolysis of acetylcholine into choline and acetic acid has been completed, it can be imagined that the membrane units will again enter complex formation with the acetylcholinesterase molecules, thus shutting off the ion fluxes by restoration of selective membrane permeability. The key to such a control mechanism for the ion fluxes would thus reside in the possession by acetylcholinesterase of a higher affinity for acetylcholine than for the membrane units but of a higher affinity for the membrane units than for choline and acetic acid—the cleavage products of acetylcholine. It is to be stressed, however, that none of these affinities need necessarily be of a particularly high order of magnitude and that affinities for acetylcholinesterase as measured *in vitro* may bear no relationship to those pertaining *in vivo*.

The isolation of a ribonucleoprotein from human skeletal muscle which, in addition to being precipitated from saline solution by (+)-tubocurarine in concentrations of the same order as will produce complete neuromuscular block *in vivo* [with this precipitation being inhibited or reversed by pharmacological antagonists of (+)-tubocurarine], also showed potent acetylcholinesterase activity (*280, 281, 467, 468*) would give further support for identity of one of the receptor constituents with acetylcholinesterase, but once again the *in vitro* preparation can not be expected (*37*) to possess the complete properties shown by the *in vivo* system. Interestingly, treatment of artificial lipid membranes with acetylcholinesterase from bovine erythrocytes gives a system having a number of the properties which would be expected of the cholinergic receptor (*185*).

Further evidence supporting the involvement of acetylcholinesterase as a unit of the cholinergic receptor is the observation that the ability of different alkyltrimethylammonium ions to accelerate the inhibition of acetylcholinesterase by methanesulfonyl fluoride (*37a, 37b*) almost exactly parallels their relative potencies at the receptor level (*598a*), a correlation which also exists with respect to the polymethonium depolarizing neuromuscular blocking agents (*37b*), and that the antidepolarizing neuromuscular blocking agents, in marked contrast to the depolarizers, retard the inhibition of the enzyme by methanesulfonyl fluoride (*37b*) thus reflecting exactly their different modes of action at the receptor. Similarly alkyltrimethylammonium ions accelerate the inhibition of acetylcholinesterase by carbamylating agents (*371a, 450a*) while antidepolarizing neuromuscular blocking agents accelerate the decarbamylation of the carbamylated enzyme (*371a*).

The ability of acetylcholine to promote incorporation of inorganic phosphate into phospholipids, particularly phosphatidylinositol and its biogenetic precursor, phosphatidic acid, has led to the proposal (*199a*) that increased permeability of the endplate results from acetylcholine-induced phosphodiesteric cleavage of membrane phosphatides, rather than simply from conformational changes in the membrane molecules, with the membrane-bound diglyceride then undergoing conversion into phosphatidylinositol. This phosphodiesteric cleavage could conceivably be initiated by the dissociation of the acetylcholinesterase from the membrane by acetylcholine.

In addition to detailed studies of the bonding characteristics of acetylcholine and related drugs (e.g., *126, 254*) attempts have been made to explain the interaction of acetylcholine with the receptor system in terms of the interactions present in acetylcholine in the crystalline state (*117, 119*) and to define the conformation adopted by acetylcholine at its binding site (*138a, 139, 444, 543a, 564*).*

D. Biosynthesis and Storage of Acetylcholine

Once acetylcholine has been inactivated by hydrolysis the liberated choline is believed to be taken up via an active "choline-carrier" mechanism (*432*) by the nerve terminals and reacetylated to acetylcholine which is bound in a physiologically inactive form in the vesicles awaiting release in response to a subsequent nerve impulse, thus completing the cycle uptake, synthesis,

* See Addendum, p. 530.

storage, release, distribution, initiation of postsynaptic events, and hydrolytic inactivation.

There would seem to be some dubiety as to whether acetylcholine synthesis occurs within the presynaptic vesicles or takes place in the cytoplasm of the nerve ending but work with brain tissue has indicated (428) that the enzyme responsible for choline acetylation, choline acetyl transferase, has a subcellular distribution in this situation which apparently varies according to species—being present in high concentrations in the cytoplasm in the case of the guinea pig and pigeon but being mainly associated with the vesicular fraction in the case of the rat or the rabbit. However, it is generally believed (243a) that choline acetylation probably occurs in the soluble cytoplasm of the nerve endings, after which the acetylcholine presumably passes through the vesicle membrane by some type of active transport mechanism. The acetyl group necessary for the acetylation of the choline is provided by acetyl coenzyme A (417, 460, 462) and it is the step involving transfer of the "active acetyl" from acetyl coenzyme A to choline which is specifically catalyzed by choline acetyl transferase (304).

IV. Mechanisms of Neuromuscular Blockade

From the foregoing synopsis it is immediately apparent that there are a number of potential points—both prejunctional and postjunctional—at which it should be theoretically possible to achieve a disruption of the normal events at the neuromuscular junction so as to produce neuromuscular blockade, and indeed drugs are now known which do, in fact, appear to achieve this end result via a primary action at one or another of the various theoretically possible sites. Quite apart from species variations, the situation is complicated, however, by the fact that many drugs acting as neuromuscular blocking agents exert an influence at more than one site, both with respect to the neuromuscular junction itself and with respect to other tissues in the animal body, as is only to be expected from considerations inherent in the theory of biological relativity (442). Moreover, with drugs acting at more than one site about the neuromuscular junction a tendency to block transmission at some sites may be accompanied by a tendency to facilitation at others, as is the case in mammals with benzoquinonium which shows both anticholinesterase activity (49, 322) and postjunctional blocking activity (68). Nevertheless, a number of drugs are known for which the relative specificity is sufficiently well marked to permit a valid discussion in terms of predominant actions at different points about the neuromuscular junction and some of these drugs will now be briefly discussed in terms of their varying modes of action.

A. PREJUNCTIONAL EVENTS SUSCEPTIBLE TO INTERFERENCE RESULTING IN NEUROMUSCULAR BLOCKADE

Basically prejunctional block depends upon a reduction in the quantity of acetylcholine released in response to a nerve impulse to a level below that required to produce the threshold endplate potential at which initiation of the muscle fiber action potential occurs. The more obvious ways in which prejunctional block might be induced would seem to be:

1. Prevention of the biosynthesis of acetylcholine in the nerve endings. This could be achieved in several ways, as for example by:
   (a) inhibition of uptake of choline by the nerve terminals,
   (b) inhibition of choline acetyl transferase,
   (c) depletion of acetyl coenzyme A by various means.
2. Prejunctional accumulation of a false transmitter, which, on release in response to a nerve impulse, would interfere with postjunctional events. Such a false transmitter could conceivably be taken up and stored as such, or it could result from a competition between an exogenous molecule and choline for the acetylation process prior to storage, thus inhibiting acetylcholine synthesis as well as later interfering with postjunctional events.
3. Prevention of the release of acetylcholine. This could be achieved in several ways, as for instance by:
   (a) interference with the action potential at the nerve terminals,
   (b) interference with the links between the action potential and the release of acetylcholine, including the role played by calcium ions,
   (c) stabilization of the vesicles.
4. Depletion of acetylcholine stores brought about, for example, by drugs displacing the neurohormone from its binding site in the vesicles or effecting the complete disruption of the vesicles. Depletion of acetylcholine stores in the vesicles could also be brought about by drugs preventing uptake of the neurohormone from the cytoplasm into the vesicles.

1. Inhibition of Acetylcholine Synthesis

At the present time the only known drugs which show a reasonable specificity for the neuromuscular junction while acting predominantly prejunctionally via an inhibition of acetylcholine synthesis would seem to be compounds which prevent the uptake of choline by the nerve terminals. Until recently (128a, 546a) no drug was known which acted as a direct specific choline acetyl transferase inhibitor, although nonspecific inhibition of this enzyme is doubtlessly brought about to some extent together with the inhibition of other enzymes by various drugs acting as general enzyme inhibitors. At the same time recent work (304a) has shown that the pharmacological activity of the styrylpyridine choline acetyl transferase inhibitors can not be attributed solely to inhibition of this enzyme alone.

Drugs capable of preventing acetylcholine synthesis through a depletion of acetyl coenzyme A by lowering the concentration of any of the various substances essential to the formation of the coenzyme including ATP, glucose, or oxygen, might reasonably be expected to inhibit acetyl coenzyme A formation in many situations throughout the body and so, in the absence of any selective affinity for the terminals of the motor nerves innervating striated muscle, would be so nonspecific in their pharmacological effects as to warrant no specific recognition as neuromuscular blocking agents. So far no drug inhibiting acetyl coenzyme A formation and at the same time showing the requisite specific affinity for the motor nerve terminals has been discovered.

The first compounds to be recognized as inducing neuromuscular blockade via a selective depression of the uptake of choline by the nerve terminals (585)—an action also exerted in minced brain tissue (259, 433) and ganglia (48)—were a series of tetracyclic bisquaternary ammonium salts derived from α,α'-dibromo-4,4'-bisacetophenone (422, 537) known as the hemicholiniums —the most active of the series being HC-3 which has structure VI. Although they also exert an action at the neuroeffector junction of autonomic cholinergic

VI

nerves (633), these drugs in moderate doses produce a neuromuscular block which is characteristically slow in onset and only follows upon a high frequency of stimulation of the nerve (76, 77, 135, 223, 226, 421, 507, 510, 537, 625) since it is dependent upon prior depletion of existing acetylcholine stored in the nerve endings. The block is readily reversed by choline (271, 511), and more slowly by choline esters which are first hydrolyzed to liberate free choline. In high doses, however, the hemicholiniums also exert a postjunctional action. It has also been suggested (432a) that HC-3 is transported to intracellular sites by combination with the choline carrier mechanism and may then compete with acetylcholine for intracellular binding sites.

Reinvestigation (72, 74, 75, 77–79, 103, 104, 223, 447, 531) of the triethyl analog of choline (VII), the effects of which were previously known to be reversed by choline (365), then showed that this compound exhibits similar

$$\overset{+}{Et_3N}—CH_2CH_2OH \quad .X^-$$

VII

actions to HC-3 at the neuromuscular junction, although it is less potent than HC-3, shows a relatively weaker postjunctional component to its actions, and is more readily reversed by choline than is HC-3. There is also some evidence that the triethyl analog of choline could be being acetylated in place of choline by choline acetyl transferase (*105, 500*) [although other workers (*173, 305*) have failed to detect acetylation of this compound by various preparations of choline acetyl transferase]* but the transmission failure appears to be the result of the absence of acetylcholine rather than the liberation of a false transmitter since the triethyl analog of acetylcholine is devoid of either stimulant or blocking activity at motor endplates in any concentration that could conceivably be liberated from the nerve endings (*74, 321*). However, since the diminished output of acetylcholine induced by the triethyl analog of choline appears to be first preceded by an initial increase in the amount of acetylcholine released in response to nerve impulses (*72*) and is then accompanied by an increased output of choline (*531*) it would appear that not only is the triethyl compound transported into the nerve endings in place of choline, but once there it displaces preformed acetylcholine and previously transported choline from intracellular binding sites as well, thus exhibiting a neurohormone depleting component to its overall actions.

Other drugs now known to exhibit a prejunctional interference with acetylcholine metabolism, although this may be of less importance in the production of neuromuscular blockade than their postjunctional actions, include decamethylene bis(hydroxyethyl)dimethylammonium salts (**VIII**) (*73*), bretylium tosylate (**IX**) (*76*), ethyl-2-(3,4,5-trimethoxybenzoyloxy)ethyl pyridinium iodide (*44*), 3,6-bis(3-diethylaminopropoxy)pyridazine bismethiodide (*263*), and hexamethonium (*76*). Many other quaternary ammonium compounds

$$HOCH_2CH_2 \overset{CH_3}{\underset{CH_3}{\overset{+}{N}}} (CH_2)_{10} \overset{CH_3}{\underset{CH_3}{\overset{+}{N}}} CH_2CH_2OH \cdot 2X^-$$

VIII

$$Me \overset{+}{N} \overset{Et}{\underset{Me}{}}$$

IX

also appear to possess a prejunctional component to their actions at the neuromuscular junction, apparently involving an inhibition of acetylcholine synthesis, and intensive studies of the prejunctional actions of such compounds constitute an active field at the present time (*76, 440*).

---

* Recent work (*305a*) has in fact confirmed that choline acetyl transferase can acetylate the triethyl analog of choline.

2. Other Prejunctional Sites of Attack by Drugs Giving Rise to Neuromuscular Blockade

At the present time there would seem to be no known drug which functions predominantly as a false transmitter at the neuromuscular junction. Similarly, although acetylcholine release can be brought about by cobra venom lecithinase (*87, 261*), high concentrations of the higher alkali metal ions (*94, 230*), or carbachol (*436, 512*), there appears to be no drug which specifically and selectively depletes acetylcholine stores in the motor nerve terminals at the neuromuscular junction in analogous fashion to the way in which reserpine-like drugs achieve depletion of dopamine, noradrenaline, and serotonin from their various storage depots. It may be noted, however, that atropine and hyoscine and similar drugs have been shown (*33, 43, 264, 265, 320, 456, 565*) to deplete acetylcholine levels in the brain. Prevention of acetylcholine release from the nerve terminals at the neuromuscular junction, on the other hand, is brought about by *Cl. botulinus* toxin (*7, 91, 92, 106, 544b, 579*) via a primary action on the mechanism linking acetylcholine release to the nerve impulse, and by lack of calcium ions or excess of magnesium ions (*177, 178, 186, 222, 325, 350, 437*), with the latter presumably acting via competition for the calcium ion carrier mechanism.* Interestingly, the neuromuscular blockade induced by high doses of the sugar-derived antibiotics streptomycin (*88, 353*), dihydrostreptomycin (*353*), and neomycin (*151, 253, 499*) has characteristics similar to the blockade produced by an excess of magnesium ions and is at least partially relieved by calcium ions (*88, 151, 353*). This is highly suggestive of an influence of the sugar units comparable to the well-known ability of inositol to complex with calcium ions and to a possible complexing of calcium ions by the sugar units of the gangliosides which could be a key factor in the release of acetylcholine from the prejunctional vesicles.

Recent studies (*439a*) on the neuromuscular blocking action of 2-(4-phenyl-piperidino)cyclohexanol (AH 5183) have led to the suggestion that this compound penetrates to intraneuronal sites where it competes with newly synthesized acetylcholine for a carried mechanism which is presumed to be necessary for the transport of acetylcholine from the cytoplasm to the inside of the vesicles. Thus it would appear that this drug represents the first example of a compound having the ability to interfere with the passage of acetylcholine across the vesicle membrane.

Of the remaining methods listed earlier as possible means of achieving prejunctional neuromuscular blockade, none would seem of practical application at the present time on account of the low specificity of the drugs concerned for the motor nerve terminals. This is particularly true of a number of drugs

---

* Recent work (*196c*) has indicated that the action of *Cl. botulinus* toxin seems to be quite independent of the calcium ion transporting mechanisms of nerve endings.

such as general anesthetics (596), local anesthetics (296, 297, 518, 543, 563), barbiturates (518), meprobramate (516), and diphenylhydantoin (506) which show a depressant action on the fine nonmyelinated nerve endings of the neuromuscular junction, thus inhibiting transmission; and of the cardiac glycosides which in high concentrations will abolish the nerve action potential in the nerve endings.

B. NEUROMUSCULAR BLOCKING AGENTS ACTING POSTJUNCTIONALLY

Although in his classic demonstration of the locus of action of curare as the neuromuscular junction Claude Bernard (40, 41) suggested that it was the nerve terminals which were affected, the weight of evidence now available leads to the generally accepted conclusion, despite some dissension (e.g., 553), that preparations of curare, in common with all the neuromuscular blocking agents at present employed clinically, act predominantly postjunctionally. Unfortunately, lack of detailed knowledge of postjunctional events prevents the pinpointing of specific sites susceptible to attack in an analogous manner to that applicable in the case of prejunctional events. The difficulties besetting attempts to rationalize the complexities occurring during the course of the interactions of postjunctionally active neuromuscular blocking agents in terms of simple models, without any clear understanding of the full sequence of molecular events involved, have been emphasized by Taylor and Nedergaard (575). Such attempts, based on the law of mass action, include the approach based on the dual concepts of affinity and intrinsic activity (13, 597) as described in Volume I of this treatise, and the approach based on kinetic theory introduced by Paton (481, 485, 486).

Thus, without prejudice to the ultimate mechanisms involved, it is usual to divide neuromuscular blocking agents acting predominantly postjunctionally into two main groups according to the observed characteristics of the pharmacological response. The rather arbitrary nature of this classification, based as it is on superficial rather than fundamental differences, is underlined by the existence of a number of compounds showing characteristics of both groups so that one group merges into the other without clear demarcation (11). Moreover, other compounds, most notably prodeconium may be deserving of being placed in a third separate category (599). The two groups of postjunctionally active neuromuscular blocking agents commonly distinguished are, respectively, those which produce blockade without any depolarization of the motor endplate and those which produce blockade with depolarization of the endplate, even if such depolarization is only a transient phase, with the second group exhibiting different modes of action in different species or even in different muscles of the same species. The depolarizing groups are frequently termed agonists, while the antidepolarizing groups are considered as antagonists of acetylcholine. Intermediate cases may then be classed as partial agonists.

1. *Curariform or Antidepolarizing Neuromuscular Blocking Agents*

As is apparent from the introduction, the author prefers to restrict the term "curariform drug" to designate this group of neuromuscular blocking agents, but unfortunately other authors have used this term in the wider sense as being synonymous with "neuromuscular blocking agent." Of the other names, "antidepolarizing," "nondepolarizing," and "competitive" neuromuscular blocking agents, which have been applied to the group, the first-mentioned is probably the next best choice on the grounds that these compounds all share the common property of actively preventing depolarization of the postjunctional membrane, not only by acetylcholine but also by the depolarizing neuromuscular blocking agents, no matter what the ultimate mechanisms of action of the different members of the group may be (cf. *181, 343, 575*). Thus the term "antidepolarizing" drug (*236*) would seem preferable to the more passive term "nondepolarizing" drug, provided it is accepted that it is completely without significance as regards mechanism at the molecular level. The much less desirable term "competitive" neuromuscular blocking agent was introduced (*494*) on the grounds that the action of these drugs is readily reversed by an increased concentration of acetylcholine, as occurs, for example, in the presence of an antiacetylcholinesterase drug such as neostigmine (*513*), but the word "competitive" has too many connotations with respect to events at the molecular level to be acceptable. That there is no necessity for the antidepolarizing drugs to compete with acetylcholine for its postjunctional binding sites has already been stressed.

Characteristically, under the influence of increasing concentrations of an antidepolarizing neuromuscular blocking agent, the endplate potentials produced by successive nerve impulses rapidly diminish in size and duration until they are completely abolished (*227*), at which time acetylcholine can exert no influence on the muscle endplate at all. Neuromuscular blockade sets in at the stage when the amplitude of the endplate potential falls below that necessary to trigger the muscle action potential (*203, 390*), and consequently it is possible to achieve a reversal of an antidepolarizing neuromuscular block by reducing the threshold endplate potential through addition of potassium ions (*504*) or by passing a cathodal current (*109*). At the height of the block, conduction in the motor nerve and the response of the muscle to direct ionic and electrical stimulation remain unimpaired (*227, 327, 482*), the muscle being electrically normal (*479*) with no apparent changes in the membrane resting potential or in its ionic permeability. Nor is the output of acetylcholine from the nerve terminals significantly reduced (*169*).

As well as blocking the transmission from the motor nerve terminals to the muscle endplate, the antidepolarizing neuromuscular blocking agents also block transmission from the γ-efferent nerves to the muscle spindles and many show other side effects, the most prominent of which are usually blockade of autonomic ganglia and inhibition of acetylcholinesterase.

Among the best known of the antidepolarizing neuromuscular blocking agents are the active principles of the various curare mixtures constituting the arrow poisons prepared by some South American Indians from varied crude extracts obtained from plants of the species *Strychnos* and *Chondodendron*, and it is on this account that the antidepolarizing group may be accurately referred to as the "curariform" group. Examples of the active principles of different curares are toxiferine-I (**X**) from calabash curare and (+)-tubocurarine (**XI**) from tube curare. In addition, many synthetic compounds including

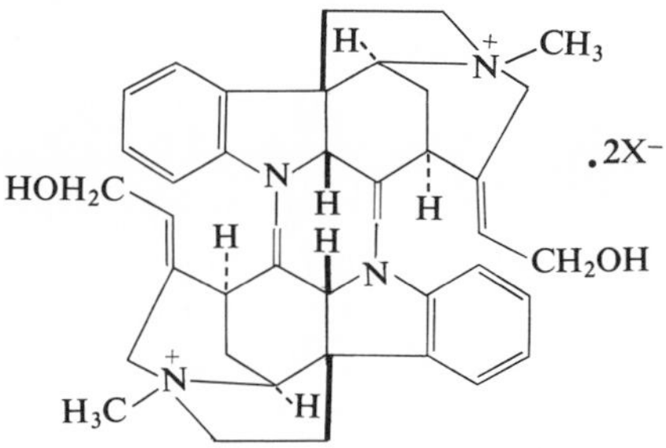

X

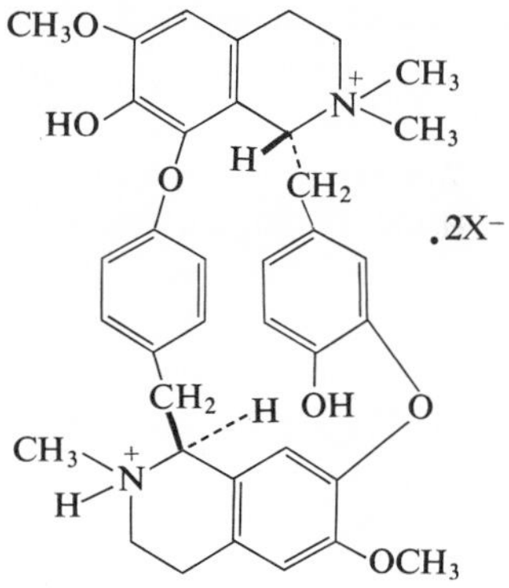

XI

the dimethyl ether of (+)-tubocurarine and gallamine triethiodide (**XII**) both of which have seen clinical application, also belong to the antidepolarizing group. Further characteristics of these compounds are that their separate effects summate when different representatives of the group are administered together, that they prevent the development of a sustained tetanus on high-frequency stimulation of the motor nerve, and that their effects are antagonized by drugs producing neuromuscular blockade by a depolarizing mechanism (*339*).

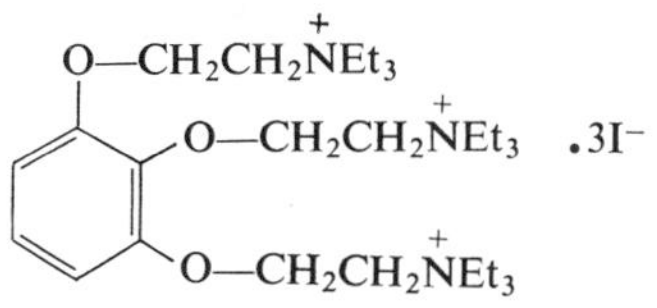

XII

In the case of (+)-tubocurarine, injection of low concentrations into the interior of the muscle fiber behind the endplate has no effect on transmission (*181*), in direct contrast to the block induced by its application to the exterior thus indicating that, as for acetylcholine, the points at which it exerts its influence are situated on the exterior of the endplate. At the same time there is evidence (*31, 414, 415, 465, 466, 518*) that (+)-tubocurarine, like acetylcholine, has a prejunctional component to its actions.

2. *Depolarizing Neuromuscular Blocking Agents*

For the purposes of the present chapter this group is taken to include all neuromuscular blocking agents which characteristically produce a depolarization of the motor endplate, whether this be the final effect or whether it be a preliminary effect which is later overcome to give a final block similar in nature to that produced by the antidepolarizing group. In some instances some members of the group would seem to act as antidepolarizing compounds in some species and as depolarizing compounds in others. Moreover, cases can be expected where the initial depolarization is of very brief duration so that experimentally the block induced is not readily distinguishable from a typical antidepolarizing block. Thus assignment of a compound to this group must be made with a certain elasticity of interpretation. Typical representatives of the depolarizing group include decamethonium bromide (**XIII**), suxamethonium dichloride dihydrate (**XIV**), suxethonium chloride (**XV**), and carbolonium dibromide (**XVI**).

In the main, these compounds would seem to act in the same way as do high concentrations of acetylcholine (*19, 639*) (either endogenous or exogenous) when suitably protected against inactivation by acetylcholinesterase and so they produce flaccid paralysis only in muscles composed solely or almost exclusively of focally innervated fibers. Muscles containing a high percentage of multiply innervated fibers enter a state of sustained contracture (*115, 123, 138*) and the production of a sustained contracture in the muscles of species such as the chicken provides a useful means of distinguishing compounds acting as depolarizing neuromuscular blocking agents from antidepolarizing neuromuscular blocking agents, since in mammals both groups give rise to a flaccid paralysis.

Muscles containing multiply innervated fibers are much more sensitive to intravenously injected depolarizing drugs than are those containing only focally innervated fibers. The explanation for this probably lies in the fact that after the drug has become distributed throughout the extracellular fluid bathing the muscle fiber surfaces, a much higher proportion of the membrane surface will be sensitive to its action in the case of the multiply innervated fibers, thus increasing the probability of inducing response. The order of paralysis of different muscles in the body thus closely parallels the proportion of multiply innervated fibers in the muscle.

A further feature of the depolarizing neuromuscular blocking agents is that the response of focally innervated muscles can vary in its finer details with respect to different species and even with respect to different muscles in the same animal. Thus, with the skeletal muscles of healthy human beings (*120, 143*) and most skeletal muscles of the cat (*28, 488–491, 493, 494, 639*), as has been well demonstrated with respect to decamethonium, after a brief period of fasciculation and potentiation of maximal twitch tension the muscle enters a protracted period of relaxation which has been shown (*109*), as is the case with acetylcholine, to result not directly from the depolarization of the motor endplates per se but from the depolarization of a small area of the muscle fiber membrane surrounding the endplates which creates a barrier to the propagation of any muscle action potential from the endplates. However, action potentials inducing contraction can still be triggered by electrical means from other points on the muscle fiber membrane. Characteristically a depolarization block is not reversed by anticholinesterase drugs, but is antagonized by antidepolarizing neuromuscular blocking agents given both prior to (*640*) and after (*109, 172*) the administration of the depolarizing compound.

However, the limb muscles of other mammals, including the monkey, hare, and dog, show a somewhat different type of response to depolarizing neuromuscular blocking agents (*640*) and there is some evidence (*10, 89, 142, 160, 242, 277, 282, 311, 312, 501, 530, 623*), which is not universally accepted (e.g., *69, 140, 641*), that the type of block exhibited in these species may also occur in some muscles of unhealthy human beings. Here, after initial muscle fasciculations and potentiation of the maximal twitch tension indicating a depolarizing action by the drugs, the block appears (*16, 577, 578, 582*) to pass through a relatively short phase similar to that just described for the situation in healthy human beings and most of the skeletal muscles of the cat, in which there is depolarization of the muscle fiber membrane around the endplate, before passing on through a period in which the membrane becomes repolarized to a second prolonged phase of paralysis exhibiting characteristics similar to those produced by the antidepolarizing neuromuscular blocking agents. This last stage is reversed by neostigmine and increased by small doses of (+)-tubocurarine (*349*), although prior administration of curare will prevent its development (*472*). Accordingly the two phases observed in these species are sometimes termed phase I and phase II blocks (*575*). These effects occur in the guinea pig (*287*), the rabbit (*348, 349*), the soleus muscle of the cat (*352*), and the muscles of human beings suffering from myasthenia gravis (*143, 541*).

The situation is further complicated by differences in the effects observed with intact animals and with isolated nerve–muscle preparations (*640a, 640b*) and by the influence of foreign anions (*294a*) in the latter. It would appear that motor endplate desensitization (*521a, 578*) and/or depression of transmitter release (*247, 247a*) could also be playing an important role.

There is evidence (*109, 161, 435, 470, 570–574, 610, 611*) that the development of phase II block is accompanied by an entry of the molecules of depolarizing neuromuscular blocking agents into the muscle fiber, and that this process is blocked by the molecules of antidepolarizing compounds such as (+)-tubocurarine. Such a diffusion of the depolarizing drugs could well underlie the fact that it is not possible to attain a steady state of partial paralysis with depolarizing drugs (*349*) as it is with antidepolarizing drugs (*319*).

As with the antidepolarizing drugs, the depolarizing group show a prejunctional component to their actions (*247, 552*).

Since the different pharmacological methods used in the assessment of neuromuscular blocking agents (*69, 70, 410*), the influence on their activities of the anesthetic agent employed (*69*) and the important bearing of species variation (*411*) on these assessments have been well reviewed elsewhere, they will not be discussed in this chapter.

In terms of the possible identity of acetylcholinesterase as a unit of the cholinergic receptor as depicted in Fig. 2, those neuromuscular blocking agents having an antidepolarizing action might be expected to be adsorbed in such a way that there was retention of a good fit between the membrane and the hydrolytically unfunctional enzyme molecule, thus maintaining selective membrane permeability and polarization of the endplate. With the depolarizing neuromuscular blocking agents, however, adsorption might be expected to occur in such a way as to prevent a good fit between the membrane and enzyme thus preventing attainment of selective membrane permeability.

Change of a phase I block to a phase II block could depend on changes in the type of adsorption, while penetration of depolarizers into the muscle fiber itself might play a role in the changing adsorption phenomena. Indirect support for differing adsorption patterns as between depolarizers and anti-depolarizers is provided by the fact that these two groups would seem to be adsorbed at different allosteric sites of purified acetylcholinesterase (37b).

V. Clinically Desirable Features in a Neuromuscular Blocking Agent

Obviously the clinically desirable features in a neuromuscular blocking agent will depend to some extent upon the particular use to which it will be put. At the present time, although these drugs have other minor applications in the control of the convulsive seizures of tetanus, in the treatment of certain spastic states (108), in the prevention of trauma in electroshock therapy (39), in orthopedics (372a), and in ocular surgery (524), their major application is in the production of muscular relaxation during surgical anesthesia, where their use obviates the need for the high doses of the anesthetic agent which would otherwise be required for the dual purpose of relieving pain and pre-paring the skeletal muscles, particularly those of the abdomen, for facile manipulation. Indeed the introduction of these agents in this capacity some twenty-five years ago (168, 279) produced a major revolution in surgical and anesthetic techniques since once the dual role of the anesthetic agent was eliminated and it could be used solely for the purpose of elimination of pain through the induction of unconsciousness, lower doses of anesthetic could be employed with consequent gain in safety margin. At the same time the way was opened to modern anesthetic procedures involving intravenous induction followed by maintenance of the anesthesia by closed-circuit techniques.

Apart from the need for a low toxicity and a high chemical stability so as to facilitate presentation in sterile condition, for the purposes just listed the major requirements of a clinically suitable neuromuscular blocking agent are:

1. A high specificity for the neuromuscular junction with freedom from side effects resulting from actions at other sites in the body
2. A rapid, reliable and reproducible onset of action
3. A relatively short duration of action
4. A ready reversibility of action
5. A rapid elimination from the body
6. A freedom from aftereffects

However, a long rather than a short duration of action would be best suited for the treatment of spastic conditions.

Since, by and large, the above requirements, especially 4 and 6, are best met by the antidepolarizing or curariform group, a rational approach to the design of new compounds involves the intentional search for drugs falling into this category.

Apart from their lack of ready reversibility, if this should suddenly be required, most depolarizing drugs are too long-acting to be well suited for application as muscle relaxants in surgical anesthesia, although suxamethonium is an exception on account of its usual ready hydrolysis by the nonspecific serum esterases into inactive products (590, 622). However, as a result of certain hereditary differences (404), some human beings possess an atypical cholinesterase incapable of effecting rapid hydrolysis of the drug (354) with the result that patients possessing this particular genetic makeup remain paralyzed for prolonged periods of time. It is established that only 1 individual in about 4,000 possesses this atypical cholinesterase while 97 % of the population have normal cholinesterase and the remainder possess an intermediate type. It would appear (294) that at least three genes are involved in these hereditary differences. Interestingly, suxamethonium is resistant to hydrolysis by plasma esterases in the domestic fowl (50).

Other drawbacks to the clinical use of suxamethonium include a tendency to the production of deep muscle pain as an aftereffect (238), which possibly arises from the initial fasciculations (480) and from damage to the muscle spindles (505), and an increase in intraocular pressure (318, 416) arising from the extreme sensitivity to this compound of the external rectus and oblique muscles of the eye with their multiply innervated fibers.

Drawbacks to the use of (+)-tubocurarine include its marked propensity to induce histamine release (548) and ganglion blockade (238), while the production of tachycardia (519) by gallamine triethiodide can be a disadvantage to the use of this agent in some instances. The need for superior neuromuscular blocking agents of the antidepolarizing group which would be free from these undesirable side effects and at the same time show a much shorter duration of action (69, 141, 237) has, in fact, been the main driving force behind the recent intensive search for new neuromuscular blocking drugs, the rational elements of which form the underlying theme of this chapter.

However, another line of research capable of rational development within the neuromuscular blocking field would seem to be the intentional search for new drugs, of which no satisfactory representatives have so far been discovered, having useful clinical application in the suppression of the symptoms of Parkinson's disease. At present the chemotherapeutic approach to the treatment of this condition, which originates in the development of various lesions in the midbrain and basal ganglia, is confined to the use of drugs acting on the central nervous system, but another point of attack to prevent the tremor and muscular rigidity characterizing the disease would seem to be at the neuromuscular junction or the muscle spindles. Here the need is for a long-acting, highly specific agent, having little or no activity at other cholinergic sites, which would abolish the response of the skeletal muscle to all but intentional nerve impulses. The more promising type of drug would seem to be one which partially reduced the acetylcholine output of the nerve terminals in direct proportion to dose so that a satisfactory dosage level could be found at which voluntary control persisted but involuntary contractions were abolished, at the same time minimizing the pronounced muscular atrophy known to accompany denervation of striated muscle. Such a drug might well be one inhibiting the prejunctional uptake of choline in the manner characteristic of the hemicholiniums, although a much higher specificity for the neuromuscular junction than is present in the hemicholiniums would be necessary, but a new approach would be the intentional development of a specific anticholine acetyl transferase drug (cf. *128a*, *546a*) using the concept of active-site-directed irreversible enzyme inhibition which is currently being applied in many other situations (*22*).

VI. Relationships between Chemical Constitution and Neuromuscular Blocking Activity

Once an appreciation has been gained of the normal functioning of the neuromuscular junction, the ways in which this may be disrupted, and the criteria which must be met before a neuromuscular blocking agent is acceptable clinically, the next key step in the development of a rational approach to the synthesis of superior compounds is to consider structural features present in the molecules of established neuromuscular blocking agents in order to uncover any underlying relationships between the biological properties required and the presence of specific chemical groupings.

The first intimation that there might be a valid general correlation between neuromuscular blocking activity and certain molecular features of the drugs displaying it was revealed over one hundred years ago by the classic experiments of Crum Brown and Fraser. These workers, prompted by the realization that biologically active curare extracts contained quaternary ammonium salts (of as then undetermined chemical structure), first (*164*) examined the pharmacological actions of the methiodides derived from brucine, codeine, morphine, nicotine, strychnine, and thebaine and then (*165*, *166*) extended their investigations to various quaternary salts derived from atropine and coniine to give clear demonstration that, in marked contrast to the highly individualistic pharmacological properties of the parent alkaloids, the quaternary compounds all share the common property of inducing a paralysis of voluntary muscle even though this action is not necessarily the only one displayed. Moreover, the paralysis was found to be similar in its gross manifestations to that produced by the extracts of curare. Further extension of this correlation between the quaternary ammonium function and neuromuscular blocking activity (which, in fact, represents the first generally valid structure–action relationship to be established) so as to include various other positively charged organic molecules then followed from the work of Renshaw (38, 333) and of Ing and Wright (343, 344) who showed that neuromuscular blocking properties were also associated with tertiary sulfonium, quaternary phosphonium, quaternary arsonium, and quaternary stibonium groups with the order of potency among the isosteres falling off in the sequence $N^+ > S^+ > P^+ > As^+$. This work also revealed a relative lack of dependence of the neuromuscular blocking activity upon either the nature of the substituents at the onium center or the anion associated with it (341), although later studies have revealed that appreciable differences in biological properties do, in fact, result from variations in the degree of localization of the cationic charge [as has been emphasized in at least two reviews (128, 556)] and in other physicochemical characteristics, particularly the hydrophilic to lipophilic balance in the molecule (128). That neuromuscular blocking activity is also exhibited by various large inorganic cations was demonstrated by Beccari (34) and by Dwyer et al. (200).

From these studies and others it is now firmly established that neuromuscular blockade is intimately associated with the presence within a molecule of a positively charged center, which may ultimately owe its activity to an ability to influence ordered water molecules (35–37), giving rise to an observed mimicry or antagonism of the normal physiological actions of acetylcholine. The relative lack of specificity for the neuromuscular junction shown by many quaternary ammonium compounds also finds rationalization in this interference with the normal functioning of acetylcholine, since it would be expected a priori that compounds capable of interfering with the actions of the neurohormone at one site should also be capable of similar activity at other sites. With normal routes of administration the "blood–brain barrier" usually ensures that quaternary ammonium salts, which are fully ionized, do not gain access to sites of action of acetylcholine within the central nervous system, but, depending upon the lipophilic to hydrophilic ratio of the particular molecule in question, certain quaternary ammonium salts do gain access to autonomic ganglia or to the neuroeffector junctions of autonomic cholinergic nerves so as to exert effects at these sites, including effects on acetylcholinesterase located there. Generally speaking, nicotinic sites appear to lack the same degree of lipid protection as is afforded to other cholinergic sites and so are the more selectively influenced the greater the hydrophilic nature of the quaternary salt. Conversely, an increase in the lipophilic character of the molecule tends to enhance activity at "muscarinic" sites, but other factors also come into play.

As with most generalizations there are a number of exceptions, and an appreciable degree of neuromuscular blocking activity has been discovered in a number of compounds lacking an onium center, although in some cases at least, a degree of protonation of the nitrogen atom of an amino function may in fact be occurring at physiological pH so as to generate a cationic center *in vivo*. Another possibility is that with sterically hindered amines the degree of hydration is lower than with other amines, thus making them somewhat more akin to quaternary ammonium compounds which per se are unable to hydrogen-bond to water. Prominent among the nononium neuromuscular blocking agents are the tertiary amine, dihydro-β-erythroidine (*195, 288, 345, 532, 591*), which is now known (*293*) to have the absolute stereochemistry shown in **XVII**, and some of its closely related analogs (*403, 532, 591*). These compounds act as antidepolarizing agents. On the other hand, other tertiary bases, such as certain of the pyrrolizidine alkaloids, can act as depolarizing compounds (*257*). Further examples of nononium neuromuscular blocking agents are a number of 2-halogenoalkylamines, including **XVIII** (*276*), but here there is a strong possibility that the actual active molecular species is a cyclic ethyleneimonium ion (cf. *528*). Reference to the neuromuscular blocking activity of the sugar-derived antibiotics, streptomycin, dihydrostreptomycin, and neomycin, has already been made.

More recently the alkaloid, emetine, which has both a secondary and tertiary nitrogen atom in its molecule, has been shown to exhibit anti-depolarizing neuromuscular blocking properties (*531a, 531b*).

XVII   XVIII

A. Molecular Features Associated with High Potency and High Specificity in Neuromuscular Blocking Agents

With the isolation in pure form of (+)-tubocurarine, the most active component of tube curare, and the long-held belief that it was a bisquaternary ammonium compound (*368, 369, 371, 587, 632*) [the correct constitution as the monoquaternary ammonium salt, **XI**, being established (*226a*) only in 1970] the inference was drawn that high neuromuscular blocking potency was most probably correlated with a bisonium structure. Despite the fallacious manner in which it arose, this correlation has nevertheless proved to have a certain validity and indeed all the highly active principles of calabash curare which include toxiferine I (**X**), *C*-dihydrotoxiferine I, *C*-curarine I, and *C*-alkaloids E, G, and H, are in fact bisquaternary ammonium salts (*601*). Moreover, a bisquaternary structure tends to give a high selectivity for nicotinic sites and, where the interonium distance is of the order of 10 Å, to confine activity to the neuromuscular junction. The presence of ganglion-blocking properties in (+)-tubocurarine (*238*) which appeared anomalous in terms of its former erroneous portrayal as a bisquaternary salt becomes fully explicable in the light of its true structure.

The generalization that bisonium salts of suitable constitution tend to show high potency as neuromuscular blocking agents, as well as a high specificity for the neuromuscular junction, has been reconfirmed many times over with reference to a large number of synthetic compounds, and it must be considered the fundamental premise upon which nearly all rational approaches to the synthesis of new neuromuscular blocking agents are based.

It is well established that optical isomerism, both with respect to asymmetric carbon atoms and asymmetric nitrogen atoms, has a marked influence (*405, 569*) upon neuromuscular blocking potency, as is well exemplified by certain configurational isomers having a tubocurarine-like structure (*370, 631*), and at the present time detailed correlation of potency with absolute configuration in neuromuscular blocking agents is an active field (e.g., *406, 441, 557*).

B. MOLECULAR FEATURES ASSOCIATED WITH SPECIFIC MODES OF ACTION AT THE NEUROMUSCULAR JUNCTION

Although at the present time there would seem no clear indication of any underlying relationship between molecular structure and mode of action for those neuromuscular blocking agents acting prejunctionally, there would seem to be a generally valid structure–action relationship for bisonium neuromuscular blocking agents acting postjunctionally. In mammals at least, bulky or compacted molecules (whether the bulk be in the molecular unit bearing the two onium centers or in the substituents on the onium centers) tend to be antidepolarizing compounds, whereas long attenuated molecules tend to be depolarizing compounds. This generalization, which is subject to a certain elasticity of interpretation in the light of factors such as species variations and the absence of a clear-cut distinction between depolarizing and antidepolarizing compounds (*11, 171*), was first pointed out by Bovet (*60*) who applied the term "pachycurares" to the compact antidepolarizing group and "leptocurares" to the thin depolarizing group which are those apparently capable (*575*) of penetrating the muscle endplate. Certainly for maximal effective depolarizing activity the onium head should bear substituents of minimal steric bulk and it is well established that a change from a depolarizing action to an antidepolarizing action accompanies progressive increase in size of the substituents on the onium centers in many instances (*149, 285, 400, 439, 584, 598*), although potency usually decreases at the same time.

C. MOLECULAR FEATURES ASSOCIATED WITH SHORT DURATION OF ACTION IN A NEUROMUSCULAR BLOCKING AGENT

Obviously any molecular feature rendering a neuromuscular blocking agent susceptible to ready *in vivo* conversion into inactive products via any of the normal general biotransformation pathways of the body will tend to produce a short-acting drug, but at the present time, with one or two exceptions, attention would seem to have been focused almost exclusively on the incorporation of ester functions following the discovery that suxamethonium in most human beings is readily hydrolyzed by the nonspecific serum esterases (*590, 622*). Succinyldicholine dichloride was actually first synthesized in 1906 (*334*) but its neuromuscular blocking action was not discovered until 1949 (*64, 498*) when it was intentionally reinvestigated in a rational search for short-acting drugs based on an expected ready hydrolysis in the body as it was anticipated that the hydrolytic products succinyl monocholine and choline would not themselves exhibit potent neuromuscular blocking activity, which, in fact, proved to be the case (*240, 241*). Carbamyl esters, unlike simple esters, are insusceptible to hydrolysis by cholinesterases and so short-acting compounds are not to be found within this class of compound.

An *in vivo* equivalent of the Hofmann elimination undergone *in vitro* by quaternary ammonium salts on heating with strong base does not appear to exist. Certainly acetylcholine itself is not degraded *in vivo* by extrusion of trimethylamine, and the absence of such an elimination process probably explains the extreme stability *in vivo* of quaternary ammonium compounds lacking groups readily susceptible to hydrolysis, hydroxylation, etc.

VII. Rational Applications of Structure–Action Relationships to the Synthesis of New Neuromuscular Blocking Agents

With the realization that the neuromuscular blockade associated with various quaternary ammonium salts resulted from some sort of interference with the normal physiological action of acetylcholine, early attention was inevitably focused on structural alterations to the molecule of acetylcholine in the quest for new agents. Although these exercises in molecular manipulation, in common with those in other areas of drug research, have been criticized on the grounds that they lack intellectual inspiration, such criticism is unjust. In the absence of any logical alternative approach it was obviously necessary to start somewhere, and it is largely as a result of the accumulated information obtained as a result of such tedious studies, pedestrian as they may be, that the more sophisticated approaches now available have been made possible. Certainly a degree of retrospective justification (443) for these structural modification studies can be made in terms of the receptor theory of drug action [where mimicry or antagonism can be related to the intrinsic activity of the compound (13), whatever the ultimate significance of this term], the theory of metabolite displacement (634), the concept of allosterism (457), the supporting moiety theory (124, 125) and the concept of bioisosterism (248, 534); while it is only after a sufficient number of structural variations have already been made available that it is possible to apply regression analyses (e.g., 246, 251, 252, 289–292, 547) in the quest for reliable predictions as to which particular structure within a related series should possess the most favorable activity.

The acetylcholine molecule has been subjected to a wide range of structural modifications involving all manner of alterations to the cationic head, the ester function, and the dimethylene chain, and these studies have produced compounds variously showing mimicry or antagonism of the actions of acetylcholine at nicotinic and/or muscarinic sites as well as compounds acting as anticholinesterase drugs. Of the compounds prepared from these considerations, which have been the subject of a number of detailed surveys (25, 63, 128, 159, 342, 513, 556), some, including the higher n-alkyltrimethylammonium salts (170, 172, 496, 497), in appropriate doses act as depolarizing neuromuscular blocking agents, but, apart from suxamethonium (XIV), which can be regarded as a "bisacetylcholine," and the corresponding N-ethyl analog, suxethonium (XV), none has been of more than academic interest.

A. Bisonium Structure as a Basis for Design of Neuromuscular Blocking Agents

Following the isolation and assignment of structure to (+)-tubocurarine by King (368, 369) several groups of workers paid intensive attention to the preparation of synthetic bisquaternary ammonium salts. The group headed by Bovet (62, 65) prepared a number of aryl and heterocyclic bisquaternary salts meeting the criteria of pachycurares, while Barlow and Ing (27, 28) and Paton and Zaimis (488, 490, 492) in their studies with the polymethylene α,ω-bistrimethylammonium series discovered the prototype leptocurare in decamethonium, which was to lead to the subsequent distinction between antidepolarizing and depolarizing neuromuscular blocking agents.

Structural modifications on the molecule of (+)-tubocurarine itself (*369*) gave rise to the dimethyl ether which has seen a limited amount of clinical application (*174, 309, 559, 560*) on account of its greater potency (*592*), shorter duration of action (*495*), and the lesser histamine-liberating and autonomic effects (*148, 626*) than the parent compound, while combination of benzyl-tetrahydroisoquinoline moieties similar to those present in (+)-tubocurarine with the decamethylene chain of decamethonium gave rise to laudexium methylsulfate, (**XIX**), which at one time also saw some clinical application (*46, 57, 199, 336, 480, 637*). Laudexium methylsulfate has about half the potency of (+)-tubocurarine in anesthetized patients but the onset of action

XIX

is slower and the duration of action considerably longer. Although reversible by neostigmine in accordance with its curariform nature its persistence in the body may give rise to recurarization, so laudexium methylsulfate has been displaced from clinical use.

Replacement of the benzyltetrahydroisoquinoline units of laudexium by 9-fluorenylamino units and shortening of the polymethylene chain to six carbon atoms give rise to hexafluorenium which is used in anesthesia in combination with suxamethonium, where it is claimed (*116a, 128b, 233a*) that complete muscle relaxation can be secured without the occurrence of postoperative muscle pains.

Further variants on the structural modification theme with respect to the molecules of (+)-tubocurarine and decamethonium have given rise to a large diversity of compounds showing varying degrees of neuromuscular blocking potency. As illustrative examples of the varied compounds so prepared may be cited the series of substituted derivatives of *N,N*-dimethyl-1,10-decamethyl-enebistetrahydroquinolinium (**XX**) (*149, 576*); cyclomethone (**XXI**) (*427, 602*); compounds of types **XXII** (*508*), **XXIII** (*301, 302*), and **XXIV** (*323*); 9-(*p*-methoxyphenyl)fluorene-2,7-bistrimethylammonium (**XXV**) (*449*); compounds of type **XXVI** (*445, 476, 529*); and diplacine (**XXVII**) (*399, 450*). These compounds, of which benzoquinonium chloride (**XXIV**, R = —Et, R' = —CH$_2$Ph, $n = 3$, X = Cl) saw brief clinical application (*14, 198, 235, 335*) before rejection on account of its lack of ready reversibility by neostigmine (*68*), together with many other bisquaternary ammonium salts prepared from essentially the same considerations have been subjected to detailed discussion in terms of the influence of chemical structure on biological activity by several authors (*128, 556, 569*). In the light of the existence of these surveys, and since too detailed an analysis of structure–activity relationships is completely unwarranted where there is no knowledge of events at the postjunctional sites, these compounds will not be further considered here.

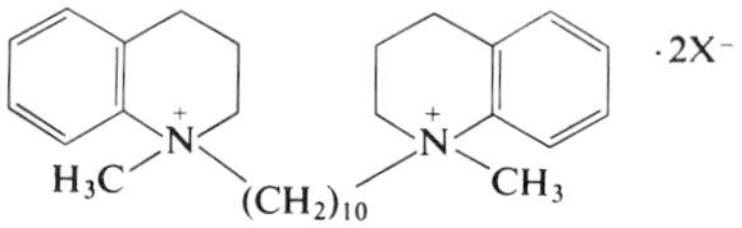

XX

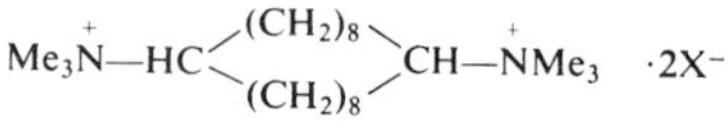

XXI

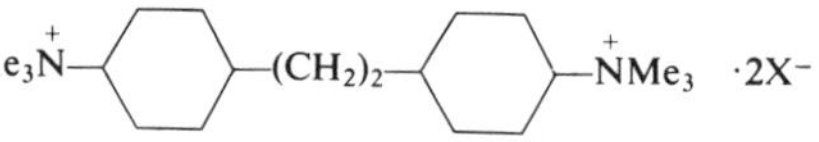

XXII

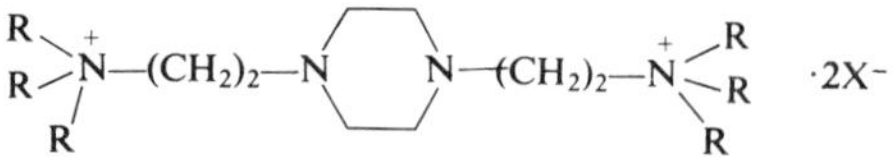

XXIII

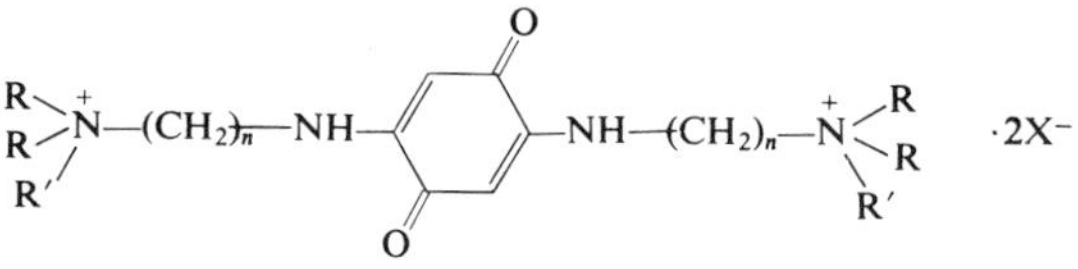

XXIV

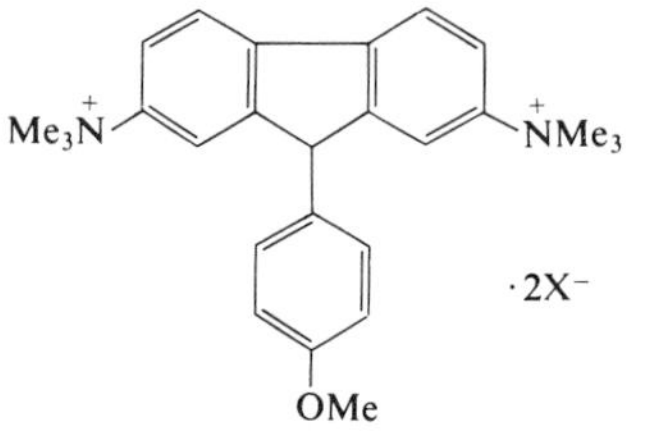

XXV

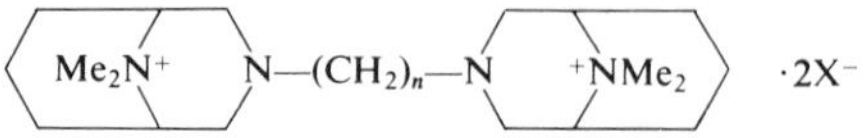

XXVI

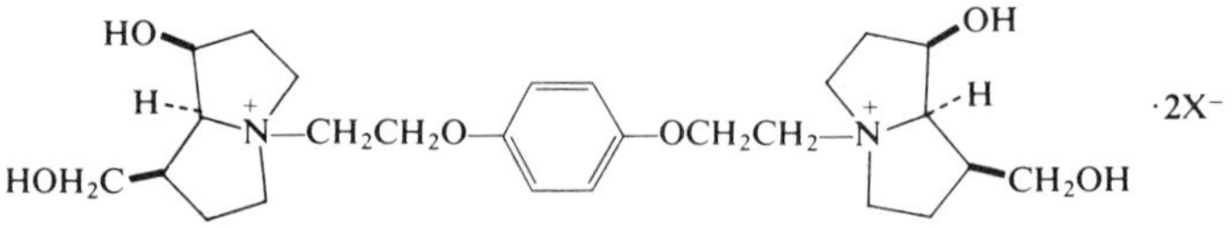

XXVII

In order to rationalize the high potency displayed by bisquaternary ammonium compounds, such as decamethonium, when compared with the potencies of N,N-dimethyldecamethylenediamine monomethiodide (**XXVIII**) (*26*) or N,N-dimethyldecylamine methiodide (**XXIX**) (*170*), it has been proposed (*24*) that the postjunctional membrane could carry a lattice of regularly spaced

$$\overset{+}{\text{Me}_3\text{N}}\text{—(CH}_2)_{10}\text{—NH}_2 \quad \cdot \text{I}^- \qquad \overset{+}{\text{Me}_3\text{N}}\text{—(CH}_2)_9\text{—CH}_3 \quad \cdot \text{I}^-$$

$$\textbf{XXVIII} \qquad\qquad\qquad\qquad \textbf{XXIX}$$

anionic groupings responsible for the binding of acetylcholine, and that bisquaternary ammonium salts having the appropriate interonium distances might be interacting with two adjacent anionic groupings to give a "two-point attachment," thus exerting their actions in a "pharmacologically bivalent" manner. Apart from species differences, that the lattices in ganglia and at the neuromuscular junction were probably different in their spatial arrangements was implied from the fact that, whereas in most species decamethonium is the most potent neuromuscular blocking agent of the polymethylene-α,ω-bis-trimethylammonium salts, the corresponding hexamethylene compound shows the most pronounced ganglion blocking activity. Indeed, it would appear that, as a generalization, bisquaternary ammonium compounds with shorter interonium distances tend to show ganglion blocking properties rather than neuromuscular blocking activity.

With disregard for the differences in the modes of action of the two drugs it was further suggested (*28, 490*) that the spacing of the anionic groupings on the muscle endplate might be of the order of 13–15 Å apart, since in certain conformations an intercharge distance of this value, which is a quadruple identity distance (*422*), can be discerned within the molecules of both decamethonium and (+)-tubocurarine. However, these molecules are conformationally flexible, permitting considerable variations in intercharge distance and, as was stressed by Alauddin and Martin-Smith (*3*), any deductions from molecules which are conformationally nonrigid are fraught with uncertainties. Cavallito and Gray (*128*) have suggested alternative possibilities to the classic two-point attachment, and Loewe and Harvey (*420*) have proposed that the high potency in bisquaternary ammonium salts could arise not from a two-point attachment but from a one-point attachment in which the bulk of the molecule may well shield the binding site, the so-called "adumbration theory." Should the bisquaternary salt be occupying actual acetylcholine binding sites, which as emphasized earlier in this chapter is by no means established, it is conceivable that the second quaternary ammonium function, not involved in the binding of the molecule to the membrane of the muscle endplate, might exert an electrostatic repulsion on incoming molecules of acetylcholine, thus hindering ready displacement of the bisquaternary molecule from the immediate vicinity of the binding site and contributing to its prolonged action, whether this be ultimately due to an "occupation" mechanism or a "dynamic" mechanism in accordance with the rate theory of Paton (481).

That the original estimate of the membrane interanionic site distance as 13–15 Å (based on the assumption that decamethonium was binding to the postjunctional sites in its fully extended, fully staggered conformation) was almost certainly incorrect soon became apparent from the fact that certain compounds, in which a molecular interonium distance as large as this is not possible, exhibit potent neuromuscular blocking activity (65, 67, 284, 427). Further circumstantial evidence against the 13–15 Å distance was then provided by conductimetric studies on decamethonium iodide (225) which showed that the conformations adopted by the molecule in aqueous or ethanolic solution are such as to give a mean interonium distance of around 9.5 Å.

In order to reduce the ambiguities inherent in studies employing conformationally flexible molecules and particularly in the transfer of knowledge concerning their preferred conformations in the crystalline state or in solution to the situation pertaining at binding sites, Martin-Smith and his colleagues decided to employ the steroid nucleus as a supporting moiety upon which to append two quaternary ammonium groups in various positions so as to give a series of compounds with different interonium distances but at the same time having essentially the same physicochemical properties. For each compound in the series the spatial relationship between the two onium centers would be expected to be fixed within narrow limits, a certain amount of flexibility being possible through conformational variations in ring A. That these compounds would possess a suitable hydrophilic to lipophilic ratio was indicated by the discovery of neuromuscular blocking activity comparable to that of (+)-tubocurarine in the steroidal alkaloid malouetine (**XXX**) (346, 503) and its configurational isomers at C-3 and C-20 (367), all of which show an increased degree of variation in interonium distance over that occurring in steroids where both quaternary ammonium groups are directly attached to the nucleus, owing to free rotation of the side chain. The first compounds synthesized by Martin-Smith et al. (2) were a series of 3α,17α-bis(quaternary ammonium)-5α-androstanes (**XXXI**). These compounds were chosen since

XXX   XXXI

inspection of models revealed the interonium distance to fall within the apparently favorable range of 9.2–10.6 Å (according to the conformation adopted by ring A) if bond angle distortions arising from substituent effects are ignored. The α-configuration for the appended quaternary ammonium functions at C-3 and C-17 was chosen in order to eliminate any possible steric hindrance to postjunctional binding by the β-face angular methyl groups on C-10 and C-13, but it later transpired (23, 116) that 3β,17β-bisdimethylamino-5α-androstane dimethiodide showed the same order of potency as the compounds having the onium centers in the α-configuration, all of which showed roughly the same order of potency as (+)-tubocurarine in different assays and exhibited typical antidepolarizing activity (2).

Independently several other groups also instigated investigations on steroidal bisquaternary ammonium salts. The Glaxo group (113) investigated bisquaternary salts of general type **XXXII** derived from the alkaloid conessine and related steroids, all of which have an interonium distance of 10.1 Å as

XXXII

revealed by molecular models, while the compounds prepared by the May and Baker group (23, 45), like those of the Glasgow group, were 3,17-bisquaternary ammonium androstanes. An interesting observation made by the M and B workers was that in addition to configurational isomerism at C-3 and C-17 having relatively little effect on the activity displayed, potent activity was present in 3α,17β- and 3β,17α-bisquaternary ammonium salts where the onium centers lie on opposite sides of the general plane of the steroid nucleus. Unless the molecules of these compounds are approaching adjacent anionic sites in an edge-on manner along the staggered chain of carbon atoms constituting positions 3, 2, 1, 10, 9, 11, 12, 13, and 17 of the steroid nucleus, it might seem that the adumbration theory (420) or the pore concept of Waser (606) represent more acceptable models of postjunctional events than the anionic lattice concept. However, investigation (409) of a series of monoquaternary ammonium salts derived from various 2β- and 3α-aminosteroids having androstane or pregnane skeletons and related in structure to acetylcholine through possession of an acetoxyl or hydroxyl substituent on a nuclear carbon atom adjacent to that holding the quaternary nitrogen atom, revealed them to have low neuromuscular blocking potency only, thus militating against the one-point attachment theory. The considerably higher potencies observed with a number of monoquaternary ammonium salts derived from conessine (113) which have been advanced as support for a one-point attachment are not open to simple interpretation since the possibility exists that the second nitrogen atom could become protonated *in vivo* giving rise to a second cationic center.

From these studies with steroidal bisquaternary ammonium salts it would appear that within certain limits interonium distance per se could be relatively unimportant (2, 23) and that other factors, particularly the number of weak bonding contacts possible between the postjunctional membrane and the molecular units separating the onium centers of the bisquaternary ammonium compound, could be exerting a dominant influence as has been proposed in the case of decamethonium, where in the crystalline state the nitrogen atoms are disposed on opposite sides of the carbon chain (423), and in the case of (+)-tubocurarine and related compounds (441).

Steroidal bisquaternary ammonium salts have been reported as having a much shorter duration of action than (+)-tubocurarine on the cat sciatic nerve–gastrocnemius muscle preparation but an analogous brief duration of action does not occur in man. Indeed, it has been stated (113, 458) that with steroidal neuromuscular blocking agents the monkey is a more suitable animal than the cat for indicating duration of action in human beings, although factors such as the pulse width of the sciatic nerve stimulation could have been affecting the results obtained in the experiments with the cat. Despite the lack of any marked superiority over (+)-tubocurarine as regards their duration of action in man, the steroidal compounds have little or no propensity to cause histamine release and have little or no action at ganglia or on the heart rate and several of these compounds, including dipyrandium chloride (**XXXIII**) (458), *N,N'*-dimethylconessine (**XXXII**), R = R' = —Me (600), and pancuronium bromide (**XXXIV**) (21, 59, 99–101, 163, 542, 561)

XXXIII   **XXXIV**

have shown promise on clinical trial, thus representing a notable success for the rational approach to drug synthesis. X-ray crystallographic studies (*233*) with pancuronium bromide have revealed the actual interonium distance in the solid state to be 11.1 Å as against the 10.6 Å calculated from Dreiding models.

As with the monoonium compounds, neuromuscular blocking potency falls off in the order $N^+ > S^+ > P^+ > As^+$ in the bisonium series and 1,10-bis-(dimethylsulfonium)decane (**XXXV**) is appreciably less active than decameth-

$$CH_3\overset{+}{\underset{\underset{\displaystyle CH_3}{|}}{S}}-(CH_2)_{10}-\overset{+}{\underset{\underset{\displaystyle CH_3}{|}}{S}}-CH_3$$

XXXV

onium while the mixed ammonium–sulfonium derivative exhibits intermediate potency (*603*). The disulfonium analog of suxamethonium has about one-tenth the potency of its prototype and is resistant to the action of cholinesterases (*188, 189*). The bishydrazinium analogs of decamethonium (*538*), and suxamethonium (*245*), like certain polymethylene *S*-linked bisisothiouronium salts (*137, 187, 624*), show only weak neuromuscular blocking activity. Neuromuscular blocking activity is completely absent from polymethylene bis-*N*-oxides (*351*).

B. POLYONIUM COMPOUNDS

A logical extension of the studies with bisquaternary ammonium salts, especially within the context of the postjunctional anionic lattice theory, was to ascertain the effect of the presence within a molecule of 3, 4, 5, and more onium centers on neuromurcular blocking activity, although, as pointed out by Cavallito and Gray (*128*), the introduction of more than two onium centers would not only be expected to produce critical changes in the hydrophilic to lipophilic balance of a molecule, but also to reduce the probability of securing optimal spatial relationships between all groups involved in the crucial interactions with the postjunctional membrane. If cationic groups were to be wrongly situated spatially they could even act as points of repulsion from, rather than attraction to, the binding sites on the motor endplate, should the latter contain positively charged groups in addition to the proposed anionic lattice.

One of the first polyonium compounds to be prepared, although it was synthesized more from considerations of means of increasing the neuromuscular blocking potency of various aliphatic choline ethers (*544*) than from the anionic lattice concept which at that time had not been formally proposed, was gallamine triethiodide (**XII**) (*66, 67*) which proved to be more potent than the analogous monoquaternary compound, **XXXVI**, and the analogous bisquaternary compound, **XXXVII** (*102*). Indeed gallamine triethiodide has seen considerable clinical success as an antidepolarizing neuromuscular blocking agent (*459*). It has relatively low ganglion blocking activity, but shows pronounced ability to block the effects of vagal stimulation of the heart

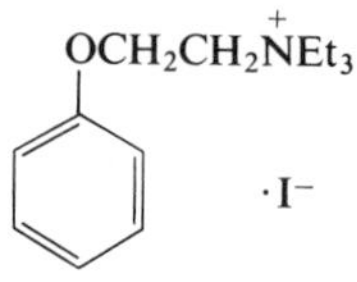

$$OCH_2CH_2\overset{+}{N}Et_3$$

·I⁻

XXXVI

$$OCH_2CH_2\overset{+}{N}Et_3$$
$$OCH_2CH_2\overset{+}{N}Et_3$$

·2I⁻

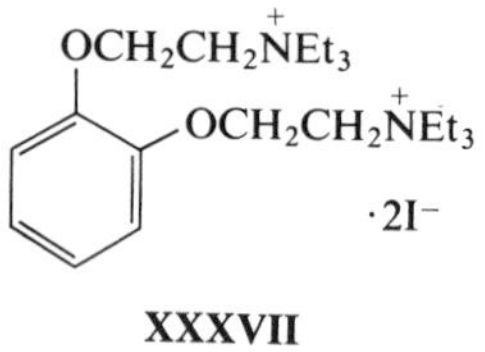

XXXVII

(*519*), a property shown to a lesser degree by (+)-tubocurarine (*448*). However, gallamine triethiodide has no activity at other muscarinic sites, and in the absence of complicating circumstances, such as the presence of coronary disease or hyperthyroidism, the tachycardia produced in the majority of patients receiving the drug is no real disadvantage to its use, and may even be advantageous in counteracting the bradycardia frequently produced by cyclopropane when this agent is used as the anesthetic.

Trisonium compounds of general formula **XXXVIII**, $n = 2,3,4$ (*364*) show maximum neuromuscular blocking potency at $n = 4$, R $= $ —Et, but the longer

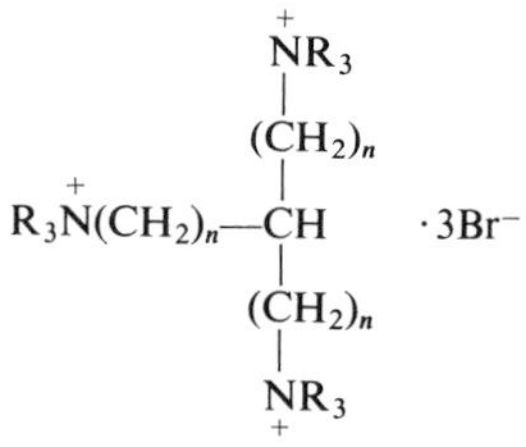

$$\overset{+}{N}R_3$$
$$|$$
$$(CH_2)_n$$
$$|$$
$$R_3\overset{+}{N}(CH_2)_n—CH \qquad ·3Br^-$$
$$|$$
$$(CH_2)_n$$
$$|$$
$$\underset{+}{N}R_3$$

XXXVIII

polymethylene chain compounds of this series which might be expected to be more potent do not seem to have been investigated, although structurally similar compounds of type **XXXIX** were subsequently investigated (*207*). All members of this series proved to be antidepolarizing compounds and the compound with R = R′ = —Et was found to be the most active in the majority of species examined, having 80 % of the potency of (+)-tubocurarine in the cat. Compound **XL** (*363*) exhibits weak decamethonium-like properties but also shows muscarinic properties, while compound **XLI** has been reported (*8*) to have antidepolarizing properties and to be slightly more potent than (+)-tubocurarine.

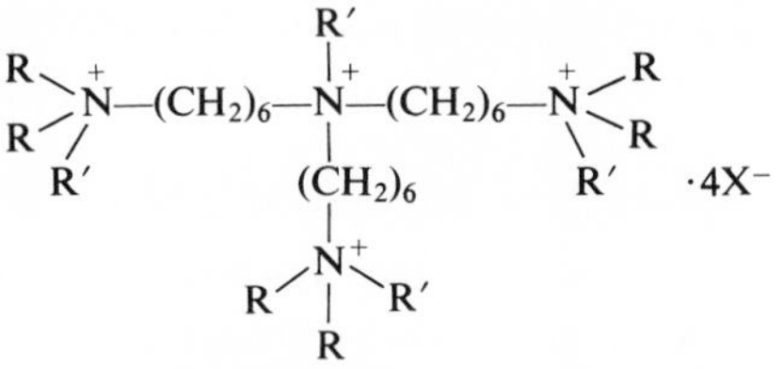

XXXIX

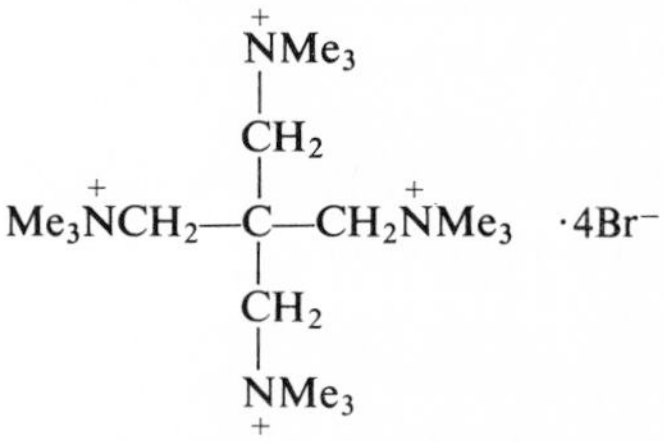

XL

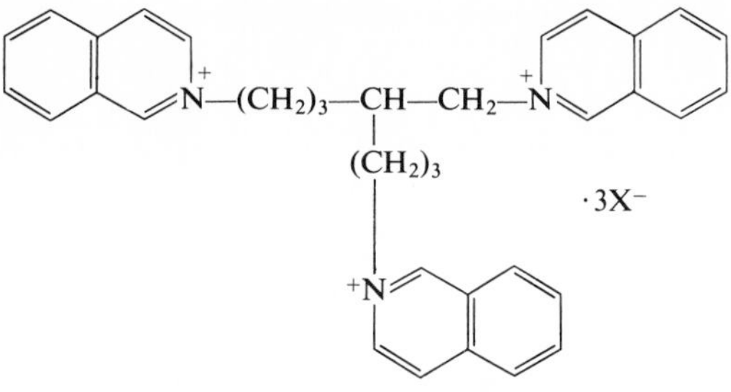

XLI

Linear trisquaternary ammonium salts of type **XLII**, in which n is 5 to 10, together with analogous compounds containing four onium centers and three

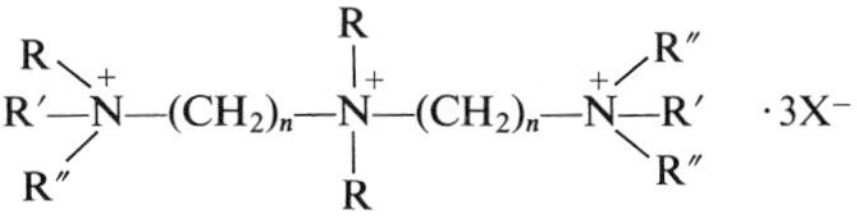

XLII

polymethylene chains, were first examined by Edwards, Lewis, Stenlake, and Zoha (*210*). A large number of variations on the same general pattern were also reported by the same group (*121, 122, 208, 209, 211*), including N,S,N-trisonium compounds (*121, 209*), N,N,S,N,N-pentaonium compounds, and the N,N,N,N,N,N-hexaonium compound (**XLIII**) (*208*). Considerable species variation was observed both with respect to potency and with respect to mode of action within these linear compounds (where replacement of N by S had relatively insignificant effects) but among the compounds bearing only ethyl groups on the onium centers curariform activity tends to predominate when

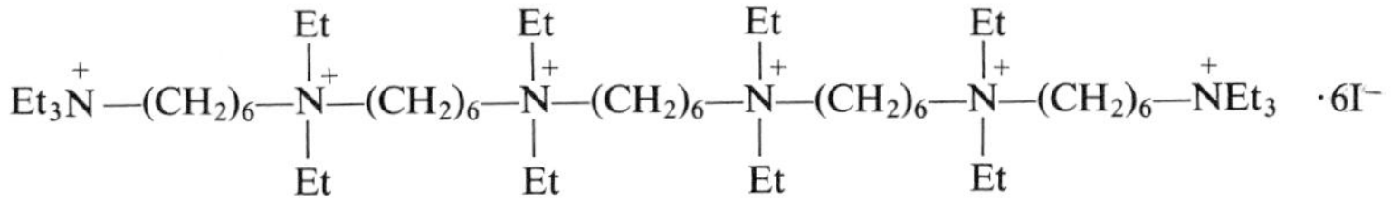

XLIII

the onium groups are separated by five or six methylene groups while depolarizing activity tends to predominate when the onium groups are separated by ten methylene groups. These observations thus serve to support the application of the pachycurare and leptocurare concept as a means of predicting the type of neuromuscular blockade associated with a given chemical structure since the fewer the methylene groups the less attenuated the molecule. Among the hexamethylene-separated ethonium compounds potency tends to increase with the number of onium groups present, but some anomalies occur. Nevertheless the overall picture of activity within the series as a whole would not be inconsistent with a repeating arrangement of anionic binding sites on the motor endplate.

Replacement of a methylene group in the interonium polymethylene chains by an ether oxygen atom tends to produce a drop in potency (*208, 407, 408, 502, 595*).

Certain polymeric quaternary ammonium compounds have been claimed to exhibit neuromuscular blocking and anticholinesterase activities (*278, 539*), but, as has been pointed out by Cavallito and Gray (*128*), caution must be exercised in the interpretation of results obtained with polymerized material where the size of all molecular species present has not been determined.

C. Rational Approaches to Shorter-Acting Neuromuscular Blocking Agents

As already indicated, by far the greatest attention in the search for short-acting neuromuscular blocking agents has been focused upon the incorporation of carboxylic ester functions within the molecular structure in order to secure ready hydrolysis by the esterases of the body. A large number of variants of the suxamethonium structure have been studied, including a variety of compounds of general structures **XLIV, XLV**, and **XLVI** (*64, 255, 285*) and related trisonium compounds (*440*), as well as derivatives of camphoric acid of type **XLVII** (*535*) and various compounds of type **XLVIII** (*439*) which incorporate the norbornane skeleton. Comprehensive reviews of compounds of this type have appeared elsewhere (*60, 61, 96*) and so they need not be further considered here, other than to draw attention to suxethonium (**XV**) and prodeconium, (**XLIX**) both of which have seen some clinical application. Suxethonium is significantly less potent than suxamethonium (*593*) as well as being hydrolyzed by the plasma esterases more readily (*480*), thus showing a shorter duration of action. It has also been claimed (*286*) that postoperative pain is less severe with suxethonium than with suxamethonium. Prodeconium which shows characteristics somewhat different from both the depolarizing and the antidepolarizing drugs (*599*), also exhibits neuromuscular blocking activity of short duration (*337*).

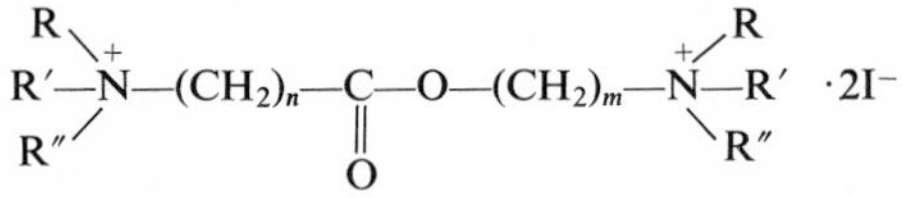

$$\underset{R''}{\overset{R}{\diagdown}}N^{+}-(CH_2)_n-\underset{\underset{O}{\parallel}}{C}-O-(CH_2)_m-N^{+}\underset{R''}{\overset{R}{\diagup}}R' \quad \cdot 2I^{-}$$

XLIV

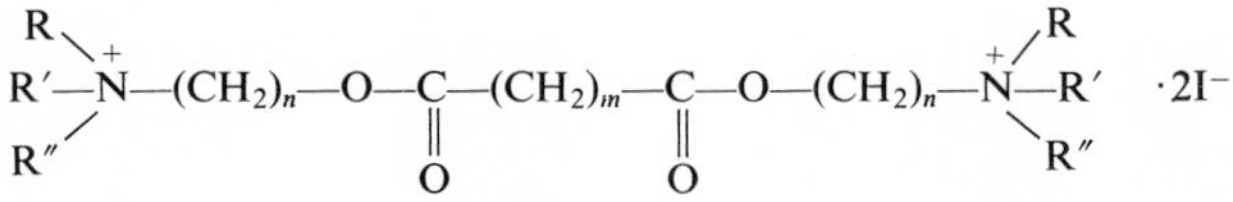

$$\underset{R''}{\overset{R}{\diagdown}}N^{+}-(CH_2)_n-O-\underset{\underset{O}{\parallel}}{C}-(CH_2)_m-\underset{\underset{O}{\parallel}}{C}-O-(CH_2)_n-N^{+}\underset{R''}{\overset{R}{\diagup}}R' \quad \cdot 2I^{-}$$

XLV

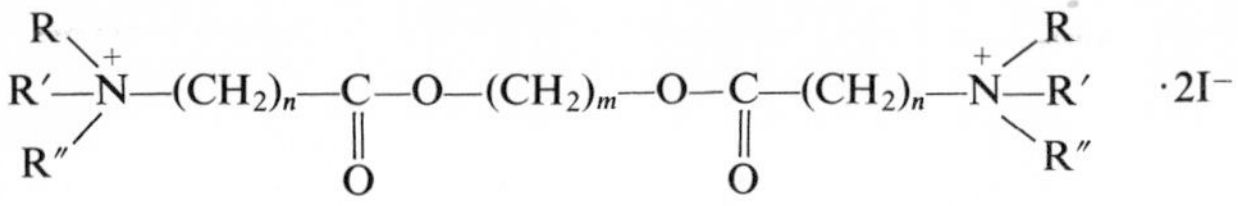

$$\underset{R''}{\overset{R}{\diagdown}}N^{+}-(CH_2)_n-\underset{\underset{O}{\parallel}}{C}-O-(CH_2)_m-O-\underset{\underset{O}{\parallel}}{C}-(CH_2)_n-N^{+}\underset{R''}{\overset{R}{\diagup}}R' \quad \cdot 2I^{-}$$

XLVI

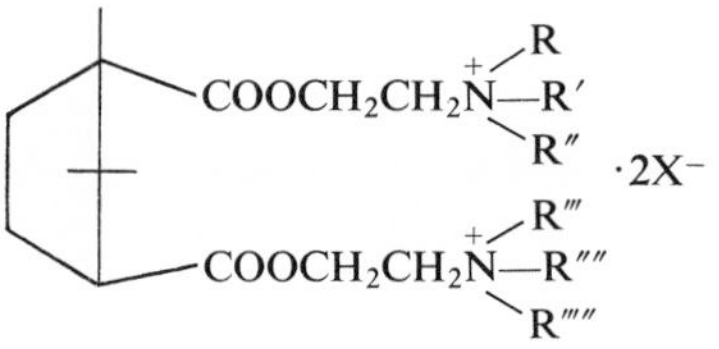

COOCH₂CH₂N⁺—R′/R″ ... ·2X⁻

COOCH₂CH₂N⁺—R‴/R‴′

XLVII

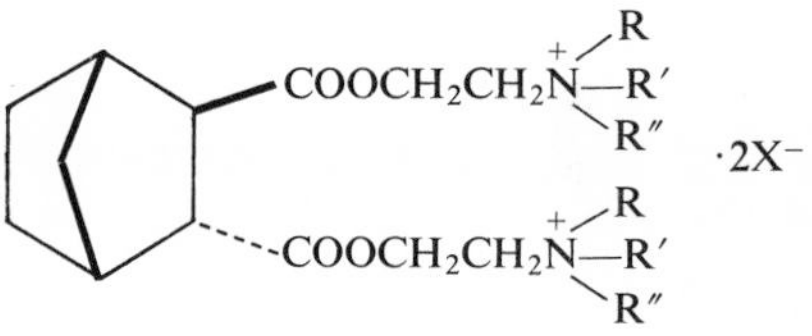

COOCH₂CH₂N⁺—R′/R″ ·2X⁻

COOCH₂CH₂N⁺—R/R′... R″

XLVIII

$$Me_2\overset{+}{N}\!-\!(CH_2)_2\!-\!O\!-\!(CH_2)_{10}\!-\!O\!-\!(CH_2)_2\!-\!\overset{+}{N}Me_2 \quad \cdot 2Br^{-}$$

with CH₂ groups and C—O—CH₂CH₂CH₃ / CH₃CH₂CH₂—O—C ester groups

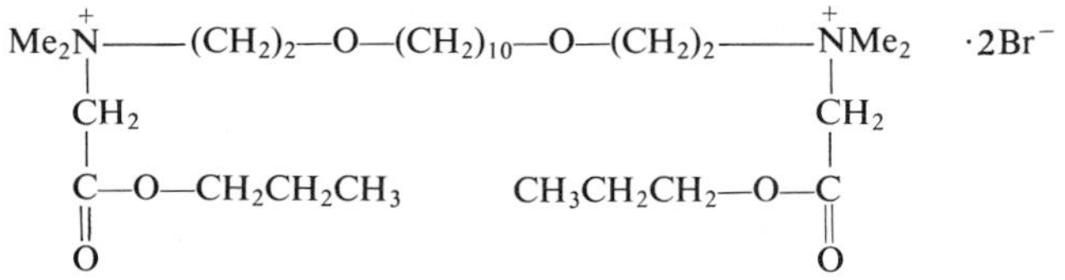

XLIX

The bischoline esters of carbonic acid and oxalic acid are essentially without neuromuscular blocking activity (*96*).

A completely different approach toward securing a shorter-acting neuro-muscular blocking agent was adopted in the case of alcuronium chloride(**L**). Here, clinical trials with toxiferine I (**X**) (*243, 613*) and the related alkaloid, curarine I (*613*) revealed these compounds to be too long-acting (*604*) for satisfactory application, while metabolic studies (*605, 615*) revealed that biotransformation was negligible. Thus structural modification studies were undertaken, and in view of the known drastic change in the biological properties of morphine brought about by replacement of the *N*-methyl group by an *N*-allyl group, coupled with the possibility of the allylic function acting as a potential site of biotransformation, one of the compounds obviously

L

warranting consideration as a modification of the toxiferine molecule was
N,N'-diallybisnortoxiferine, now known as alcuronium chloride (**L**). A ready
route to this compound is available from the Wieland-Gumlich aldehyde
which is obtainable from strychnine, and alcuronium has now gained an
established place in several countries as the muscle relaxant of choice in
surgery. It is relatively short-acting, produces a typical antidepolarizing
neuromuscular block readily reversed by neostigmine, and does not procure
histamine release (*20, 114, 175, 197, 239, 338, 418, 425, 540, 614*).

Another possible line of approach, as yet apparently unexplored, to new
short-acting neuromuscular blocking agents is perhaps suggested by work
carried out in the author's laboratories on the constitution of the alkaloid
petaline (**LI**) (*431*) which is an unusual benzyltetrahydroisoquinoline alkaloid
in that it possesses a 7,8-dioxygenated pattern. In the course of the chemical
studies it was observed that petaline underwent an extremely facile Hofmann
elimination reaction to yield the corresponding methine base, leonticine (**LII**),
passage of a solution of petaline reineckate down an IRA-400 (OH) ion
exchange resin being sufficient to achieve quantitative conversion. Further
studies on this ready elimination reaction (*430*) have revealed it to be characteristic of benzyltetrahydroisoquinolines having a free —OH group in the 6- or
8-positions, where formation of the phenolic anion can be seen to be a means

LI   **LII**

of electronically promoting cleavage of the 1–2 bond. Although, as is to be expected of a monoquaternary compound, petaline itself shows only weak neuromuscular blocking potency (*1*, *98*), giving 50% blockade in the cat sciatic–gastrocnemius preparation at a dose of ~4.5 mg/kg as the iodide [(+)-tubocurarine = 0.08 mg/kg] (*98*), a remarkable feature of the alkaloid is its potent convulsant activity. In mice it produces tonic convulsions at an $ED_{50} = 5.5$ mg/kg (*98*), and in view of the unusual occurrence of convulsant activity in a quaternary salt it was considered that petaline might be displaying this activity through an *in vivo* conversion into leonticine promoted by alkaline pH (cf. *14*). That this may not be so, however, has now been shown by the fact that the ED_{50} of leonticine, in the production of tonic convulsions in mice, is ~33.2 mg/kg (*98*), although the possibility of marked differences in transport characteristics of the two compounds affecting the issue can not be disregarded.

Nevertheless, this work does suggest the possibility of synthesizing bisquaternary ammonium salts with various built-in features serving to promote *in vivo* Hofmann eliminations as a means of securing short duration of action in neuromuscular blocking agents, and it remains to be seen whether this potential rational approach will meet with successful fulfilment.

VIII. Conclusion

From the foregoing it is readily apparent that the successful development of a number of new neuromuscular blocking agents represents a considerable triumph for the rational approach to drug design. This may be further emphasized by briefly listing the factors which were taken into consideration in the rational design of pancuronium bromide. These were as follows.

1. Choice of quaternary nitrogen atoms over other onium groups since these give greatest neuromuscular blocking potency.

2. Choice of a bisquaternary ammonium structure since this has greater potency than a monoquaternary ammonium structure and at the same time eliminates the difficulties in securing optimal spatial relationships of all bonding groups in higher polyonium salts.

3. Choice of a relatively fixed interonium distance of the order of 10.5 Å as this would appear to fall within the optimal range of neuromuscular blocking activity, and be too great for ganglion blocking activity.

4. Choice of a bulky molecule upon which to append the quaternary ammonium functions so as to produce antidepolarizing rather than depolarizing activity.

5. Choice of bulky substituents on the nitrogen atoms so as to further promote antidepolarizing activity.

6. Insertion of carboxylic ester functions so as to give a ready means of biotransformation.

7. Insertion of the ester functions adjacent to the onium centers so as to permit biotransformation parallel to the conversion of acetylcholine into choline, since the latter compound is devoid of any marked neuromuscular blocking activity, and at the same time permit pancuronium bromide the maximum chance of having affinity for acetylcholine binding sites.

As more and more compounds are screened for neuromuscular blocking activity and the more subtle molecular modifications favoring a given mode of action become more readily apparent, particularly the influence of absolute configuration, it may be confidently anticipated that still further rational guidelines to the synthesis of superior agents will become available. A major breakthrough would be the complete elucidation of the molecular ecology of the receptor system and the complete chemical characterization of all molecular species present, as this can then be expected to open new horizons in rational drug design.* Similarly, full elucidation of the biochemical phenomena involved in the prejunctional liberation of acetylcholine can be expected to permit new rational approaches to the design of agents specifically suited to the treatment of the symptoms of Parkinson's disease. Work with active-site-directed irreversible enzyme inhibitors with a view to producing new anticholine acetyl transferase drugs can be expected to play a role in this area, as can perhaps work directed toward the preparation of compounds interfering with the role of gangliosides.

In terms of the progress so far achieved, it is apparent that a rational approach to the design of new neuromuscular blocking agents is already well developed, and there would appear to be great promise for the future.

* See Addendum, p. 530.

REFERENCES

1. K. Ahmad and J. J. Lewis, *J. Pharm. Pharmacol.* **12**, 163 (1960).
2. M. Alauddin, B. Caddy, J. J. Lewis, M. Martin-Smith, and M. F. Sugrue, *J. Pharm. Pharmacol.* **17**, 55 (1965).
3. M. Alauddin and M. Martin-Smith, *J. Pharm. Pharmacol.* **14**, 325 (1962).
4. D. Albe-Fessard, C. Chagas, and H. Martins Ferreira, *An. Acad. Brasil. Cilnc.* **23**, 327 (1951).
5. R. W. Albers and G. J. Koval, *Biochim. Biophys. Acta* **60**, 359 (1962).
6. E. X. Albuquerque, M. D. Sokoll, B. Sonesson, and S. Thesleff, *Euro. J. Pharmacol.* **4**, 40 (1968).
7. N. Ambache and A. W. Lessin, *J. Physiol.* (*London*) **127**, 449 (1955).
8. H. Andersag and F. Bossert, *Naturwissenschaften* **42**, 46 (1955).
9. E. Andersson-Cedergren, *J. Ultrastruct. Res.* Suppl. 1, 1 (1959).
10. D. E. Argent, O. P. Dimick, and F. Hobbiger, *Brit. J. Anaesth.* **27**, 24 (1955).

11. E. J. Ariëns and W. M. de Groot, *Arch. Int. Pharmacodyn. Ther.* **99**, 193 (1954).
12. E. J. Ariëns and A. M. Simonis, *in* "Quantitative Methods in Pharmacology" (H. De Jonge, ed.), p. 286. North-Holland Publ., Amsterdam, 1961.
13. E. J. Ariëns, J. M. Van Rossum, and A. M. Simonis, *Pharmacol. Rev.* **9**, 218 (1957).
14. J. G. Arrowood, *Anesthesiology* **12**, 753 (1951).
15. K. B. Augustinsson, *Acta Physiol. Scand.* Suppl. 15, 1 (1948).
16. J. Axelsson and S. Thesleff, *Acta Physiol. Scand.* **43**, 15 (1958).
17. J. Axelsson and S. Thesleff, *J. Physiol. (London)* **147**, 178 (1959).
18. P. Bach-y-Rita and F. Ito, *J. Gen. Physiol.* **49**, 1177 (1966).
19. Z. M. Bacq and G. L. Brown, *J. Physiol. (London)* **89**, 45 (1937).
20. H. P. Baechtold, F. Fornasari, and A. Huerlimann, *Helv. Physiol. Pharmacol. Acta* **22**, 70 (1964).
21. W. L. M. Baird and A. M. Reid, *Brit. J. Anaesth.* **39**, 775 (1967).
22. B. R. Baker, "Design of Active-Site-Directed Irreversible Enzyme Inhibitors. The Organic Chemistry of the Enzymic Active-Site." Wiley, New York, 1967.
23. D. G. Bamford, D. F. Biggs, M. Davis, and E. W. Parnell, *Brit. J. Pharmacol.* **30**, 194 (1967).
24. R. B. Barlow, *Biochem. Soc. Symp.* **19**, 46 (and refs. cited) (1960).
25. R. B. Barlow, "Introduction to Chemical Pharmacology," 2nd ed. Methuen, London, 1964.
26. R. B. Barlow, H. Blaschko, J. M. Himms, and U. Trendelenburg, *Brit. J. Pharmacol.* **10**, 116 (1955).
27. R. B. Barlow and H. R. Ing, *Nature (London)* **161**, 718 (1948).
28. R. B. Barlow and H. R. Ing, *Brit. J. Pharmacol.* **3**, 298 (1948).
29. E. A. Barnard and A. W. Rogers, *Ann. N.Y. Acad. Sci.* **144**, 584 (1967).
30. R. J. Barrnett, *J. Cell Biol.* **12**, 247 (1962).
31. J. A. B. Barstad, *Experientia* **18**, 579 (1962).
31a. E. Bartels, *Biochem. Pharmacol.* **17**, 945 (1968).
32. L. Bass and W. J. Moore, *Proc. Nat. Acad. Sci. U.S.* **55**, 1214 (1966).
33. L. Beani, C. Bianchi, and P. Megazzini, *Experientia* **20**, 677 (1964).
34. E. Beccari, *Arch. Sci. Physiol.* **3**, 611 (1949).
34a. A. H. Beckett, *Ann. N.Y. Acad. Sci.* **144**, 675 (1967).
35. B. Belleau, *J. Med. Chem.* **7**, 776 (1964).
36. B. Belleau, *Advanc. Drug Res.* **2**, 89 (1965).
37. B. Belleau, *Ann. N.Y. Acad. Sci.* **144**, 705 (1967).
37a. B. Belleau, *in* "Physico-Chemical Aspects of Drug Actions" (E. J. Ariëns, ed.), p. 207. Pergamon Press, Oxford, 1968.
37b. B. Belleau, V. Di Tullio, and Y. H. Tsai, *Mol. Pharmacol.* **6**, 41 (1970).
38. I. Bencowitz and R. R. Renshaw, *J. Amer. Chem. Soc.* **47**, 1904 (1925).
39. A. E. Bennett, *Amer. J. Psychiat.* **97**, 1040 (1941).
40. C. Bernard, *C. R. Soc. Biol.* **2**, 195 (1851).
41. C. Bernard, *C. R. Acad. Sci.* **43**, 825 (1856).
42. J. Bernstein, *Arch. Gesamte Physiol. Menschen Tiere* **92**, 521 (1902).
43. J. F. Berry and E. Starz, *Quart. J. Stud. Alc.* **17**, 190 (1956).
44. S. P. Bhatnager, A. Lane, and J. D. McColl, *Nature (London)* **204**, 485 (1964).
45. R. S. Biggs, M. Davis, and R. Wien, *Experientia* **20**, 119 (1964).
46. R. Binning, *Anaesthesia* **8**, 268 (1953).
47. R. I. Birks, B. Katz, and R. Miledi, *J. Physiol. (London)* **150**, 145 (1960).
48. R. I. Birks and F. C. MacIntosh, *Can. J. Biochem. Physiol.* **39**, 787 (1961).
49. L. C. Blaber and W. C. Bowman, *Arch. Int. Pharmacodyn. Ther.* **138**, 90 (1962).

50. L. C. Blaber and W. C. Bowman, *Arch. Int. Pharmacodyn. Ther.* **138**, 185 (1962).
51. L. C. Blaber and W. C. Bowman, *Brit. J. Pharmacol.* **20**, 326 (1963).
52. L. C. Blaber and W. C. Bowman, *Int. J. Neuropharmacol.* **2**, 1 (1963).
53. L. C. Blaber and A. W. Cuthbert, *Biochem. Pharmacol.* **11**, 113 (1962).
54. M. P. Blaustein, *Biochim. Biophys. Acta* **135**, 653 (1967).
55. M. P. Blaustein and D. E. Goldman, *J. Gen. Physiol.* **49**, 1043 (1966).
56. D. Bodian, *Physiol. Rev.* **22**, 146 (1942).
57. R. I. Bodman, H. J. V. Morton, and W. D. Wylie, *Lancet* **2**, 517 (1952).
58. S. Bogoch, *Biochem. J.* **68**, 319 (1958).
59. I. L. Bonta, E. M. Goorissen, and F. H. Derkx, *Euro. J. Pharmacol.* **4**, 83 (1968).
60. D. Bovet, *Ann. N.Y. Acad. Sci.* **54**, 407 (1951).
61. D. Bovet, *in* "Curare and Curare-like Agents" (D. Bovet, F. Bovet-Nitti, and G. B. Marini-Bettolo, eds.), p. 252. Elsevier, Amsterdam, 1959.
62. D. Bovet and F. Bovet-Nitti, *Experientia* **4**, 325 (1948).
63. D. Bovet and F. Bovet-Nitti, "Medicaments du système nerveux végétatif." Karger, Basel, 1948.
64. D. Bovet, F. Bovet-Nitti, S. Guarino, V. G. Longo, and M. Marotta, *Rend. Ist Super. Sanita* **12**, 106 (1949).
65. D. Bovet, S. Courvoisier, R. Ducrot, and R. Horclois, *C. R. Acad. Sci.* **223**, 597 (1946).
66. D. Bovet, F. Depierre, S. Courvoisier, and Y. de Lestrange, *Arch. Int. Pharmacodyn. Ther.* **80**, 172 (1949).
67. D. Bovet, F. Depierre, and Y. de Lestrange, *C. R. Acad. Sci.* **225**, 74 (1947).
68. W. C. Bowman, *Brit. J. Pharmacol.* **13**, 521 (1958).
69. W. C. Bowman, *Progr. Med. Chem.* **2**, 88 (1962).
70. W. C. Bowman, *in* "Evaluation of Drug Activities: Pharmacometrics" (D. R. Laurence and A. L. Bacharach, eds.), Vol. 1, p. 325. Academic Press, New York, 1964.
71. W. C. Bowman, *in* "Physiology of the Domestic Fowl" (C. Horton-Smith and E. C. Amoroso, eds.), p. 249. Oliver & Boyd, Ltd., Edinburgh and London, 1966.
72. W. C. Bowman and B. A. Hemsworth, *Brit. J. Pharmacol.* **24**, 110 (1965).
73. W. C. Bowman and B. A. Hemsworth, *Brit. J. Pharmacol.* **25**, 392 (1965).
74. W. C. Bowman, B. A. Hemsworth, and M. J. Rand, *Brit. J. Pharmacol.* **19**, 198 (1962).
75. W. C. Bowman, B. A. Hemsworth, and M. J. Rand, *J. Pharm. Pharmacol.* **14**, 37T (1962).
76. W. C. Bowman, B. A. Hemsworth, and M. J. Rand, *Ann. N.Y. Acad. Sci.* **144**, 471 (1967).
77. W. C. Bowman and M. J. Rand, *Brit. J. Pharmacol.* **17**, 176 (1961).
78. W. C. Bowman and M. J. Rand, *Lancet* **1**, 480 (1961).
79. W. C. Bowman and M. J. Rand, *Int. J. Neuropharmacol.* **1**, 129 (1962).
80. W. C. Bowman, M. J. Rand, and G. B. West, "Textbook of Pharmacology," p. 660. Blackwell, Oxford, 1968.
81. W. C. Bowman and C. Raper, *Nature (London)* **201**, 160 (1964).
82. I. A. Boyd, *J. Physiol. (London)* **140**, 14P (1958).
83. I. A. Boyd, *J. Physiol. (London)* **145**, 55P (1959).
84. I. A. Boyd, *Phil. Trans. Roy. Soc. London, Sr. B* **245**, 81 (1962).
85. I. A. Boyd and A. R. Martin, *J. Physiol. (London)* **132**, 74 (1956).
86. P. J. Boyle and E. J. Conway, *J. Physiol. (London)* **100**, 1 (1941).
87. B. M. Braganca and J. H. Quastel, *Nature (London)* **169**, 695 (1952).
88. O. V. Brazil and A. P. Corrado, *J. Pharmacol. Exp. Ther.* **120**, 452 (1957).
89. H. J. Brennan, *Brit. J. Anaesth.* **28**, 159 (1956).
90. E. Brodkin and K. A. C. Elliot, *Amer. J. Physiol.* **173**, 437 (1953).

91. V. B. Brooks, *J. Physiol. (London)* **123**, 501 (1954).
92. V. B. Brooks, *J. Physiol. (London)* **151**, 598 (1960).
93. G. L. Brown, H. H. Dale, and W. J. Feldberg, *J. Physiol. (London)* **87**, 394 (1936).
94. G. L. Brown and W. Feldberg, *J. Physiol. (London)* **86**, 290 (1936).
95. G. L. Brown and A. M. Harvey, *J. Physiol. (London)* **93**, 285 (1938).
96. F. Brücke, *Pharmacol. Rev.* **8**, 265 (1956).
97. F. Buchthal and J. Lindhard, *Acta Physiol. Scand.* **4**, 136 (1942).
98. W. R. Buckett, personal communication (1968).
99. W. R. Buckett and I. L. Bonta, *Fed Proc., Fed. Amer. Soc. Exp. Biol.* **25**, 718 (1966).
100. W. R. Buckett, C. L. Hewett, and D. S. Savage, *Chim. Ther.* **2**, 186 (1967).
101. W. R. Buckett, C. E. B. Marjoribanks, F. A. Marwick, and M. B. Morton, *Brit. J. Pharmacol.* **32**, 671 (1968).
102. E. Bülbring and F. Depierre, *Brit. J. Pharmacol.* **4**, 22 (1949).
103. G. Bull and B. A. Hemsworth, *Nature (London)* **199**, 487 (1963).
104. G. Bull and B. A. Hemsworth, *Brit. J. Pharmacol.* **25**, 228 (1965).
104a. A. J. Buller, *Endeavour* **29**, 107 (1970).
105. A. S. V. Burgen, G. Burke, and M. L. Desbarats-Schonbaum, *Brit. J. Pharmacol.* **11**, 308 (1956).
106. A. S. V. Burgen, F. Dickens, and L. S. Zatman, *J. Physiol. (London)* **109**, 10 (1949).
107. W. Burke and B. L. Ginsborg, *J. Physiol. (London)* **132**, 599 (1956).
108. M. S. Burman, *J. Bone Joint Surg.* **20**, 754 (1938).
109. B. D. Burns and W. D. M. Paton, *J. Physiol. (London)* **115**, 41 (1951).
110. R. M. Burton and J. M. Gibbons, *Biochim. Biophys. Acta* **84**, 220 (1964).
111. R. M. Burton and R. E. Howard, *Ann. N.Y. Acad. Sci.* **144**, 411 (1967).
112. R. M. Burton, R. E. Howard, S. Baer, and Y. M. Balfour, *Biochim. Biophys. Acta* **84**, 441 (1964).
113. D. Busfield, K. J. Child, A. J. Clarke, B. Davis, and M. G. Dodds, *Brit. J. Pharmacol.* **32**, 609 (1968).
114. G. H. Bush, *Proc. Roy. Soc. Med.* **58**, 633 (1965).
115. G. A. H. Buttle and E. J. Zaimis, *J. Pharm. Pharmacol.* **1**, 991 (1949).
116. B. Caddy, M. Martin-Smith, and T. C. Muir, unpublished results (1964).
116a. F. N. Campbell and M. Swerdlow, *Brit. J. Anaesth.* **41**, 962 (1969).
117. F. G. Canepa, *Nature (London)* **195**, 573 (1962).
118. F. G. Canepa, *Nature (London)* **201**, 184 (1964).
119. F. G. Canepa, *Ann. N.Y. Acad. Sci.* **144**, 918 (1967).
120. T. H. Cannard and E. J. Zaimis, *J. Physiol. (London)* **149**, 112 (1959).
121. F. M. Carey, D. Edwards, J. J. Lewis, and J. B. Stenlake, *J. Pharm. Pharmacol.* Suppl. 11, 70T (1959).
122. F. M. Carey, C. I. Furst, J. J. Lewis, and J. B. Stenlake, *J. Pharm. Pharmacol.* Suppl. 16, 89T (1964).
123. R. F. Carlyle, *Brit. J. Pharmacol.* **18**, 612 (1962).
123a. L. D. Carnay and W. H. Barry, *Science* **165**, 608 (1969).
124. G. Cavallini, *Farmaco Ed. Sci.* **10**, 644 (1955).
125. G. Cavallini and E. Massarani, *J. Med. Pharm. Chem.* **1**, 365 (1959).
126. C. J. Cavallito, *Ann. N.Y. Acad. Sci.* **144**, 900 (1967).
127. C. J. Cavallito, *Fed. Proc., Fed. Amer. Soc. Exp. Biol.* **26**, 1647 (1967).
128. C. J. Cavallito and A. P. Gray, *Progr. Drug Res.* **2**, 135 (1960).
128a. C. J. Cavallito, H. S. Yun, J. C. Smith, and F. F. Foldes, *J. Med. Chem.* **12**, 134 (1969).
128b. D. Cecconello, G. L. Franchiotti, and A. Giussani, *Acta Anaesthesiol. Scand.* **12**, 31 (1968).

129. C. Chagas, *An. Acad. Brasil. Cienc.* **19**, 113 (1947).

130. C. Chagas, *Ann. N.Y. Acad. Sci.* **81**, 345 (1959).

131. C. Chagas, in "Curare and Curare-like Agents" (D. Bovet, F. Bovet-Nitti, and G. B. Marini-Bettolo, eds.), p. 327. Elsevier, Amsterdam, 1959.

132. C. Chagas, E. Penna-Franca, A. Hassón, C. Crocker, K. Nishie, and E. J. Garcia, *An. Acad. Brasil. Cienc.* **29**, 53 (1957).

133. C. Chagas, E. Penna-Franca, K. Nishie, and E. J. Garcia, *Arch. Biochem. Biophys.* **75**, 251 (1958).

134. C. Chagas, E. Penna-Franca, K. Nishie, C. Crocker, and M. Miranda, *C. R. Acad. Sci.* **242**, 2671 (1956).

134a. C. C. Chang, S. E. Lu, P. N. Wang, and S. T. Chuang, *Euro. J. Pharmacol.* **11**, 195 (1970) and refs. cited therein.

135. V. Chang and M. J. Rand, *Brit. J. Pharmacol.* **15**, 588 (1960).

136. J. P. Changeux, *Sci. Amer.* **212**, No. 4, 36 (1965).

136a. J. P. Changeux, *Mol. Pharmacol.* **2**, 369 (1966).

137. J. Cheymol P. Chabrier, F. Bourillet, and K. Smarzewska, *Therapie* **8**, 929 (1953).

138. K. J. Child and E. J. Zaimis, *Brit. J. Pharmacol.* **15**, 412 (1960).

138a. C. Chothia, *Nature (London)* **225**, 36 (1970).

139. C. Chothia, *Nature (London)* **227**, 1355 (1970).

140. T. H. Christie, R. P. Wise, and H. C. Churchill-Davidson, *Lancet* **2**, 648 (1959).

141. H. C. Churchill-Davidson, *Brit. Med. Bull.* **14**, 31 (1958).

142. H. C. Churchill-Davidson and T. H. Christie, *Brit. J. Anaesth.* **31**, 290 (1959).

143. H. C. Churchill-Davidson and A. T. Richardson, *Nature (London)* **170**, 617 (1952).

144. S. Ciani and C. Edwards, *J. Pharmacol. Exp. Ther.* **142**, 21 (1963).

145. C. Cöers and A. L. Woolf, "The Innervation of Muscle. A Biopsy Study." Thomas, Springfield, Illinois, 1959.

146. J. A. Cohen, R. A. Oosterbaan, H. S. Jansz, and F. Berends, *J. Cell. Comp. Physiol.* **54**, 231 (1959).

147. W. V. Cole, *J. Comp. Neurol.* **102**, 671 (1955).

148. H. O. J. Collier, *Brit. Med. J.* **1**, 1293 (1950).

149. H. O. J. Collier and E. P. Taylor, *Nature (London)* **164**, 491 (1949).

150. E. J. Conway, R. P. Kernan, and J. A. Zadunaisky, *J. Physiol. (London)* **155**, 263 (1961).

151. A. P. Corrado, A. O. Ramos, and C. T. De Escobar, *Arch. Int. Pharmacodyn. Ther.* **121**, 380 (1959).

152. R. Couteaux, *Rev. Can. Biol.* **6**, 563 (1947).

153. R. Couteaux, *C. R. Soc. Biol.* **147**, 1974 (1953).

154. R. Couteaux, *Int. Rev. Cytol.* **4**, 335 (1955).

155. R. Couteaux, *Exp. Cell. Res.* Suppl. **5**, 294 (1958).

156. R. Couteaux, in "The Structure and Function of Muscle" (G. H. Bourne, ed.), Vol. 1, p. 337. Academic Press, New York, 1960.

157. R. Couteaux and D. Nachmansohn, *Proc. Soc. Exp. Biol. Med.* **43**, 177 (1940).

158. R. Couteaux and J. Taxi, *Arch. Anat. Microsc. Morphol. Exp.* **41**, 352 (1952).

159. L. E. Craig, *Chem. Rev.* **42**, 285 (1948).

160. R. Creese, J. B. Dillon, J. Marshall, P. B. Sabawala, D. J. Schneider, and D. B. Taylor, *J. Pharmacol. Exp. Ther.* **119**, 485 (1957).

161. R. Creese, D. B. Taylor, and B. Tilton, *J. Pharmacol. Exp. Ther.* **139**, 8 (1963).

162. J. Crossland, *J. Pharm. Pharmacol.* **12**, 1 (1960).

163. J. F. Crul, *Excerpta Med.* ICS No. 168. *4th World Congr. Anaesthesiol.* p. 135 (1968).

164. A. Crum Brown and T. R. Fraser, *Trans. Roy. Soc. Edinburgh* **25**, 151 (1868).

165. A. Crum Brown and T. R. Fraser, *Proc. Roy. Soc. Edinburgh* **6**, 556 (1869).

166. A. Crum Brown and T. R. Fraser, *Trans. Roy. Soc. Edinburgh* **25**, 693 (1869).
167. B. Csillik, "Functional Structure of the Post-Synaptic Membrane in the Myoneural Junction," Akadémiai Kiadó, Budapest, 1965.
168. S. C. Cullen, *Surgery* **14**, 261 (1943).
169. H. H. Dale, W. J. Feldberg, and M. Vogt, *J. Physiol. (London)* **86**, 353 (1936).
170. M. J. Dallemagne and E. Philippot, *Arch. Int. Pharmacodyn. Ther.* **87**, 127 (1951).
171. M. J. Dallemagne and E. Philppot, *Arch. Int. Physiol.* **59**, 407 (1951).
172. M. J. Dallemagne and E. Philippot, *Brit. J. Pharmacol.* **7**, 601 (1952).
173. W. C. Dautermann and K. N. Mehrotra, *J. Neurochem.* **10**, 113 (1963).
174. N. Davis and M. Karp, *Curr. Res. Anesth. Analg.* **30**, 47 (1951).
175. M. T. de Cournaut, B. Dupuy, and J. Jaquenoud, *Agressologie* **3**, 627 (1961).
176. E. Dee and R. P. Kernan, *J. Physiol. (London)* **165**, 550 (1963).
177. J. Del Castillo and L. Engbaek, *J. Physiol. (London)* **120**, 54P (1953).
178. J. Del Castillo and L. Engbaek, *J. Physiol. (London)* **124**, 370 (1954).
179. J. Del Castillo and B. Katz, *J. Physiol. (London)* **128**, 157 (1955).
180. J. Del Castillo and B. Katz, *Progr. Biophys. Biophys. Chem.* **6**, 121 (1956).
181. J. Del Castillo and B. Katz, *Proc. Roy. Soc., Ser. B* **146**, 339 (1957).
182. J. Del Castillo and B. Katz, *Proc. Roy. Soc., Ser. B.* **146**, 357 (1957).
183. J. Del Castillo and B. Katz, *Proc. Roy. Soc., Ser. B.* **146**, 369 (1957).
184. J. Del Castillo and B. Katz, *Collog. Int. Cent. Nat. Rech. Sci.* **67**, 245 (1957).
185. J. Del Castillo, A. Rodriguez, and C. A. Romero, *Ann. N.Y. Acad. Sci.* **144**, 803 (1967).
186. J. Del Castillo and L. Stark, *J. Physiol. (London)* **116**, 507 (1952).
187. D. Della Bella and R. Villani, *Boll. Soc. Ital. Biol. Sper.* **31**, 703 (1955).
188. D. Della Bella, R. Villani, and G. F. Zuanazzi, *Arch. Exp. Pathol. Pharmak.* **229**, 536 (1956).
189. D. Della Bella, R. Villani, and G. F. Zuanazzi, *Boll. Soc. Ital. Biol. Sper.* **32**, 483 (1956).
190. E. D. P. De Robertis, *Exp. Cell Res.* Suppl. **5**, 347 (1958).
191. E. D. P. De Robertis, *Int. Rev. Cytol.* **8**, 61 (1959).
192. E. D. P. De Robertis and H. S. Bennett, *J. Biophys. Biochem. Cytol.* **1**, 47 (1955).
193. E. D. P. De Robertis, G. Rodriguez De Lores Arnaiz, L. Salganicoff, A. Pellegrino De Iraldi, and L. M. Zieher, *J. Neurochem.* **10**, 225 (1963).
194. J. E. Desmedt, *J. Physiol. (London)* **121**, 191 (1953).
195. V. Deulofeu, *in* "Curare and Curare-like Agents" (D. Bovet, F. Bovet-Nitti, and G. B. Marini-Bettolo, eds.), p. 163. Elsevier, Amsterdam, 1959.
196. J. Diamond and R. Miledi, *J. Physiol. (London)* **162**, 393 (1962).
196a. V. di Carlo, *Nature (London)* **213**, 833 (1967).
196b. F. A. Dodge and R. Rahaminoff, *J. Physiol. (London)* **193**, 419 (1967).
196c. D. B. Drachman and B. L. Fanburg, *J. Neurochem.* **16**, 1633 (1969).
197. R. Droh and J. Hoerst, *Anaesthesist* **14**, 275 (1965).
198. J. W. Dundee, T. C. Gray, and G. J. Rees, *Anaesthesia* **7**, 134 (1952).
199. J. W. Dundee, T. C. Gray, and J. E. Riding, *Brit. J. Anaesth.* **26**, 13 (1954).
199a. J. Durell, J. T. Garland, and R. O. Friedel, *Science* **165**, 862 (1969).
200. F. P. Dwyer, E. C. Gyarfas, R. D. Wright, and A. Schulman, *Nature (London)* **179**, 425 (1957).
201. J. C. Eccles, *Arch. Sci. Physiol.* **3**, 567 (1949).
202. J. C. Eccles, "The Physiology of Synapses." Springer, Berlin, 1964.
203. J. C. Eccles, B. Katz, and S. W. Kuffler, *J. Neurophysiol.* **4**, 362 (1941).
204. J. C. Eccles, B. Katz, and S. W. Kuffler, *Biol. Symp.* **3**, 349 (1941).
205. J. C. Eccles, B. Katz, and S. W. Kuffler, *J. Neurophysiol.* **5**, 211 (1942).
206. J. C. Eccles and M. V. Macfarlane, *J. Neurophysiol.* **12**, 59 (1949).
207. D. Edwards, J. J. Lewis, and G. Marren, *J. Pharm. Pharmacol.* **18**, 670 (1966).

208. D. Edwards, J. J. Lewis, D. E. McPhail, T. C. Muir, and J. B. Stenlake, *J. Pharm. Pharmacol.* Suppl. 12, 137T (1960).
209. D. Edwards, J. J. Lewis, J. B. Stenlake, and M. S. Zoha, *J. Pharm. Pharmacol.* **9**, 1004 (1957).
210. D. Edwards, J. J. Lewis, J. B. Stenlake, and M. S. Zoha, *J. Pharm. Pharmacol.* Suppl. 10, 106T and 122T (1958).
211. D. Edwards, J. B. Stenlake, J. J. Lewis, and F. Stothers, *J. Med. Pharm. Chem.* **3**, 369 (1961).
212. S. Ehrenpreis, *Fed. Proc., Fed. Amer. Soc. Exp. Biol.* **18**, 220 (1959).
213. S. Ehrenpreis, *Science* **129**, 1613 (1959).
214. S. Ehrenpreis, *Biochim. Biophys. Acta* **44**, 561 (1960).
215. S. Ehrenpreis, *Int. J. Neuropharmacol.* **1**, 273 (1962).
216. S. Ehrenpreis, *Nature (London)* **194**, 586 (1962).
217. S. Ehrenpreis, *Proc. 1st Int. Pharmacol. Meet., 1961* Vol. 7, p. 119 (1962).
218. S. Ehrenpreis, *Nature (London)* **201**, 887 (1964).
219. S. Ehrenpreis, *J. Cell. Comp. Physiol.* **66**, 159 (1965).
220. S. Ehrenpreis, *Ann. N.Y. Acad. Sci.* **144**, 720 (1967).
221. S. Ehrenpreis, *in* "Drugs Affecting The Peripheral Nervous System" (A. Burger, ed.), Vol. 1, p. 1. Arnold, London, 1967.
221a. S. Ellis and S. B. Beckett, *J. Pharmacol. Exp. Ther.* **112**, 202 (1954).
222. D. Elmqvist and D. S. Feldman, *J. Physiol. (London)* **181**, 487 (1965).
223. D. Elmqvist and D. M. J. Quastel, *J. Physiol. (London)* **177**, 463 (1965).
224. D. Elmqvist and S. Thesleff, *Rev. Can. Biol.* **21**, 229 (1962).
225. P. H. Elworthy, *J. Pharm. Pharmacol.* Suppl. 15, 137T (1963).
226. E. R. Evans and H. Wilson, *Brit. J. Pharmacol.* **22**, 441 (1964).
226a. A. J. Everett, L. A. Lowe, and S. Wilkinson, *Chem. Commun.* p. 1020 (1970).
227. P. Fatt and B. Katz, *J. Physiol. (London)* **115**, 320 (1951).
228. P. Fatt and B. Katz, *J. Physiol. (London)* **117**, 109 (1952).
228a. M. R. Fedde, *J. Gen. Physiol.* **53**, 624 (1969).
229. M. B. Feinstein, *J. Gen. Physiol.* **48**, 357 (1964).
230. W. Feldberg, *Physiol. Rev.* **25**, 596 (1945).
231. W. Feldberg, A. Fessard, and D. Nachmansohn, *J. Physiol. (London)* **97**, 3 (1940).
232. T. P. Feng and T. H. Li, *Chin. J. Physiol.* **16**, 37 (1941).
233. G. Ferguson, personal communication (1968).
233a. M. Figueroa, *South. Med. J.* **61**, 808 (1968).
234. J. Folch, A. Meath, and S. Arsove, *J. Biol. Chem.* **191**, 819 (1951).
235. F. F. Foldes, *Ann. N.Y. Acad. Sci.* **54**, 503 (1951).
236. F. F. Foldes, *Brit. J. Anaesth.* **26**, 394 (1954).
237. F. F. Foldes, "Muscle Relaxants in Anesthesiology." Thomas, Springfield, Illinois, 1957.
238. F. F. Foldes, *Clin. Pharmacol. Ther.* **1**, 345 (1960).
239. F. F. Foldes, I. M. Brown, J. N. Lunn, J. Moore, and D. Duncalf, *Curr. Res. Anesth. Analg.* **42**, 177 (1963).
240. F. F. Foldes, P. G. McNall, and J. H. Birch, *Brit. Med. J.* **1**, 967 (1954).
241. F. F. Foldes and F. I. Tsuji, *Fed. Proc., Fed. Amer. Soc. Exp. Biol.* **12**, 321 (1953).
242. F. F. Foldes, A. L. Wnuck, R. J. H. Hodges, S. Thesleff, and E. J. de Beer, *Curr. Res. Anesth. Analg.* **36**, 23 (1957).
243. F. F. Foldes, O. Wolfram, and M. D. Sokoll, *Anaesthesist* **10**, 210 (1961).
243a. F. Fonnum, *Biochem. J.* **103**, 262 (1967).
244. B. Frankenhaeuser and A. L. Hodgkin, *J. Physiol. (London)* **137**, 218 (1957).
245. T. Fredriksson, *Acta Pharmacol. Toxicol.* **13**, 86 (1957).
246. S. M. Free and J. M. Wilson, *J. Med. Chem.* **7**, 395 (1964).

247. S. E. Freeman, *Brit. J. Pharmacol.* **32**, 546 (1968).
247a. S. E. Freeman, *J. Pharmacol. Exp. Ther.* **162**, 10 (1968).
248. H. L. Friedman, *Nat. Acad. Sci.—Nat. Res. Counc., Publ.* **206** (1951).
249. S. L. Friess, *Ann. N.Y. Acad. Sci.* **144**, 839 (1967).
250. S. L. Friess, R. C. Durant, J. B. Chenley, and T. Mezzetti, *Biochem. Pharmacol.* **14**, 1237 (1965).
251. T. Fujita, *J. Med. Chem.* **9**, 797 (1966).
252. T. Fujita and C. Hansch, *J. Med. Chem.* **10**, 996 (1967).
253. E. Fulchiero, M. R. Turcotte, and S. J. Martin, *Proc. Soc. Exp. Biol. Med.* **99**, 537 (1958).
254. R. F. Furchgott and P. Bursztyn, *Ann. N.Y. Acad. Sci.* **144**, 882 (1967).
255. R. Fusco, G. Palazzo, S. Chiavarelli, and D. Bovet, *Gazz. Chim. Ital.* **79**, 836 (1949).
256. P. W. Gage and D. M. J. Quastel, *Nature (London)* **206**, 625 (1965).
257. C. H. Gallagher and J. H. Koch, *Nature (London)* **183**, 1124 (1959).
258. D. B. Gammack, *Biochem. J.* **88**, 373 (1963).
259. J. E. Gardiner, *Biochem. J.* **81**, 297 (1961).
260. J. E. Garvin and M. L. Karnovsky, *J. Biol. Chem.* **221**, 211 (1956).
261. J. Gautrelet and E. Corteggiani, *C. R. Acad. Sci.* **131**, 951 (1939).
262. M. A. Gerebtzoff, "Cholinesterases." Pergamon Press, Oxford, 1959.
263. R. M. Gesler and J. O. Hoppe, *Fed. Proc., Fed. Amer. Soc. Exp. Biol.* **20**, 587 (1961).
264. N. J. Giarman and G. Pepeu, *Brit. J. Pharmacol.* **19**, 226 (1962).
265. N. J. Giarman and G. Pepeu, *Brit. J. Pharmacol.* **23**, 123 (1964).
266. A. G. Ginetzinsky and N. M. Shamarina, *Usp. Sovrem. Biol.* **15**, 283 (1942).
267. B. L. Ginsborg, *J. Physiol. (London)* **150**, 707 (1960).
268. B. L. Ginsborg, *J. Physiol. (London)* **154**, 581 (1960).
269. B. L. Ginsborg and B. Mackay, *J. Physiol. (London)* **153**, 19P (1960).
270. B. L. Ginsborg and B. Mackay, *Bibl. Anat.* **2**, 174 (1961).
271. J. F. Giovinco, *Bull. Tulane Univ. Med. Fac.* **16**, 177 (1957).
272. D. E. Goldman, *Biophys. J.* **4**, 167 (1964).
273. H. Göpfert and H. Schaefer, *Pfluegers Arch. Gesamte Physiol. Menschen Tiere* **239**, 597 (1938).
274. G. L. A. Graff, A. J. Hudson, and K. P. Strickland, *Biochim. Biophys. Acta* **104**, 543 (1965).
275. M. A. Grafius and D. B. Millar, *Biochemistry* **6**, 1034 (1967).
276. J. D. P. Graham and G. W. L. James, *J. Med. Pharm. Chem.* **3**, 489 (1961).
277. G. Grant, *Brit. Med. J.* **1**, 1352 (1952).
278. E. N. Greenblatt and R. K. Thomas, *Arch. Int. Pharmacodyn. Ther.* **117**, 364 (1958).
279. H. R. Griffith and G. E. Johnson, *Anesthesiology* **3**, 418 (1942).
280. D. Grob and T. Namba, *Fed. Proc., Fed. Amer. Soc. Exp. Biol.* **22**, 215 (1963).
281. D. Grob, T. Namba, N. A. Solomon, and D. S. Feldman, *J. Clin. Invest.* **41**, 1363 (1962).
281a. H. Grundfest, *Progr. Biophys. Biophys. Chem.* **7**, 1 (1957).
282. S. M. Guerier and R. Huxley-Williams, *Anaesthesia* **9**, 213 (1954).
283. P. G. Günther, *Anat. Anz.* **97**, 175 (1949).
283a. L. Guth, *Physiol. Rev.* **48**, 645 (1968).
284. C. G. Haining and R. G. Johnston, *Brit. J. Pharmacol.* **18**, 275 (1962).
285. C. G. Haining, R. G. Johnston, and J. M. Smith, *Nature (London)* **183**, 542 (1959).
286. G. E. Hale-Enderby, *Brit. J. Anaesth.* **31**, 530 (1959).
287. R. A. Hall and M. W. Parkes, *J. Physiol. (London)* **122**, 274 (1953).
288. C. Hanna, W. H. MacMillan, and P. B. McHugo, *Arch. Int. Pharmacodyn. Ther.* **124**, 445 (1960).
289. C. Hansch, *Accounts Chem. Res.* **2**, 232 (1969).
289a. C. Hansch and T. Fujita, *J. Amer. Chem. Soc.* **86**, 1616 (1964).
290. C. Hansch, P. P. Maloney, T. Fujita, and R. M. Muir, *Nature (London)* **194**, 178 (1962).

291. C. Hansch, A. R. Steward, S. M. Anderson, and D. Bently, *J. Med. Chem.* **11**, 1 (1968).
292. C. Hansch, A. R. Steward, J. Iwasa, and E. W. Deutsch, *Mol. Pharmacol.* **1**, 205 (1965).
293. A. W. Hanson, *Acta Crystallogr.* **16**, 939 (1963).
294. H. Harris and M. Whittaker, *Nature (London)* **191**, 496 (1961).
294a. J. B. Harris and G. H. D. Leach, *Brit. J. Pharmacol.* **38**, 517 (1970).
295. J. I. Harris and R. N. Perham, *Nature (London)* **219**, 1025 (1968).
296. A. M. Harvey, *Bull. Johns Hopkins Hosp.* **65**, 223 (1939).
297. A. M. Harvey, *Bull. Johns Hopkins Hosp.* **66**, 52 (1940).
298. A. Hassón, *Biochim. Biophys. Acta* **65**, 275 (1962).
299. A. Hassón and C. Chagas, *Biochim. Biophys. Acta* **36**, 301 (1959).
300. A. Hassón and C. Chagas, *in* "Bioelectrogenesis" (C. Chagas and A. Paes de Carvalho, eds.), p. 362. Elsevier, Amsterdam, 1961.
301. R. Hazard, J. Cheymol, P. Chabrier, E. Corteggiani, and F. Nicolas, *Arch. Int. Pharmacodyn. Ther.* **84**, 237 (1950).
302. R. Hazard, J. Cheymol, P. Chabrier, E. Corteggiani, and F. Nicolas, *Bull. Soc. Chim. Fr.* p. 209 (1951).
303. C. O. Hebb, K. Krnjević, and A. Silver, *J. Physiol (London)* **171**, 504 (1964).
304. C. O. Hebb and B. H. Smallman, *J. Physiol. (London)* **134**, 385 (1956).
304a. B. A. Hemsworth and F. F. Foldes, *Euro. J. Pharmacol.* **11**, 187 (1970).
305. B. A. Hemsworth and D. Morris, *J. Neurochem.* **11**, 793 (1964).
305a. B. A. Hemsworth and J. C. Smith, *J. Neurochem.* **17**, 171 (1970).
306. A. Hess, *J. Physiol. (London)* **157**, 221 (1961).
307. A. Hess, *Rev. Can. Biol.* **21**, 241 (1962).
308. A. Hess and G. Pilar, *J. Physiol. (London)* **169**, 780 (1963).
309. D. W. Hesselschwerdt, E. L. Rushia, and S. C. Cullen, *Anesthesiology* **12**, 14 (1951).
310. J. C. Hinsey, *Physiol. Rev.* **14**, 514 (1934).
311. R. J. H. Hodges, *Brit. J. Anaesth.* **27**, 484 (1955).
312. R. J. H. Hodges and F. F. Foldes, *Lancet* **2**, 788 (1956).
313. R. J. H. Hodges and F. F. Foldes, *Lancet* **1**, 373 (1957).
314. A. L. Hodgkin, *Biol. Rev.* **26**, 339 (1951).
315. A. L. Hodgkin, *Proc. Roy. Soc., Ser. B.* **148**, 1 (1958).
316. A. L. Hodgkin and R. D. Keynes, *J. Physiol. (London)* **128**, 28 (1955).
317. A. L. Hodgkin and R. D. Keynes, *J. Physiol. (London)* **138**, 253 (1957).
318. H. Hofmann and H. Holzer, *Klin. Monatsbl. Augenheilk.* **123**, 1 (1953).
319. P. E. B. Holmes, D. J. Jenden, and D. B. Taylor, *J. Pharmacol. Exp. Ther.* **103**, 382 (1951).
320. B. Holmstedt, *Ann. N.Y. Acad. Sci.* **144**, 433 (1967).
321. P. Holton and H. R. Ing, *Brit. J. Pharmacol.* **4**, 190 (1949).
322. J. O. Hoppe, *Ann. N.Y. Acad. Sci.* **54**, 395 (1951).
323. J. O. Hoppe, J. E. Funnell, and H. Lape, *J. Pharmacol. Exp. Ther.* **115**, 106 (1955).
324. R. E. Howard and R. M. Burton, *Biochim. Biophys. Acta* **84**, 435 (1964).
325. J. I. Hubbard, *J. Physiol. (London)* **159**, 507 (1961).
326. J. I. Hubbard, S. F. Jones, and E. M. Landau, *Ann. N.Y. Acad. Sci.* **144**, 459 (1967).
327. J. I. Hubbard and R. F. Schmidt, *Nature (London)* **196**, 378 (1962).
328. J. I. Hubbard and R. F. Schmidt, *J. Physiol. (London)* **166**, 145 (1963).
329. J. I. Hubbard, R. F. Schmidt, and T. Yokota, *J. Physiol. (London)* **181**, 810 (1965).
330. J. I. Hubbard and W. D. Willis, *Nature (London)* **193**, 1294 (1962).
331. C. C. Hunt and S. W. Kuffler, *J. Physiol. (London)* **113**, 283 (1951).
332. C. C. Hunt and S. W. Kuffler, *J. Physiol. (London)* **126**, 293 (1954).
333. R. Hunt and R. R. Renshaw, *J. Pharmacol. Exp. Ther.* **25**, 315 (1925).
334. R. Hunt and R. M. de Taveau, *Brit. Med. J.* **2**, 1788 (1906).
335. A. R. Hunter, *Anaesthesia* **7**, 145 (1952).

336. A. R. Hunter, *Brit. J. Anaesth.* **27**, 73 (1955).
337. A. R. Hunter, *Anaesthesist* **8**, 82 (1959).
338. A. R. Hunter, *Brit. J. Anaesth.* **36**, 466 (1964).
339. O. F. Hutter and J. E. Pascoe, *Brit. J. Pharmacol.* **6**, 691 (1951).
340. A. F. Huxley, *Ann. N.Y. Acad. Sci.* **81**, 221 (1959).
341. H. R. Ing, *Physiol. Rev.* **16**, 527 (1936).
342. H. R. Ing, *Science* **109**, 264 (1949).
343. H. R. Ing and W. M. Wright, *Proc. Roy. Soc., Ser. B* **109**, 337 (1931).
344. H. R. Ing and W. M. Wright, *Proc. Roy. Soc., Ser. B* **114**, 48 (1933).
345. R. L. Irwin and E. G. Trams, *J. Pharmacol. Exp. Ther.* **137**, 242 (1962).
346. M. M. Janot, F. Lainé, and R. Goutarel, *Ann. Pharm. Fr.* **18**, 673 (1960).
347. L. W. Jarcho, C. Eyzaguirre, B. Berman, and J. L. Lilienthal, *Amer. J. Physiol.* **168**, 446 (1952).
348. D. J. Jenden, K. Kamijo, and D. B. Taylor, *J. Pharmacol. Exp. Ther.* **103**, 348 (1951).
349. D. J. Jenden, K. Kamijo, and D. B. Taylor, *J. Pharmacol. Exp. Ther.* **111**, 229 (1954).
350. D. H. Jenkinson, *J. Physiol. (London)* **138**, 438 (1957).
351. D. Jerchel and G. Jung, *Chem. Ber.* **85**, 1130 (1952).
352. P. A. Jewell and E. J. Zaimis, *J. Physiol. (London)* **124**, 417 (1954).
353. M. N. Jindal and V. R. Desphande, *Brit. J. Pharmacol.* **15**, 506 (1960).
353a. S. F. Jones and S. Kwanbunbumpen, *Life Sci.* **7**, 1251 (1968).
353b. S. F. Jones and S. Kwanbunbumpen, *J. Physiol. (London)* **207**, 31 (1970).
354. W. Kalow, *Biochem. Hum. Genet., Ciba Found. Symp.* pp. 39–56 (1959).
355. V. M. Karassik, *Usp. Sovrem. Biol.* **21**, 1 (1946).
356. A. Karlin, *J. Theor. Biol.* **16**, 306 (1967).
356a. A. Karlin, *Biochim. Biophys. Acta* **139**, 358 (1967).
357. B. Katz, *Bull. Johns Hopkins Hosp.* **102**, 275 (1958).
358. B. Katz, *Rev. Mod. Phys.* **31**, 524 (1959).
359. B. Katz, *Proc. Roy. Soc., Ser. B* **155**, 455 (1962).
360. B. Katz, "Nerve, Muscle, and Synpase." McGraw-Hill, New York, 1966.
361. B. Katz and R. Miledi, *Proc. Roy. Soc., Ser. B* **161**, 453 (1965).
362. B. Katz and S. Thesleff, *J. Physiol. (London)* **138**, 63 (1957).
363. C. J. Kensler, H. Langemann, and C. L. Zirkle, *J. Pharmacol. Exp. Ther.* **110**, 127 (1954).
364. C. J. Kensler, C. L. Zirkle, A. Matallana, and G. Condouris, *J. Pharmacol. Exp. Ther.* **112**, 210 (1954).
365. A. S. Keston and S. B. Wortis, *Proc. Soc. Exp. Biol. Med.* **61**, 439 (1946).
366. R. D. Keynes and G. W. Maisel, *Proc. Roy. Soc., Ser. B* **142**, 383 (1954).
367. F. Khuong Huu-Lainé and W. Pinto-Scognamiglio, *Arch. Int. Pharmacodyn. Ther.* **147**, 209 (1964).
368. H. King, *Nature (London)* **135**, 469 (1935).
369. H. King, *J. Chem. Soc.* p. 1381 (1935).
370. H. King, *J. Chem. Soc.* p. 936 (1947).
371. H. King, *J. Chem. Soc.* p. 265 (1948).
371a. R. J. Kitz, L. M. Braswell, and S. Ginsburg, *Mol. Pharmacol.* **6**, 108 (1970).
371b. R. J. Kitz and L. T. Kremzner, *Mol. Pharmacol.* **4**, 104 (1968).
372. E. Klenk and W. Gielen, *Hoppe-Seyler's Z. Physiol. Chem.* **319**, 283 (1960).
372a. F. Koch and O. Lundskog, *Nord. Med.* **44**, 1211 (1950).
373. G. B. Koelle, *J. Pharm. Pharmacol.* **14**, 65 (1962).
374. G. B. Koelle, *in* 'Handbuch der experimentellen Pharmakologie" (A. Heffter and H. Heubner, eds.), Vol. 15, p. 187. Springer, Berlin, 1963.
375. G. B. Koelle, R. Davis, and C. G. Gromadzki, *Ann. N.Y. Acad. Sci.* **144**, 613 (1967).
376. *cf.* D. E. Koshland, *Proc. Nat. Acad. Sci. U.S.* **44**, 98 (1958).
376a. D. E. Koshland, *J. Cell. Comp. Physiol.* **54**, Suppl. 1, 245 (1959).

376b. D. E. Koshland, *Science* **142**, 1533 (1963).
377. D. E. Koshland, *Fed. Proc.*, *Fed. Amer. Soc. Exp. Biol.* **23**, 719 (1964).
378. D. E. Koshland and K. E. Neet, *Ann. Rev. Biochem.* **37**, 359 (1968).
379. L. T. Kremzner and I. B. Wilson, *Biochemistry* **3**, 1902 (1964).
380. K. Krnjevič and R. Miledi, *Nature (London)* **182**, 805 (1958).
381. K. Krnjevič and J. F. Mitchell, *Nature (London)* **186**, 241 (1960).
382. K. Krnjevič and J. F. Mitchell, *J. Physiol. (London)* **155**, 246 (1961).
383. P. Krüger, *Experientia* **6**, 75 (1950).
384. P. Krüger, "Tetanus und Tonus der quergestreiften Skelettmuskeln der Wierbeltiere und des Menschen." Akad. Verlagsges., Leipzig, 1952.
385. P. Krüger and P. G. Günther, *Acta Anat.* **28**, 135 (1956).
386. P. Krüger and P. G. Günther, *Acta Anat.* **33**, 325 (1958).
387. R. M. Krupka, *Biochemistry* **5**, 1988 (1966).
388. R. M. Krupka, *Biochemistry* **6**, 1183 (1967).
389. R. M. Krupka and K. J. Laidler, *J. Amer. Chem. Soc.* **83**, 1458 (1961).
390. S. W. Kuffler, *J. Neurophysiol.* **5**, 18 (1942).
391. S. W. Kuffler, *J. Neurophysiol.* **6**, 99 (1943).
392. S. W. Kuffler, *J. Neurophysiol.* **8**, 77 (1945).
393. S. W. Kuffler, *Arch. Sci. Physiol.* **3**, 585 (1949).
394. S. W. Kuffler and R. W. Gerrard, *J. Neurophysiol.* **10**, 383 (1947).
395. S. W. Kuffler and E. M. Vaughan-Williams, *J. Physiol. (London)* **121**, 289 (1953).
396. S. W. Kuffler and E. M. Vaughan-Williams, *J. Physiol. (London)* **121**, 318 (1953).
397. R. Kuhn and H. Wiegandt, *Chem. Ber.* **96**, 866 (1963).
398. C. Küpfer, *J. Physiol. (London)* **153**, 522 (1960).
399. A. D. Kuzovkov, M. D. Mashkovskii, A. V. Danilova, and G. P. Men'shikov, *Dokl. Akad. Nauk SSSR* **103**, 251 (1955); *Chem. Abstr.* **50**, 5695 (1956).
400. A. M. Lands and C. J. Cavallito, *J. Pharmacol. Exp. Ther.* **110**, 369 (1954).
401. H. C. Lawler, *Biochim. Biophys. Acta* **81**, 280 (1964).
402. R. Ledeen, *J. Amer. Oil Chem. Soc.* **43**, 57 (1966).
403. A. J. Lehman, *Proc. Soc. Exp. Biol. Med.* **33**, 501 (1935).
404. H. Lehmann and E. Ryan, *Lancet* **2**, 124 (1956).
405. E. Lesser, *J. Pharm. Pharmacol.* **13**, 703 (1961).
406. E. Lesser, *J. Pharm. Pharmacol.* **18**, 408 (1966).
407. J. J. Lewis, D. E. McPhail, T. C. Muir, and J. B. Stenlake, *J. Pharm. Pharmacol.* **13**, 543 (1961).
408. J. J. Lewis, M. Martin-Smith, and T. C. Muir, *Brit. J. Pharmacol.* **20**, 307 (1963).
409. J. J. Lewis, M. Martin-Smith, T. C. Muir, and H. H. Ross, *J. Pharm. Pharmacol.* **19**, 502 (1967).
410. J. J. Lewis and T. C. Muir, *Lab. Pract.* **8**, 364 and 404 (1959).
411. J. J. Lewis and T. C. Muir, *in* "Drugs Affecting The Peripheral Nervous System" (A. Burger, ed.), Vol. 1, p. 327. Arnold, London, 1967.
412. A. W. Liley, *J. Physiol. (London)* **132**, 650 (1956).
413. A. W. Liley, *J. Physiol. (London)* **133**, 571 (1956).
414. G. Lilleheil and K. Naess, *Experientia* **16**, 550 (1960).
415. G. Lilleheil and K. Naess, *Acta Physiol. Scand.* **52**, 120 (1961).
416. H. A. Lincoff, C. H. Ellis, A. G. De Voe, E. J. Beer, D. J. de Impestato, S. Berg, L. Orkin, and H. Magda, *Amer. J. Ophthalmol.* **40**, 501 (1955).
417. F. Lipmann and N. O. Kaplan, *J. Biol. Chem.* **162**, 743 (1946).
418. J. Lissac, R. Herenberg, J. Vallois, J. C. Pocidalo, and F. Liot, *C. R. Soc. Biol.* **157**, 61 (1963).
419. D. P. C. Lloyd, *J. Neurophysiol.* **5**, 153 (1942).
420. S. Loewe and S. C. Harvey, *Arch. Exp. Pathol. Pharmakol.* **214**, 214 (1952).

421. J. P. Long and N. Reitzel, *J. Pharmacol. Exp. Ther.* **122**, 44 (1958).
422. J. P. Long and F. W. Schueler, *J. Amer. Pharm. Ass., Sci. Ed.* **43**, 79 (1954).
423. K. Lonsdale, H. J. Milledge, and L. M. Pant, *Acta Crystallogr.* **19**, 827 (1965).
424. J. V. Luco and P. Sanchez, *in* "Curare and Curare-like Agents" (D. Bovet, F. Bovet-Nitti, and G. B. Marini-Bettolo, eds.), p. 405. Elsevier, Amsterdam, 1959.
425. I. Lund and J. Stovner, *Acta Anaesthesiol. Scand.* **6**, 85 and 161 (1962).
426. H. C. Lüttgau and R. Niedergerke, *J. Physiol. (London)* **143**, 486 (1958).
427. A. Lüttringhaus, L. Kerp, and H. Preugschas, *Arzneim.-Forsch.* **7**, 222 (1957).
428. R. E. McCaman, G. Rodriguez De Lores Arnaiz, and E. De Robertis, *J. Neurochem.* **12**, 927 (1965).
429. L. P. McCarty, *Ann. N.Y. Acad. Sci.* **144**, 407 (1967).
430. N. J. McCorkindale, personal communication (1968).
431. N. J. McCorkindale, D. S. Magrill, M. Martin-Smith, S. J. Smith, and J. B. Stenlake, *Tetrahedron Lett.* p. 3841 (1964).
432. F. C. MacIntosh, *Can. J. Biochem. Physiol.* **37**, 343 (1959).
432a. F. C. MacIntosh, *Fed. Proc., Fed. Amer. Soc. Exp. Biol.* **20**, 562 (1961).
433. F. C. MacIntosh, R. I. Birks, and P. B. Sastry, *Nature (London)* **178**, 1181 (1956).
434. A. R. McIntyre, R. E. King, and A. L. Dunn, *J. Neurophysiol.* **8**, 297 (1945).
435. D. Mackay, *Nature (London)* **197**, 1171 (1963).
436. D. N. McKinstry, E. Koenig, W. A. Koelle, and G. B. Koelle, *Can. J. Biochem. Physiol.* **41**, 2599 (1963).
437. J. Mambrini and P. R. Benoit, *C. R. Soc. Biol.* **158**, 1454 (1964).
438. A. Marnay and D. Nachmansohn, *J. Physiol. (London)* **92**, 37 (1938).
439. I. G. Marshall, *Brit. J. Pharmacol.* **34**, 56 (1968).
439a. I. G. Marshall, *Brit. J. Pharmacol.* **38**, 503 (1970).
440. I. G. Marshall, *Euro. J. Pharmacol.* **2**, 258 (1968).
441. I. G. Marshall, J. B. Murray, G. A. Smail, and J. B. Stenlake, *J. Pharm. Pharmacol.* Suppl. 19, 53S (1967).
442. G. J. Martin, *J. Chem. Educ.* **33**, 204 (1956).
443. M. Martin-Smith, *Pharm. J.* **197**, 557 (1966).
444. M. Martin-Smith, G. A. Smail, and J. B. Stenlake, *J. Pharm. Pharmacol.* **19**, 561 (1967).
445. M. D. Mashkovskii and B. A. Medvedev, *Farmakol. Toksikol. (Moscow)* **23**, 493 (1960); *Chem. Abstr.* **55**, 14723 (1961).
446. R. L. Masland and R. S. Wigton, *J. Neurophysiol.* **3**, 269 (1940).
447. E. K. Mathews, *Proc. Can. Fed. Biol. Soc.* **6**, 40 (1963).
448. H. Mautner and A. Luisada, *J. Pharmacol. Exp. Ther.* **72**, 386 (1941).
449. C. Medesan and M. Stoica, *Commun. Acad. Rep. Pop. Rom., Inst. Biochim. Stud. Cercet Biochim.* **3**, 417 (1960); *Chem. Abstr.* **55**, 11647 (1961).
450. G. P. Men'shikov, A. V. Danilova, A. D. Kuzovkov, and M. I. Garina. Russ. Pat. 118, 205 (1959); *Chem. Abstr.* **53**, 19313 (1959).
450a. H. P. Metzger and I. B. Wilson, *J. Biol. Chem.* **238**, 3432 (1963).
451. I. A. Michaelson, *Ann. N.Y. Acad. Sci.* **144**, 387 (1967).
452. H. O. Michel and S. Krop, *J. Biol. Chem.* **190**, 119 (1951).
453. R. Miledi, *J. Physiol. (London)* **151**, 24 (1960).
454. R. Miledi, *J. Physiol. (London)* **154**, 190 (1960).
455. R. Miledi, *Nature (London)* **199**, 1191 (1963).
456. J. F. Mitchell, *J. Physiol. (London)* **165**, 98 (1963).
456a. W. F. H. M. Mommaerts, *Physiol. Rev.* **49**, 427 (1969).
457. J. Monod, J.-P. Changeux, and F. Jacob, *J. Mol. Biol.* **6**, 306 (1963).
458. W. W. Mushin and W. W. Mapleson, *Brit. J. Anaesth.* **36**, 761 (1964).
459. W. W. Mushin, R. Wien, D. F. J. Mason, and G. T. Langston, *Lancet* **1**, 726 (1949).
460. D. Nachmansohn, *Ann. N.Y. Acad. Sci.* **47**, 395 (1946).

461. D. Nachmansohn, "Chemical and Molecular Basis of Nerve Activity." Academic Press, New York, 1959.
462. D. Nachmansohn and A. L. Machado, *J. Neurophysiol.* **6**, 397 (1943).
463. D. Nachmansohn and M. A. Rothenberg, *J. Biol. Chem.* **158**, 653 (1945).
464. D. Nachmansohn and I. B. Wilson, *Advan. Enzymol.* **12**, 259 (1951).
465. K. Naess, *Acta Pharmacol. Toxicol.* **8**, 400 (1952).
466. K. Naess, *Acta Pharmacol. Toxicol.* **9**, 196 (1953).
467. T. Namba and D. Grob, *Ann. N.Y. Acad. Sci.* **144**, 772 (1967).
468. T. Namba and D. Grob, *Biochem. Pharmacol.* **16**, 1135 (1967).
469. W. L. Nastuk, *Fed. Proc., Fed. Amer. Soc. Exp. Biol.* **12**, 102 (1953).
470. W. L. Nastuk, *Ann. N.Y. Acad. Sci.* **81**, 317 (1959).
471. W. L. Nastuk, *Fed. Proc., Fed. Amer. Soc. Exp. Biol.* **26**, 1639 (1967).
472. O. A. Nedergaard and D. B. Taylor, *Fed. Proc., Fed. Amer. Soc. Exp. Biol.* **22**, 310 (1963).
473. K. E. Neet and S. L. Friess, *Arch. Biochem. Biophys.* **99**, 484 (1962).
474. H. Neurath, *Sci. Amer.* **211**, No. 6, 68 (1964).
475. M. Nickerson, *Nature (London)* **178**, 697 (1956).
476. E. S. Nikitskaya, V. S. Usovskaya, and M. V. Rubtsov, *Zh. Obshch. Khim.* **30**, 3306 (1960); *Chem. Abstr.* **55**, 18743 (1961).
477. G. E. Palade, *Anat. Rec.* **118**, 335 (1954).
478. S. L. Palay, *J. Biophys. Biochem. Cytol.* **2**, 193 (1956).
479. W. D. M. Paton, *Ann. N.Y. Acad. Sci.* **54**, 347 (1951).
480. W. D. M. Paton, *Anesthesiology* **20**, 453 (1959).
481. W. D. M. Paton, *Proc. Roy Soc., Ser. B.* **154**. 21 (1961).
482. W. D. M. Paton, *Can. J. Biochem. Physiol.* **41**, 2637 (1963).
483. W. D. M. Paton, *Ann. N.Y. Acad. Sci.* **144**, 869 (1967).
484. W. D. M. Paton and H. P. Rang, *Proc. Roy. Soc., Ser. B.* **163**, 1 (1965).
485. W. D. M. Paton and D. R. Waud, *Brit. J. Anaesth.* **34**, 251 (1962).
486. W. D. M. Paton and D. R. Waud, *in* "Curare and Curare-like Agents" (A. V. S. de Reuck, ed.), p. 34. Churchill, London, 1962.
487. W. D. M. Paton and D. R. Waud, *J. Physiol. (London)* **191**, 59 (1967).
488. W. D. M. Paton and E. J. Zaimis, *Nature (London)* **161**, 718 (1948).
489. W. D. M. Paton and E. J. Zaimis, *Nature (London* **162**, 810 (1948).
490. W. D. M. Paton and E. J. Zaimis, *Brit. J. Pharmacol.* **4**, 381 (1949).
491. W. D. M. Paton and E. J. Zaimis, *Lancet* **2**, 568 (1950).
492. W. D. M. Paton and E. J. Zaimis, *Brit. J. Pharmacol.* **6**, 155 (1951).
493. W. D. M. Paton and E. J. Zaimis, *J. Physiol. (London)* **112**, 311 (1951).
494. W. D. M. Paton and E. J. Zaimis, *Pharmacol. Rev.* **4**, 219 (1952).
495. E. W. Pelikan, K. R. Unna, D. W. MacFarlane, R. J. Cazort, M. S. Sadove, and J. T. Nelson, *J. Pharmacol. Exp. Ther.* **99**, 215 (1950).
496. E. Philippot and M. J. Dallemagne, *Arch. Int. Physiol.* **59**, 357 (1951).
497. E. Philippot and M. J. Dallemagne, *Arch. Exp. Pathol. Pharmakol.* **220**, 100 (1953).
498. A. P. Phillips, *J. Amer. Chem. Soc.* **71**, 3264 (1949).
499. C. B. Pittinger and J. P. Long, *Antibiot. Chemother. (Washington, D.C.)* **8**, 198 (1958).
500. L. T. Potter, *Ann. N.Y. Acad. Sci.* **144**, 482 (1967).
501. H. Poulsen and W. Hougs, *Acta Anaesthesiol. Scand.* **1**, 15 (1957).
502. M. Protiva and J. Pliml, *Collect. Czech. Chem. Commun.* **18**, 836 (1953).
502a. R. Quarles and J. Folch-Pi, *J. Neurochem.* **12**, 543 (1965).
503. A. Quévauviller and F. Lainé, *Ann. Pharm. Fr.* **18**, 678 (1960).
504. J. P. Quilliam and D. B. Taylor, *Nature (London)* **160**, 603 (1947).
505. P. M. H. Rack and D. R. Westbury, *J. Physiol. (London)* **186**, 698 (1966).
505a. R. Rahaminoff, *J. Physiol. (London)* **195**, 471 (1968).

506. A. Raines and F. G. Standaert, *J. Pharmacol. Exp. Ther.* **153**, 361 (1966).
507. M. J. Rand and V. Chang, *Nature (London)* **188**, 858 (1960).
508. L. O. Randall, E. Giuliano, B. Kappell, and E. Allen, *J. Pharmacol. Exp. Ther.* **105**, 7 (1952).
509. M. Randić and D. W. Straughan, *J. Physiol. (London)* **173**, 130 (1964).
509a. G. N. Reeke, J. A. Hartsuck, M. L. Ludwig, F. A. Quiocho, T. A. Steitz, and W. N. Lipscomb, *Proc. Nat. Acad. Sci. U.S.* **58**, 2220 (1967).
510. N. L. Reitzel and J. P. Long, *Arch. Int. Pharmacodyn. Ther.* **119**, 20 (1959).
511. N. L. Reitzel and J. P. Long, *J. Pharmacol. Exp. Ther.* **127**, 15 (1959).
512. R. R. Renshaw, D. Green, and M. Ziff, *J. Pharmacol. Exp. Ther.* **62**, 430 (1938).
513. W. Riker, *Pharmacol. Rev.* **5**, 1 (1953).
514. W. F. Riker, *J. Pharmacol. Exp. Ther.* **152**, 397 (1966).
515. W. F. Riker, J. Roberts, F. G. Standaert, and H. Fujimori, *J. Pharmacol. Exp. Ther.* **121**, 286 (1957).
516. W. F. Riker and F. G. Standaert, *Ann. N.Y. Acad. Sci.* **135**, 164 (1966).
517. W. F. Riker, G. Werner, J. Roberts, and A. Kuperman, *Ann. N.Y. Acad. Sci.* **81**, 328 (1959).
518. W. F. Riker, G. Werner, J. Roberts, and A. Kuperman, *J. Pharmacol. Exp. Ther.* **125**, 150 (1959).
519. W. F. Riker and W. C. Wescoe, *Ann. N.Y. Acad. Sci.* **54**, 373 (1951).
520. J. M. Ritchie, *Ann. N.Y. Acad. Sci.* **144**, 504 (1967).
521. J. M. Ritchie and C. Armett, *J. Pharmacol. Exp. Ther.* **139**, 201 (1963).
521a. D. V. Roberts and S. Thesleff. *Acta Anaesthiol Scand.* **9**, 165 (1965).
522. J. D. Robertson, *J. Biophys. Biochem. Cytol.* **2**, 369 (1956).
523. J. D. Robertson, *J. Biophys. Biochem. Cytol.* **3**, 1043 (1957).
524. J. R. Roche, *Amer. J. Ophthalmol.* **33**, 91 (1950).
525. M. H. Roepke, *J. Pharmacol. Exp. Ther.* **59**, 264 (1937).
526. E. Rojas and J. M. Tobias, *Biochim. Biophys. Acta* **94**, 394 (1965).
527. A. Rosenberg and E. Chargaff, *J. Biol. Chem.* **232**, 1031 (1958).
528. W. C. J. Ross, "Biological Alkylating Agents." Butterworth, London and Washington, D.C., 1962.
529. M. V. Rubtsov, M. D. Mashkovskii, E. C. Nikitskaya, B. A. Medvedev, and V. S. Urovskaya, *J. Med. Pharm. Chem.* **3**, 441 (1961).
530. P. B. Sabawala and J. B. Dillon, *Acta Anaesthesiol. Scand.* **3**, 83 (1959).
531. J. K. Saelens and W. R. Stoll, *Fed. Proc., Fed. Amer. Soc. Exp. Biol.* **24**, 675 (1965).
531a. L. A. Salako, *J. Pharm. Pharmacol.* **22**, 69 (1970).
531b. L. A. Salako, *Euro. J. Pharmacol.* **11**, 342 (1970).
532. S. Salama and S. Wright, *Brit. J. Pharmacol.* **6**, 459 (1951).
533. F. Sanger, *Proc. Chem. Soc.* p. 76 (1963).
534. V. B. Schatz, *in* "Medicinal Chemistry" (A. Burger, ed.), 2nd ed., p. 72. Wiley (Interscience), New York, 1960.
535. M. Schilling and J. G. A. Pedersen, *Arch. Exp. Pathol. Pharmakol.* **228**, 371 (1956).
536. F. O. Schmitt and P. F. Davison, *Neurosci. Res. Program. Bull.* **3**, No. 6, 55 (1965).
537. F. W. Schueler, *J. Pharmacol. Exp. Ther.* **115**, 127 (1955).
538. F. W. Schueler and C. Hanna, *J. Amer. Chem. Soc.* **74**, 2112 (1952).
539. F. W. Schueler and H. H. Keasling, *J. Amer. Pharm. Ass., Sci. Ed.* **45**, 792. (1956).
540. R. Seeger, F. Ahnefeld, and E. Hauenschild, *Anaesthesist* **11**, 37 (1962).
541. B. A. Sellick, *Lancet* **2**, 822 (1950).
542. B. A. Sellick, *Excerpta Med.* ICS No. 168. *4th World Congr. Anaesthesiol.* p. 125 (1968).
543. A. M. Shanes, *Pharmacol. Rev.* **10**, 59 (1958).
543a. E. Shefter and D. J. Triggle, *Nature (London)* **227**, 1354 (1970).
544. A. Simonart, *J. Pharmacol. Exp. Ther.* **6**, 147 (1914).

544a. L. L. Simpson, *J. Pharm. Pharmacol.* **20**, 889 (1968).
544b. L. L. Simpson and J. T. Tapp, *Int. J. Neuropharmacol.* **6**, 485 (1967).
545. J. C. Skou, *Acta Pharmacol. Toxicol.* **10**, 325 (1954).
546. J. C. Skou, *Biochim. Biophys. Acta* **31**, 1 (1959).
546a J. C. Smith, C. J. Cavallito, and F. F. Foldes, *Biochem. Pharmacol.* **16**, 2438 (1967).
547. W. R. Smithfield and W. P. Purcell, *J. Pharm. Sci.* **56**, 577 (1967).
548. W. Sniper, *Brit. J. Anaesth.* **24**, 232 (1952).
549. M. D. Sokoll, B. Sonesson, and S. Thesleff, *Euro. J. Pharmacol.* **4**, 179 (1968).
550. M. D. Sokoll and S. Thesleff, *Euro. J. Pharmacol.* **4**, 71 (1968).
551. F. G. Standaert, *J. Pharmacol. Exp. Ther.* **143**, 181 (1964).
552. F. G. Standaert and J. E. Adams, *J. Pharmacol. Exp. Ther.* **149**, 113 (1965).
553. F. G. Standaert and W. F. Riker, *Ann. N.Y. Acad. Sci.* **144**, 517 (1967).
554. E. Stedman, E. Stedman, and L. H. Easson, *Biochem. J.* **26**, 2056 (1932).
555. H. B. Steinbach, *Symp. Soc. Exp. Biol.* **8**, 438 (1954).
556. J. B. Stenlake, *Progr. Med. Chem.* **3**, 1 (1963).
557. J. B. Stenlake, *Ann. Pharm. Fr.* **26**, 185 (1968).
558. R. P. Stephenson, *Brit. J. Pharmacol.* **11**, 379 (1956).
559. V. K. Stoelting, J. P. Graf, and Z. Vieira, *Proc. Soc. Exp. Biol. Med.* **69**, 565 (1948).
560. V. K. Stoetling, J. P. Graf, and Z. Vieira, *Curr. Res. Anesth. Analg.* **28**, 130 (1949).
561. J. Stovner and I. Lund, unpublished observations (1968).
562. D. W. Straughan, *Brit. J. Pharmacol.* **15**, 417 (1960).
563. D. W. Straughan, *J. Pharm. Pharmacol.* **13**, 49 (1961).
564. M. Sundaralingham, *Nature (London)* **217**, 35 (1968).
565. J. C. Szerb, *Can. J. Physiol. Pharmacol.* **42**, 303 (1966).
566. A. Takeuchi and N. Takeuchi, *J. Physiol. (London)* **154**, 52 (1960).
567. N. Takeuchi, *J. Physiol. (London)* **167**, 128 and 141 (1963).
568. I. Tasaki and K. Mizutani, *Jap. J. Med. Sci. & Biol.* **10**, 237 (1944).
569. D. B. Taylor, *Pharmacol. Rev.* **3**, 412 (1951).
570. D. B. Taylor, *Anesthesiology* **20**, 439 (1959).
571. D. B. Taylor, *in* "Curare and Curare-like Agents" (A. V. S. de Reuck, ed.), p. 21. Churchill, London, 1962.
572. D. B. Taylor, R. Creese, T. C. Lu, and R. Case, *Ann. N.Y. Acad. Sci.* **144**, 768 (1967).
573. D. B. Taylor, R. Creese, O. A. Nedergaard, and R. Case, *Nature (London)* **208**, 901 (1965).
574. D. B. Taylor, R. Creese, and N. W. Scholes, *J. Pharmacol. Exp. Ther.* **144**, 293 (1964).
575. D. B. Taylor and O. A. Nedergaard, *Physiol. Rev.* **45**, 523 (1965).
576. E. P. Taylor and H. O. J. Collier, *Nature (London)* **165**, 602 (1950).
577. S. Thesleff, *Acta Physiol. Scand.* **34**, 218 and 286 (1955).
578. S. Thesleff, *Acta Anaesthesiol. Scand.* **2**, 69 (1958).
579. S. Thesleff, *J. Physiol. (London)* **151**, 598 (1960).
580. S. Thesleff, *Physiol. Rev.* **40**, 734 (1960).
581. S. Thesleff, *Progr. Neurobiol.* **5**, 1 (1963).
582. S. Thesleff, *in* "The Structure and Function of Muscle" (G. H. Bourne, ed.), Vol. 3, p. 1. Academic Press, New York, 1961.
583. S. Thesleff and E. X. Albuquerque, *Ann. N.Y. Acad. Sci.* **144**, 534 (1967).
584. S. Thesleff and K. Unna, *J. Pharmacol. Exp. Ther.* **111**, 99 (1954).
585. R. E. Thies, *Physiologist* **5**, 220 (1962).
586. O. W. Tiegs, *Physiol. Rev.* **33**, 90 (1953).
587. M. Tomita and J. Kunitomo, *J. Pharm. Soc. Jap.* **82**, 734 (1962).
588. E. G. Trams and C. J. Lauter, *Biochim. Biophys. Acta* **60**, 350 (1962).
589. E. G. Trams and C. J. Lauter, *Biochim. Biophys. Acta* **83**, 296 (1964).
590. F. I. Tsuji and F. F. Foldes, *Fed. Proc., Fed. Amer. Soc. Exp. Biol.* **12**, 374 (1953).

591. K. R. Unna, M. Kniazuk, and J. G. Greslin, *J. Pharmacol. Exp. Ther.* **80**, 39 (1944).
592. K. R. Unna, E. W. Pelikan, D. W. MacFarlane, R. J. Cazort, M. S. Sadove, J. T. Nelson, and A. P. Drucker, *J. Pharmacol. Exp. Ther.* **98**, 318 (1950).
593. P. Valdoni, *Rend. Ist Super. Sanita* **12**, 255 (1949).
594. C. Van der Meer and E. Meeter, *Acta Physiol. Pharmacol. Neer.* **4**, 454 (1956).
595. M. Vaněček, Z. Votava, J. Šramková, and H. Šrajerová, *Physiol. Bohemoslov.* **4**, 220 (1955).
596. A. Van Poznak, *Fed. Proc., Fed. Amer. Soc. Exp. Biol.* **22**, 390 (1963).
597. J. M. Van Rossum, *J. Pharm. Pharmacol.* **15**, 285 (1963).
598. J. M. Van Rossum and E. J. Ariëns, *Arch. Int. Pharmacodyn. Ther.* **118**, 393 (1959).
598a. J. M. Van Rossum and E. J. Ariëns, *Arch. Int. Pharmacodyn. Ther.* **118**, 418 (1959).
599. J. M. Van Rossum, E. J. Ariëns, and G. H. Linssen, *Biochem. Pharmacol.* **1**, 193 (1958).
600. I. R. Verner, *Proc. Roy. Soc. Med.* **60**, 1280 (1967).
600a. D. Vincent and M. Parant, *C.R. Soc. Biol.* **150**, 444 (1956).
601. W. von Philipsborn, H. Schmid, and P. Karrer, *Helv. Chim. Acta* **39**, 913 (1956).
602. Z. Votava and J. Metyšová-Srankova, *Physiol. Bohemoslov.* **8**, 431 (1955).
603. J. Walker, *J. Chem. Soc.* p. 193 (1950).
604. P. G. Waser, *Helv. Physiol. Pharmacol. Acta* **8**, 342 (1950).
605. P. G. Waser, *Helv. Physiol. Pharmacol. Acta* Suppl. VIII, 1 (1953).
606. P. G. Waser, *in* "Curare and Curare-like Agents" (D. Bovet, F. Bovet-Nitti, and G. B. Marini-Bettolo, eds.), p. 219. Elsevier, Amsterdam, 1959.
607. P. G. Waser, *J. Pharm. Pharmacol.* **12**, 577 (1960).
608. P. G. Waser, *in* "Bioelectrogenesis" (C. Chagas and A. P. de Carvalho, eds.), p. 353. Elsevier, Amsterdam, 1961.
609. P. G. Waser, *Enzymes Drug Action, Ciba Found. Symp.* p. 206 (1962).
610. P. G. Waser, *Pfluegers Arch. Gesamte. Physiol. Menschen Tiere* **274**, 431 (1962).
611. P. G. Waser, *Proc. 1st Int. Pharmacol. Meet., 1961* Vol. 7, p. 101 (1962).
612. P. G. Waser, *Ann. N.Y. Acad. Sci.* **144**, 737 (1967).
613. P. G. Waser and P. Harbeck, *Anaesthesist* **8**, 193 (1959).
614. P. G. Waser and H. Harbeck, *Anaesthesist* **11**, 33 (1962).
615. P. G. Waser, H. Schmid, and K. Schmid, *Arch. Int. Pharmacodyn. Ther.* **96**, 386 (1954),
616. J. C. Watkins, *J. Theor. Biol.* **9**, 37 (1965).
617. G. Werner, *J. Neurophysiol.* **23**, 171 (1960).
618. G. Werner, *J. Neurophysiol.* **23**, 453 (1960).
619. G. Werner, *J. Neurophysiol.* **24**, 401 (1961).
620. V. P. Whittaker, I. A. Michaelson, and R. J. Kirkland, *Biochem. Pharmacol.* **12**, 300 (1963).
621. V. P. Whittaker, I. A. Michaelson, and R. J. Kirkland, *Biochem. J.* **90**, 293 (1964).
622. V. P. Whittaker and S. Wijesundera, *Biochem. J.* **52**, 475 (1952).
623. K. Wiemers and W. Overbeck, *Brit. J. Anaesth.* **32**, 607 (1960).
624. A. R. Williams, J. Hidalgo, and I. F. Halverstadt, *J. Amer. Pharm. Ass., Sci. Ed.* **45**, 423 (1956).
625. H. Wilson and J. P. Long, *Arch. Int. Pharmacodyn. Ther.* **120**, 343 (1959).
626. H. B. Wilson, H. E. Gordon, and A. W. Raffan, *Brit. Med. J.* **1**, 1296 (1950).
627. *cf.* I. B. Wilson, *Ann. N.Y. Acad. Sci.* **144**, 664 (1967).
628. I. B. Wilson, F. Bergman, and D. Nachmansohn, *J. Biol. Chem.* **186**, 781 (1950).
629. I. B. Wilson and E. Cabib, *J. Amer. Chem. Soc.* **78**, 202 (1956).
630. I. B. Wilson and M. A. Harrison, *J. Biol. Chem.* **236**, 2292 (1961).
631. O. Wintersteiner, *in* "Curare and Curare-like Agents" (D. Bovet, F. Bovet-Nitti and G. B. Marini-Bettolo, eds.), p. 160. Elsevier, Amsterdam, 1959.
632. O. Wintersteiner and J. D. Dutcher, *Science* **97**, 467 (1943).
633. K. C. Wong and J. P. Long, *J. Pharmacol. Exp. Ther.* **133**, 211 (1961).

634. D. W. Woolley, *Progr. Drug Res.* **2**, 613 (1960).
635. M. Wurzel, *Experientia* **15**, 430 (1959).
636. M. Wurzel, *Ann. N.Y. Acad. Sci.* **144**, 694 (1967).
637. G. M. Wyant and M. S. Sadove, *Curr. Res. Anesth. Analg.* **33**, 178 (1954).
638. S. I. Zacks, "The Motor End Plate." Saunders, Philadelphia, Pennsylvania, 1964.
639. E. J. Zaimis, *J. Physiol. (London)* **112**, 176 (1951).
640. E. J. Zaimis, *J. Physiol. (London)* **122**, 238 (1953).
640a. E. J. Zaimis, *in* "Curare and Curare-like Agents" (A. V. S. de Reuck, ed.), p. 75. Churchill, London, 1962.
640b. E. J. Zaimis, *in* "Disorders of Voluntary Muscle" (J. N. Walton, ed.), Chap. 4. Churchill, London, 1964.
641. E. J. Zaimis, "Quantitative Methods in Human Pharmacology and Therapeutics," p. 24. Pergamon Press, Oxford, 1959.
642. A. O. Župančič, *Acta Physiol. Scand.* **29**, 63 (1953).
643. A. O. Župančič, *Ann. N.Y. Acad. Sci.* **144**, 689 (1967).
644. A. O. Župančič, *Biochim. Biophys. Acta* **99**, 325 (1965).

Addendum

A most elegant model of the acetylcholine receptor has recently been proposed [J. R. Smythies, *Euro. J. Pharmacol.* **14**, 268 (1971)] which may be expected to open up the further rational approaches to the design of neuromuscular blocking agents anticipated on p. 514. This model of the acetylcholine receptor was derived from consideration of molecular models and proposes that the receptor consists of a complex of protein, nucleotides, phospholipids, prostaglandins and calcium ions, thus accommodating the concept of "molecular ecology" (p. 471) and permitting the intercession of conformational perturbations (p. 473) as well as phosphodiesteric cleavages [J. T. Garland and J. Durell, *Intern. Rev. Neurobiol.* **13**, 159 (1970)]. In particular it is proposed that a protein strand in the β-form is linked by Watson–Crick-like ion–dipole bonds with guanine and cytosine units of nucleotides via glutamate and arginine units and that this complex then forms hydrogen bonds to prostaglandin molecules. The nucleotide units can be covalently bound to lipid while calcium ions act as stabilizers of the whole complex through interaction with phosphate anions. The action of acetylcholine is then postulated to be via disruption of one of the ion–dipole bonds linking the polypeptide to the nucleophospholipid leading to a cooperative disruption of the whole complex. The protein component could then take on the role of acetylcholinesterase. The role of the prostaglandins is postulated as providing highly specific accessory binding sites. The molecular models also indicate how muscarinic agents and nicotinic agents find different binding sites and rationalize the differences between pachycurares and leptocurares.

Chapter 13   The Design of Tumor-Inhibitory Alkylating Drugs

J. A. Stock

I. Introduction

The biological alkylating agents have been widely explored and used in cancer research and treatment, experimental and clinical. Whatever may be thought of their virtues or vices as anticancer drugs, no one can dispute the innumerable man-hours consumed in their synthesis and study. A 1963 survey (*1*) lists well over 2000 nitrogen mustards alone, and two years later, the same agency issued over 1500 pages of close-packed pharmacological data on alkylating agents (*2*).

The first study of the biological action of an alkylating agent seems to be that of Ehrlich, who, in 1898, investigated the effects of ethyleneimine (*3*). However, the proposition that compounds of this type may have application in the control of cancer derived from much later work on potential war gases, which led to the discovery of the clinical value of a nitrogen mustard, di-(2-chloroethyl)methylamine (HN2; **I**; $R = CH_3$; hydrochloride) in Hodgkin's disease and certain related conditions (*4*). From that time, organic chemists busied themselves with synthetic variants of almost every shape and size. These many derivatives were not, on the whole, profound exercises in drug design, but this is hardly surprising; knowledge of the normal and malignant cellular processes was—and is—insufficient for the writing down, in advance, of the formula of a sure winner, therapeutically speaking. Congeners were therefore prepared "either on the basis of an empirical gap-filling philosophy or the belief that a specific 'carrier group' would in one way or another improve antitumor activity" (*5*). Most alkylating agents have been made without any precise clinical aim as to what kind of malignancy they might ultimately be useful for. As a rule, the tumor-inhibitory alkylating agents suppress the blood elements and are potential candidates for clinical trial in leukemic as well as other neoplastic conditions. Individual compounds may nevertheless show very different effects. For example, busulfan, an alkylating agent of the sulfonic ester type, gives a blood response pattern unlike that of chlorambucil, an aromatic nitrogen mustard, and these drugs are consequently used in quite different kinds of leukemia (Section IV). Although some limited guidance may on occasion be given to the clinician from blood studies in the experimental animal, the treatment of solid human tumors develops empirically. It is probable, however, that we can look forward to an improvement in this situation as we come to learn more of the biochemical nature of human tumors and their specific drug-metabolizing capabilities, so that alkylating agents, unless they have been superseded by then, can be tailored, as it were, to the tumor. At present a clinical assessment cannot be made with any confidence at the drug design stage.

The same is largely true, for that matter, of the drug activity seen in the experimental animal tumor screens. The same alkylating compound (or other type of drug) can be a very good agent in one tumor system, and a very poor or inactive drug in another screen. The reason for such differences is generally not clear, but it can on occasion be related to biochemical and metabolic features of the host or tumor.

It is not possible, in the space of a short review, to attempt anything approaching a comprehensive coverage of alkylating agents. More detailed information may be gleaned from extensive reviews (e.g., 6, 7), and from the excellent assemblages of data (e.g., 1, 2, 8) published under the auspices of the Cancer Chemotherapy National Service Center, U.S. Public Health Service. But we can, perhaps, pick out certain general features and give some consideration to agents designed to take advantage of possible metabolic differences, even though, in practice, such advantages frequently, alas, turn out to be not much in evidence. It might be pertinent here to define alkylation. Briefly, the term is used to describe the process of transferring an alkyl group to another molecule. For example, the acetate ion can be converted to ethyl acetate by reaction with ethyl iodide:

$$CH_3CO_2^- + C_2H_5I \rightarrow CH_3CO_2C_2H_5 + I^-$$

Here, ethyl iodide is the alkylating (ethylating) agent. Biological alkylating agents are characterized by their ability to react under physiological conditions, and the alkyl group transferred is commonly more complex than ethyl. The subsequent discussion will be restricted to such agents.

II. Types of Alkylating Groups

For all practical purposes alkylating agents of current interest as tumor inhibitors fall into four classes.

A. Chloroethylamines and Haloethyl Sulfides

The nitrogen mustards, of which HN2 (**I**; $R = CH_3$) is an example, are of this type. Almost all of them can be represented by formula **I**. In the case of the aliphatic compounds (**I**; $R = alkyl$), alkylation in aqueous solution has

$$RN(CH_2CH_2Cl)_2$$

I

been shown to be preceded by a relatively fast unimolecular conversion to a cyclic immonium ion. This ion (**II**) can alkylate nucleophilic centers (A^-) in the cell by a bimolecular (S_N2) mechanism and at a rate dependent upon the effective concentration of these centers (*6, 9*) (Scheme 1). The aromatic nitrogen

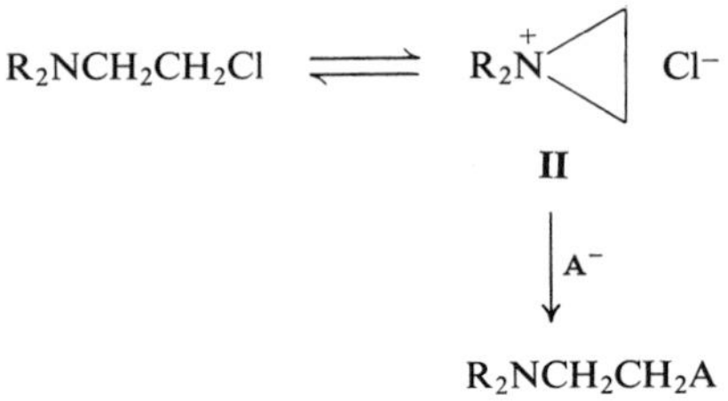

$$R_2NCH_2CH_2Cl \rightleftharpoons R_2\overset{+}{N}\!\!\triangleleft \quad Cl^-$$

II

$$\downarrow A^-$$

$$R_2NCH_2CH_2A$$

Scheme 1

mustards (**I**; R = aryl) have posed a more complex problem. It has been proposed that here the lower basicity of the nitrogen atom precludes the formation of a stable cyclic ion of type **II**; instead, the agents may be considered as reacting via a carbonium ion (**III**), formed relatively slowly by unimolecular loss of chloride (S_N1 reaction) (*6, 9*) (Scheme 2). It is likely that

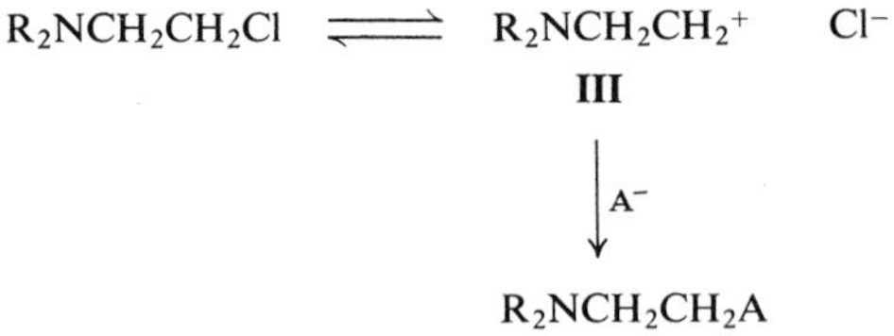

$$R_2NCH_2CH_2Cl \rightleftharpoons R_2NCH_2CH_2^+ \quad Cl^-$$

III

$$\downarrow A^-$$

$$R_2NCH_2CH_2A$$

Scheme 2

ion **III** is not linear but forms a carbonium ion–nitrogen dipole of type **IV** (*10*). This is a modification of an earlier view (*11*) that the aromatic nitrogen mustards behave in aqueous solution entirely like the aliphatic ones, forming a fully cyclic immonium ion. In this connection, evidence has recently been presented

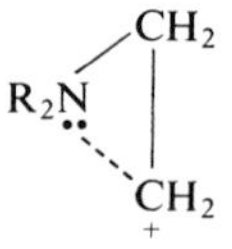

$$R_2\overset{..}{N}\begin{array}{c} {}^{CH_2} \\ | \\ {}_{CH_2^+} \end{array}$$

IV

(*12*) that chlorambucil forms an aziridinium ring of type **II**. However, although there may be exceptions, the aromatic nitrogen mustards in general differ from their aliphatic congeners in that their rates of reaction are independent of substrate concentration, although the presence of chloride ion will increase the back reaction rate and hence effectively slow down the ionization process. The reactivity of nitrogen mustards is suppressed if the pH of the solution falls to the point where the weakly basic nitrogen atom becomes protonated, because the presence of a positive charge on the nitrogen inhibits the expulsion of the negative chloride ion.

Although they have been widely used experimentally, haloethyl sulfides (sulfur mustards), such as mustard gas (bis-2-chloroethyl sulfide) are of little therapeutic importance. A recent exception is a fast-reacting bisbromoethyl derivative (CB 1850), described in Section X.

B. ETHYLENEIMINES AND ETHYLENEIMIDES

This type of structure (**V**) is reminiscent of the aziridinium intermediates mentioned above. Most cytotoxic agents of this kind are ethyleneimides (**V**;

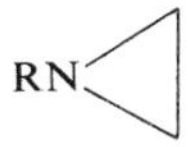

$$RN\triangleleft$$

V

R = R′CO or R′R″PO); these are chemically more reactive than uncharged *N*-alkyl ethyleneimines because electron withdrawal by the acyl group renders the methylene groups more susceptible to nucleophilic attack (Scheme 3).

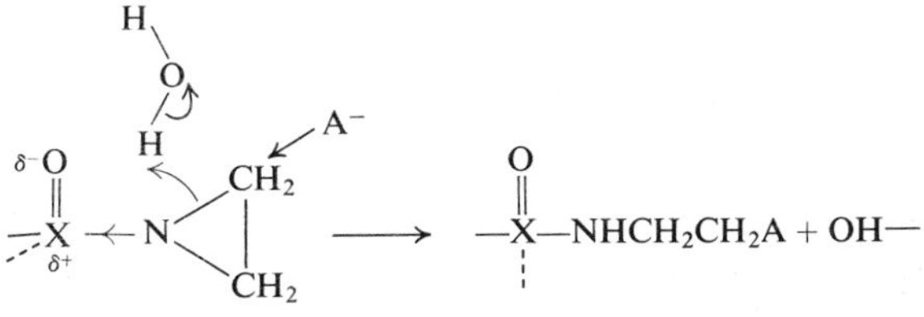

(X = C or P)

Scheme 3

Protonation of the nitrogen has a similar activating effect, hence the increased reactivity, particularly of *N*-alkylethyleneimines, under acid conditions. Compounds of type **V** react by an S_N2 mechanism, the reaction rate being dependent upon substrate concentration (*6*).

C. Epoxides

Reaction of epoxides (**VI**) with nucleophilic centers (e.g., A^-) occurs by a bimolecular (S_N2) mechanism (Scheme 4). Almost all the carcinostatic

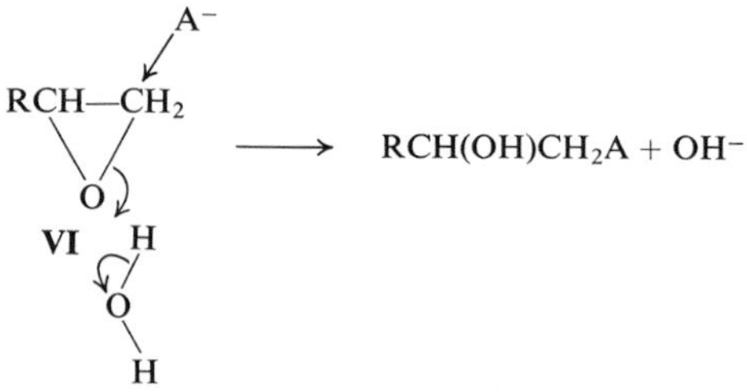

$$RCH(OH)CH_2A + OH^-$$

Scheme 4

epoxides contain an unsubstituted methylene group on each epoxide ring. Substitution markedly lowers both chemical and biological activity (*6*). Work with methanesulfonates of sugar alcohols has led to a renewed interest in the epoxide agents as we shall see (Section VI,B).

D. Sulfonic Acid Esters

These esters (**VII**) alkylate by an S_N1 or S_N2 mechanism (or by both mechanisms) depending upon the nature of the ester group R; O—R fission occurs and the alkyl group R is transferred to the substrate (*6*).

$$R'SO_2OR$$

VII

III. Sites of Reaction and Correlation with Biological Effects

Ross (*6*) has extensively discussed the types of reaction alkylating agents may undergo, both *in vitro* and *in vivo*. There is no doubt that many different kinds of sites in the cell are potentially reactive. For example, carboxyl, phosphate and thiol groups, in the anionic form, uncharged amino groups and imidazole groups are candidates.

In recent years attention has focused on the reaction of alkylating agents, especially nitrogen mustards, with DNA. There are several lines of evidence indicating that DNA is the biologically significant site of action in the cell and the work has been well reviewed (*6, 7, 13, 14*). Here again, more than one kind of reaction doubtless occurs, but interstrand linking between the N^7

atoms of near-opposite guanine residues in the twin helix has been described, and proposed as the principle cause of mitotic inhibition (*15, 16*). This may well be true, at least in certain cases, but it is also possible that other sites on the DNA molecule are involved. For example, it has been shown that ethyl methane sulfonate (EMS) is mutagenic in T-even phage systems while the analogous methyl methanesulfonate is not. Furthermore, each of these compounds reacts with deoxyguanosine *in vitro* to form N^7-alkyldeoxyguanosine but only EMS gives, in addition, O^6-alkyldeoxyguanosine. This work suggests a correlation between *O*-alkylation and mutagenesis (*17*). It would be premature to draw any general conclusions, particularly with regard to tumor inhibition by alkylating agents, until further work is done. The antitumor activity of dimethanesulfonoxymethane, discussed below, nevertheless reopens the whole cross-linking question; and the antitumor activity of 1-bromo-4-methanesulfonoxy-*n*-butane (*18*) inevitably leads one to wonder whether crosslinking between nucleic acid and, say, thiol groups in nucleoprotein might not turn out to be a mechanism of growth inhibition. The cross-linking potential of certain bifunctional alkylating agents, particularly epoxides, has recently been discussed by Van Duuren (*18a*).

IV. General Structural Considerations

A. Nitrogen Mustards

The aromatic nitrogen mustards began to be studied in a search for agents which could be administered orally (*19*). HN2 and related compounds need to be given intravenously because of their powerful vesicant action. The reactivity of a nitrogen mustard depends upon the separation of the halogen atom as an anion, and this process is dependent upon the electron-releasing capacity (basicity) of the nitrogen atom. Since aromatic amines are in general less basic than aliphatic ones, it was reasonable to suppose that their N,N-bis-2-chloroethyl derivatives would be less reactive than the aliphatic analogs. In the event, compounds were developed which were active against tumors, yet mild enough to be given by mouth.

The aromatic ring system has the advantage of being amenable to substitution by groups which can increase or reduce the basicity of an amino substituent. It was thus possible to synthesize aromatic nitrogen mustards of graded reactivity, and it became clear that there was a correlation between chemical reactivity and experimental antitumor potency (*6, 9*). The biological assessment was not quantitative so that one cannot say how close was the correlation. Moreover, structural changes in the molecule can affect other properties, such

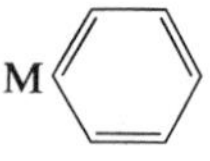

M⟨⟩

VIII

M⟨⟩CO₂C₂H₅

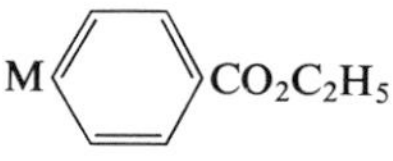

IX

as lipid solubility or transport. Nevertheless, the biological potency is susceptible to structural variation. For example, aniline mustard [**VIII**; M =
$(ClCH_2CH_2)_2N$, here and in subsequent formulas] inhibited the Walker rat
tumor while its p-ethoxycarbonyl derivative (**IX**) did not; the extent of hydrolysis of these compounds under defined conditions was 20% and less than 1%,
respectively (9). Although a minimum degree of reactivity is necessary for
useful biological activity, a relatively very high reactivity is undesirable where
systemic administration is intended because reaction at therapeutically
irrelevant sites could consume the agent before it reaches the tumor. It may,
however, be possible to make use of such a compound by special administration techniques (Section X).

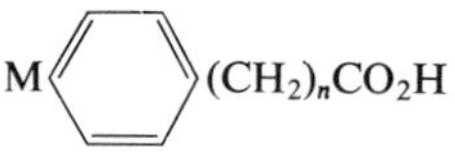

M⟨⟩$(CH_2)_nCO_2H$

X

Alterations in biological potency can sometimes be brought about by
structural changes which have little or no effect upon chemical reactivity.
For example, the introduction of an acidic side chain into aniline mustard led
to a series of derivatives (**X**) in which antitumor activity was found to be
highest where $n = 3$; chemical reactivity, on the other hand, was essentially
the same from $n = 1$ to $n = 4$ (6). This work led to chlorambucil (**X**; $n = 3$),
now widely used in the treatment of chronic lymphocytic leukemia. In the
form of the anion (in which it will largely exist under physiological conditions)
chlorambucil has certain surface-active properties and solubility characteristics which no doubt affect its transport, both extra- and intracellular. It is
likely that it diffuses through cell membranes as the undissociated acid (in
equilibrium with the more abundant anionic form) at physiological pH, since
anions do not normally pass through such membranes (20). Indeed, derivatives
which carry a strong acid group fully dissociated around pH 7 are likely to
be inactive. A recent example is compound **XI** (R = SO_3H); this was almost

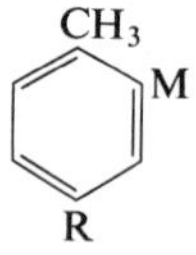

CH₃

M

R

XI

inactive against the Jensen sarcoma (21), contrasting with the highly active carboxylic analog (**XI**; R = CO$_2$H) (22).

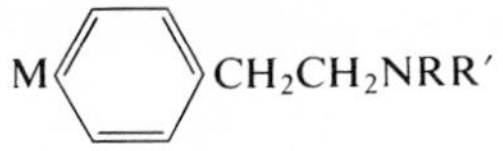

$$M\text{—}\langle\bigcirc\rangle\text{—}CH_2CH_2NRR'$$

XII

Similar considerations seem to apply to basic derivatives. Compounds **XII** where R = R' = H and R = H, R' = CH$_3$, were active; compound **XII**, where R = R' = CH$_3$, was less active; while the fully ionized quaternary derivative (**XIII**) and its noranalog were inactive against the Walker tumor (23). Other carriers of more "biological" character are discussed later.

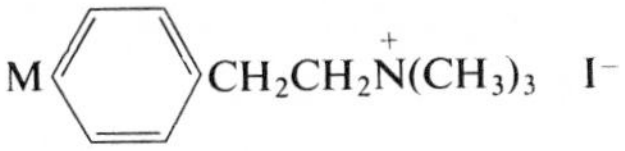

$$M\text{—}\langle\bigcirc\rangle\text{—}CH_2CH_2\overset{+}{N}(CH_3)_3 \quad I^-$$

XIII

Increased biological potency alone is not necessarily of any special virtue in an antitumor drug. What matters more is selectivity of action. It is therefore unfortunate that an increase in antitumor potency usually goes hand in hand with an increase in host toxicity, but there are exceptions.

The study of aromatic nitrogen mustards was extended to condensed ring systems, but these are not of any current importance. It might be mentioned in passing, however, that the mustard derived from β-naphthylamine (Erysan or CB 1048) was one of the first aromatic mustards to be used clinically (6).

Substitution, in aromatic nitrogen mustards, of bromine for chlorine, leads to an increased reactivity, but the introduction of iodine has the opposite effect (6). Most of the effective nitrogen mustards contain chlorine as the reactive halogen, but bromine has on occasion replaced it to advantage, at least as measured in experimental tumor systems. An example is the thiol derivative (**XIV**). This compound was more reactive chemically and, more

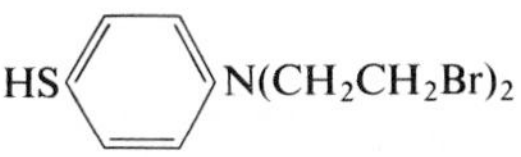

$$HS\text{—}\langle\bigcirc\rangle\text{—}N(CH_2CH_2Br)_2$$

XIV

importantly, had a substantially higher therapeutic index *in vivo* against the Walker rat tumor (10). Iodomustards have proved of little interest biologically (6). Fluoronitrogen mustards have been examined to a limited extent. Some years ago the clinical application of ftorpan (**XV**) was described (24). Since then, several reports have appeared on the preparation and properties of mustards in which one or both reactive halogens are fluorine. Bis-2-fluoro-

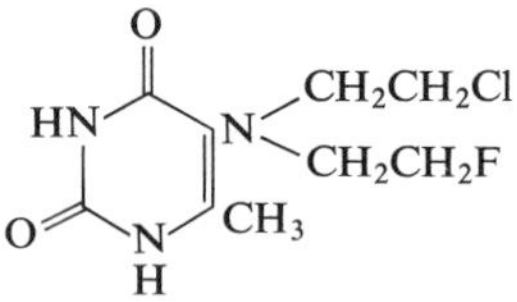

XV

ethylamine hydrobromide (**XVI**) had a degree of activity against the Walker rat tumor at toxic levels (*25*), but some *N,N*-bis-2-fluoroethylanilines, corresponding to various active aromatic chloromustards, were essentially inactive

$$HBr \cdot HN(CH_2CH_2F)_2$$

XVI

against experimental tumors (*26*). So, too, were fluoro analogs (**XVII**, X = Y = F; or X = Cl, Y = F) of cyclophosphamide (*27*). In summary, one can say that, although bromine can very occasionally replace chlorine to advantage, fluoro- and iodomustards do not seem at present to hold out much promise.

The length of the halo side chain is critical because the activating effect of the nitrogen atom upon the halogen atom is lost when the separation is more than two carbon atoms. For example, while aniline mustard (**VIII**) gave a

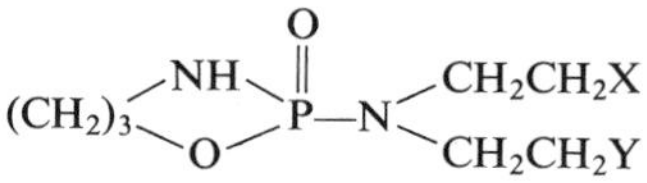

XVII

hydrolysis figure of 20 % under standard conditions and was tumor-inhibitory, the *n*-propyl analog (**XVIII**) hydrolyzed to a much more limited extent (<1 %) and was biologically inactive. 2-Chloro-*n*-propyl side chains are, on the other hand, more reactive than the standard ethyl analogs, although the alkylating capacity toward centers other than water is reduced and one may not therefore necessarily gain a biological advantage (*6*).

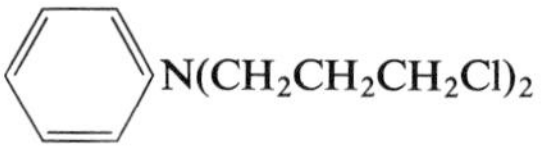

XVIII

In almost all active nitrogen mustards, the 2-chloroethyl groups are attached to the same nitrogen atom. This condition is not, however, essential for biological activity. For example, derivatives of type **XIX**, where *n* = 2 or 3, were active. Antitumor potency was nevertheless reduced when *n* was greater than 3 (*28*).

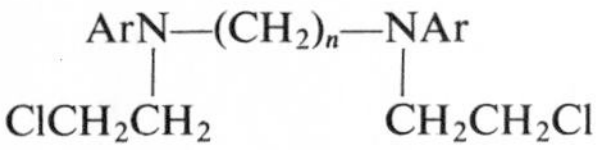

$$\begin{array}{c} \text{ArN---(CH}_2)_n\text{---NAr} \\ | \qquad\qquad | \\ \text{ClCH}_2\text{CH}_2 \qquad \text{CH}_2\text{CH}_2\text{Cl} \end{array}$$

XIX

One modification of the nitrogen mustards was the replacement of nitrogen by phosphorus, but neither bis-2-chloroethylphenylphosphine oxide nor the phosphorus analog (**XX**) of HN2 displayed "mustard-like" biological activity (*29, 30*).

$$CH_3P(CH_2CH_2Cl)_2 \cdot HCl$$

XX

B. ETHYLENEIMINES

Little need be said here in any general sense, but we shall see later how attempts have been made to improve the selectivity of action of compounds of this type. A typical derivative is triethylenemelamine (TEM; **XXI**), used in the textile industry long before it was found to have antitumor activity.

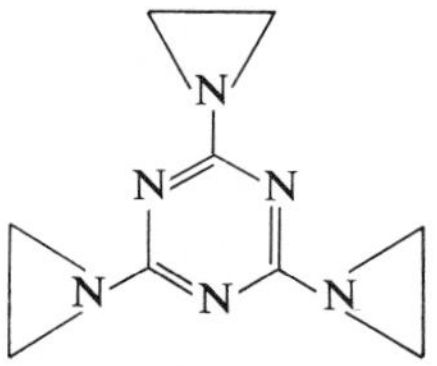

XXI

Its polyfunctional structure and its ability to react with wool fibers under mild conditions attracted the attention of biological investigators and it has been used clinically quite extensively, both orally and intravenously. As would be expected (see earlier discussion) TEM is more reactive under acid conditions (*31, 32*) and this fact has been taken advantage of, at least experi-

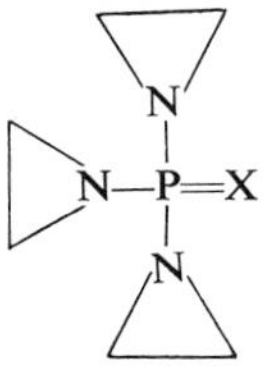

XXII

mentally (see below). It was seen earlier that ethyleneimines are rendered more reactive by attachment of the nitrogen atom to an electron-withdrawing group. It was therefore natural that the effect of an attached phosphoryl group should be explored. The two best known derivatives of this type are triethylenephosphoramide (TEPA; **XXII**, X = O) and the thio analog (thio-TEPA; **XXII**, X = S). Both TEPA (*33*) and thioTEPA (*34*) have been used extensively, experimentally and clinically. Other ethyleneimine derivatives are discussed below.

C. DIEPOXIDES

As we saw above, an important feature of the biologically active epoxides is that the carbon atoms involved in alkylation are unsubstituted. Among the first diepoxides to be examined was diepoxybutane (*35*). This was prepared as the racemic mixture (dianhydro-DL-threitol; **XXIII**) and as the *meso*-isomer (dianhydroerythritol; **XXIV**) although antitumor tests have often been done with mixtures of **XXIII** and **XXIV**. The racemic form was a more potent inhibitor of the Walker tumor than the *meso* (*36*) and the clinical use of the latter was abandoned because of side effects (*37*). In general, the tumor-inhibitory and lethal doses in the series of diepoxides tested were close and

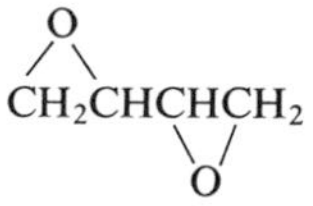

$$CH_2CHCHCH_2$$

with epoxide oxygens bridging.

XXIII

it was felt that this type of compound was unlikely to be of much clinical value (*36*). Nevertheless, some interest in the epoxides as therapeutic agents continued, and one of the products which has undergone fairly extensive study, experimentally (*38*) and clinically (*39*), is triethyleneglycol diglycidyl

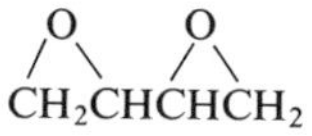

$$CH_2CHCHCH_2$$

XXIV

ether (Epodyl; **XXV**). This compound exemplifies the fact that the antitumor activity of diepoxides is not precluded by an extended link between the alkylating centers.

Acid catalysis of the reaction of epoxides is not apparent in most cases at physiological pH because protonation will not generally occur to a significant

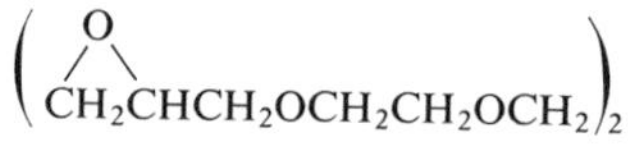

$$\left(CH_2CHCH_2OCH_2CH_2OCH_2 \right)_2$$

XXV

extent under these conditions (6). In a series of basic derivatives it was found that basicity, rate of reaction with phosphate ion, and activity against mouse leukemia P1534 went roughly hand in hand (40). Moreoever, the rate of reaction increased with acidity, presumably largely a result of protonation of the base. Such compounds are doubtless protonated *in vivo*, the extent depending upon the basicity of the molecule and the pH of the environment. This situation could form the basis of increased selectivity of action provided the pH of the tumor cells is lower than that of normal tissues (6). This approach, which tries to exploit pH differences, is discussed later. One of the most active members of the group of basic diepoxides was the dipiperidyl derivative (**XXVI**; Eponate); it has been used clinically (41).

Recent interest in epoxides centers upon their possible formation from tumor-inhibitory methanesulfonic esters of sugar alcohols (Section VI,B).

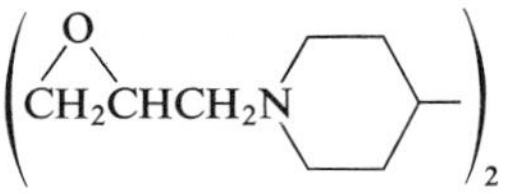

XXVI

D. METHANESULFONATES

Most of the synthetic work in this field was carried out in the 1950s, and a 1960 survey (42) includes most of the known compounds. The best known agent of this group is busulfan (Myleran; **XXVII**; $n = 4$), used clinically in

$$CH_3SO_2O(CH_2)_nOSO_2CH_3$$

XXVII

the treatment of chronic myelocytic leukemia. Experimentally it was one of the most active of a series (43). This work originated from a study of sulfonic esters, first made as analogs of the aromatic nitrogen mustards. It was the tumor-inhibitory effects of such compounds as **XXVIII**, and their relatively

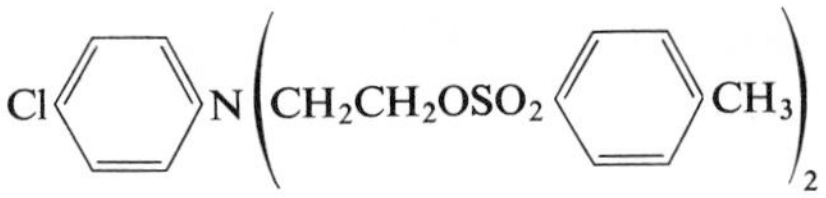

XXVIII

low bone marrow toxicity, which led to the preparation of busulfan and its congeners. The choice of busulfan for clinical trial against chronic myelocytic leukemia arose from the fact that it had a specially pronounced depressing action upon the granulocytes in the rat (44), although most members (**XXVII**; $n = 3$ to 9) of the series inhibited the Walker rat tumor (43). Compound **XXVII** ($n = 18$) had no significant activity against this tumor (45). The extent of separation of the alkylating groups is therefore of some importance. Of a series of branched-chain sulfonates (**XXIX**), "dimethyl–Myleran" (**XXIX**;

$$CH_3SO_2OCH(CH_2)_nCHOSO_2CH_3$$

with CH_3 groups on each CH

XXIX

$n = 2$) was the most active of its congeners as a neutrophil-depressing agent and was rather quicker acting than the unbranched analogs. Unlike busulfan, it had no effect upon the Walker tumor. This difference may be related to the fact that compounds of type **XXIX** react by an S_N1 mechanism; busulfan reacts mainly by S_N2 (46). In both the branched and unbranched series the fall in biological activity with increasing chain length correlated with a fall in the water–ether solubility ratios, but although such partition factors may play a part they do not explain the fact that the highest activity is seen with a separation of 4 carbon atoms between the functional groups. A cyclization process has been suggested, because greater ring stability would be expected when $n = 4$ or 5, than when $n = 2$ or 3 (**XXVII**). When $n = 6$ to 10, ring formation would be slower (46). Busulfan certainly undergoes a cyclization reaction with thiols *in vivo* (47) but it is not known what relevance this reaction has to the biological activity. All that can be said is that the metabolic end product, 3-hydroxytetrahydrothiophen-1,1-dioxide (**XXX**) and its precursor, tetra-

XXX

hydrothiophen-1,1-dioxide, did not show busulfan-like effects. Hence, if the cyclization reaction is related to the biological action, it is likely to be so by virtue of the desulfurization process (47). Whether busulfan can act as a crosslinking agent to an extent sufficient to account for its effects is not known. Although the nonane derivative (**XXVII**; $n = 9$) is less potent than busulfan in its depressing action on neutrophils (46) it appears to be the more active of the two compounds in some experimental tumor systems (48). This is again a reflection of the fact that structure–activity relationships may show different patterns with different biological systems. The busulfan analog (**XXVII**; $n = 2$) was inactive, against both the Walker tumor and the circulating neutrophils in the rat (43, 46). It is therefore perhaps surprising that bismethanesulfonoxymethane [methylene dimethanesulfonate (MDMS), after Fox (*49*); **XXVII**, $n = 1$] was highly active—much more so than busulfan—against the Walker and Yoshida tumors in the rat. MDMS differs from its higher homologs in that it may be regarded as a potential source of formaldehyde. Whether this has any bearing on the biological activity remains to be seen. The biological effects very closely resemble those of typical alkylating agents, and cross resistance to TEM (**XXI**) was observed (*49, 50*). MDMS clearly cannot undergo cyclization reactions as busulfan can. Furthermore, studies made by Dr. M. Jarman of this Institute, this author, and Dr. W. Fuller of King's College, University of London, with the use of the latter's accurate space-filling molecular models, indicated that MDMS (or formaldehyde) is unable to form intrastrand links in DNA between adjacent bases. Interstrand cross-linking is possible but only (on the assumption the model is at all times valid) between the following three pairs of atoms, assuming electron shifts equivalent to enolization:

Guanine-N^2—Cytosine-O^2
Guanine-O^6—Cytosine-N^4
Adenine-N^6—Thymine-O^4

These are pairs of atoms which are hydrogen-bonded in the core of the DNA twin helix. It may be that these sites would react with MDMS or formaldehyde only in regions where the DNA is single-stranded or the helix partially un-wound. It is known that formaldehyde reacts with native single-stranded and denatured DNA, but not with double-stranded DNA (*51*). Interstrand linkage of DNA by MDMS might thus be favored during certain periods in the mitotic cycle, but there is no possibility of crosslinking with the N^7 atoms of DNA guanine as can occur (*15, 16*) with other alkylating agents. It is conceivable that reaction with nucleophilic centers (such as thiols) in protein or nucleo-protein might be important. This possibility finds some reinforcement in the finding that a busulfan analog (**XXXI**), prepared very recently, is active against

$$Br(CH_2)_4OSO_2CH_3$$

XXXI

the Walker rat tumor (unlike 1,4-dibromo-*n*-butane) and appears to have, in the initial study, a reasonably good therapeutic index, unlike busulfan (*18*). Thiol groups, rather than DNA purine bases, are the more likely candidates for reaction with the halogen end of the molecule. It must be borne in mind, however, that if the molecule is anchored by reaction at one end, the other alkylating end may be held in a position favoring reaction with what may, in the ordinary way, be considered to be a less likely site. Moreoever, as we shall see, some monosulfonates have shown antitumor activity. However, that busulfan and compound **XXXI** are different in their modes of action is suggested by the fact that the peripheral blood pattern of the bromo compound resembles that of the *N*-mustards (*52*).

Another type of compound being studied is a series of mixed functional agents (**XXXII** and the bromo analogs). Such compounds would be capable of alkylating neighboring groups but not of cross-linking them (*18*). Studies of this kind may throw further light on the significant biological reactions of alkylating agents.

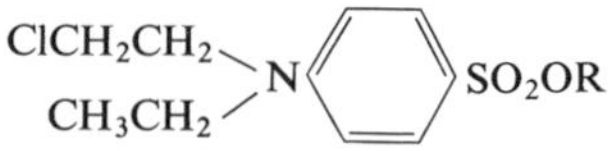

$$\text{ClCH}_2\text{CH}_2\diagdown \atop \text{CH}_3\text{CH}_2\diagup \text{N}\diagup\hspace{-0.3em}\bigcirc\hspace{-0.3em}\diagdown \text{SO}_2\text{OR}$$

XXXII

V. Number of Reactive Centers

With very few exceptions, antitumor activity is not shown by alkylating agents having less than two functional groups, while the presence of more than two does not commonly confer any advantage (*6*). This is not to say that monofunctional agents are devoid of biological activity. On the contrary, they may display carcinogenic and mutagenic properties, as well as general toxic effects. Sometimes, indeed, the mutational activity of a monofunctional compound in certain systems exceeds that of its bifunctional analog (*53*). However, where growth inhibition is concerned, polyfunctionality is generally necessary. This is well exemplified among the nitrogen mustards, although an interesting exception is the monofunctional acridine derivative, ICR-170 (**XXXIII**; R = H) which was almost as active against various ascites tumors *in vivo* as the difunctional analog (**XXXIII**; R = Cl) (*54*). Several active monofunctional nitrogen and sulfur mustards of this type are now known (*55*).

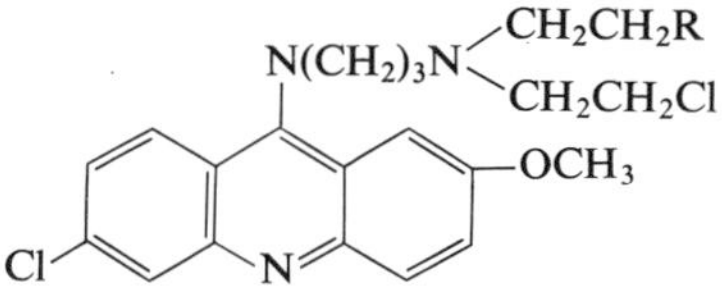

$$\text{N(CH}_2)_3\text{N}\diagup \text{CH}_2\text{CH}_2\text{R} \atop \diagdown \text{CH}_2\text{CH}_2\text{Cl}$$

XXXIII

This kind of agent perhaps represents a special case in that the acridine part of the molecule may bind strongly to DNA by a process of intercalation between adjacent nucleotides (*56*).

A second type of active monofunctional *N*-mustard is the bromoethyl derivative (**XXXIIIa**), prepared (*57*) as a result of an earlier study (*58*) of a series of bisbromoethyl derivatives of aryl sulfonamides in which it was suggested that activity may be related to alkylation of a folate-utilizing enzyme. Compound (**XXXIIIa**) caused complete regression of the Murphy-Sturm rat lymphosarcoma, and was more potent on a molar basis than the dibromo analog. It was proposed that the high activity is due to adsorption at a specific receptor. It is of interest that the analog in which bromine is replaced by chlorine was completely inactive at tolerated doses (*57*).

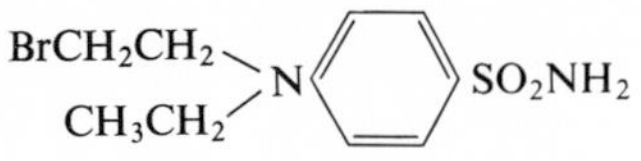

$$BrCH_2CH_2 \diagdown N \diagup SO_2NH_2$$
$$CH_3CH_2 \diagup$$

XXXIIIa

A one-armed *N*-mustard derivative of D-glucose which was reported to be more active *in vivo* than the bifunctional analog is described later (Section VI,B).

Following a suggestion (*59*) regarding irreversible enzyme inhibition, a series of monochloroethylamino derivatives of 3 lactic acid dehydrogenase inhibitors—phenoxyacetic, oxanilic, and salicylic acids—was made (*60*). None showed significant activity against the Walker tumor or L1210 mouse leukemia. It is not known whether this failure was due to inadequate enzyme inhibition. It may be that other areas of Baker's extensive work (*60a*) on irreversible enzyme inhibition could be applied more fruitfully.

Among the ethyleneimines, a number of monofunctional tumor inhibitors are known. Tetramin, a mixture of isomers (**XXXIVa,b**), inhibited a number of experimental tumors and has been used clinically (*61–63*). It could be that activity is here due to oxidation of the double bond to epoxide (*6*).

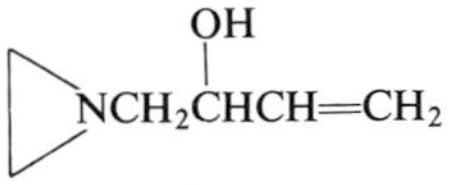

$$\overset{OH}{\underset{|}{NCH_2CHCH{=}CH_2}}$$

XXXIVa

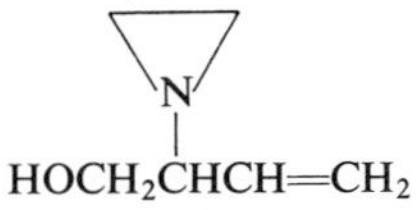

$$\overset{\diagup N \diagdown}{\underset{|}{HOCH_2CHCH{=}CH_2}}$$

XXXIVb

The monofunctional compounds (**XXXV**) and (**XXXVI**; R = NH$_2$ or OCH$_3$) are tumor-inhibiting (*5, 8*). The ethyleneimine (**XXXVII**) also has antitumor properties and its therapeutic index (~11), in the Walker rat tumor system, compares favorably with the average bifunctional agent. It seems likely that the dinitrophenyl residue binds strongly to the substrate. Such compounds produce effects comparable to TEM, but only at much larger doses (10- or 20-fold) (*6*).

XXXV   XXXVI

Very recently, in a search for water-soluble derivatives of the dinitro compound (**XXXVII**), it was found that the monofunctional benzamide (**XXXVIII**) completely inhibited the 1-day Walker rat tumor at the relatively low dose of 2 mg/kg. Moreover, the therapeutic index (LD_{50}/ED_{90}) was 70, the highest yet recorded in this system at the Chester Beatty Research Institute, bifunctional agents included. Curiously, other tumors were not affected by compound **XXXVIII**, even the PC6 plasma cell tumor which is extremely sensitive to bifunctional agents. Many analogs of compound **XXXVIII** have been made, but none showed such a high index, although several were better in this respect than the original monofunctional derivative (**XXXVII**) (*64*). This is an example of how structural modification, undertaken for a special reason, can lead to an unexpected and encouraging result not necessarily related to the original quest.

XXXVII   XXXVIII

We saw earlier that the ability of monofunctional alkyl methanesulfonates (**XXXIX**) to *O*-alkylate the base of deoxyguanosine correlated with mutagenic activity in bacteriophage (*17*). These esters (**XXXIX**, $R = CH_3$ or C_2H_5) and some related compounds also inhibited the Walker rat tumor (*65, 66*). They were studied because of the discovery that 2-chloroethyl methanesulfonate (**XXXIX**; $R = ClCH_2CH_2$) was tumor-inhibitory; this compound was

$$CH_3SO_2OR$$

XXXIX

originally made as a potential chloroethylating agent (*65*). The chloro compound was more active biologically than its congeners in the tumor tests at this institute, possibly because of conversion into a highly reactive intermediate; it forms *S*-(2-chloroethyl)cysteine, a sulfur mustard, *in vivo* (*6*). Studies carried out with 2-chloroethyl methanesulfonate using several mouse and rat tumor systems, including the Walker tumor, revealed activity only against lymphoma 8 in rats (67). In the latter system the compound was indeed more effective than a number of standard alkylating agents potent in other screens. The lack of activity against the Walker carcinoma in these American experiments is surprising. It may be related to the fact that Holtzman strain rats were used, whereas Wistar strain animals were employed both for the lymphoma 8 and the Chester Beatty-Walker tumor tests. We at any rate have here an example of the way in which a biological assessment of an anti-tumor agent in one laboratory does not always confirm the results in another, even though the test systems are superficially similar.

In spite of the work described above, difunctionality is advantageous in the sulfonic ester series, just as it is with the ethyleneimines. In general, if one were to set out to design a new antitumor alkylating agent, there would be no *a priori* case for making it monofunctional rather than difunctional; the known examples of active compounds containing only one alkylating center do not materially affect this conclusion.

VI. Naturally Occurring Compounds and Analogs as Carriers of Alkylating Groups

The presumed need of alkylating agents to permeate the cell membrane before they can exert an inhibitory action led to the exploration of carrying molecules which might assist transport into the cell and confer a greater degree of selectivity against tumors. Amino acids, peptides, proteins, carbo-hydrates, and various heterocyclic compounds have been employed to this end.

A. AMINO ACIDS, PEPTIDES, AND PROTEINS

The phenylalanine derivative (**XL**) has been prepared in the racemic (DL) form (merphalan or sarcolysin) (68–71) and in the optically active L and D forms (melphalan and medphalan) (68–70). The L-isomer, corresponding to the natural form of the amino acid, was biologically more active than the D-isomer (72). A range of experimental tumors was inhibited by these deriva-tives (73). The compounds provided an early example, in the field of alkylating agents, of the effect chirality may have upon biological activity. Melphalan

$$M\langle\bigcirc\rangle CH_2CHCO_2H$$
$$\underset{NH_2}{|}$$

XL

and sarcolysin are both used clinically (*73–75*). The *para*-substituted phenyl-alanine mustards are potent compounds, but transfer of the mustard group to the *ortho* position led to an even more powerful agent, merophan or ortho-merphalan (*75a*), now used clinically, mainly in Burkitt's lymphoma (*76*). The *meta*-substituted derivatives have also been made, so too have derivatives of β-phenyl-β-alanine. In general, the *meta* compounds were more active than the *para*, although their therapeutic indices were no better; they have not been developed clinically. The various modifications have been reviewed in some detail (*77*). Attention may perhaps be drawn to aminochlorambucil (**XLI**), a derivative of an α-amino acid not known to occur in nature. This

$$\text{M}\langle\ \rangle\text{CH}_2\text{CH}_2\underset{\underset{\text{NH}_2}{|}}{\text{C}}\text{HCO}_2\text{H}$$

XLI

compound was originally made in the racemic form (*78*). Subsequently, the two optical enantiomers were prepared (*79*). Again, one isomer was a more active tumor inhibitor than the other; optical rotatory studies showed it to be the D form (*79, 80*). Many peptide derivatives of sarcolysin and melphalan have been prepared independently by Russian and British workers, respectively, again with the hope of improving therapeutic efficacy. The two series were complementary in that the phenylalanine mustard residue was almost invariably *C*-terminal in the British work and *N*-terminal in the Russian. A detailed discussion of this field will not be attempted here. Fuller information can be found in other reviews (*77, 81–83*). Our own findings may be summed up as follows: (1) Peptides with a free primary amino group are more active (and more toxic) than peptides in which the amino group is acylated. (The same is true of free and *N*-acyl melphalan or sarcolysin.) (2) Peptide esters (e.g., **XLII**) of melphalan, in which the attached amino acids also have the L configuration, are about as active as melphalan on a molar basis (*84*). The

$$\text{H}_2\text{NCHRCONH}\underset{\underset{\text{CO}_2\text{C}_2\text{H}_5}{|}}{\text{C}}\text{HCH}_2\langle\ \rangle\text{M}$$

XLII

attachment of free or *N*-acetylated D-amino acids to melphalan ester gave products which were less potent and had a less favorable therapeutic index (*85, 86*). The comparison between α-L- and α-D-glutamylmelphalan ester (**XLII**; R = CH$_2$CH$_2$CO$_2$H) was particularly striking (*85*). Russian workers have also found that, in general, an LL configuration in dipeptides of phenyl-alanine mustard is advantageous (*87*), although the reservation should be made that the synthetic methods used by them do not preclude some racemization of asymmetric centers (81).

There is no doubt that the biological testing of peptides of phenylalanine mustard has been much more extensive in the Soviet Union. A typical product, asaline (**XLIII**), has been much studied. It has a relatively low toxicity and is reported not to cause blood changes at therapeutic doses (82, 83). Like many of the peptides synthesized in Russia, the amino acid components were used in the DL form, so asaline is a mixture of 4 isomers. Different preparations may differ in the proportions of diastereoisomers they contain, and precise biological standardization was difficult (87). It nevertheless seems clear that the antitumor spectrum and the relative intensities of antitumor action, toxicity, and blood effects depend upon the nature of the amino acids in the sarcolysin

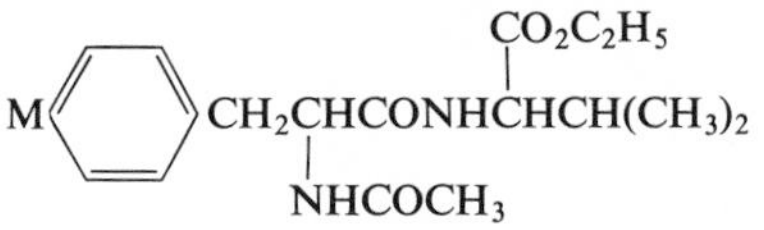

$$M\langle\text{—}\rangle CH_2CHCONHCHCH(CH_3)_2$$

with substituents $CO_2C_2H_5$ and $NHCOCH_3$

XLIII

peptides, and the configuration of the components. Polyamino acids and copolyamino acids have also been studied as carriers of melphalan ester, and the nature of the carrier again clearly determines the activity and therapeutic index in the Walker (rat) and the PC6 plasma cell (mouse) tumor systems (88).

Although phenylalanine nitrogen mustard and its derivatives have been the most extensively studied, other amino acid nitrogen mustard derivatives are known (1). The glycine and alanine derivatives (**XLIV** and **XLV**, respectively)

$$MCH_2CO_2H$$

XLIV

$$MCHCO_2H \quad \text{with } CH_3$$

XLV

were early examples (89, 90), although, in these cases, the α-amino group was itself incorporated into the mustard group and is not free to participate in possible active transport processes. The compounds were less toxic than HN2 and less vesicant. 5-Di-(2-chloroethyl)amino-DL-tryptophan (**XLVI**; M at 5) (91) was effective against experimental tumors. It has been tried clinically and may have some value (92, 93). The racemic 6- and 7-substituted analogs (**XLVI**; M at 6 or 7) have also been described. The 7-substituted

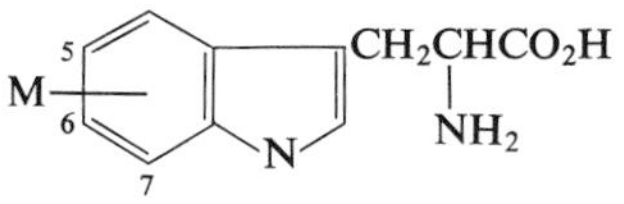

$$M\text{—indole—}CH_2CHCO_2H \quad \text{with } NH_2$$

XLVI

compound had a therapeutic index of 14 in the Walker tumor system, the highest of the three congeners (*94*).

The same laboratory has also studied an interesting group of aromatic nitrogen mustard derivatives (**XLVII–LI**), mainly of cysteine (*95*). Tests at this institute against the Walker rat tumor showed that the activity of **XLVII**, already low (probably because of *in vivo* oxidation), was abolished by oxidation to the sulfone (**XLVIII**), presumably because of chemical deactivation of the mustard group. However, when the S atom was insulated from the ring, oxidation does not reduce the inhibitory effect. Indeed, compound **L** was as potent as the sulfide (**XLIX**), but less toxic, so oxidation represented a favorable change in this case.

$$M-\langle\!\!\!\bigcirc\!\!\!\rangle-\left\{ \begin{array}{l} -S- \\ -SO_2- \\ -CH_2S- \\ -CH_2SO_2- \\ -CH_2SCH_2- \end{array} \right\} -CH_2\underset{NH_2}{CHCO_2H}$$

(**XLVII**; DL)
(**XLVIII**; DL)
(**XLIX**; D and L)
(**L**; L)
(**LI**; DL)

The ω-substituted *N*-mustard derivatives of DL-lysine and DL-ornithine have been studied (*96*). It has been observed that the L form of a mixture of α- and ε-substituted lysines was more active than the D form (*97*).

This brief summary should not be closed without reference to azaserine (**LII**) and 6-diazo-5-oxo-L-norleucine (DON, **LIII**). These are antibiotics which are monofunctional alkylating agents active against a number of

$$N_2CHCOOCH_2\underset{NH_2}{CHCO_2H}$$

LII

$$N_2CHCOCH_2CH_2\underset{NH_2}{CHCO_2H}$$

LIII

experimental tumors. DON is much more potent on a weight basis. Both have the L configuration; the synthetic D forms were much less active. The compounds may be regarded as bifunctional in the sense that they are also glutamine antagonists; their alkylating ability enables them to render irreversible their combination with transaminases (*98*). They are of little clinical value, and the elucidation of their structure has not been followed by any advance in the development of useful compounds able to act by similar mechanisms. Synthetic analogs of azaserine, in which the serine residue was replaced by other hydroxyamino acids showed no antitumor activity (*98a*). *N*-Diazoacetylglycine hydrazide was the best tumor inhibitor among a number of related glycine derivatives, but a detailed study in several species showed it to be a highly toxic compound (*98b*).

Some amino acid derivatives fall into the class of compounds with latent activity, and these will be discussed later (Section VIII).

We have seen how amino acids, peptides, and polyamino acids have been used as carriers of melphalan. Some years ago, as a model for the eventual use of tumor-specific antibodies, albumin was employed as a carrier for alkylating groups of the latent type (see below). At the time, it was thought that the combination of active nitrogen mustards with protein carriers would give unstable products; it seemed likely that the alkylating groups would react with the carrying molecules. Later work indicated that this was not necessarily the case (99). Indeed, albumin has a protective effect and slows down the rate of hydrolysis of some types of active N-mustards in aqueous solution (100, 101). Study of a series of products in which, in particular, N,N-di-(2-chloroethyl)-p-phenylenediamine was conjugated chemically to albumin, fibrinogen or globulin or their alaninated derivatives showed that such coupling sometimes led to a marked improvement, up to 8-fold, in the therapeutic index in the PC6 plasma cell mouse tumor screen. It was further discovered that chemical combination was not necessary; physical association seemed adequate (102). The reason for the improved index is not clear, but may be related to the finding that administration of radioactive albumin or fibrinogen leads to a relatively high incorporation of radioactivity into tumors (103, 104). It still remains to assess the value of protein carriers in other tumor systems.

B. CARBOHYDRATES

The study of ethyleneimino and chloroethylamino derivatives of sugar alcohols led to the discovery of 1,6-di-(2-chloroethyl)amino-1,6-dideoxy-D-mannitol (Degranol; BCM; **LIV**), reported to be superior to nitrogen mustard and other alkylating agents, particularly in its ability to suppress metastatic growth (105, 106). The carrying structure has a specific influence upon biological activity. If galactitol (dulcitol) replaces mannitol (i.e., inversion at C-2), as in compound **LV**, activity is lost. The hexane derivative (**LVI**) is also

$$
\begin{array}{cc}
\mathrm{CH_2NHCH_2CH_2Cl} & \mathrm{CH_2NHCH_2CH_2Cl} \\
| & | \\
\mathrm{HOCH} & \mathrm{HCOH} \\
| & | \\
\mathrm{HOCH} & \mathrm{HOCH} \\
| & | \\
\mathrm{HCOH} & \mathrm{HCOH} \\
| & | \\
\mathrm{HCOH} & \mathrm{HCOH} \\
| & | \\
\mathrm{CH_2NHCH_2CH_2Cl} & \mathrm{CH_2NHCH_2CH_2Cl} \\
\mathbf{LIV} & \mathbf{LV}
\end{array}
$$

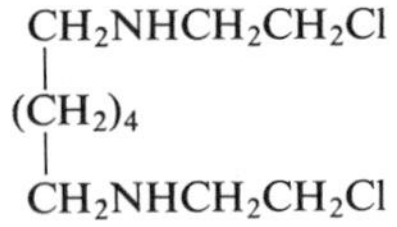

CH$_2$NHCH$_2$CH$_2$Cl
|
(CH$_2$)$_4$
|
CH$_2$NHCH$_2$CH$_2$Cl

LVI

inactive. Thus, in this type of structure, hydroxyl groups are necessary and the steric requirements are stringent (*105*). The *N*-bromomustard analog of degranol is also an effective agent (*107*). Glucose has been used as a carrier of nitrogen mustard groups. 2-(Bischloroethylamino)-2-deoxy-D-glucose had an activity similar to that of HN2 (*105*). It is surprising that the one-armed mustards (**LVII**; R = CH$_3$ or C$_2$H$_5$) derived from 6-deoxy-D-glucose showed

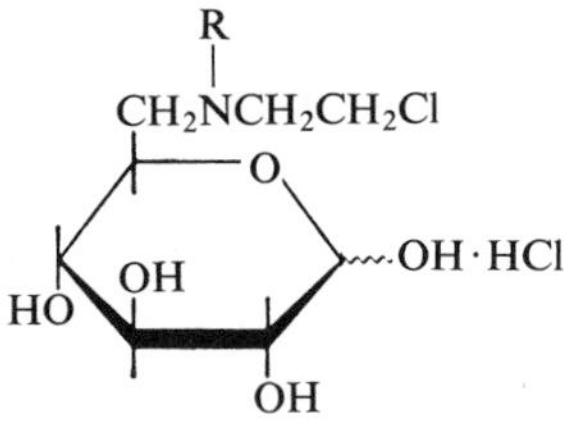

R
|
CH$_2$NCH$_2$CH$_2$Cl

LVII

substantial activity against L1210 leukemia in mice, while the two-armed analog (**LVII**; R = CH$_2$CH$_2$Cl) was barely active. Such a distinction was not seen when the carrier was D-ribose (*108*).

Carbohydrate molecules have also been used as carriers of the methanesulfonic ester group. Here again, a marked dependence of biological activity upon stereochemistry is seen (*109*). Thus, most members of a range of dimesyl derivatives of sugars and sugar alcohols investigated independently at this institute and in Hungary had no significant antitumor activity. Only 1,6-dimethanesulfonyl-D-mannitol (mannitol–Myleran; **LVIII**) showed substantial inhibitory effects; the L-isomer was inactive (*110–114*). Just why D-mannitol is especially advantageous among hexitols as a carrier for mustard groups and methanesulfonyloxy groups is not known.

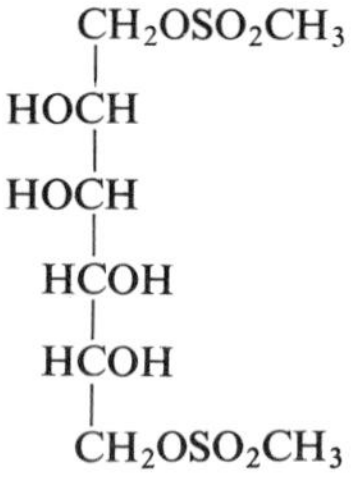

CH$_2$OSO$_2$CH$_3$
|
HOCH
|
HOCH
|
HCOH
|
HCOH
|
CH$_2$OSO$_2$CH$_3$

LVIII

Other related derivatives which have shown antitumor effects include 1,2,5,6-tetramethanesulfonyl-D-mannitol and the 1,6-diethyleneimino and 1,6-bismethanesulphonoxyethylamino derivatives of 1,6-dideoxy-D-mannitol (*115*).

The 4-carbon sugar alcohol, L-threitol, has also proved to be an effective carrier in work carried out initially in Denmark where the 1,4-dimethanesulfonyl derivative (**LIX**) was made (*116*, *117*). It was rather more effective than busulfan experimentally, but there is no indication that it would be of special clinical value (*118*). More recently, 1,4-di-(methanesulphonoxyethylamino)-1,4-dideoxyerythritol was reported to show marked inhibitory effects on several experimental tumors. Comparison with other mesylates in the treatment of L1210 mouse leukemia suggested the importance of the aminoethyl group for activity in this system (*119*).

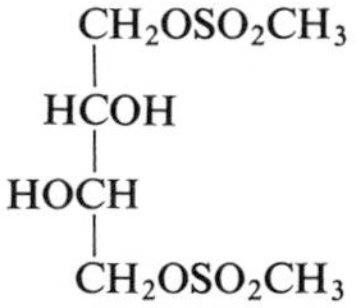

CH2OSO2CH3
HCOH
HOCH
CH2OSO2CH3

LIX

One important difference between busulfan (**XXVII**; $n = 4$) and mannitol–Myleran (**LVIII**) is that the latter can undergo elimination reactions to give anhydride structures. Recently, it has been conclusively established that the diepoxide (**LX**) is formed in aqueous solutions of mannitol–Myleran kept at pH 8 (*120*). The same compound is formed from another antitumor agent, 1,6-dibromo-1,6-dideoxy-D-mannitol (**LXI**) (Scheme 5). Furthermore, the biological effects are consistent with such a conversion occurring *in vivo* (*120*). A 2 or 3% conversion would be sufficient to account for the activity of mannitol–Myleran, because the diepoxide is a relatively very potent compound, now being studied in its own right. These findings are an extension of earlier

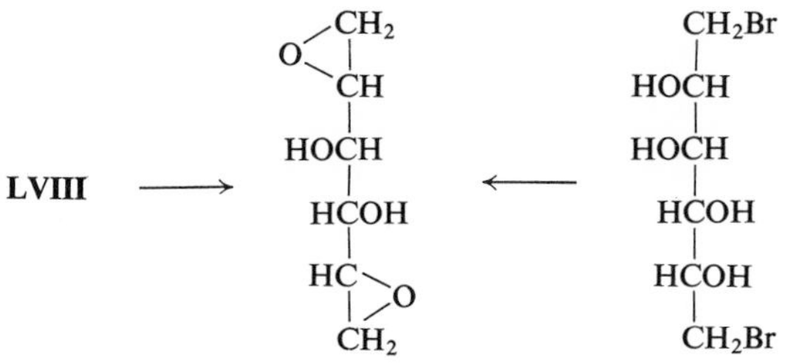

LVIII
CH2
O
CH
HOCH
HCOH
HC
O
CH2
CH2Br
HOCH
HOCH
HCOH
HCOH
CH2Br

LX **LXI**

Scheme 5

work which had also indicated that the threitol analog (**LIX**) was converted to epoxide in aqueous solution (*121*).

C. OTHER CARRYING STRUCTURES

Alkylating groups have been attached to many other kinds of molecules which normally have a metabolic function or which are analogous to such structures. The hope has clearly been, as with the classes discussed above, that some useful attribute will thereby be accorded the alkylating function. Heterocyclic compounds are well represented. Two of the best known are Dopan (**LXII**; R = CH$_3$), used mainly in the Soviet Union (*122*), and the related uracil mustard (**LXII**; R = H), developed independently in the USSR

LXII   **LXIII**

and the US (*123*). Some monofunctional derivatives of nicotinic acid have been made as potential irreversible inhibitors of glycolysis, on the grounds that many tumors derive much of their energy from glycolytic activity. Compounds **LXIII** (X = Br or Cl) and **LXIV** showed slight antitumor activity (*124*).

A compound of some interest is the hydrazone derivative (**LXV**). This

LXIV   **LXV**

compound (NSC 54012) was remarkable in that it was highly active against the Yoshida ascites tumor but inactive in other tumor systems (*125*). Agents active against only one tumor are rare. One other example, the monoethyleneimino derivative (**XXXVIII**), was described above. Tests in the United States appeared to reveal a further case of this kind which concerned esters of methanesulfonic acid (*67, 125*); but, as we saw earlier, results in the Chester Beatty Institute were at variance with the outcome of the American tests. Findings like this again make it abundantly clear that one kind of tumor test system may give the *coup de grâce* to an agent which, in another system, may show up very well. It is impossible to say how many good agents, if any, have been overlooked in such a way.

The imidazole derivative (**LXVI**) is of current interest. It was made as an extension of earlier work on nonmustard inhibitory analogs of the purine precursor, 5 (or 4)-aminoimidazole-4(or 5)-carboxamide (*126, 127*).

1,3-Bis-2-chloroethyl-1-nitrosourea (BCNU; **LXVII**) has attracted considerable clinical attention in recent years (*128*). It was evolved as an extension of a series of nitrosoguanidines and nitrosoureas, and was much more effective

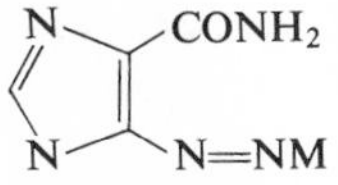

$$CICH_2CH_2NCONHCH_2CH_2Cl$$
$$NO$$

LXVI 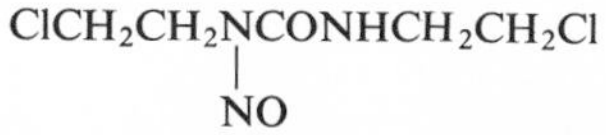   **LXVII**

in experimental leukemia than compounds containing no chloroethyl groups, or only one chloroethyl group (*129*). However, a related compound containing one chloroethyl group and one cyclohexyl residue (**LXVIII**) is being studied clinically, because of its superiority over BCNU in the L1210 leukemia screen (*130*).

Other kinds of carrier, including steroids have been discussed elsewhere (cf. *6*).

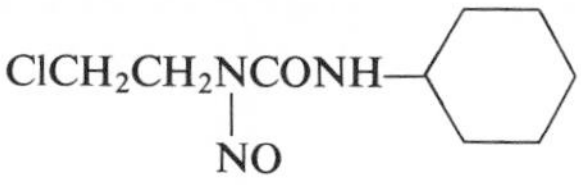

$$CICH_2CH_2NCONH-$$
$$NO$$

LXVIII

VII. Dual Antagonists

Attempts have been made to develop agents in which alkylating groups are combined chemically to other types of inhibiting groups. One of the best known of these dual antagonists is benzcarbimine (AB 103; **LXIX**), widely studied experimentally and clinically (*131, 132*). More recently, a number

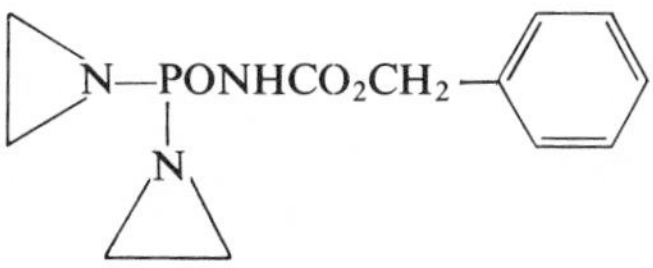

$$N-PONHCO_2CH_2-$$
$$N$$

LXIX

of arsenicals carrying the nitrogen mustard group have been made. The idea behind this approach was to combine general alkylating ability with specific sulfydryl reactivity (*133*). In general, the toxic effects of the arsenic group precluded the administration of doses large enough to inhibit the Walker tumor, although the Ehrlich ascites tumor was completely inhibited at non-toxic doses of compounds **LXX** and **LXXI**. However, there seems to be no evidence that such chemical combination of alkylating function with other antimetabolite functions has so far produced useful synergistic effects.

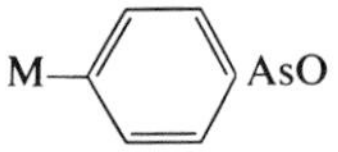

LXX 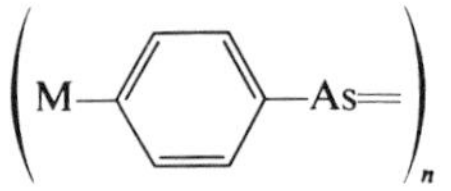   **LXXI**

VIII. Alkylating Agents Capable of Being Activated or Potentiated

The kinds of compounds discussed above are chemically reactive and able to alkylate body constituents immediately they are introduced into the organism. Some of them are nevertheless converted *in vivo* into a more effective species. A case in point is mannitol–Myleran (**LVIII**) which, as we have seen, is probably transformed *in vivo* into the more active diepoxide (**LX**). Again, aniline mustard (**VIII**) was found to be exceptionally potent against a mouse plasma cell tumor. This potency appears to be due to an initial conversion to the glucuronide (**LXXII**), with subsequent degradation to the free, toxic *p*-hydroxy derivative (**LXXIII**) (Scheme 6). The latter compound is formed

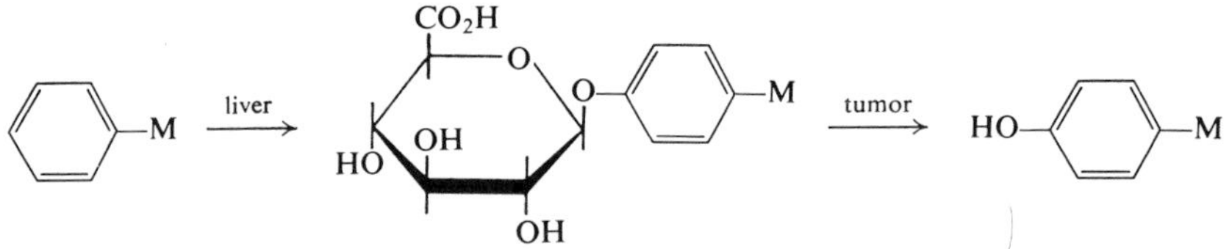

VIII   **LXXII**   **LXXIII**

Scheme 6

mainly in the tumor because this neoplasm possesses a relatively high β-glucuronidase activity (*134, 135*). One would expect the precursor (**LXXII**) to be as active chemically, but its solubility and distribution characteristics are probably very different. The therapeutic index of compound **LXXIII** is poor when it is administered systemically, but this is of little significance if the product is confined largely to the tumor. Here, then, is an active agent which is converted into a more active agent through the cooperation of both the host and the tumor. Human tumors with high glucuronidase activities may be good candidates for aniline mustard and the general principle will doubtless be exploited further.

This leads us on to consider agents, initially inactive, which have been synthesized in the hope that metabolic activation will render them selectively active.

The scientific bases of the various approaches which have been made have been discussed in some detail (6). No attempt will be made here to cover the numerous variations. Rather, a few examples will be taken as illustrations.

A. ACTIVATION BY HYDROLYSIS

Many compounds have been made in which cleavage of part of the molecule would result in increased chemical reactivity. Hydrolytic cleavage is in general the easiest type of fission to plan for, and it has been the pious hope that drugs conceived in this context would be converted into a more active form by hydrolytic enzymes residing largely in the tumor. The best known example of an agent designed to this end is cyclophosphamide, but this will be discussed later because it appears that activation in fact occurs by an oxidative process not a hydrolytic one. Cyclophosphamide, as we shall see, contains a phosphoramide mustard group. Among other structures into which this group has been incorporated with the principle of latent activity in mind may be mentioned the stereoisomeric modifications of a cyclic serine derivative (**LXXIV**) (whose structure is reminiscent of cyclophosphamide), the racemic, LL-, and DD-serylserine esters (**LXXV**; $n = 1$), and the corresponding derivatives (**LXXV**; $n = 15$ or higher) of poly-DL-, L-, and D-serine (*136*). As in the amino acid derivatives discussed earlier, the inhibitory effects of these various products were markedly dependent upon the stereochemistry. Although the mechanism of activation may be hydrolytic, no evidence is available on this point.

$$
\begin{array}{cc}
\overset{\displaystyle NH-CHCO_2H}{\underset{\displaystyle MPO\qquad CH_2}{\diagup\;\;\;\;\;\;\;\diagdown}} & \left(H-\!\!\!\overbrace{}^{}\!\!HNCHCONHCHCO\!\!\!\overbrace{}^{}\!\!-OH\right)
\end{array}
$$

NH—CHCO₂H   H—[—HNCHCONHCHCO—]—OH
MPO   CH₂   CH₂ O CH₂
      O   OPO
                                M

LXXIV   **LXXV**

Albumin has also been used as a carrier of the phosphoramide mustard group (and of a mustard carbamoylglycollic acid residue); the products were inactive biologically at the doses used (*137*). Another example of a latent alkylating agent in which an amino acid is used as the carrier is the carbamoyl mustard derivative of DL-serine (camosin; **LXXVI**; R = H), which has been used clinically (*138*). Reactivity presumably depends upon a metabolic conversion which leads, perhaps indirectly, to bis-2-chloropropylamine. The threonine analog (**LXXVI**; $R = CH_3$) was unexpectedly quite inactive against the Walker tumor (*139*).

A series of amino acid amides has been described in which the amide nitrogen atom carries one or two chloroethyl groups. The monofunctional derivatives (**LXXVII**) were more cytotoxic *in vitro* than were the bifunctional analogs, perhaps because they rearrange to a nonalkylating product less rapidly. More interesting is the observation that the cytotoxicity of compounds **LXXVII** in fact exceeded that of 2-chloroethylamine (*140*).

$$\left(\begin{array}{c} CH_3 \\ | \\ ClCHCH_2 \end{array}\right)_2 NCOOCHRCHCO_2H \qquad\qquad RCHCONHCH_2CH_2Cl$$
$$\qquad\qquad\qquad\qquad\qquad | \qquad\qquad\qquad\qquad\qquad\qquad | $$
$$\qquad\qquad\qquad\qquad\qquad NH_2 \qquad\qquad\qquad\qquad\qquad\qquad NH_2$$

LXXVI   **LXXVII**

Many latent compounds other than those of an amino acid character have been described (*6*). Considerable attention has, for instance, been given to derivatives of *p*-phenylenediamine mustard (**LXXVIII**; $R = H$) (*141*). The latter is highly reactive because of the enhancing effect of the *p*-amino group. Conversion of this amino group to, for example, a urethane (**LXXVIII**, $R = R'OCO$) reduces the reactivity. Selective cleavage within the tumor would lead to the release of the highly toxic parent (**LXXVIII**; $R = H$) (*6*). An interesting claim suggests that adaptive enzymes in the tumor can be stimulated by pretreatment with a nonmustard analog, such as the urethane (**LXXIX**). Subsequent administration of the corresponding mustard derivative [**LXXVIII**; $R = (CH_3)_2CHOCO$] was said to produce a far greater antitumor effect than a parallel experiment in which the pretreatment was omitted (*142*). Enzyme stimulation of this type in mammals does not appear to have been confirmed but the idea seems well worth pursuing.

$M\langle\bigcirc\rangle NHR$ $\qquad\qquad\qquad$ $\langle\bigcirc\rangle NHCO_2CH(CH_3)_2$

LXXVIII $\qquad\qquad\qquad\qquad\qquad\qquad$ **LXXIX**

Another urethane derivative (**LXXX**) prepared as a "damped-down" version of the phenol mustard (**LXXIII**) (*141*), is of interest in showing a relatively high therapeutic index in the Walker rat tumor system—17 as against 2.3 for the parent phenol (*10*).

Attention has been given to the selective detoxication of esters and amides containing haloacetyl groups. Of such compounds, ethylene bisiodoacetate (**LXXXI**) has been most studied experimentally and clinically (*143*). The rationale for this type of compound is that normal cells are likely to possess greater esterase activity than tumor cells, and hence a greater ability to detoxify the agent.

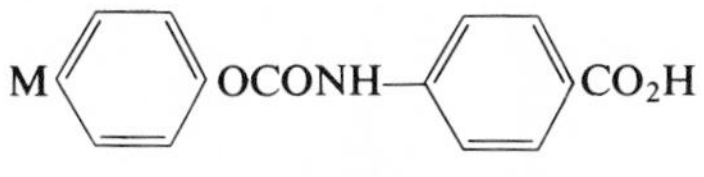

$$M\text{—}OCONH\text{—}CO_2H$$

LXXX

$$
\begin{array}{l}
CH_2OCOCH_2I \\
| \\
CH_2OCOCH_2I
\end{array}
$$

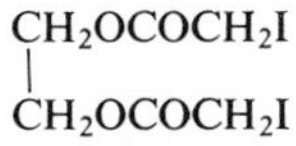

LXXXI

B. Processes of Reduction or Oxidation

At the beginning of this section we discussed the *p*-hydroxylation of aniline mustard, essentially an oxidative process. Activation and deactivation by oxidation or reduction have been considered in detail by Ross (*6*). Nitromin (**LXXXII**) and various azo mustards such as compound **LXXXIII** afford examples of reductive activation. Nitromin is probably converted into HN2, and it seems likely that xanthine oxidase is involved in the *in vivo* reduction of

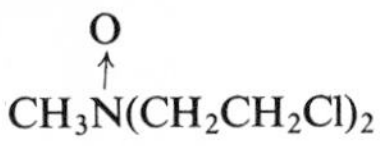

$$
\begin{array}{c}
O \\
\uparrow \\
CH_3N(CH_2CH_2Cl)_2
\end{array}
$$

LXXXII

$$\text{—N}=\text{N—}M$$
$$CO_2H \quad CH_3$$

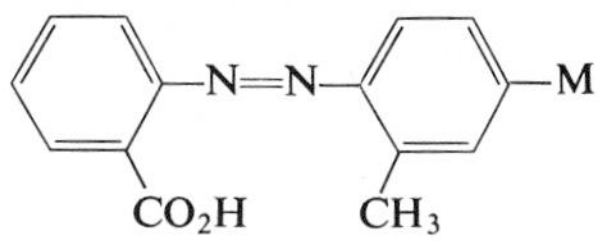

LXXXIII

the azo compounds to the corresponding active, *p*-amino aromatic mustards; tumors rich in this enzyme may be more susceptible to such azo agents (*144*).

It was mentioned earlier that the best known alkylating agent dependent upon activation is cyclophosphamide (**LXXXIV**). This compound was developed with the idea that splitting of the bond between the phosphorus

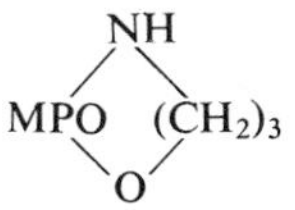

$$
\begin{array}{c}
NH \\
/ \quad \backslash \\
MPO \quad (CH_2)_3 \\
\backslash \quad / \\
O
\end{array}
$$

LXXXIV

atom and the mustard group would release the latter in an active form (*145*). A similar attempt to make use of tumor phosphoramidase activity had been described earlier (*146*). Cyclophosphamide is now a widely used drug, but it has become clear that its activity arises through unforseen processes, not yet fully described. Activation occurs in the liver, not the tumor (not, at any rate, in those neoplasms tested) and the transformation is an intracellular oxidative process (*147, 148, 148a*). More than one active alkylating metabolite is possibly formed, but bis-2-chloroethylamine, the compound which it was originally thought would be released by metabolic hydrolysis, does not, in fact seem to be important in the context of cyclophosphamide activity. Here then, is an example of an agent which happily turned out well, but in which the original design concepts were not realized.

Some attention has also been directed toward selective oxidative or reductive deactivation of agents by normal tissues. Hydroquinone mustards such as "Weatherbee mustard" (**LXXXV**) are a case in point. Oxidation to the corresponding quinone would deactivate the mustard groups. Compound **LXXXV** had an exceptionally high therapeutic index against the Ehrlich ascites tumor (*149*). This may be indicative of oxidative detoxication in normal

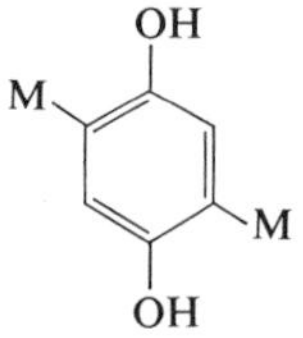

LXXXV

cells. The situation is the reverse of that with ethyleneimino derivatives of benzoquinone (*150*). Here the reduced form would be inactive, but there appears to be no evidence that selective reduction of such compounds by the host tissues occurs. We have already seen how a cysteine derivative (**XLVII**) may have a much reduced potency because of oxidative deactivation. Therapeutic advantage is, of course, only gained if the deactivation is carried out selectively, at least to a degree. Some thiol and thioether derivatives have been discussed from this point of view (*6*). For example, the very low toxicity of the tumor-inhibitory thiol (**LXXXVI**) may be due to its selective conversion by the host tissues to the inactive sulfonic acid derivative (**LXXXVII**).

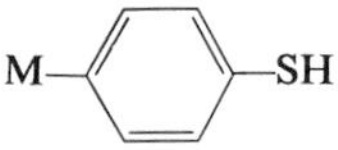

LXXXVI 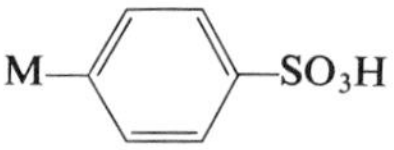 **LXXXVII**

A compound which may well undergo metabolic transformation, with consequent effects upon activity and chemical mechanism, is the nitroso derivative (**LXXXVIII**), active against many animal tumors, particularly the Dunning ascites leukemia, in which system the therapeutic index was 150 (*151*). The activity against intracerebrally implanted Dunning leukemia indicated that the agent could pass the blood–brain barrier in adequate amounts. Unlike BCNU, the nitroso compound produced no delayed deaths (*152*). Finally, it is perhaps appropriate to mention that the activity of the antibiotic, mitomycin C, evidently depends upon a reduction process *in vivo*.

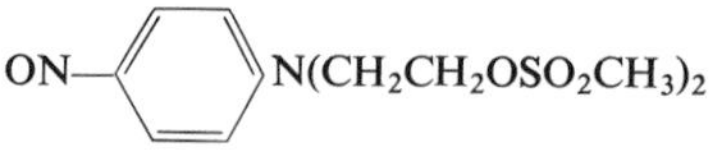

LXXXVIII

The active form of the antibiotic is an alkylating agent which is able to cross-link DNA, and this capability may form the basis of its antitumor action (*152a*).

C. ACTIVATION OF QUATERNARY NITROGEN MUSTARDS

In a new approach, several quaternary compounds (**LXXXIX**) have been made which displayed activity against an experimental mouse leukemia (*153*). These compounds were designed to be split by nucleophilic attack (by Y^- in Scheme 7) with the release of HN2. The relatively high activity of the *p*-nitro-

$$\underset{\substack{|\\ \underset{\textstyle \mathbf{LXXXIX}}{CH_3}}}{RCH_2\overset{+}{N}(CH_2CH_2Cl)_2} \quad \xrightarrow{\;Y^-\;} \quad CH_3M + RCH_2Y$$

Scheme 7

benzyl derivative (**LXXXIX**; $R = p\text{-}O_2NC_6H_4$) supports the proposed activation mechanism. It remains to be seen whether useful selectivity can be achieved in such a way.

IX. The Application of pH Differences

The pH of some experimental tumors appears to be lower than that of normal tissue, particularly in animals which have received glucose (*6*). Attempts have been made to exploit this feature in two ways: (1) by designing nitrogen mustards with basic side chains of such a pK value that the nondiffusible cationic form tends to accumulate in the more acidic (tumor) regions; and (2) by studying the effect of glucose pretreatment on the therapeutic efficiency of certain epoxides and ethyleneimines, classes of compounds which tend to be more reactive in regions of higher acidity.

It has indeed been found that the antitumor activity of certain basic aromatic *N*-mustard derivatives, such as compound **XII** ($R = R' = CH_3$) was increased by glucose administration, but further studies showed that the therapeutic index in such cases was not improved (*154, 155*). It may be recalled in passing that the aromatic nitrogen mustard group is too weakly basic to be protonated under physiological conditions. Such protonation would in any case deactivate the compound. The activity of certain basic diepoxides and their increased reactivity at lower pH were discussed earlier, but there was no indication of any enhancement, by glucose pretreatment, of the antitumor activity of a representative compound (Eponate; **XXVI**); nor was the potency of a neutral diepoxide affected, though a positive response to a reduction of pH would not be expected in this case, as we saw above. With triethylenemelamine (TEM; **XXI**), however, the antitumor activity was enhanced more than the toxicity, so a therapeutic advantage was gained (*155*). The antitumor action and toxicity of mannitol–Myleran (**LVIII**) were both increased 8-fold by glucose treatment, an exceptionally high potentiation (*156*). It turned out, however, that this was primarily a result of the antidiuretic action of glucose, and the point was made that the effect of glucose administration on the activity of TEM may be related to the neutralization by the sugar of a possible powerful diuretic action of the ethyleneimine derivative. We thus have a cautionary tale which demonstrates that, even where a biological result appears to support a theory of action, further study might reveal a quite different explanation. It is not certain whether a pH differential played a role in any of the glucose effects referred to above. It is nevertheless true that a sulfadiazine mustard derivative (**XC**) has been found to have a favorable

$$M-\!\!\!\bigcirc\!\!\!-SO_2NH-\!\!\!\left\langle\begin{array}{c}N\\ \\N\\H\end{array}\right.$$

XC

therapeutic index (24.5 as against about 11 for the average aromatic nitrogen mustard) in the Walker tumor system (*157*). This compound was the best of a series of sulfonamides designed to explore the effects of variation of p*K*. The selective deposition of the analogous sulfadiazine (**XC**; with NH_2 in place of M) in the solid Yoshida sarcoma, relatively highly sensitive to **XC**, was established and it seems a reasonable thesis that the activity of compound **XC** is due to such selective concentration (*157*).

In another attempt to make use of the alleged lower pH in tumor cells, efforts were made to prepare a diazoamino mustard of type **XCI** (X = Cl)

$$ArN\!=\!NN(CH_2CH_2X)_2$$

XCI

on the basis that such a compound would be inactive but would be susceptible to an activating cleavage under slightly acid conditions (*151*). The representative compound which was prepared was, however, unstable; two fluoro analogs (**XCI**; X = F) were more stable, but proved to be biologically inactive. It is of some interest that the related, active imidazole mustard derivative (**LXVI**) is of a similar chemical type.

It should not be forgotten in considering attempts of the above kind that not every tumor has a low pH. Often indeed, there appears to be little significant difference between the intracellular pH of normal and tumor tissue, and some tumors may even be more basic (*158*). Whether, or how widely, the approach dependent on pH differences can be applied in clinical cancer remains to be seen.

X. Compounds Designed for Intraarterial Infusion

Some attention has been given to the synthesis of alkylating agents with very short biological half-lives for introduction into an artery supplying a tumor. Such compounds are designed to react almost completely before the blood conveying them emerges from the tumor area. In this way, general toxic effects are greatly reduced (*159*). A recent example is the sulfur bromo-mustard derivative, CB 1850 (**XCII**), which has a half-life of 4.8 sec at 37°C and pH 8.3; at this pH the compound is in the anionic form (*160*). Injection of the agent (in dimethylsulfoxide solution) into the artery supplying an established Walker tumor caused significant inhibition; intraperitoneal injection had no effect (*161*). The agent has been successfully used clinically for the intraarterial infusion of tumors, particularly those of the head and neck (*162*).

$$HO_2C \quad \text{—} \quad OCH_2CHSCH_2CH_2Br$$
$$CH_2SCH_2CH_2Br$$

XCII

XI. Conclusion

In this review, we have looked at the attempts which have been made to render alkylating groups more effective against cancer. Great difficulties still remain, notably selectivity of action and the problem of drug resistance. Few would pretend that the alkylating agents are an answer to the cancer problem or that ways in which they can be materially improved are clear. We hope in due time to move on to more specific therapies, but alkylating agents are currently an important section of the drugs used in the treatment of neoplastic disease, notably the leukemias and allied conditions. In the immediate future, their value may be enhanced by the discovery of better ways of using them. Further studies on cell kinetics and on the variation of sensitivity to agents with stage of cell cycle; the ways in which resistance to alkylating

agents develops; the part played by host factors, particularly the immuno-
logical system, during drug treatment; the study of combination therapy:
these kinds of investigations may help to achieve improved responses in
individual patients. Selective protection of the host against alkylating agents
by hemopoietic tissue (*163*) may become a useful technique in due time,
although selective protection by chemical agents, such as thiols (*164*), seems
less promising. It may be, too, that the known heat sensitivity (*165, 166*) of
some tumors may be exploited as an aid to chemotherapy. We also need
better immediate ways of assessing in advance what the likely response of a
particular human tumor to an agent will be. Most of the foregoing remarks
apply, of course, not only to alkylating agents but also to other kinds of anticancer therapy. They are not, strictly speaking, relevant to drug design, but
we have to remember that the biological activity of any agent depends not
only upon its chemistry but upon the nature and condition of the host. Finally,
more rational drug design will perhaps result from studies (1) of the biochemical
characteristics of individual tumors, and (2) of the metabolism of known agents
by tumor and host.

ACKNOWLEDGMENT

The author is grateful to Professor W. C. J. Ross of this Institute for his valuable advice
and comments on a number of topics covered in this review.

REFERENCES

1. R. P. Bratzel, *Cancer Chemother. Rep.* **26**, 1 (1963).
2. L. H. Schmidt, R. Fradkin, R. Sullivan, and A. Flowers, *Cancer Chemother. Rep.*
   Suppl. 2, Parts I, II, and III (1965).
3. P. Ehrlich, *in* "The Collected Papers of Paul Ehrlich" (F. Himmelweit, ed.), Vol. 1,
   p. 612. Pergamon Press, Oxford, 1956.
4. A. Gilman and F. S. Philips, *Science* **103**, 409 (1946).
5. L. H. Schmidt, R. Fradkin, R. Sullivan, and A. Flowers, *Cancer Chemother. Rep.*
   Suppl. 2, Part I, 1 (1965).
6. W. C. J. Ross, "Biological Alkylating Agents." Butterworth, London and Washington,
   D.C., 1962.
7. M. Ochoa and E. Hirschberg, *in* "Experimental Chemotherapy" (R. J. Schnitzer and F.
   Hawking, eds.), Vol. 5, p. 1. Academic Press, New York, 1967.
8. E. Hirschberg, *Cancer Res.* **23**, Part 2, 521 (1963).
9. W. C. J. Ross, *Advan. Cancer Res.* **1**, 397 (1953).
10. T. J. Bardos, N. Datta-Gupta, P. Hebborn, and D. J. Triggle, *J. Med. Chem.* **8**, 167
    (1965).

11. D. J. Triggle, *J. Theor. Biol.* **7**, 241 (1964).
12. C. E. Williamson and B. Witten, *Cancer Res.* **27**, Part 1, 33 (1967).
13. G. P. Warwick, *Cancer Res.* **23**, Part 1, 1315 (1963).
14. G. P. Wheeler, *Cancer Res.* **22**, Part 1, 651 (1962).
15. P. Brookes and P. D. Lawley, *Brit. Med. Bull.* **20**, 91 (1964).
16. P. Brookes, *in* "Chemotherapy of Cancer" (P. A. Plattner, ed.), p. 32. Elsevier, Amsterdam, 1964.
17. A. Loveless, *Nature (London)* **223**, 206 (1969).
18. W. C. J. Ross and M. Tisdale, personal communication (1970).
18a. B. L. Van Duuren, *Ann. N.Y. Acad. Sci.* **163**, 633 (1969).
19. A. Haddow, G. A. R. Kon, and W. C. J. Ross, *Nature (London)* **162**, 824 (1948).
20. A. Albert, "Selective Toxicity," 3rd ed., p. 208. Methuen, London, 1965.
21. A. Cambanis, V. Dobre, and I. Niculescu-Duvas, *J. Med. Chem.* **12**, 161 (1969).
22. I. Niculescu-Duvas, M. Ionescu, A. Cambanis, M. Vitan, and V. Feyns, *J. Med. Chem.* **11**, 500 (1968).
23. F. Bergel, J. L. Everett, J. J. Roberts, and W. C. J. Ross, *J. Chem. Soc.* p. 3835 (1955).
24. L. F. Larionov, M. D. Chadakova, and E. I. Arkhangel'skaia, *Vop. Onkol.* **7**, 112 (1961); *Cancer Chemother. Abstr.* **2**, 872 (1961).
25. G. R. Pettit and R. L. Smith, *Can. J. Chem.* **42**, 572 (1964).
26. F. D. Popp, F. P. Silver, and D. W. Ahrani, *J. Med. Chem.* **10**, 481 (1967).
27. Z. B. Papanastassiou, R. W. Bruni, F. P. Fernandes, and P. L. Levins, *J. Med. Chem.* **9**, 357 (1966).
28. G. A. R. Kon and J. J. Roberts, *J. Chem. Soc.* p. 978 (1950).
29. T. P. Abbiss, A. H. Soloway, and V. H. Mark, *J. Med. Chem.* **7**, 763 (1964).
30. D. C. Smith, A. H. Soloway, and R. W. Turner, *J. Med. Chem.* **9**, 360 (1966).
31. S. Farber, R. Toch, E. M. Sears, and D. Pinkel, *Advan. Cancer Res.* **4**, 1 (1956).
32. W. C. J. Ross, *J. Chem. Soc.* p. 2257 (1950).
33. L. R. Duvall, *Cancer Chemother. Rep.* **8**, 156 (1960).
34. J. E. Ultmann, G. A. Hyman, C. Crandall, H. Naujoks, and A. Gellhorn, *Cancer* **10**, 902 (1967).
35. F. R. White, *Cancer Chemother. Rep.* **4**, 55 (1959).
36. J. A. Hendry, R. F. Homer, and F. L. Rose, *Brit. J. Pharmacol.* **6**, 235 (1951).
37. J. Bichel, *Abstr. 7th Int. Cancer Congr., 1958* p. 32 (1958).
38. W. A. M. Duncan and G. A. Snow, *Biochem. J.* **82**, 8P (1962).
39. J. Horton, K. B. Olson, T. J. Cunningham, and J. M. Sullivan, *Cancer* **20**, 1837 (1967).
40. K. Gerzon, J. E. Cochran, L. A. White, R. Monahan, E. V. Krumkalns, R. E. Scroggs, and J. Mills, *J. Med. Pharm. Chem.* **1**, 223 (1959).
41. D. G. Miller, H. D. Diamond, and L. F. Craver, *Clin. Pharmacol. Ther.* **1**, 31 (1960).
42. T. H. Goodridge, M. T. Flather, R. E. Harmon, and R. P. Bratzel, *Cancer Chemother. Rep.* **9**, 78 (1960).
43. A. Haddow and G. M. Timmis, *Lancet* **1**, 207 (1953).
44. L. A. Elson, "Radiation and Radiomimetic Chemicals," p. 62. Butterworth, London and Washington, D.C., 1963.
45. Chester Beatty Research Institute, *Annu. Rep. Brit. Emp. Cancer Campaign* **28**, 58 (1950).
46. G. M. Timmis and R. F. Hudson, *Ann. N.Y. Acad. Sci.* **68**, 727 (1958).
47. J. J. Roberts and G. P. Warwick, *Biochem. Pharmacol.* **6**, 217 (1961).
48. C. C. Stock, *Nat. Cancer Inst., Monogr.* No. 3, 23 (1960).
49. B. W. Fox, *Int. J. Cancer* **4**, 54 (1969).
50. T. A. Connors, personal communication (1969).

51. A. M. Michelson, "The Chemistry of Nucleosides and Nucleotides," p. 375. Academic Press, New York, 1963.
52. L. A. Elson, personal communication (1969).
53. A. Loveless, "Genetic and Allied Effects of Alkylating Agents." Butterworth, London and Washington, D.C., 1966.
54. H. J. Creech, E. Breuninger, R. F. Hankwitz, G. Polsky, and M. L. Wilson, *Cancer Res.* **20**, Part 2, 471 (1960).
55. R. M. Peck, A. P. O'Connell, and H. J. Creech, *J. Med. Chem.* **9**, 217 (1966).
56. L. S. Lerman, *J. Mol. Biol.* **3**, 18 (1961).
57. P. Hebborn and D. J. Triggle, *J. Med. Chem.* **8**, 541 (1965).
58. R. D. Hawkins, L. N. Owen, and J. F. Danielli, *J. Theor. Biol.* **5**, 236 (1963).
59. B. R. Baker, W. W. Lee, W. A. Skinner, A. P. Martinez, and E. Tong, *J. Med. Pharm. Chem.* **2**, 633 (1960).
60. M. Artico and W. C. J. Ross, *Biochem. Pharmacol.* **17**, 873 and 883 (1968).
60a. B. R. Baker, "Design of Active-Site-Directed Irreversible Enzyme Inhibitors." Wiley, New York, 1967.
61. F. R. White, *Cancer Chemother. Rep.* **4**, 52 (1959).
62. J. M. Venditti, A. Goldin, and I. Kline, *Cancer Chemother. Rep.* **11**, 73 (1961).
63. D. B. Rochlin and J. Shiner, *Cancer Chemother. Rep.* **11**, 69 (1961).
64. L. M. Cobb, T. A. Connors, L. A. Elson, A. H. Kahn, B. C. V. Mitchley, W. C. J. Ross, and M. E. Whisson, *Biochem. Pharmacol.* **18**, 1519 (1969).
65. A. Haddow and W. C. J. Ross, *Nature (London)* **177**, 995 (1956).
66. W. C. J. Ross and W. Davis, *J. Chem. Soc.* p. 2420 (1957).
67. L. H. Schmidt, *Cancer Chemother. Rep.* **9**, 56 (1960).
68. F. Bergel and J. A. Stock, *Annu. Rep. Brit. Emp. Cancer Campaign* **31**, 6 (1953).
69. F. Bergel and J. A. Stock, *J. Chem. Soc.* p. 2409 (1954).
70. F. Bergel, V. C. E. Burnop, and J. A. Stock, *J. Chem. Soc.* p. 1223 (1955).
71. L. F. Larionov, A. S. Khoklov, E. N. Shkodinskaya, O. S. Vasina, V. I. Trusheikina, and M. A. Novikova, *Lancet* **2**, 169 (1955).
72. J. A. Stock, (1958). *Amino Acids Peptides Antimetab. Activ., Ciba Found. Symp.* p. 89 (1958).
73. F. R. White, *Cancer Chemother. Rep.* **6**, 61 (1960).
74. J. A. Stock, *in* "The Biology of Cancer" (E. J. Ambrose and F. J. C. Roe, eds.), p. 176. Van Nostrand, Princeton, New Jersey, 1966.
75. L. F. Larionov, "Cancer Chemotherapy," p. 296. Pergamon Press, Oxford, 1965.
75a. T. A. Connors and W. C. J. Ross, *Chem. Ind. (London)* p. 492 (1960).
76. P. Clifford, S. Singh, J. Stjernswärd, and G. Klein, *Cancer Res.* **27**, Part 1, 2578 (1967).
77. J. M. Johnson and F. Bergel, *in* "Metabolic Inhibitors" (R. M. Hochster and J. H. Quastel, eds.), Vol. 2, p. 161. Academic Press, New York, 1963.
78. W. Davis, J. J. Roberts, and W. C. J. Ross, *J. Chem. Soc.* p. 890 (1955).
79. H. E. Smith and J. M. Luck, *J. Org. Chem.* **23**, 837 (1958).
80. F. Bergel, G. E. Lewis, S. M. D. Orr, and J. Butler, *J. Chem. Soc.* p. 1431 (1959).
81. F. Bergel, *Farmaco, Ed. Sci.* **19**, 99 (1964).
82. L. F. Larionov, "Cancer Chemotherapy," p. 307. Pergamon Press, Oxford, 1965.
83. L. F. Larionov, *Cancer Chemother. Rep.* **11**, 165 (1961).
84. L. A. Elson, A. Haddow, F. Bergel, and J. A. Stock, *Biochem. Pharmacol.* **11**, 1079 (1962).
85. M. Szekerke, R. Wade, and F. Bergel, *Acta Chim. Acad. Sci. Hung.* **44**, 159 (1965).
86. F. Bergel, J. M. Johnson, and R. Wade, *Proc. 6th Euro. Symp. Peptides 1963* p. 241 (1965).

87. Z. P. Sophina, L. F. Larionov, E. N. Shkodinskaya, O. S. Vasina, and A. J. Berlin. *Acta Unio Int. Contra Cancrum* **20**, 82 (1964).
88. M. Szekerke, R. Wade, and F. Bergel, *J. Chem. Soc.*, C p. 1792 (1968).
89. M. Ishidate, J. Sakurai, and M. Izumi, *J. Amer. Pharm. Ass.*, *Sci. Ed.* **44**, 132 (1955).
90. F. R. White, *Cancer Chemother. Rep.* **7**, 99 (1960).
91. J. DeGraw and L. E. Goodman, *J. Org. Chem.* **27**, 1395 (1962).
92. W. N. Fishbein, P. P. Carbone, A. H. Owens, M. G. Kelly, D. P. Rall, and N. Tarr, *Cancer Chemother. Rep.* **42**, 19 (1964).
93. R. N. Kyle, P. P. Carbone, J. J. Lynch, A. H. Owens, G. Costa, R. T. Silver, J. Cuttner, J. B. Harley, L. A. Leone, B. I. Schnider, and J. F. Holland, *Cancer Res.* **27**, Part 1, 510 (1967).
94. L. Goodman, R. R. Spencer, G. Casini, O. P. Crews, and E. J. Reist, *J. Med. Chem.* **8**, 251 (1965).
95. R. H. Iwamoto, E. M. Acton, L. O. Ross, W. A. Skinner, B. R. Baker, and L. Goodman, *J. Med. Chem.* **6**, 43 (1963).
96. M. Ishidate, Y. Sakurai, and I. Aiko, *Chem. Pharm. Bull.* **8**, 732 (1960).
97. L. F. Larionov and I. G. Spasskaya, *Probl. Oncol.* (*USSR*) **7**, 1629 (1961).
98. J. A. Stock, *in* "Experimental Chemotherapy" (R. J. Schnitzer and F. Hawking, eds.), Vol. 4, p. 277 and p. 288. Academic Press, New York, 1966.
98a. H. A. DeWald, D. C. Behn, and A. M. Moore, *J. Amer. Chem. Soc.* **81**, 4364 (1959).
98b. G. Brambilla, F. Mattioli, M. Cavanna, S. Parodi, and L. Baldini, *Cancer Chemother. Rep.* **53**, Part 1, 13 (1969).
99. B. Larsen, *Eur. J. Cancer* **2**, 163 (1967).
100. L. G. Israels and J. H. Linford, *Proc. Can. Cancer Res. Conf.* **5**, 399 (1963).
101. W. J. Hopwood and J. A. Stock, *Chem. Biol. Interactions* (1971) (in press).
102. R. Wade, M. E. Whisson, and M. Szekerke, *Nature* (*London*) **215**, 1303 (1967).
103. H. Busch and H. S. N. Greene, *J. Biol. Med.* **27**, 339 (1955).
104. H. Isliker, J. C. Cerottini, J. C. Jaton, and G. Magnenat, *in* "Chemotherapy of Cancer" (P. A. Plattner, ed.), p. 278. Elsevier, Amsterdam, 1964.
105. L. Vargha, *Ann. N.Y. Acad. Sci.* **68**, 875 (1958).
106. L. Németh, B. Kellner, and K. Lapis, *Ann. N.Y. Acad. Sci.* **68**, 879 (1958).
107. J. Baló, G. Kendrey, J. Juhász, and I. Besznyak, *Brit. J. Cancer* **13**, 634 (1959).
108. E. J. Reist, R. R. Spencer, M. E. Wain, I. G. Junga, L. Goodman, and B. R. Baker, *J. Org. Chem.* **26**, 2821 (1961).
109. S. S. Brown, *Advan. Pharmacol.* **2**, 243 (1963).
110. S. S. Brown and G. M. Timmis, *Annu. Rep. Brit. Emp. Cancer Campaign* **37**, 29 (1959).
111. G. M. Timmis and S. S. Brown, *Biochem. Pharmacol.* **3**, 247 (1960).
112. L. Vargha, L. Toldy, Ö. Fehér, T. Horváth, E. Kasztreiner, J. Kuszmann, and S. Lendvai, *Acta Physiol. Acad. Sci. Hung.* **19**, 305 (1961).
113. A. Haddow, G. M. Timmis, and S. S. Brown, *Nature* (*London*) **182**, 1164 (1958).
114. F. R. White, *Cancer Chemother. Rep.* **23**, 71 (1962).
115. J. Baló, J. Juhász, G. Gyenes, and M. Sellei, *Orv. Hetil.* **103**, 260 (1962); *Cancer Chemother. Abstr.* **3**, 3856 (1962).
116. P. W. Feit, *Tetrahedron Lett.* **20**, 716 (1961).
117. F. R. White, *Cancer Chemother. Rep.* **24**, 95 (1962).
118. F. S. Dietrich, *Cancer Chemother. Rep.* **52**, 603 (1968).
119. J. Sandberg, S. Brulé, and A. Goldin, *Proc. Amer. Ass. Cancer Res.* **10**, 75 (1969).
120. L. A. Elson, M. Jarman, and W. C. J. Ross, *Eur. J. Cancer* **4**, 617 (1968).
121. W. Davis and W. C. J. Ross, *Biochem. Pharmacol.* **12**, 915 (1963).
122. F. R. White, *Cancer Chemother. Rep.* **14**, 169 (1961).

123. H. G. Petering, H. H. Buskirk, E. A. Musser, and J. S. Evans, *Cancer Chemother. Rep.* **27**, 1 (1963).
124. W. C. J. Ross, *J. Med. Chem.* **10**, 257 (1967).
125. L. H. Schmidt, R. Fradkin, R. Sullivan, and A. Flowers, *Cancer Chemother. Rep.* Suppl. 2, Part I, 204 (1965).
126. F. Shealy and C. A. Krauth, *Nature (London)* **210**, 208 (1966).
127. G. Hoffman, I. Kline, M. Gang, D. D. Tyrer, J. M. Venditti, and A. Goldin, *Cancer Chemother. Rep.* **52**, Part 1, 715 (1968).
128. J. A. Stock, *in* "Experimental Chemotherapy" (R. J. Schnitzer and F. Hawking, eds.), Vol. 5, p. 386. Academic Press, New York, 1967.
129. F. M. Schnabel, T. P. Johnston, G. S. McCaleb, J. A. Montgomery, W. R. Laster, and H. E. Skipper, *Cancer Res.* **23**, Part 1, 725 (1963).
130. O. S. Selawry and H. H. Hansen, *Proc. Amer. Ass. Cancer Res.* **10**, 78 (1969).
131. T. J. Bardos, Z. B. Papanastassiou, A. Segaloff, and J. L. Ambrus, *Nature (London)* **183**, 399 (1959).
132. Pacific Veterans Administration Cancer Chemotherapy Group, *Cancer Chemother. Rep.* **33**, 15 (1963).
133. T. J. Bardos, N. Datta-Gupta, and P. Hebborn, *J. Med. Chem.* **9**, 221 (1966).
134. M. E. Whisson and T. A. Connors, *Nature (London)* **206**, 689 (1965).
135. T. A. Connors and M. E. Whisson, *Nature (London)* **210**, 866 (1966).
136. M. Szekerke, J. Czászár, and V. Bruckner, *Acta Chim. Acad. Sci. Hung.* **46**, 379 (1965).
137. F. Bergel, J. A. Stock, and R. Wade, *in* "Biological Approaches to Cancer Chemotherapy" (R. J. C. Harris, ed.), p. 125. Academic Press, New York, 1961.
138. R. Wade and F. Bergel, *J. Chem. Soc.,* C p. 592 (1967).
139. F. Bergel and R. Wade, *Annu. Rep. Brit. Emp. Cancer Campaign* **36**, 4 (1958).
140. H. Z. Sommer, C. Scher, S. Bien, G. Olsen, J. K. Chakrabarti, and O. M. Friedman, *J. Med. Chem.* **9**, 84 (1966).
141. M. H. Benn, A. M. Creighton, L. N. Owen, and G. R. White, *J. Chem. Soc.* p. 2365 (1961).
142. J. F. Danielli, K. Montague, F. Price, P. Barnard, D. Cotton, and A. Kuku, *Annu. Rep. Brit. Emp. Cancer Campaign* **36**, 527 (1958).
143. S. P. Kramer, L. E. Goodman, H. Dorfman, R. Solomon, A. M. Rutenberg, E. Pineda, L. L. Nason, A. Ulfohn, S. D. Gaby, D. Bakal, C. E. Williamson, J. I. Miller, S. Sass, B. Witten, and A. M. Seligman, *J. Nat. Cancer Inst.* **31**, 297 (1963).
144. W. C. J. Ross and G. P. Warwick, *Nature (London)* **176**, 298 (1955).
145. H. Arnold, F. Bourseaux, and N. Brock, *Naturwissenschaften* **45**, 64 (1958); *Nature (London)* **181**, 931 (1958).
146. O. M. Friedman and A. M. Seligman, *J. Amer. Chem. Soc.* **76**, 655 (1954).
147. N. Brock, *Cancer Chemother. Rep.* **51**, 315 (1967).
148. J. L. Cohen and J. Y. Jao, *Proc. Amer. Ass. Cancer Res.* **10**, 14 (1969).
148a. T. A. Connors, P. L. Grover, and A. M. McLoughlin, *Biochem. Pharmacol.* **19**, 1533 (1969).
149. H. J. Creech, E. Breuninger, R. F. Hankwitz, G. Polsky, and M. L. Wilson, *Cancer Res.* **20**, Part 2, 471 (1960).
150. G. Domagk, *Ann. N.Y. Acad. Sci.* **68**, 1197 (1958).
151. Z. B. Papanastassiou, R. J. Bruni, E. White, and P. L. Levins, *J. Med. Chem.* **9**, 725 (1966).
152. I. Wodinsky, Z. B. Papanastassiou, and C. V. Kensler, *Proc. Amer. Ass. Cancer Res.* **7**, 77 (1966).

152a. J. A. Stock, *in* "Experimental Chemotherapy" (R. J. Schnitzer and F. Hawking, eds.), Vol. 4, p. 274. Academic Press, New York, 1966.

153. Z. B. Papanastassiou, R. J. Bruni, and E. White, *Experientia* **24**, 325 (1968).

154. W. C. J. Ross, *Biochem. Pharmacol.* **8**, 235 (1961).

155. T. A. Connors, B. C. V. Mitchley, V. M. Rosenoer, and W. C. J. Ross, *Biochem. Pharmacol.* **13**, 395 (1964).

156. T. A. Connors, L. A. Elson, and C. L. Leese, *Biochem. Pharmacol.* **13**, 963 (1964).

157. N. Calvert, T. A. Connors, and W. C. J. Ross, *Eur. J. Cancer* **4**, 627 (1968).

158. W. J. Waddell and R. G. Bates, *Physiol. Rev.* **49**, 285 (1969).

159. C. E. Williamson, J. I. Miller, S. Sass, J. Casanova, S. P. Kramer, A. M. Seligman, and B. Witten, *J. Nat. Cancer Inst.* **31**, 273 (1963).

160. W. Davis and W. C. J. Ross, *J. Med. Chem.* **8**, 757 (1965).

161. L. M. Cobb, *Intn. J. Cancer* **2**, 5 (1967).

162. J. Meyza and L. M. Cobb, *Cancer* **27**, 369 (1971).

163. G. L. Floersheim, *Lancet* **1**, 228 (1969).

164. T. A. Connors, *Eur. J. Cancer* **2**, 293 (1969).

165. R. Cavaliere, E. C. Ciocatto, B. C. Giovanella, C. Heidelberger, R. O. Johnson, M. Margottini, B. Mondovi, G. Moricca, and A. Rossi-Fanella, *Cancer* **20**, 1351 (1967).

166. M. von Ardenne and P. G. Reitnauer, *Z. Naturforsch.* B **22**, 422 (1967).

Author Index

Numbers in parentheses are reference numbers and indicate that an author's work is referred to, although his name is not cited in the text. Numbers in italics show the page on which the complete reference is listed.

Subject Index

Italicized page numbers indicate page on which structure of compound is found.

A

Acetohexamide, *113*
  improving stability of, 113
Acetoxycycloheximide, 178
  as protein-synthesis inhibitor, 242
Acetphenolisatin, masking moieties in, 116
Acetrizoate, *27, 30*
  as radiopaque, 27, 30
Acetylaranotin, as antiviral agent, 269
  site of action, 262
Acetylcholine, *461, 481*
  biosynthesis and storage of, 481–482
  in design of neuromuscular blocking agents, 500
  enzyme inhibitor from, 103
  as neurohormone of neuromuscular junction, 461–465
  stabilization by vulnerable moieties, 100, 101
Acetylcholinesterase (AChE), 162
  active zone of, 215
    configuration, 180
  n-alkylammoniums as inhibitors of, 168–169
  n-alkyltrimethylammonium ion complexes of, 146
  anionic sites of, 183
  binding sites of, 167
  changes during catalysis, 179–180
  conformation of, modification, 208
  inhibitors of, *see* Anticholinesterases

Acetylcholinesterase (AChE)—*continued*
  isoenzymes of, 177–179
  reactivators for, 213–229
    kinetics for, 215–217, 219–220
    nucleophilicity of, 218–222
    pharmacokinetics of, 36
Acetyl-β-methylcholine, *103*
  as enzyme inhibitor, 103
  stability of, 101
Acetylsalicylic acid, *115*
  intestinal absorption at various pH's, 88
  masking moieties in, 114, 115
Acids, gastric absorption at various pH's, 88, 89
Acriflavine, as protein-synthesis inhibitor, 238
  amebicidal activity, 239
ACTH, depot preparations of, 70
Actinomycin, as antiviral agent, 270
  site of action, 262
Active site (active zone), of cholinesterases, 164–180
α-(Acylaminosuccinimido)carboxylic acids, *300*
  antibacterial activity of, 300
N-Acylaziridines, in antibacterial drug design, 299–300
N-(Acylglycyl)-α-(acylaminosuccinimido) carboxylic acids, *300*
  antibacterial activity of, 300
N-(Acylglycyl)-5,5-dimethyl-2-oxothiazolidine-4-carboxylic acids, *300*
  antibacterial activity of, 300

U

U-12, 504, *113*
  stability of, 113
U-17, 835, stability of, improvement, 113
Ultracorten solubile, solubilizing moiety of, 79
Uracil mustard, *50*
  as antitumor agent, 556
  as cytostatic, pharmacokinetics of, 49, 50
Urethanes
  bioactivation of, 59, 62
  derivatives of, *560*
    as antitumor agents, 560
Uric acid, metabolism
  control of, 135, 136
  in gout, 135–136
Urine, pH of, effect on drug excretion, 89–90

V

Vaccinia virus
  adsorption and penetration of, 263
  inhibition of, 271
  mRNA of, 264
Vasopressin(s)
  analogs
    antagonists as, 377, 379, 382
    enzyme-resistant, 390, 393
    evolutionary aspects, 398
    hormonogens as, 395–397
    immunoreactivity suppression, 376
    of increased potency and selectivity, 371–373
    by peptide changes in, 334, 363
    by side-chain modification, 337, 339–340, 342, 346, 347, 360, 363
  arginine-containing, *see* Arginine vasopressin
  depot preparations of, 70
  lysine-containing, *see* Lysine vasopressin
  physiological activity of, 324
  structure-activity relationship of, 322
Vasotocin, *324*
  analogs of, 379
  evolutionary aspects, 398
  physiological activity of, 324
Viadril, *82*
  solubilizing moiety of, 82
Virus(es)
  adsorption and penetration of, 263
    inhibition of, 266–267

Virus(es)—*continued*
  agents used for treatment of, *see* Antiviral agents
  assembly and release of, inhibition, 272
  inhibition of host cell functions by, 263
  mRNA of, attachment and function of, 264
    inhibition of, 267–268
  nucleic acids of biosynthesis, 264–265
    inhibition of, 270–271
  proteins of, biosynthesis, 265–266
    inhibition, 271
  replication of, 261–266
    scheme for, 262
  tRNA of, inhibition, 271–272
Vitamin A
  increasing stability of, 107
  introduction of disposable moieties into, 110–111
Vitamin B_{12}, depot preparations of, 70
Vitamin K, derivatives of, in tumor diagnosis, 49
Vitamin K_4, *75*
  solubilizing moieties for, 82
Vitamins
  disposable moieties in, use to promote stability, 110–111
  esters of, for prolonged action, 73
  water-soluble, modulation of pharmacokinetics of, 37
Vulnerable moieties of drugs, 10, 11
  pharmacokinetics of, 57–58, 91–114

W

Water, as acetylcholinesterase reactivator, 216
Weatherbee mustard, *562*
  antitumor activity of, 562
Weed killers, *see* Herbicides
Wy-5256, *423*
  and derivatives, as diuretics, 422–424

X

Xanthine oxidase
  in activation of antitumor agents, 561
  allopurinol as inhibitor of, 134–135
  alloxanthine as inhibitor of, 136
  irreversible inhibitors of, 156
X-ray, contrast media for, pharmacokinetics of, 25, 26

Y

Yoshida sarcoma, drug therapy of, 564